Expert | CONSULT

Activate your access at
expertconsult.com

1 REGISTER

- Visit **expertconsult.com.**
- Click **"Register Now."**
- Fill in your **user information.**
- Click **"Create Account."**

2 ACTIVATE YOUR BOOK

- Scratch off your **Activation Code** below and enter it into the **"Add a title"** box.
- **You're done!** Click on the book's title under **"My Titles."**

For technical assistance, email **online.help@elsevier.com** or call **800-401-9962** (inside the US) or **+1-314-995-3200** (outside the US).

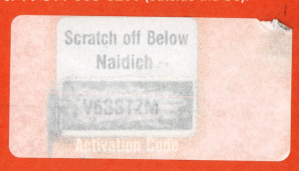

Scratch off Below
Naidich

V63STZM

Activation Code

Imaging of the Spine

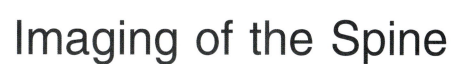

Imaging of the Spine

Editors

Thomas P. Naidich, MD, FACR

Professor of Radiology
Professor of Anatomy and Functional Morphology
Professor of Neurosurgery
Mount Sinai School of Medicine
New York, New York

Mauricio Castillo, MD

Professor of Radiology
Chief and Program Director, Neuroradiology
University of North Carolina at Chapel Hill
Chapel Hill, North Carolina

Soonmee Cha, MD

Associate Professor of Radiology
University of California, San Francisco
Attending Neuroradiologist
University of California, San Francisco Medical Center
San Francisco, California

Charles Raybaud, MD, FRCPC

Professor of Radiology
University of Toronto
Division Head of Neuroradiology
Hospital for Sick Children
Toronto, Ontario
Canada

James Smirniotopoulos, MD

Professor of Radiology and Radiological Sciences
Uniformed Services University of the Health Sciences
Bethesda, Maryland

Spyridon Kollias, MD

Professor of Radiology
Chief of Magnetic Resonance Imaging and MR Research
Institute of Neuroradiology
University Hospital Zurich
Zurich, Switzerland

George M. Kleinman, MD

Associate Professor of Pathology
Mount Sinai School of Medicine
New York, New York

SAUNDERS

ELSEVIER

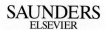

1600 John F. Kennedy Blvd.
Ste 1800
Philadelphia, PA 19103-2899

IMAGING OF THE SPINE   ISBN: 978-1-4377-1551-4

Library of Congress Cataloging-in-Publication Data
Imaging of the spine / Thomas P. Naidich . . . [et al.].—1st ed.
    p. ; cm.
    Includes bibliographical references.
    ISBN 978-1-4377-1551-4
    1. Spine—Imaging.   2. Spine—Imaging—Atlases.   I. Naidich, Thomas P.
[DNLM: 1. Spine—pathology—Atlases.   2. Diagnostic Imaging—Atlases.   3. Spinal Cord Diseases—diagnosis—Atlases.   4. Spinal Cord Injuries—diagnosis—Atlases.   5. Spinal Diseases—Diagnosis—Atlases.   6. Spinal Injuries—diagnosis—Atlases. WL 17 I31 2010]
    RD768.I45 2010
    617.5′60754—dc22

                                                                         2009053174

Acquisitions Editor: Rebecca Gaertner
Developmental Editor: Jennifer Shreiner
Publishing Services Manager: Tina Rebane
Project Manager: Norm Stellander
Design Direction: Steve Stave

Printed in China

Last digit is the print number: 9 8 7 6 5 4 3 2 1

Contributors

Krisztina Baráth, MD
Senior Staff Neuroradiologist, Institute of Neuroradiology, University Hospital Zurich, Zurich, Switzerland

David Mark Capper, MD
Department of Neuropathology, Institute of Pathology, Ruprecht-Karls University, Heidelberg, Germany

Francis Michael Castellano, MD
Neuroradiology Fellow, Department of Radiology, University of North Caroline at Chapel Hill, Chapel Hill, North Carolina

Mauricio Castillo, MD
Professor and Chief of Neuroradiology, Department of Radiology, University of North Carolina at Chapel Hill School of Medicine and University of North Carolina Hospital, Chapel Hill, North Carolina

Cynthia T. Chin, MD
Associate Professor of Radiology and Neurosurgery, University of California at San Francisco, San Francisco, California

Tanvir Fiaz Choudhri, MD
Assistant Professor of Neurosurgery, Department of Surgery, and Co-Director, Neurosurgery Spine Program, Mount Sinai School of Medicine, New York, New York

David L. Daniels, MD
Professor of Radiology, Medical College of Wisconsin, Milwaukee, Wisconsin

Bradley Neil Delman, MD
Associate Professor of Radiology and Director of Radiology Quality and Performance Improvement, Mount Sinai School of Medicine, New York, New York

Girish Manohar Fatterpekar, MBBS, DNB, MD
Assistant Professor of Radiology, James J. Peters Veterans Administration Medical Center, Mount Sinai Medical Center, New York, New York

Mary Elizabeth Fowkes, MD, PhD
Assistant Professor, Division of Neuropathology, Department of Pathology, Mount Sinai Hospital, New York, New York

Sosikhan Geibprasert, MD
Lecturer, Neuroradiology, Mahidol University; Staff, Neuroradiology, Ramathibodi Hospital, Bangok, Thailand

Ronit Gilad, MD
Resident, Mount Sinai School of Medicine, New York, New York

Yakov Gologorsky, MD
Resident, Department of Neurosurgery, Mount Sinai School of Medicine, New York, New York

Serap Gultekin, MD
Faculty of Medicine, Department of Radiology, Gazi University School of Medicine, Ankara, Turkey

Victor M. Haughton, MD
Professor, Department of Radiology, University of Wisconsin; Radologist, University of Wisconsin Hospitals and Clinics, Madison, Wisconsin

Michael Christian Hollingshead, MD
Neuroradiology Fellow, Department of Radiology, University of North Carolina at Chapel Hill, Chapel Hill, North Carolina

Sundar Jayaraman, MD
Clinical Assistant Professor, Department of Radiology, State University of New York-Upstate Medical University, Binghamton; Attending Radiologist, Department of Radiology, Wilson Regional Medical Center, Johnson City, New York

David M. Johnson, MD
Associate Professor of Radiology and Neurosurgery, Fletcher Allen Health Care, University of Vermont, Burlington, Vermont

Spyros S. Kollias, MD
Professor of Radiology (Neuroradiology), Department of Medical Radiology, and Chief of Neuro-MRI, Institute of Neuroradiology, University of Zurich, Zurich, Switzerland

Timo Krings, MD, PhD
Professor of Neuroradiology, Toronto Western Hospital, University Health Network, Toronto, Ontario, Canada

Pierre L. Lasjaunias, MD, PhD†
Professor of Neuroradiology, University Paris Sud, University Hospital Bicetre, Le Kremlin-Bicetre, Paris, France

Patrick A. Lento, MD
Associate Professor, Departments of Pathology, Internal Medicine, and Medical Education, Mount Sinai Medical Center, New York, New York

Kenneth Michael Lury, MD
Assistant Professor, Department of Radiology, Medical University of South Carolina, Charleston, South Carolina

Kenneth R. Maravilla, MD
Professor, Radiology and Neuroradiology, and Director, MR Research Laboratory, University of Washington, Seattle, Washington

Michel Guy André Mittelbronn, MD
Institute of Brain Research, University of Tuebingen, Tuebingen, Germany

Thomas Paul Naidich, MD, FARC
Professor of Radiology and Neurosurgery, Irving and Dorothy Regenstreif Research Professor of Neuroscience (Neuroimaging); Director of Neuroradiology, Mount Sinai School of Medicine, New York, New York

Matthew F. Omojola, MB, FRCPC
Professor, Section of Neuroradiology, Department of Radiology, University of Nebraska Medical Center, Omaha, Nebraska

Irina Oyfe, BS, MS Eng
Post Processing Analyst, Department of Radiology, Mount Sinai Medical Center, New York, New York

Paola Carmina Valbuena Parra, MD
Institute of Neuroradiology, University Hospital Zurich, Zurich, Switzerland

Aman B. Patel, MD
Associate Professor, Department of Neurosurgery and Radiology, Mount Sinai School of Medicine, New York, New York

Sumit Pruthi, MD, DNB
Assistant Professor, Department of Radiology, University of Washington; Attending, Children's Hospital and Regional Medical Center, Seattle, Washington

Joy S. Reidenberg, PhD
Professor, Center for Anatomy and Functional Morphology, Mount Sinai School of Medicine, New York, New York

Jose Conrado Rios, MD
Neuroradiology Fellow, Department of Radiology, Mount Sinai Medical Center, New York, New York

Nadja Saupe, MD
Department of Radiology, University Hospital Balgrist, Zurich, Switzerland

Marta Martínez Schmickrath, MD
Staff Neuroradiologist, La Paz Hospital, Madrid, Spain

J. Keith Smith, MD, PhD
Associate Professor, Department of Radiology, University of North Carolina at Chapel Hill School of Medicine, Chapel Hill, North Carolina

Maria Vittoria Spampinato, MD
Assistant Professor, Department of Radiology, Medical University of South Carolina, Charleston, South Carolina

Evan Gary Stein, MD
Resident, Neuroradiology Division, Department of Radiology, Mount Sinai Medical Center, New York, New York

Jeffrey Stone, MD
Associate Professor of Radiology, Mayo Clinic, Rochester, Minnesota

E. Turgut Tali, MD
Professor and Director, Division of Neuroradiology, Department of Radiology, Gazi University School of Medicine, Ankara, Turkey

Cheuk Ying Tang, PhD
Assistant Professor, Mount Sinai School of Medicine; Director, Neurovascular Imaging Research, Translational and Molecular Imaging Institute, Departments of Radiology and Psychiatry; Director, In Vivo molecular Imaging SRF, Mount Sinai Medical Center, New York, New York

Armin K. Thron, MD
Professor, Department of Radiology, University Hospital Aachen, Aachen, Germany

Carrie L. Tong, MD
Faculty Lecturer, Department of Radiology, Mount Sinai School of Medicine; Attending Radiologist, Good Samaritan Hospital, Suffern, New York

Donald J. Weisz, PhD
Associate Professor, Department of Neurosurgery, Mount Sinai School of Medicine, New York, New York

---

†Deceased.

Preface

Over the years, the imaging of spinal disease has evolved from plain film diagnosis and polytomography to advanced computed tomography (CT) and magnetic resonance (MR) imaging (I). Year by year, what is considered to be "modern imaging" morphs from *advanced techniques* to *basic diagnostic tests* to *quaint old studies*. Year by year, cruder and more invasive procedures are replaced by safer, faster, and more precise methods for detecting and characterizing spinal disease.

Through all of these changes, however, the constants of medical diagnosis have remained the anatomy, physiology, and pathology of the spinal column and cord. The human body has evolved more slowly than the techniques used to display it, so the anatomy, physiology, and pathology of the spine remain the foundation of all medical diagnosis.

To be useful, the data derived from the imaging studies need to be communicated concisely and effectively to the clinicians who care for the patient. Too often, imaging reports are cluttered with technical details about the study but limited in their discussion of the key pathophysiologic data needed to direct patient management toward one or another path. The generations-long debate: "Who reads the studies better, the clinician or the imager?" is resolved when it is appreciated that these physicians read the studies for two fundamentally different sets of data. *Useful interpretation* of the images provides the pertinent positive and negative data clinicians need to make their management decisions as well as the detailed physical data imagers need to reach their diagnoses and to understand the limitations of their studies.

In successive chapters, therefore, this text addresses imaging techniques for the spine, the paraspinal soft tissues, the normal anatomy of the spinal column and cord, age-related changes of the spine, degenerative disorders of the spine, the normal vascularization of the spinal cord, spinal ischemia and vascular malformations, spinal trauma, spinal tumors and cysts, metabolic disorders of the spine, inflammation and infection of the spine, preoperative mapping of spinal pathology, intraoperative monitoring of spinal physiology, vertebroplasty-kyphoplasty, and the complications of surgery for decompressing spinal stenosis and disc disease. Three final chapters address the brachial plexus, the sacral plexus, and peripheral nerve compression at the carpal tunnel. The congenital malformations of the spine will be presented in a companion volume on pediatric neuroimaging.

In successive chapters, this text also provides strategies for efficiently analyzing spinal images and includes sample reports to illustrate one way to convey key findings to the clinicians and achieve "useful reporting" of our studies.

The increasingly sophisticated imaging techniques require of us increasingly sophisticated knowledge of how to perform the studies effectively, how to recognize their limitations, and how to interpret them to understand the state of the patient in health and disease. For this volume, therefore, the editors have selected a group of highly skilled physician-authors who know their subject and who can present it concisely and thoroughly. These authors specifically include neuropathologists, whose contributions underlie our imaging appreciation of neuropathology.

This volume, then, is intended to provide a concise but thorough review of the imaging diagnosis of spinal disease. It emphasizes the constant anatomy and physiology of the spinal column and cord in the detail that is now required to understand "modern" imaging. It illustrates how pathology affects the spine and reviews which patterns of pathology lead to secure imaging diagnosis. It also deliberately includes selected data that we feel may aid us in interpreting the "modern" imaging of the future.

We hope that the readers will enjoy learning about the spine as much as we have in researching this text and in making the anatomic and pathologic images that illustrate the text. It is hoped further, that the readers may discern defects in our knowledge, be stimulated by them to pursue their own investigations, and thus join us to *"Perform an act whereof what's past is prologue; what to come, [is] in your and my discharge."* **William Shakespeare, The Tempest Act 2, scene 1, 245-254.**

THOMAS P. NAIDICH

Contents

Introduction

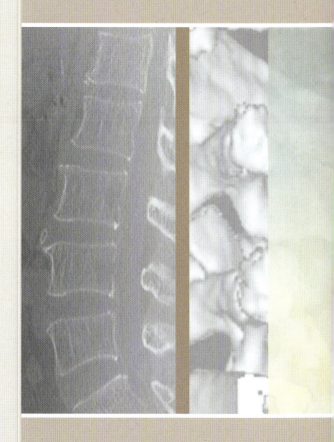

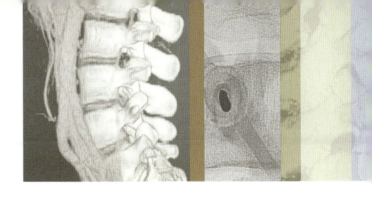

CHAPTER 1

Imaging Techniques in the Adult Spine

Jeffrey Stone

Imaging of the adult spine is typically accomplished using CT and MRI. Although conventional radiography may play a role in the evaluation of spinal disorders, the sensitivity, specificity, availability, and trends in medical practice have resulted in a paradigm shift to the use of cross-sectional imaging. CT is frequently used to study spinal fractures. Multidetector CT (MDCT) is significantly faster than routine CT, so it is very useful for evaluating the unstable or elderly patient who may not be able to hold still for lengthier examinations. MDCT significantly reduces artifacts related to beam hardening, so it also is useful for evaluating bone adjacent to surgical hardware.

MRI is used for evaluation of suspected degenerative disc disease, infection, tumor, and soft tissue trauma, including suspected spinal cord injury or spinal canal hemorrhage. MRI is motion sensitive, so adequate image resolution can be a challenge in the claustrophobic or elderly patient. Such patients may require the use of sedation. The recent availability of 3-T MRI has presented new opportunities for spinal imaging and may allow better functional and dynamic imaging of the spinal column.

Conventional contrast myelography has seen a decrease in use over the past decade mostly in response to better MRI. Myelography is useful in evaluating extrinsic compression of the neural elements in and around the spinal canal. It is typically performed when there is a contraindication to MRI. The increased use of non-ferromagnetic implants and medical devices has reduced the number of such patients. Contrast myelography may also be considered in a patient whose symptoms or physical findings are not explained on CT or MRI. MR myelography is an alternative approach to evaluation and can be performed without the injection of a contrast agent. MR myelography has the advantage of not being dependent on spine curvature, effects of gravity, dilution of contrast, or size of the thecal sac. It is, however, more sensitive to motion and may not permit imaging the patient in the symptomatic position.

PHYSICAL PRINCIPLES

MRI relies on the spin of unpaired protons around the atomic nucleus. The spin of the unpaired proton of hydrogen is typically utilized due to the abundance of hydrogen in the body. Hydrogen protons spin or precess around the axis of the applied magnetic field used in MRI. The frequency of precession is proportional to (1) the strength of the applied magnetic field (typically 0.7 to 3 T for diagnostic MRI) and (2) an intrinsic property of the nucleus referred to as the gyromagnetic ratio. The base magnetic field results in a slightly greater number of hydrogen protons becoming aligned parallel with the magnetic field (longitudinal magnetization) versus antiparallel and a resultant net magnetization of the tissue.

Once the protons are aligned, a radiofrequency (RF) pulse is applied to tilt the axes of spin away from their alignment with the applied magnetic field. This creates a net magnetization in the plane perpendicular to the original axis (transverse magnetization). Once the RF pulse is removed, these protons (1) begin to realign parallel to the applied magnetic field in exponential fashion and (2) emit a weak signal that can be detected by a receiver coil. The time after the RF pulse that 63% of the original magnetization has returned to its alignment with the applied magnetic field is a constant that depends on the anatomic environment of the proton. This constant is referred to as T1. The applied RF pulse also causes the precession of the individual protons to synchronize with each other. This synchrony of precession is lost exponentially on removal of the RF pulse. The loss of synchronization results from the effect of the local environmental on each proton and from interactions among adjacent protons (spin-spin interaction). Protons lose transverse magnetization exponentially as they return parallel to the magnetic field. The time at which protons have lost 63% of their transverse magnetization is a second constant referred to as T2.

The weak signal emitted by the spins as they realign with the main magnetic field can be made detectable as an "echo" by applying an additional 180-degree RF pulse. The echo is created when the dephased protons come back into phase. The echo occurs after the 180-degree pulse at a time equal to the time between the 90-degree pulse and 180-degree pulse. The echo time (TE) equals the time between the initial RF pulse and the time at which the echo is detectable. Spatial information is encoded in these echoes by using gradient coils to vary the magnetic field strength across the applied magnetic field. Frequency encoding along an excited slice (x-axis) provides spatial resolution between slices. It is achieved by applying a magnetic gradient along one direction of the region being sampled. This gradient causes the protons in each slice to precess at a frequency slightly different from the protons in the adjacent slice. Phase encoding allows spatial resolution within a slice. It is achieved by applying an additional magnetic gradient along the tangential axis (y-axis) of an excited slice at a time between the RF pulse and the sampling of the signal. This new applied pulse causes the spins in each row of the selected slice to precess at a slightly different frequency than the spins in an adjacent row. The raw data collected during scanning of each slice are then used to generate an image by filling in the k-space. The k-space is a mathematical construct—a matrix that provides a graphical representation of the raw data obtained within a slice. The amplitude of the signal detected at time points during the echo is used to assign a specific numerical value to each point in the k-space matrix. By repeating the process for each phase-encoding gradient applied to the slice being imaged, a matrix consisting of rows and columns is created with each number representing the signal strength. The data acquired at one phase-encoding gradient are represented by a single row, and the data obtained at different times of the echo are contained within a single column. 2D Fourier transformation is then used to generate an image.

MR myelography takes advantage of the intrinsic contrast between cerebrospinal fluid (CSF) and soft tissue structures such as the spinal cord, nerves, and fat within the epidural space. Echoplanar imaging (EPI) is especially suited for MR myelography and allows image acquisition in seconds. It decreases the effects of patient motion and is an easy addition to routine imaging protocols. EPI is accomplished by using a rapid series of gradient reversals in the frequency-encoding phase to continuously fill k-space. The resultant short repetition time (TR) allows very rapid acquisition of images in the 100- to 200-ms range. Whereas EPI is sensitive to chemical shift and magnetic susceptibility artifacts, this is not critical when imaging larger structures such as the spinal column. However, these effects may degrade resolution when EPI is used to display the spinal cord.

CT uses x-ray radiation to acquire and reconstruct thin, cross-sectional images of an object. Measurements of attenuation are obtained throughout a defined thickness of the object being imaged, and the data are used to reconstruct a cross-sectional image. Each pixel within the image represents a measurement of the mean attenuation within the voxel (volume of tissue) that extends through the thickness of the section. The attenuation measurement quantifies the amount of radiation removed from the beam as the beam traverses the voxel. This reduction in beam strength is expressed as an average attenuation coefficient. Many rays from many different rotational angles are used to calculate the average attenuation coefficient. The CT number, or Hounsfield unit (HU), is then calculated by normalizing the average attenuation coefficient of a voxel to the value of water (water = 0). Voxels that contain material that attenuates the x-ray beam more than water (i.e., muscle, bone) have positive values. Voxels that contain material that attenuates the x-ray beam less than water (i.e., fat, air) have negative values. The attenuation of water is obtained at the time the CT scanner is calibrated. The absolute CT number of materials other than air or water may vary with changes in x-ray tube potential and between different manufacturers. A HU may be assigned between −1000 and 1000. Only a limited number of all HU are actually presented on the display monitor used for interpretation. The window width is the range of HU displayed on the monitor, whereas the window level represents the central HU of all the numbers within that window width.

CT scanners have quickly evolved from single-row detector configurations to helical scanners and more recently to multiple-row or multislice scanning technology. By increasing detectors along the z-axis, multiple image slices can be acquired simultaneously. Therefore, large volumes of tissue can be rapidly scanned with near-isotropic resolution even when the slices are very thin. This results in an image that is equally sharp in any plane within the scanned volume. From these image data, multiplanar reformatted images and 3D reconstructions can be performed at amazingly high resolution and with reduction in artifact.

IMAGING
Parameters/Protocols

Protocols for MRI of the spine include T1-weighted (T1W) and T2-weighted (T2W) imaging in the axial and sagittal planes. Coronal imaging may be used to evaluate coronal imbalances such as scoliosis. T1W images provide excellent spatial resolution and are very useful for evaluating the bone marrow, ligaments, and soft tissue structures. T2W images are excellent for displaying the spinal cord and the CSF within the spinal canal. Fast spin-echo (FSE) techniques are usually used to obtain sagittal T2W images. Because FSE techniques are subject to degradation by CSF pulsation, however, FSE sequences may not provide excellent *axial* images of the cervical and thoracic spine. Instead, gradient-recalled-echo (GRE) sequences may be used for axial imaging of the cervical and thoracic regions. The GRE sequences allow for rapid imaging with a very

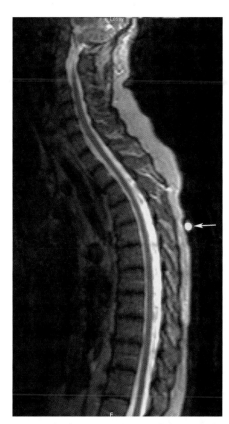

■ **FIGURE 1-1** Sagittal T2W MR image of the cervical and thoracic spine used for localization. A vitamin B_{12} external marker (*arrow*) has been placed on the back to allow accurate correlation as to vertebral level on axial and smaller field-of-view sagittal images of the thoracic spine.

short TR. A 3D low flip angle GRE sequence may be used for axial T2W images of the cervical spine. A 2D GRE sequence may be better for T2W axial imaging of the thoracic spine or if motion artifact is present at either site. Both spoiled GRE and steady-state GRE sequences are available. Steady-state GRE sequences provide very good "myelographic" effect when used in tissues with long TR such as CSF.

Phased-array coils may be used in the thoracic and lumbar regions to provide high-resolution images. Anterior and posterior neck coils and a large imaging matrix (512 or 256) are typically used to image the cervical spine. Anterior saturation bands should be employed to reduce artifacts from respiratory and bowel motion. Imaging of the thoracic spine should include an external marker to allow identification of the correct spine level (Fig. 1-1).

Gadolinium (Gd)-chelate contrast enhancement is used to evaluate suspected infection, tumor, arteriovenous malformation, and diseases of the leptomeninges. It is also used to evaluate the postoperative lumbar spine but is usually not needed in patients with uncomplicated cervical spine surgery. At least one of the Gd-enhanced imaging sequences should be obtained with fat suppression to better evaluate fat-containing structures such as the bone marrow and epidural space. In the spine, both frequency-selected and spectrally selected fat-suppression techniques are susceptible to artifact, so short-tau inversion recovery

(STIR) techniques may be used instead. The dose of Gd-chelate contrast agent is based on the patient's weight.

A typical lumbar spine protocol employs a spin-echo T1W sagittal sequence and a FSE T2W sagittal sequence. Additional axial FSE T1W and T2W images are obtained from the thoracolumbar junction to include the conus medullaris through at least the S1 level of the sacrum. Axial T2W FSE images are optimal in the lumbar region because CSF pulsation artifact is not as significant a problem as in the cervical and thoracic spine. Additional inversion recovery sequences are useful for trauma and are very sensitive for edema and hemorrhage. At least one of the axial imaging sequences should provide a series of *contiguous* images to properly assess the facet and ligamentous structures. Oblique axial images oriented with the disc space may be added.

The cervical and thoracic spine are often imaged using sagittal and axial FSE techniques, but a multiplanar gradient-echo axial sequence may substitute for or be used in addition to FSE technique to obtain high resolution and contrast while reducing CSF pulsation artifact. Sagittal images should extend sufficiently far laterally to include the neural foramen and proximal portions of the exiting spinal nerve.

Fast fluid-attenuated inversion recovery (FLAIR) is a T2W spin-echo sequence that suppresses the high signal of CSF. It has the potential advantage of displaying subtle edema or demyelination of the spinal cord, particularly near the surface of the cord. It is not limited by the CSF motion artifacts seen on T2W FSE images and can be performed rapidly using FSE techniques. Despite these inherent advantages, the literature has reported varying sensitivities that may result from (1) variations in the specific techniques used to acquire this sequence and (2) the decrease in lesion contrast that occurs with heavily T2W sequences. Additional FLAIR sagittal images are often useful when there is a suggestion of demyelinating disease such as multiple sclerosis.

3-T MRI has the theoretical advantage of doubling the signal-to-noise ratio (SNR) over imaging on a 1.5-T system (Fig. 1-2). Eight-channel phased-array coils are currently available for high-quality spinal imaging at 3 T. Long echo train, high-bandwidth acquisitions provide high resolution and can be achieved with shorter acquisition times than 1.5 T. Conventional T2W FSE sequences usually provide high quality images at 3 T. FSE or turbo spin-echo sequences are necessary for best image contrast. Free induction decay related artifacts may be reduced by using a greater number of acquisitions or flow compensation techniques. However, a challenge inherent to 3-T spine imaging is the increase in T1 relaxation time of tissue at the higher magnetic field strength. This increased T1 relaxation time requires increased time for image acquisition.

MR myelography can be performed using FSE techniques such as rapid acquisition with relaxation enhancement (RARE) and 3D fast imaging with steady-state precession (FISP) but is best accomplished using EPI. We have modified a single-shot turbo spin-echo technique described by Demaerel and colleagues to improve resolution (Fig. 1-3).[1] Each image is acquired in 8 seconds using the following parameters: TE 199.5 ms, TR 8000 ms,

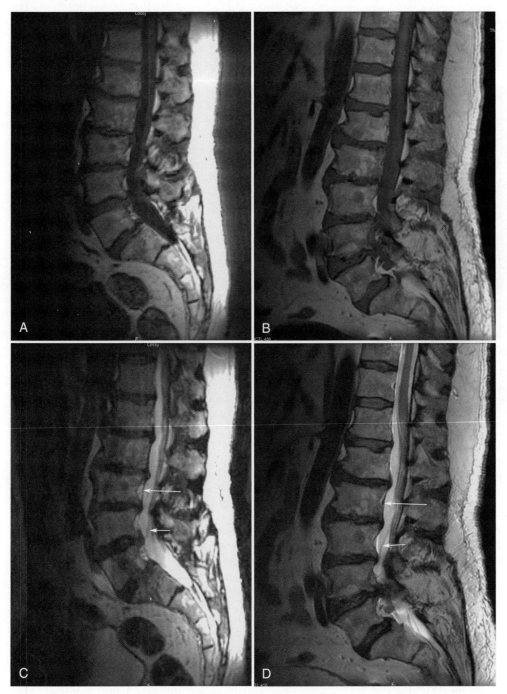

■ **FIGURE 1-2** Sagittal T1W images acquired on 1.5-T (**A**) and 3-T (**B**) MRI systems and sagittal T2W images acquired at 1.5 T (**C**) and 3 T (**D**). These studies were acquired 2 years apart. One can easily see, however, the increased signal-to-noise ratio on 3-T images by comparing similar structures on both T1W and T2W images. Note the increased definition of the bone marrow, nerve roots (*short arrows*), and longitudinal ligaments (*long arrows*).

256 × 256 matrix, 1 acquisition, 200 × 200-mm field of view (FOV), and 20-mm slice thickness. A presaturation fat pulse is used to improve resolution.

CT of the spine is performed in the axial plane using thin contiguous sections. Multislice scanners can image very thin slices very rapidly over substantial lengths of tissue. The resulting data loads are often very large, particularly if the images are obtained with near isotropic resolution. The most important imaging parameters for MDCT are section collimation, table feed per rotation, and pitch.

Slice thickness is typically 0.625 mm, with axial images reconstructed at 1.25-mm thickness for cervical spine and 2.5-mm thickness for the thoracic and lumbar spine. Sagittal and coronal reformatted images are usually used for interpretation. The 3D reconstructions and oblique reformatted images may be reconstructed at the workstation to assist in interpretation.

Intravascular contrast is not routinely utilized for spine CT. It may be administered in cases of suspected tumor or infection. Intrathecal contrast is typically used when CT myelography is performed and allows greater contrast between CSF within the thecal sac and structures of the spinal canal. This is useful in the evaluation of spinal cord or nerve compression (Fig. 1-4). Nonionic contrast agent that is specifically formulated without preservatives

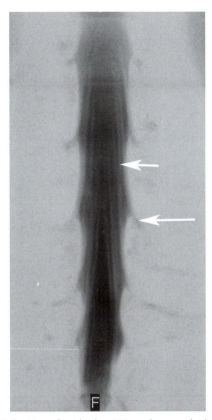

■ **FIGURE 1-3** Frontal projection MR myelogram obtained using 3D fast imaging with steady-state precession. This rapid technique uses the natural contrast effects of CSF to produce a myelographic effect. The descending nerve roots (*short arrow*) are easily identified, including the CSF-filled nerve root sleeve (*long arrow*).

for safe use in myelography is administered through a standard lumbar puncture or cervical puncture at the C1-2 level. Because the dense myelographic contrast will flow through the CSF by gravity before becoming mixed with and diluted by the CSF, consideration must be given to (1) the relative positions of the puncture site, the site of expected pathology, and the specific curvature of the patient's spine and (2) the volume of contrast administered versus the volume of the spinal canal. Correct assessment of both factors will bring the contrast to the site of the pathologic process in proper concentration to demonstrate the lesion. Imaging the patient in the prone or symptomatic position may assist in revealing the cause of neural compression.

Postprocessing of the images on a workstation improves CT of the spine, because varying the window levels and widths provides optimal image review. Bone is typically reviewed with a level of 300 and width of 3000, whereas soft tissue is viewed with a level of 50 and width of 350. By manually adjusting the contrast and window levels at the workstation one can accentuate the differences in tissue densities and detect subtle abnormalities such as small disc protrusions. Curved plane reconstructions can display lengths of the spinal column, canal, and cord that make interpretation easier in patients with kyphoscoliosis or other deformities.

NORMAL APPEARANCE

CSF and fat act as natural contrast agents in spinal MRI. They provide excellent contrast for outlining the spinal cord, the thecal sac, and the nerve roots and veins within the neural foramina. CSF has low signal characteristics on T1W images and high signal on T2W images. The spinal cord has intermediate signal on T1W images in part owing to the abundance of myelinated fiber tracts (lipid) within the cord substance. It has very low signal on T2W images because of the predominance of dense fiber tracts and low water content (Fig. 1-5). Fat has high signal on T1W images and low signal on T2W images. On contrast-enhanced images, the high signal from the fat may obscure the high signal, resulting from contrast enhancement. Therefore, fat-suppression techniques are commonly used to eliminate the high signal from fat and thereby display the high signal from contrast enhancement in stark relief. These fat suppression techniques aid in detecting enhancement within the epidural space and within the spinal cord.

Normal adult bone marrow has intermediate to slightly increased signal intensity on T1W images owing to the presence of fatty marrow. Intermediate to slightly low signal is seen on T2W images in part from the fast imaging techniques used to acquire these images. The facet joints are easily evaluated on both sagittal and axial imaging. Sagittal imaging best illustrates the full articulation between the superior and inferior facets, but axial T1W imaging is best to evaluate the integrity of the articular hyaline cartilage. The structures within the neural foramen are easily evaluated on parasagittal images.

The cartilaginous endplates of the vertebral body are best evaluated in the sagittal or coronal planes using a fat-suppressed 3D spoiled-gradient-echo sequence.[2] This technique may detect subtle morphologic abnormalities of the endplate, including cartilaginous thinning, irregularity, erosions, defects, and Schmorl's nodes. These lesions are the earliest findings seen with degeneration of the intervertebral disc and may be a source of axial back pain. The normal cartilaginous endplate has slightly hypointense to isointense signal on spin-echo T1W images and hypointensity on fast spin-echo T2W images when compared with the normal intervertebral disc. High signal is observed within the cartilage on fat-suppressed spoiled GRE images.

CT excels at delineating bony detail of the spine and adjacent soft tissues (Fig. 1-6). The bone cortex is very dense and easily evaluated. The underlying trabeculae of the medullary bone can also be easily identified on CT. CT clearly displays early reactive or reparative changes such as sclerosis, subchondral cyst formation, and osteophytosis. Parasagittal images are useful for evaluating the integrity of the neural foramen, facet alignment, and the effect of bone remodeling (Fig. 1-7). The posterior bony structures of the spine including the pedicle, lamina, and spinous and transverse processes are easily defined on CT.

The spinal cord is difficult to evaluate on CT, given the inherent contrast limitations. The addition of intrathecal contrast during myelography allows evaluation of spinal cord size and morphology. It also permits adequate evaluation of the intradural nerve roots.

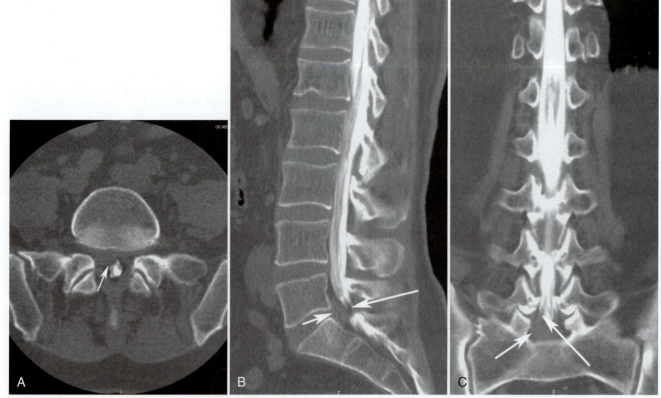

■ **FIGURE 1-4**   CT with intrathecal contrast (myelogram) in a patient with right leg S1 radiculopathy and pacemaker. Axial image (**A**) shows compression of the right anterior thecal sac and nerve roots by a soft tissue lesion consistent with protruding disc (*arrow*). Sagittal reformatted image (**B**) shows continuity of large, mushroom-shaped disc protrusion (*short arrows*) with L5-S1 intervertebral disc. There is compression of the right descending S1 nerve root (*long arrows*) confirmed on the coronal reformatted image (**C**).

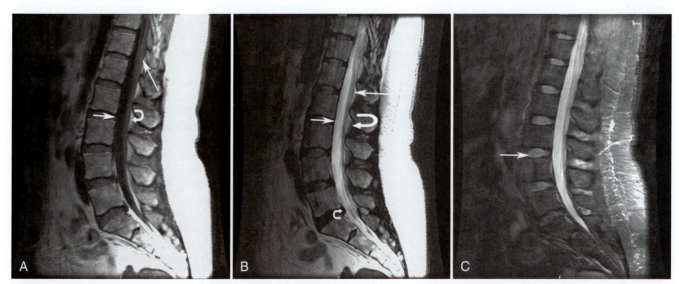

■ **FIGURE 1-5**   **A,** T1W midsagittal MR image shows low signal of CSF (*short arrow*) and intermediate signal of spinal cord/nerve roots (*long arrow*) due to water and fat content. The epidural fat (*curved arrow*) has high signal. Normal adult bone marrow has moderately high signal on T1W images owing to the presence of fatty marrow. **B,** T2W midsagittal MR image shows high signal of CSF (*short arrow*) and low signal of spinal cord (*long arrow*) from intrinsic water content. The epidural fat has low signal (*large curved arrow*), and there is decreased signal of the bone marrow due to fatty marrow. The intervertebral discs show slightly high signal owing to the high water content within the nucleus pulposus, except at L5-S1 where there is disc desiccation and a small disc protrusion (*small curved arrow*). **C,** Inversion recovery midsagittal MR image with fat saturation pulse shows greater T2 weighting; therefore, fluid-containing structures have higher signal and fatty structures show very low signal. Note the greater signal within the intervertebral disc owing to its high water content (*arrow*).

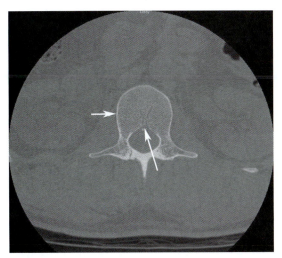

■ FIGURE 1-6 Normal axial CT image through a lumbar vertebral body. The integrity of the very dense, mineralized cortex (*short arrow*) and the underlying heterogeneous trabeculated medullary bone is well seen. The canal for the basivertebral venous plexus that drains the bone marrow into the epidural plexus is also clearly identified (*long arrow*).

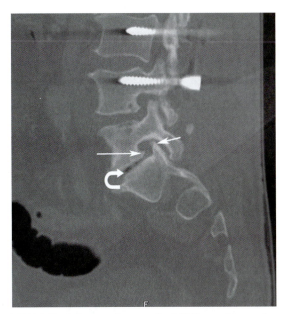

■ FIGURE 1-7 Reformatted parasagittal CT image in a patient after L3-4 fusion shows mild widening of L5-S1 and sclerosis/osteophytosis of the superior S1 facet (*short arrow*). There is also a foraminal osteophyte arising from the L5 inferior endplate (*long arrow*) where Sharpey's fibers from the annulus of the disc insert. These reactive bone changes are easily seen on CT and often are seen due to increased dynamic stress on the facet joint concomitant with degenerative disc disease. Associated disc space narrowing, vacuum phenomenon, and anterior osteophytosis are also seen in this patient (*curved arrow*).

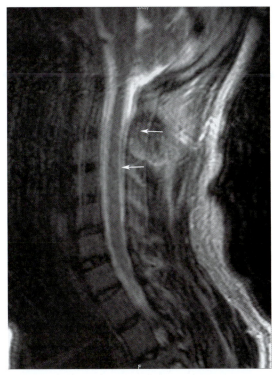

■ FIGURE 1-8 Sagittal T2W MR image degraded by blurring and ghost artifacts (*arrows*) as a result of patient motion during image acquisition.

ARTIFACTS

MRI is susceptible to many artifacts due to the magnetic field and the time required for imaging. Motion artifact is a frequent occurrence, because the phase-encoding gradient cannot predictably compensate for all tissue motion. The appearance of motion artifact is dependent on the direction and speed of motion as well as the magnetic gradient applied. Random motion tends to result in indistinct and blurred anatomic structures, whereas periodic motion results in ghost artifacts (Fig. 1-8).[3] Respiratory motion results in ghost artifact along the phase-encoding direction and is most prevalent with smaller fields of view and later echoes due to decreased signal strength. Pulsatile flow within blood vessels or aneurysms may result in pulsation artifact (phase shift) with multiple linear ghost images along the phase-encoding plane. CSF pulsation also can cause ghost artifacts within and around the spinal cord particularly on T2W images and appear as linear parallel regions of flow void (Fig. 1-9). Bright curvilinear ghost artifacts may occur over the spine due to swallowing (Fig. 1-10).

Motion-related artifacts may be reduced at the time of imaging. One simple method is to increase the number of signals acquired, but this increases overall imaging time. Respiratory and cardiac gating can also be used to synchronize image acquisition but do lengthen the time required for imaging. CSF gating techniques have been described and may be used in cases with significant CSF artifact.[4] Gradient moment nulling may be used to reverse all dephasing and completely refocus the transverse magnetization at the echo time.[3]

Nonuniformity of the magnetic field results in image distortion, dropout, or bright signal artifact. This type of artifact occurs when the different tissues being imaged do not respond in the same way to the applied read gradient. The difference may be due to different magnetic properties (magnetic susceptibility) of the different tissues within the magnetic field or to highly magnetic materials being placed within the magnetic field. Implants, foreign bodies,

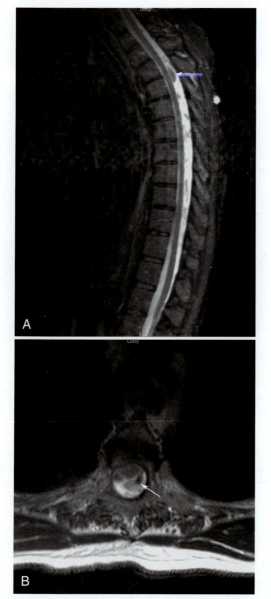

■ FIGURE 1-9 T2W sagittal (**A**) and axial (**B**) images in a patient with a large spinal canal and resultant high CSF flow dynamics. Linear CSF flow voids are seen (*arrows*) and should not be misinterpreted for the serpentine vascular flow voids seen with spinal vascular malformations.

or extrinsic material on the patient that contains iron, cobalt, or nickel results in significant distortion of the magnetic field and acquired images. Stainless steel also may produce significant artifact, but MRI is becoming more feasible as surgical implants switch to titanium. Titanium results in very focal signal dropout adjacent to the implant but acceptable signal outside the immediate region of the implant (Fig. 1-11). All patients should be screened for metallic objects and implants before being positioned within the magnetic field.

There is a significant variation of magnetic susceptibility at interfaces between tissues of the spine. Trabecular bone with intervening blood channels may result in a mottled, hypointense appearance on gradient-echo images.[3] The abrupt interface between cortical bone of

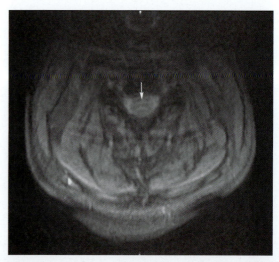

■ FIGURE 1-10 Inversion recovery MR image with ghost artifact (*arrow*) seen as high signal bands superimposed on the spinal cord. These have a well-defined linear appearance and should not be misinterpreted as edema or demyelination of the spinal cord.

the vertebrae and the epidural fat and lateral soft tissues may also result in signal loss. These artifacts are most prevalent on gradient-echo imaging and can be minimized by using a shorter TR or TE and a smaller flip angle. 3D gradient-echo imaging may also provide higher resolution images when using gradient-echo techniques for spine imaging. High signal intensity may be seen at fat/air interfaces when using frequency-selective fat saturation. The transition between fat and air causes a shift in the subcutaneous fat resonance that falls outside the bandwidth used for fat saturation and is most severe when the fat/air interface is perpendicular to the static magnetic field.[3]

Several avoidable artifacts can be seen on MRI and are the result of the imaging protocol used. If simultaneous angled images of the spine are acquired, the area of RF pulse overlap is excited multiple times and may result in signal loss called saturation artifact. Phase wraparound artifact may occur when too small an FOV is used and signal from tissue outside the FOV is superimposed on tissue within the FOV. Gibb's phenomenon is seen as a band of low or high signal along the phase-encoding plane due to the use of insufficient phase-encoding steps and is known as truncation artifact. It can mimic a pathologic process (e.g., syrinx) when superimposed over the spinal cord (Fig. 1-12). This artifact can be avoided by increasing the number of phase-encoding steps, decreasing FOV, or switching the direction of the phase- and frequency-encoding steps.[3] The use of surface coils in spine imaging is susceptible to shading artifact and results in decreased brightness of structures that are farthest (deepest) from the surface coil (Fig. 1-13).

Both MRI and CT are susceptible to partial volume averaging. This artifact occurs when the voxel being imaged contains two different tissues of different densities or MR properties and the image represents an average of this density or signal. It is increased with increasing slice thickness and seen most often between vertebra and disc on spine imaging (Fig. 1-14). Size distortion may

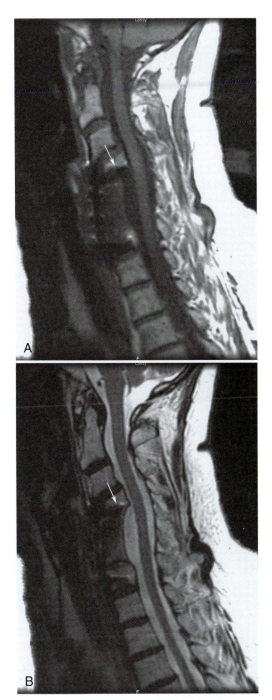

■ FIGURE 1-11 Sagittal T1W (**A**) and T2W (**B**) MR images of a patient with anterior spinal fusion titanium plate and screws. Focal signal dropout is seen immediately adjacent to the hardware (*arrows*) but no significant posterior signal degradation is seen, allowing good evaluation of the thecal sac and spinal cord.

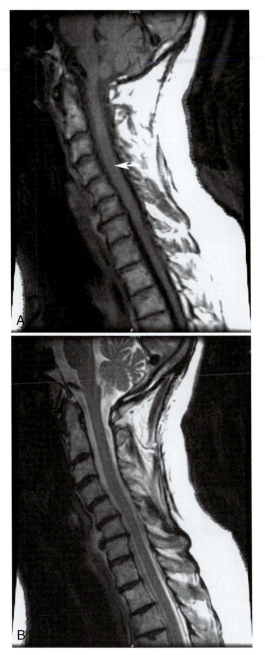

■ FIGURE 1-12 **A,** Sagittal T1W image with linear low signal overlying spinal cord (*arrow*) due to insufficient phase-encoding steps. This should not be mistaken for syringomyelia. **B,** T2W image shows no abnormal fluid-filled structure within the spinal cord substance.

also result with MRI where higher signal objects appear larger and lower signal objects appear smaller than actual size.

CT also has its own inherent susceptibility to artifacts. Beam hardening artifacts occur because low-energy photons are absorbed more rapidly than higher-energy photons. This can result in cupping artifact or streaks/dark bands on the acquired image. The asymmetry of the bony spinal canal is prone to beam hardening as more low

energy photons are absorbed by the beam passing through the thickest portions of bone, such as the vertebral body, or tangential through the posterior elements (Fig. 1-15). The presence of surgical hardware also results in significant beam hardening artifact because the density of metal is outside the normal range of Hounsfield units (Fig. 1-16). This is becoming less of a problem as titanium hardware and multislice scanners are increasingly used. Beam hardening artifact from surgical hardware can also be reduced by tilting the gantry. Any extrinsic metal on the patient should also be removed before imaging. An increase in kilovoltage may help when nonremovable metal is in the region being imaged.

CT is also susceptible to partial volume averaging as discussed for MRI. This can be reduced by using thin-slice acquisition and multislice technology. Photon starvation may cause significant streak artifact if the arms are positioned within the region being imaged. Streak artifacts also occur with patient motion due to misregistration. The use of positioning aids and adequate padding for comfort may help reduce voluntary movement.

Multislice imaging leads to more complicated axial image distortion that has a windmill appearance (Fig. 1-17).[5] This results from the intersection of several rows of detectors along the plane of reconstruction during the course of each rotation. Z-filter helical interpolators are frequently used on multislice scanners to reduce this artifact. The use of non-integer pitch values relative to detector acquisition width may also reduce windmill artifact.[5]

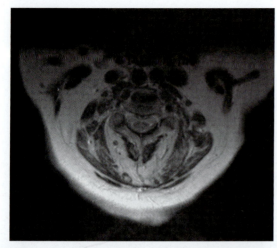

■ **FIGURE 1-13** Axial T2W MR image of the cervical spine obtained with posterior phased-array coil. Note the shading artifact of anterior structures because there is greater distance between the object being imaged and the surface coil.

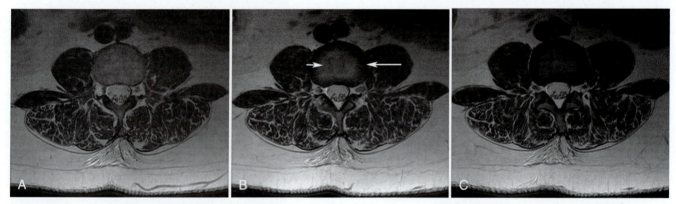

■ **FIGURE 1-14** Sequential, axial, 4-mm thick T2W images obtained through vertebral body (**A**), transition between vertebral body and intervertebral disc (**B**), and through intervertebral disc (**C**). On B, there is volume averaging with the high signal of the superior bone (*short arrow*) surrounded by the low signal of the dehydrated disc below (*long arrow*). This occurs because the selected slice thickness results in a voxel that includes portions of both the vertebral body and intervertebral disc. The resultant image is an average of the signals detected from the voxel being imaged.

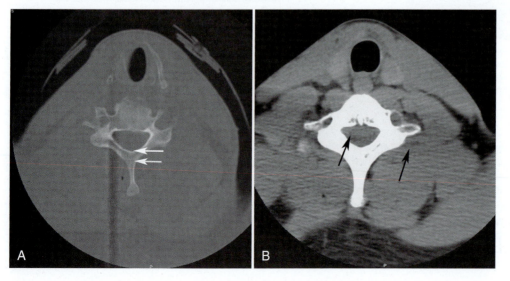

■ **FIGURE 1-15** Axial CT images reproduced with bone (**A**) and soft tissue (**B**) algorithms show a beam-hardening artifact. The linear areas of low attenuation (*arrows*) are the result of absorption of a greater number of low-energy photons along the x-ray beam that cross the thickest portion of high density structure such as bone.

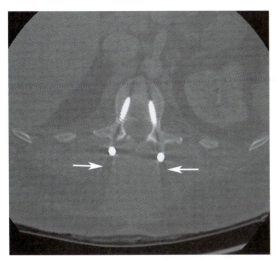

■ **FIGURE 1-16** Axial CT image of the lumbar spine of a patient with bilateral stainless steel pedicle fixation screws. Significant beam-hardening artifact is seen (*arrows*) along the trajectory of the screw.

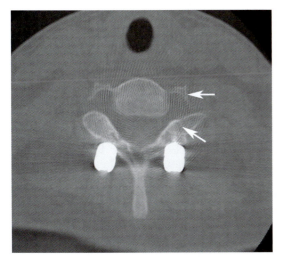

■ **FIGURE 1-17** Axial CT image of the cervical spine obtained on a multislice (64-slice) scanner of a patient with posterior hardware. The multiple rows of detectors used during each rotation results in complex patterns of beam-hardening artifact (*arrows*) that has been referred to as a windmill artifact.

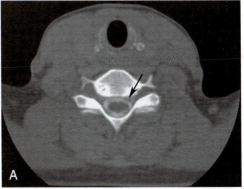

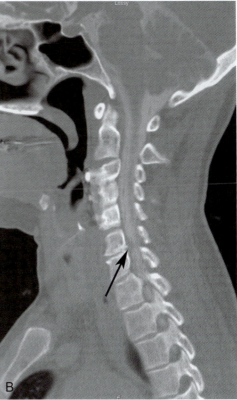

■ **FIGURE 1-18** **A,** Axial CT image after injection of intrathecal contrast agent in a patient after C3-C5 cervical fusion with progressive left C7 radiculopathy and an inconclusive MRI. There is subtle indentation of the thecal sac at the left C6-C7 neural foramen (*arrow*) that may be related to a small disc protrusion. **B,** Sagittal reformatted image shows the associated osteophytosis (*arrow*) and disc protrusion at the C6-7 level that may account for the patient's symptoms.

SPECIFIC USES

MRI of the spine is most commonly used to evaluate local pain or radicular symptoms. The multiplanar imaging capabilities, ability to image small soft tissue structures such as the spinal cord and nerves, and lack of radiation exposure make it particularly useful in this regard. The status of the intervertebral disc, facet joint, ligamentum flavum, posterior longitudinal ligament, and neural foramen are easily evaluated and often reveal the source of a patient's pain. Each study should specifically identify and describe any disc protrusions, osteophytes, and synovial cysts. Symptomatic lesions may be difficult to distinguish from nonsymptomatic lesions on imaging studies, so the imaging features should be correlated with the patient's clinical presentation when interpreting these studies. Lesions that directly compress a nerve root are more likely to be symptomatic, so the spinal canal, bilateral neural foramina, and descending nerve roots should be assessed carefully and sequentially at each level to detect any such compression.[6] In patients with suspected degenerative spine disease, CT may help to assess any osseous pathologic process such as spurring and degenerative bone remodeling that may be difficult to detect on MRI. Selected cases may require CT after injection of a myelographic contrast agent to assess compression of nerve roots more precisely (Fig. 1-18). CT is also very useful for evaluating the success of bone fusion in the postoperative patient (Figs. 1-19 and 1-20).

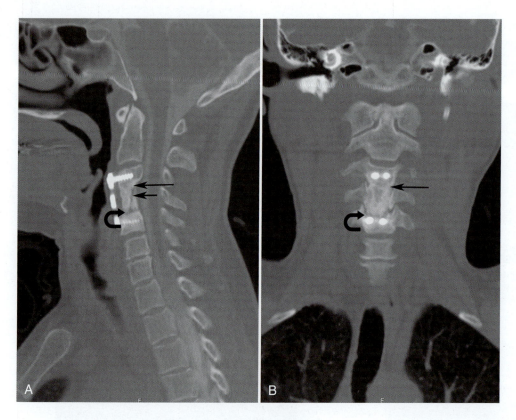

■ **FIGURE 1-19** Sagittal (A) and coronal (B) reformatted CT images of a patient after C4 corpectomy and C3-C5 fusion with strut graft shows fragmentation of the posterior graft (*short arrow*). There is bony fusion of the graft to the C3 vertebral body (*long arrows*) but nonunion at the inferior aspect of the graft (*curved arrows*). CT is very useful for evaluation of the presence of graft fusion.

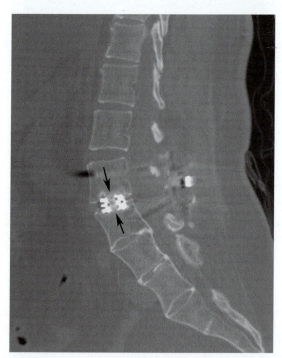

■ **FIGURE 1-20** Sagittal reformatted image of a patient after interbody fusion with a Cage at the L2-3 disc space. There is continuity of the internal bone material with the L2 and L3 vertebral endplates (*arrows*), indicating bony fusion and incorporation of the graft.

Whether using CT or MRI it is important to examine the thecal sac and spinal cord for signs of compression, keeping in mind that compression may be dynamic and seen only with certain positions. Subtle changes such as asymmetry of the hemicord may suggest the presence of intermittent compression (Figs. 1-21 and 1-22). Whenever possible, placing the patient in the symptomatic position during imaging helps to assess for direct neural compression. It is also necessary to rule out other causes of low back pain and radiculopathy, including infection and neoplasm.

MRI is used to evaluate tumors of the spinal cord or nerve root as well as benign and malignant bone tumors of the spine. It is useful for initial diagnosis, for selecting proper therapy, and for monitoring the response to treatment. Intravenous gadolinium contrast should be administered whenever a spinal column tumor is suspected. MRI aids in the differential diagnosis of spinal column tumors by localizing tumor to the intramedullary, extramedullary-intradural, or extradural compartment. Tumors involving the spinal cord (intramedullary) result in cord expansion and typically show high signal on T2W imaging. The pattern of enhancement may aid in diagnosis, as in the case of hemangioblastoma presenting as a cystic intramedullary lesion with nodular enhancement.

Tumors of the vertebral body and pedicle result in replacement of the normal fatty bone marrow. This results in decreased bone marrow signal on T1W images and variable signal on T2W images. Abnormal enhancement of the bone marrow is typical, but sensitivity is dependent on adequate fat-saturation of the normal bone marrow fat. Benign hemangiomas of the vertebrae also are frequent and often easily identified by their high signal characteristics on both T1W and T2W imaging sequences. These lesions will demonstrate significant enhancement, and an increase in coarse vertical trabeculae may be seen on both MRI and CT.

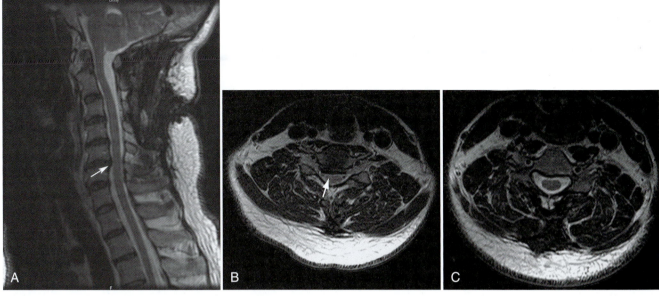

■ **FIGURE 1-21** **A,** Sagittal T2W MR image of a patient with intermittent symptoms of cord impingement. There is suspicion for impingement at the C5-6 level (*arrow*). **B,** Axial T2W MR image at this level shows a broad-based disc protrusion with mild flattening of the anterior spinal cord (*arrow*) particularly on the left. **C,** Comparison with axial T2W image from superior C4-5 disc level shows normal spinal cord size and morphology. The findings at the C5-6 disc level (see **B**) are suggestive of intermittent compression of the spinal cord.

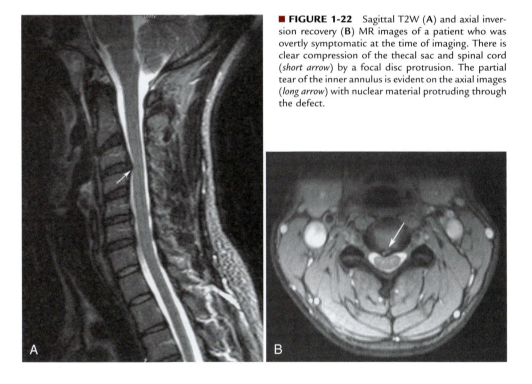

■ **FIGURE 1-22** Sagittal T2W (**A**) and axial inversion recovery (**B**) MR images of a patient who was overtly symptomatic at the time of imaging. There is clear compression of the thecal sac and spinal cord (*short arrow*) by a focal disc protrusion. The partial tear of the inner annulus is evident on the axial images (*long arrow*) with nuclear material protruding through the defect.

MR spectroscopy (MRS) has had limited success in the spine region because of the small size of the spinal cord, physiologic motion, and magnetic field inhomogeneity. High field strength imaging may overcome some of these limitations, and the feasibility of cervical spine MRS has been demonstrated at 3-T imaging.[7] Its utility in differentiating benign from malignant spine tumors has yet to be proven.

CT is frequently used to evaluate spinal column tumors that arise from the posterior elements. The full extent of

bone destruction is more clearly evaluated on CT. Destruction of cortex by tumor infiltration is also easily seen using CT. Intravenous administration of a contrast agent is generally not required but may be useful when a hypervascular tumor is suggested or there is a contraindication to MRI.

Spine CT is routinely used for the initial evaluation of suspected traumatic injury because it is very sensitive for identification of fractures. The access to multislice CT has resulted in a paradigm shift in traumatic spine imaging,

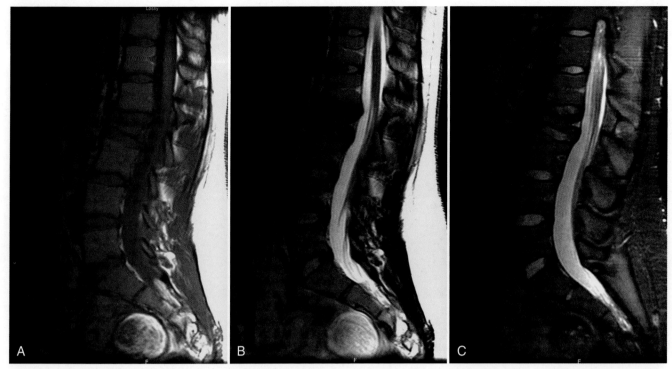

■ **FIGURE 1-23** **A,** Sagittal T1W of a patient with chronic low back pain and an L2 vertebral compression fracture seen on plain radiography. No definite sclerosis was seen. There is slightly low signal of the L2 bone marrow that might be related to bone marrow edema. T2W (**B**) and inversion recovery (**C**) sagittal images do not show increased signal to suggest bone marrow edema, indicating that this is likely an old compression fracture and not related to the patient's pain. A radionuclide bone scan showed no abnormal uptake at this level, and the patient subsequently improved with physical therapy.

and CT is now routinely used for screening of high-risk patients. This is particularly true for cervical spine imaging, when despite not having a randomized controlled trial there appears to be ample evidence that CT significantly outperforms plain radiography as a screening test for high-risk patients.[8] A meta-analysis by Holmes and Akkinepalli showed a pooled sensitivity of 52% for plain radiography and 98% for CT.[8] In properly selected patients with moderate to high probability of injury, CT screening of the cervical spine is also cost effective.[9]

MRI is used in trauma to evaluate for traumatic disc rupture, ligamentous or spinal cord injury, and intraspinal hematoma. It is also sensitive to bone marrow edema and may be used to evaluate occult fractures by CT and the acuity of a fracture in indeterminate cases. This is especially valuable for evaluating benign compression fractures (Fig. 1-23). Inversion recovery imaging is especially useful for the detection of subtle edema of the bone marrow and ligaments, and T2* GRE images may be used to increase sensitivity for hemorrhagic shear injury of the cord. T2W images with adequate fat saturation are used to evaluate the ligaments and annulus of the intervertebral disc. Inversion recovery sequences are useful to evaluate for the presence of spinal cord edema (Fig. 1-24). T1W images aid in evaluating the integrity of the ligamentous structures, particularly the anterior and posterior longitudinal ligaments. They are also useful for identification of epidural hematoma (Fig. 1-25). MR angiography and fat-suppressed T1W images of the neck should be performed if there is suspicion of vascular injury. MRI is often used in the unconscious trauma patient, in a patient with per-

sistent neurologic deficit, and before treatment of a significant injury identified on CT.

MRI should also be considered in patients with suspected spinal column infection. Osteomyelitis-discitis is a difficult diagnosis that can be confirmed by the presence of abnormal increased T2W signal within the intervertebral disc and the presence of enhancement, particularly of the intervening disc and adjacent vertebral endplates. Clinical presentation and laboratory studies aid in the diagnosis because inflammatory changes from degenerative disc disease can have a similar appearance to infection. MRI is very sensitive for epidural extension of infection and abscess formation. DWI may be used to confirm the diagnosis because epidural abscess will result in diffusion restriction.[10] DWI may also be used to evaluate postoperative paraspinal fluid collections, because simple seromas should not cause diffusion restriction, whereas abscesses do. CT is less sensitive than MRI for evaluation of suspected spine infection. It occasionally assists in evaluating the degree of bone destruction but should not be the first line of imaging in these patients.

MRI is also frequently used for evaluation of inflammatory disorders such as multiple sclerosis, sarcoidosis, and transverse myelitis. MRI is typically used to evaluate the presence of spinal cord edema (acute inflammation) or demyelination (chronic inflammation). Fast short-tau inversion recovery (STIR) sequences or magnetization transfer techniques may be used to increase sensitivity of intra-medullary inflammatory processes (Fig. 1-26). MRI findings are typically not specific but help to detect cord lesions and define their extent and morphology. Gadolin-

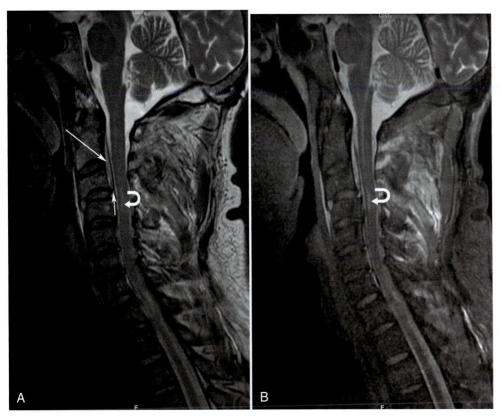

■ **FIGURE 1-24 A,** Sagittal T2W MR image of a patient with neurologic deficit after a motor vehicle accident. There is mild anterolisthesis of C3 on C4 and posterior disc protrusion with elevation of the posterior longitudinal ligament (*short arrow*) as well as associated epidural hematoma (*long arrow*). There also appears to be focal increased signal within the spinal cord (*curved arrow*), suggesting cord contusion. **B,** Sagittal inversion recovery MR image confirms the presence and extent of spinal cord edema (*curved arrow*).

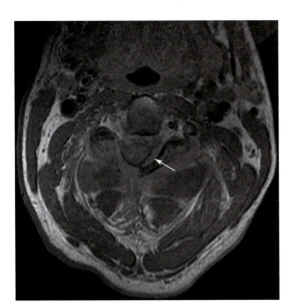

■ **FIGURE 1-25** Axial T1W MR image of the same patient in Figure 1-24 shows intermediate signal of a posterior epidural hemorrhage (*arrow*) replacing the normal high signal of the epidural fat.

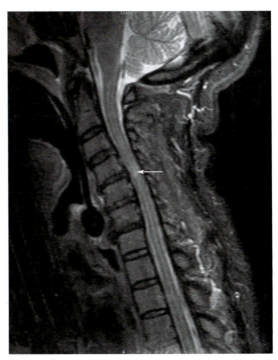

■ **FIGURE 1-26** Inversion recovery sagittal MR image of a patient with clinical myelopathy. Focal increased signal is detected within the spinal cord (*arrow*). The patient was subsequently diagnosed with multiple sclerosis by brain MRI and CSF analysis.

ium is often useful to evaluate acuity of such lesions. Newer techniques such as multiple-echo recombined gradient-echo (MERGE) or periodically overlapping parallel lines with enhanced reconstruction (PROPPELER) may serve to increase lesion detection by improving gray matter/white matter differentiation and reducing CSF pulsation artifact. Higher field strength imaging on 3-T systems may also increase identification of these lesions by increas-

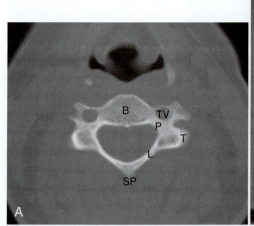

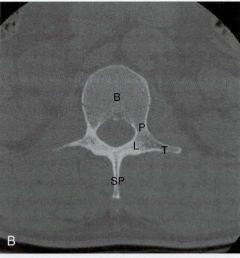

■ **FIGURE 1-27** Axial CT images of a cervical (**A**) and lumbar (**B**) vertebral body demonstrate the normal bony anatomy. B, vertebral body; P, pedicle; L, lamina; T, transverse process; SP, spinous process; TV, transverse foramen. The vertebral artery courses through the transverse foramen.

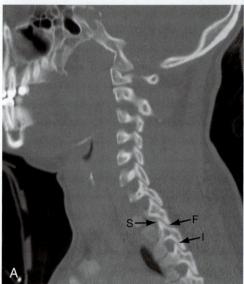

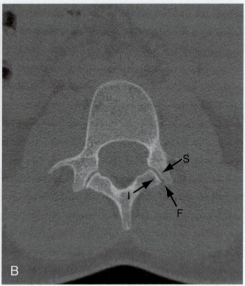

■ **FIGURE 1-28** Sagittal reformatted CT image of the cervical spine (**A**) and axial CT image of the lumbar spine (**B**) demonstrate the normal anatomic relationship of the superior and inferior facets. The superior facet lies anterior to the posterior facet with the synovial-lined facet joint between the two bony processes. S, superior facet; I, inferior facet; F, facet joint.

ing SNR and decreasing imaging time and resultant patient motion. MRS may also play a future role in spinal cord assessment and has shown a reduced N-acetyl aspartate in patients with multiple sclerosis as compared to healthy controls.[11]

ANALYSIS

It is useful to have a systematic approach to interpret spinal imaging studies. Multiplanar images should be used whether imaging with CT or MRI. Each anatomic structure should be evaluated in at least two planes, keeping in mind that images obtained perpendicular to the anatomic structure under review are often most useful.

The individual elements of the vertebra should be evaluated, including the vertebral body, pedicle, and superior and inferior facets (including the articulation with the facet above and below), lamina, and the transverse and spinous processes (Fig. 1-27). It is important to remember the ligamentous structures that attach between each vertebral body, particularly the anterior and posterior longitudinal ligaments and the posterior ligament complex.

These structures may be involved in traumatic, inflammatory, or degenerative spine disease.

The intervertebral disc should be assessed including the signal/density and morphology of the nucleus and annulus. The annulus is firmly attached to the bony margins of the vertebral body by Sharpey's fibers. The central vertebral endplate is lined with cartilage that is tightly interwoven with the annulus. The anterior and posterior longitudinal ligaments provide additional structural support to the anterior and posterior disc annulus, respectively.

The spinal cord and thecal sac should be scrutinized for compression and abnormal morphology. The full lateral extent of the thecal sac should be visualized as well as the characteristics of the surrounding epidural fat. The presence or absence of enhancement should be noted, particularly in cases of suspected tumor or infection and in patients with a prior surgical history. The signal characteristics of the spinal cord should also be assessed when reviewing MR images.

The superior facet joint is located anterior to the inferior facet joint (Fig. 1-28). The facet joint is lined with

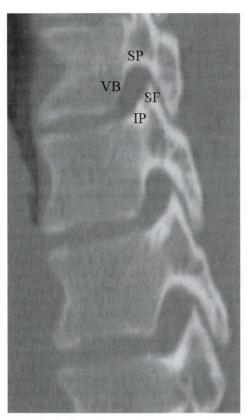

■ FIGURE 1-29 Sagittal reformatted CT image demonstrates the normal anatomic structures that form the neural foramen. SP, superior pedicle; SF, superior facet; IP, inferior pedicle; VB, vertebral body.

hyaline cartilage and should be evaluated for integrity and evidence of reparative change. The ligamentum flavum is V shaped on axial images and lies immediately deep (anterior) to the lamina. It provides additional support to the anterior facet joint capsule. The posterior facet joint capsule extends posterior and lateral along the margin of the posterior facet. The hyaline cartilage does not extend into this portion of the facet capsule. The widest portion of the facet capsule is at the superior and inferior recesses.

The neural foramen is formed by four bony structures (Fig. 1-29). The superior margin of the neural foramen is formed by the inferior surface of the pedicle of the vertebra above and the inferior margin by the superior surface of the pedicle below. The posterior margin of the neural foramen is formed by the superior facet of the vertebra below and the anterior margin by the posterior surface of the vertebra above. The dorsal and ventral nerve roots exit the neural foramen and fuse to form the spinal nerve. The spinal nerves then course anterior and inferior away from the spinal column. The radiculomedullary artery and vein also course through the neural foramen (Fig. 1-30). Both are typically anterior to the nerve, with the artery within the superior recess and the vein within the inferior recess of the foramen. These structures are surrounded by adipose tissue that is continuous with the epidural space until fusion of the dura to the spinal nerve to form the epineurium.

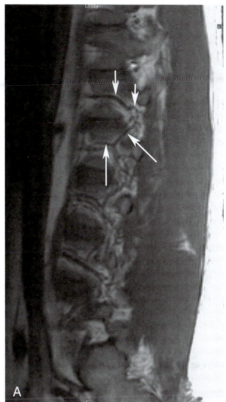

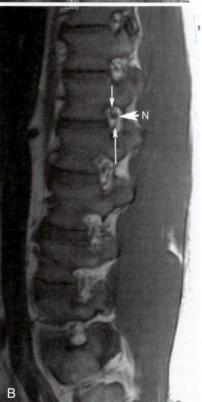

■ FIGURE 1-30 Parasagittal T1W MR images from lateral (**A**) to medial (**B**) show the radiculomedullary artery (*short arrows*) and vein (*long arrows*) arising from the lumbar artery and coursing through the neural foramen. N, spinal nerve.

Finally, the paraspinal musculature should be evaluated. Any atrophy should be noted and may be seen as loss of bulk and increase in fat density on CT or fat signal on T1W MR images. The paraspinal muscles should also be evaluated for the presence of edema or fluid collection. The erector spinae muscles are the largest group of muscles along the posterior aspect of the spinal canal. The longus colli muscles lie anterior to the cervical vertebrae, and the psoas muscles lie anterolateral to the lumbar vertebrae.

Sample reports are shown in Boxes 1-1 and 1-2.

CURRENT RESEARCH AND FUTURE DIRECTION

Parallel imaging is becoming more readily available on MRI systems and shows promise for rapid evaluation of the entire spinal axis. It takes advantage of the inherent spatial information in phased-array RF coils to reduce acquisition time while improving spatial resolution and SNR. These parallel methods are typically applied to T2W turbo spin-echo sequences. Combined head and spine arrays now allow imaging of the brain and entire spine without changing coils or repositioning the patient. This can be accomplished with a stepwise table or by merely repositioning the patient on the table. Generalized auto-calibrating partially parallel acquisition (GRAPPA) and modified sensitive encoding (mSENSE) are two such parallel imaging techniques. In the spine, GRAPPA imaging may provide very fast imaging with higher SNR than mSENSE, with no increase in alias artifacts and with an SNR similar to standard T2W turbo spin-echo sequences.[12]

BOX 1-1 MRI of the Adult Spine

PATIENT HISTORY

A 43-year-old man with chronic lumbar back pain not responsive to conventional therapy presented with a history of prior lumbar discectomy.

TECHNIQUE

Sagittal and axial T1W spin-echo and T2W fast spin-echo images were acquired from T11 through the sacrum. The risks and benefits of intravenous administration of a contrast agent were explained to the patient and written informed consent was obtained. Based on the patient's weight, 20 mL of gadolinium was administered.

FINDINGS

The bone marrow signal is normal for age. The intervertebral disc signal is normal without bulge or protrusion. The facet joints are normal, and there is no narrowing of the neural foramina. There is no compression of the thecal sac or neural elements. No abnormal enhancement is noted.

IMPRESSION

This is a normal MRI of the lumbar spine.

BOX 1-2 CT of the Adult Spine

PATIENT HISTORY

A 25-year-old woman complaining of cervical spine tenderness presented after being hit by a car.

TECHNIQUE

Contiguous axial 0.625-mm CT images were acquired and reconstructed at 1.5-mm slice thickness. Bone and soft tissue algorithm images were reviewed; sagittal and coronal reformatted images were performed at the workstation and used for interpretation.

FINDINGS

There is normal cervical lordosis and no prevertebral soft tissue swelling. No fracture or subluxation is seen. The dens is intact on axial and reformatted images. The facet alignment is normal.

IMPRESSION

This is a normal CT of the cervical spine.

Diffusion tensor imaging (DTI) of the spinal cord has many technical challenges but holds promise for future clinical use. The size of the spinal cord requires very small voxel size with decreased SNR. Local field inhomogeneities and motion due to CSF pulsation and breathing may further degrade image quality. Faster imaging acquisition techniques may compensate for these limitations. DTI and fiber tractography have been used to evaluate infiltration and displacement of spinal cord fiber tracts by tumor.[13] DTI also shows potential use for the evaluation of spondylosis and the effects of cord compression. Signal intensity changes on T2W images typically appear late after symptoms of myelopathy have developed. The imaging is further complicated by the common positional nature of cord compression, which may be minimized or relieved in the supine position used for image acquisition. DTI has been used in the evaluation of white matter tract integrity in spondylosis.[14] Animal studies have suggested that an increase in minor eigen-values may be seen with demyelination, increased axonal diameter, and changes in protein integrity.[15] DTI may therefore have a future role in predicting patients who have the most likelihood for improvement after decompression surgery.

MRI of the spine has the inherent limitation of imaging patients in the recumbent (supine) position. Most spine-mediated pain is encountered during physiologic stress or loading on the spine, which typically occurs with motion, sitting, or standing. Imaging in the position of pain generation has obvious advantages but has been slow to advance in clinical imaging. There are devices available that add axial load to the lumbar spine during imaging. This technique may improve the ability to detect symptomatic lesions.[16] Dynamic-kinetic imaging or upright weight-bearing imaging of the spine may also serve this purpose. Upright MRI systems allow imaging in both the recumbent and upright positions and permit graded degrees of axial load to be applied.[17] They also permit kinetic movements of the patient's body to image the spine in the position that replicates the clinical syndrome.

KEY POINTS

- Both CT and MRI are frequently used imaging modalities for the evaluation of degenerative spine disease, spinal tumors, trauma, infection, and inflammation.
- CT uses axial thin-section images and reformatted images in the sagittal and coronal planes for definitive interpretation. MRI typically uses both T1W and T2W sequences in the sagittal and axial planes, with occasional addition of coronal plane imaging. When MRI is contraindicated, CT myelography may be used to better delineate spinal anatomy and any compression of neural elements.

- Limitations and artifacts associated with spinal imaging are often due to the small size of the spinal cord and nerves and to edge effects at the bony spinal canal that surrounds them. The physics of spine imaging are important to consider in developing protocols that reduce inherent artifacts and produce the best diagnostic images possible.
- As 3-T imaging continues to become more readily available, newer techniques of spinal cord imaging are being developed, including diffusion tensor imaging and functional MRI of the spinal cord.

SUGGESTED READINGS

Castillo M (ed). Spinal Imaging: State of the Art. Philadelphia, Hanley and Belfus, 2001.

Chawla S. Multidetector computed tomography imaging of the spine. J Comput Assist Tomogr 2004; 28:S28-S31.

Lane B. Practical imaging of the spine and spinal cord. Top Magn Reson Imaging 2003; 14:438-443.

Phalke VV, Gujar S, Quint DJ. Comparison of 3.0 T versus 1.5 T MR: Imaging of the spine. Neuroimag Clin North Am 2006; 16:241-248.

Ross JS. Newer sequences for spinal MR imaging: smorgasbord or succotash of acronyms? AJNR Am J Neuroradiol 1999; 20:361-373.

Stone JA. MR myelography of the spine and MR peripheral nerve imaging. Magn Reson Imaging Clin North Am 2003; 11:543-558.

Vertinsky AT, Krasnokutsky MV, Augustin M, Bammer R. Cutting-edge imaging of the spine. Neuroimaging Clin North Am 2007; 17:117-136.

REFERENCES

1. Demaerel P, Bosmans H, Wilms G, et al. Rapid lumbar spine MR myelography using rapid acquisition with relaxation enhancement. AJR Am J Roentgenol 1997; 168:377-378.

2. Kakitsubata Y, Theodorou DJ, Theodorou SJ, et al. Cartilaginous endplates of the spine: MRI with anatomic correlation in cadavers. J Comput Assist Tomogr 2002; 6:933-940.

3. Taber KH, Herrick RC, Weathers SW, et al. Pitfalls and artifacts encountered in clinical MR imaging of the spine. RadioGraphics 1998; 18:1499-1521.

4. Rubin JB, Enzmann DR, Wright A. CSF-gated MR imaging of the spine: theory and clinical implementation. Radiology 1987; 163:784-792.

5. Barrett JF, Keat N. Artifacts in CT: recognition and avoidance. Radio-Graphics 2004; 24:1679-1691.

6. Phirrmann CW, Dora C, Schmid M, et al. MR image–based grading of lumbar nerve root compromise due to disk herniation: reliability study with surgical correlation. Radiology 2004; 230:583-588.

7. Marliani AF, Clementi V, Albini-Riccioli L, et al. Quantitative proton magnetic resonance spectroscopy of the human cervical spinal cord at 3 Tesla. Magn Reson Med 2007; 57:160-163.

8. Holmes JF, Akkinepalli R. Computed tomography versus plain radiography to screen for cervical spine injury: a meta-analysis. J Trauma 2005; 58:902-905.

9. Blackmore CC, Mann FA, Wilson AJ. Helical CT in the primary trauma evaluation of the cervical spine: an evidence based approach. Skeletal Radiol 2000; 29:632-639.

10. Eastwood JD, Vollmer RT, Provenzale JM. Diffusion-weighted imaging in a patient with vertebral and epidural abscesses. AJNR Am J Neuroradiol 2002; 23:496-498.

11. Kendi AT, Tan FU, Kendi M, et al. MR spectroscopy of cervical cord in patients with multiple sclerosis. Neuroradiology 2004; 46:764-769.

12. Ruel L, Brugieres P, Luciani A, et al. Comparison of in vitro and in vivo MRI of the spine using parallel imaging. AJR Am J Roentgenol 2004; 182:749-755.

13. Ducreux D, Lepeintre JF, Fillard P, et al. MR diffusion tensor imaging and fiber tracking in 5 spinal cord astrocytomas. AJNR Am J Neuroradiol 2006; 27:214-216.

14. Facon D, Ozanne A, Fillard P, et al. MR diffusion tensor imaging and fiber tracking in spinal cord compression. AJNR Am J Neuroradiol 2005; 26:1587-1594.

15. Schwartz ED, Cooper ET, Chin CL, et al. Ex vivo evaluation of ADC values within the spinal cord white matter tracts. AJNR Am J Neuroradiol 2005; 26:390-397.

16. Willen J, Danielson B, Gaulitz A. Dynamic effects on the lumbar spinal canal: axially loaded CT myelography and MRI in patients with sciatica and/or neurogenic claudication. Spine 2001; 26:2601-2606.

17. Jinkins JR, Dworkin JS, Damadian RV. Upright, weight bearing, dynamic-kinetic MRI of the spine: initial results. Eur Radiol 2005; 15:1815-1825.

Paraspinal Structures

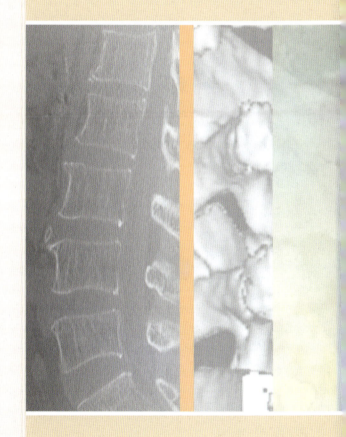

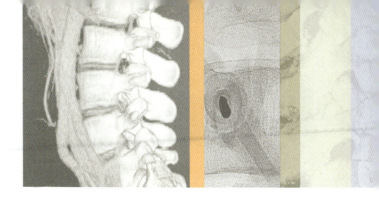

CHAPTER

2

Paraspinal Soft Tissues

Carrie L. Tong

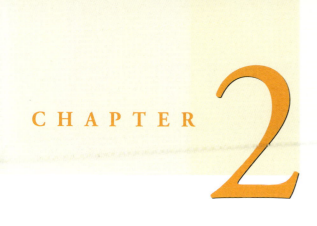

The paraspinal soft tissues consist predominantly of musculature. The area may be defined as the paraspinal muscles, the fascia that envelops them, and the vessels, lymphatics, and nerves that traverse and supply them. In the neck, this includes the anterior and lateral vertebral muscles as well as the posterior cervical musculature. In the trunk and back, the paraspinal muscles include the superficial scapular muscles and latissimus dorsi as well as the vertebral column extensors medially and the iliopsoas anterolaterally.

GROSS ANATOMY

Musculature

The Dorsal Muscles

The dorsal paraspinal muscles may be divided into the superficial group, which help move the shoulder girdle; the deep group, which extend and rotate the vertebral column; and the suboccipital group, which move the head.

Superficial Group

The most superficial of the paraspinal muscles of the neck is the *trapezius* muscle, which originates posteriorly from the occipital bone, the ligamentum nuchae, and the thoracic spinous processes. It inserts on the acromion, the lateral clavicle, and the spine of the scapula (Figs. 2-1 to 2-3). Deeper and more anterior is the *levator scapulae,* which spans from cervical spine to medial scapula. Both of these muscles are innervated by anterior rami of mid-cervical spinal nerves. The trapezius also receives additional innervation from cranial nerve XI.

Superficially in the back are found the *rhomboid minor* and *rhomboid major,* which are both innervated by the dorsal scapular nerve. They originate from the spinous processes of the upper thoracic spine and the ligamentum nuchae to attach to the medial border of the scapula. The *latissimus dorsi* is a large, flat muscle that arises from a lumbar aponeurosis (with additional slips originating from the iliac crest and lower ribs) and inserts on the humerus. It is innervated by the thoracodorsal nerve.[1-4]

Deep Group

The deep muscles weave around each other in a plait down the spinal column, maintaining the normal curves of the vertebral column.

Posterior to the levator scapulae lies the *splenius capitis,* originating from the ligamentum nuchae and the upper thoracic spinous processes and inserting on the occipital bone and mastoid. Lying underneath it is the *splenius cervicis,* which originates from the upper thoracic spinous processes to insert upon the upper cervical transverse processes (Figs. 2-3 to 2-6). Deep to this lie the *semispinalis capitis, cervicis,* and *thoracic,* originating from the transverse processes of the thoracic spine and inserting on the spinous processes of the cervical and upper thoracic spine, as well as on the occiput. Also beneath the large splenius capitis lies the *longissimus capitis,* which, along with the semispinalis, is a major extensor of the head and neck.[2,4]

Deeper still lies the column rotator muscles, the multifidi, which originate from the lateral masses of each vertebral body, spanning two or three bodies to insert on the spinous processes above.

Suboccipital Group

A series of suboccipital muscles helps to move the head. The *oblique capitis superior* originates from the transverse process of C1 to insert on the occipital bone. The *oblique capitis inferior* muscle originates from the spine of C2, inserting on the transverse process of C1.[2-4]

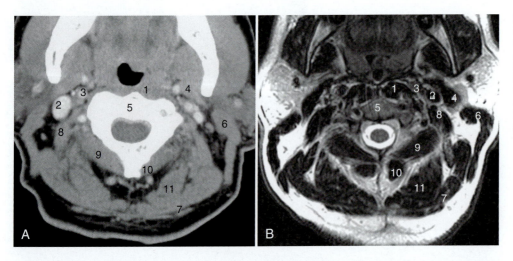

■ **FIGURE 2-1** Axial scans at an upper cervical level. **A,** CT image. **B,** T2W MR sequence. 1, longus capitis and colli; 2, jugular vein; 3, internal carotid artery; 4, posterior belly of digastric; 5, vertebral body; 6, sternocleidomastoid; 7, trapezius; 8, levator scapulae; 9, oblique capitis inferior; 10, semispinalis; 11, splenius.

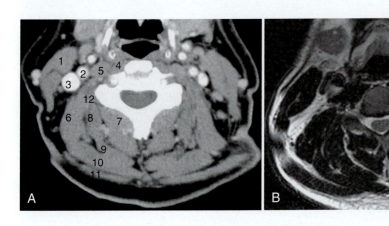

■ **FIGURE 2-2** Axial scans at a middle cervical level. **A,** CT image. **B,** T2W MR sequence. 1, sterno-cleidomastoid; 2, carotid artery; 3, jugular vein; 4, longus colli; 5, longus capitis; 6, levator scapulae; 7, multifidus; 8, longissimus capitis; 9, semispinalis; 10, splenius capitis; 11, trapezius; 12, splenius cervicis.

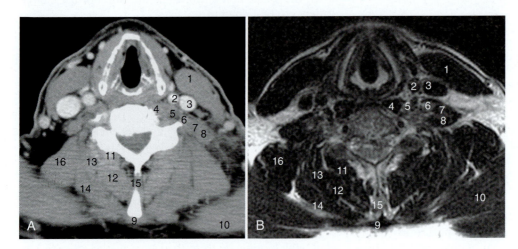

■ **FIGURE 2-3** Axial scans at a lower cervical level. **A,** CT image. **B,** T2W MR sequence. 1, sterno-cleidomastoid; 2, carotid artery; 3, jugular vein; 4, longus colli; 5, longus capitis; 6, anterior scalene; 7, middle scalene; 8, posterior scalene; 9, ligamentum nuchae; 10, trapezius; 11, multifidus; 12, semispinalis; 13, longissimus capitis; 14, splenius capitis; 15, interspinalis; 16, levator scapulae.

The Ventral Muscles

The flexor, or prevertebral, muscles lie anterior to the spinal column. The *rectus capitis* originates from the C1 and C2 to insert upon the occiput. It receives innervation from C1-C2. The *longus colli* lies anterior to the vertebral column, originating from the midcervical and upper thoracic spine and inserting upon the vertebral bodies of the upper cervical spine. Lateral to the longus colli lies the *longus capitis* with its broad superior insertion on the occipital bone and its narrow origin from the lower cervical spine. The longus colli receives innervation from C2 through C7, whereas the longus capitis is innervated by C1 to C3.

Anterolaterally in the deep neck span the *scalene* muscles, which originate from the cervical transverse

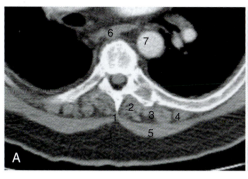
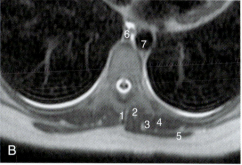

■ **FIGURE 2-4** Axial scans through a middle thoracic level. **A,** CT image. **B,** T2W MR sequence. 1, interspinalis; 2, multifidus; 3, spinalis thoracis; 4, longissimus; 5, trapezius; 6, esophagus; 7, aorta.

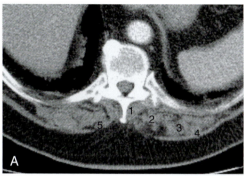
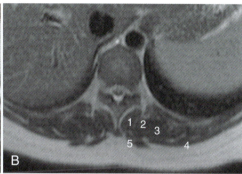

■ **FIGURE 2-5** Axial scans through a lower thoracic level. **A,** CT image. **B,** T2W MR sequence. 1, multifidus; 2, semispinalis; 3, longissimus; 4, latissimus dorsi; 5, trapezius.

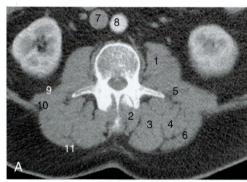
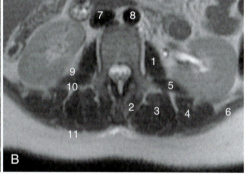

■ **FIGURE 2-6** Axial scans through an upper lumbar level. **A,** CT image. **B,** T2W MR sequence. 1, psoas; 2, multifidus; 3, longissimus; 4, iliocostalis; 5, quadratus lumborum; 6, internal and external oblique; 7, inferior vena cava; 8, aorta; 9-11, thoracolumbar fascia; 9, anterior layer; 10, middle layer; 11, posterior layer.

processes and insert anterolaterally on the first two ribs. They are innervated by the posterior rami of C5 to C8. The brachial plexus passes between the anterior and middle scalene muscles.

The Deep Muscles

The Long Set

In the deep back, posterolateral to the spinal column, are *erector spinae* or *sacrospinalis* muscles. These comprise the more superficial group of the deep muscles of the back. From lateral to medial, they consist of the *iliocostalis*, spanning from the iliac crest to the upper ribs; the *longissimus dorsi*, spanning from the sacrum to the transverse processes of the entire spine; and the *spinalis*, which originates and inserts on the spinous processes and is intimately intertwined with the longissimus dorsi (Figs. 2-4 to 2-10).

The Intervertebral Set

A series of muscles connect adjacent vertebrae. These include the *rotatores* that originate from transverse processes to insert on the spinous processes of adjacent vertebrae. These, along with the multifidi and semispinalis, comprise the intermediate oblique muscles of the deep back musculature. The deepest muscles include the *interspinalis*, which connects the apices of adjoining spinous processes from C2 to L5, and the *intertransversarii*, which connect adjacent transverse processes.

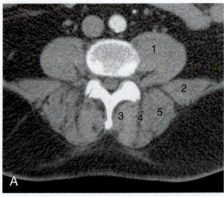
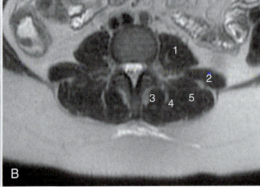

■ **FIGURE 2-7** Axial scans through a lower lumbar level. **A,** CT image. **B,** T2W MR sequence. 1, psoas; 2, quadratus lumborum; 3, multifidus; 4, longissimus; 5, iliocostalis.

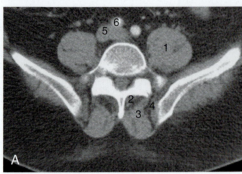
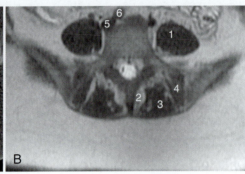

■ **FIGURE 2-8** Axial scans at the lumbosacral junction. **A,** CT image. **B,** T2W MR sequence. 1, psoas; 2, multifidus; 3, longissimus; 4, iliocostalis; 5, iliac vein; 6, iliac artery.

The Lateral Set

In the lumbar level, the *psoas muscles* are lateral and adjacent to the spinal column and functionally serve as lower extremity flexors (see Figs. 2-6 to 2-8). They originate from the anterolateral lumbar spine and insert on the lesser trochanter of the femur. The *quadratus lumborum* is a thin broad muscle that arises from the iliac crest to insert on the 12th rib and the lumbar transverse processes.[1,2,4]

Although the paraspinal muscles are described in great detail in the anatomic literature, they are rarely described individually in radiology, with the exception of the neck. This may be in part due to difficulties in resolution and also to their tendency to be affected en bloc by pathology. However, as advancements in imaging continue, higher resolution and functional studies may shed new light on this relatively unstudied region.

Arteries

The cervical structures are supplied from branches of the *occipital, vertebral, deep cervical,* and *ascending cervical* arteries. The occipital artery originates from the external carotid artery and can be found beneath the sternocleidomastoid, splenius capitis, longissimus capitis, and semispinalis capitis muscles, among others, on its tortuous path to the posterior scalp.

The vertebral artery is the first branch of the subclavian artery. It first runs upward and backward between the longus colli and the anterior scalene. It then ascends

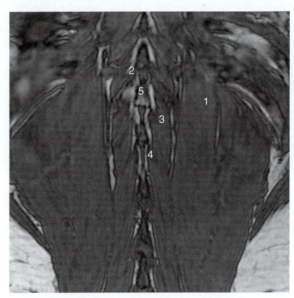

■ **FIGURE 2-9** Coronal scan at the thoracolumbar junction, posterior. 1, longissimus thoracis; 2, multifidus; 3, semispinalis thoracis; 4, spinalis thoracis; 5, spinous process.

within the transverse foramina of the upper six cervical vertebrae, passing behind the superior facet of the atlas to enter the foramen magnum.

The deep cervical artery most frequently arises from the costocervical trunk. It passes backward between the

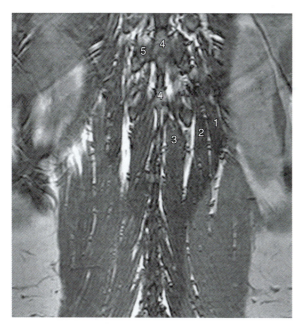

■ **FIGURE 2-10** Coronal scan at the thoracolumbar junction, just ventral to the image in Figure 2-9. 1, longissimus thoracis; 2, spinalis thoracis; 3, multifidus and rotatores; 4, spinous process; 5, lamina.

transverse process of C7 and the first rib to run cephalad between the semispinalis capitis and colli.

The ascending cervical artery arises from the inferior thyroid artery, running up on the transverse processes of the cervical vertebral bodies between the anterior scalene and the longus capitis. The ascending cervical sends branches to the muscles of the neck that anastomose with branches of the vertebral artery.[1,2]

In the thoracic region, the *posterior rami* of the *intercostal arteries* supply the structures of the back. Before terminating in muscular and cutaneous branches, these rami supply a spinal branch that enters the vertebral canal to supply the cord, membranes, and vertebrae.

In the lumbar region, the arterial supply streams from branches of the *subcostal and lumbar arteries.* Both sets of arteries arise from the posterior aspect of the aorta to run posterolaterally along the lumbar vertebral bodies. On the right they pass behind the inferior vena cava, and on both sides they pass beneath the tendinous origin of the psoas major, cross the quadratus lumborum, and continue between the abdominal wall musculature.

The *iliolumbar and lateral sacral arteries,* both branches of the posterior trunk of the internal iliac artery, supply the sacral musculature. The iliolumbar artery turns cephalad from its origin to run behind the external iliac vessels, following the posteromedial border of the psoas major muscle, where it splits into lumbar and iliac branches. There are usually two lateral sacral arteries on each side, a superior and an inferior, that supply the contents of the sacral canal as well as the skin and muscles on the dorsal surface of the sacrum.[1,2]

Veins

Complicated venous plexuses span from the skull to the coccyx to drain the structures of the back. The veins surrounding the vertebral column form the *external vertebral venous plexus.* The veins lining the interior surface of the vertebral canal form the *internal vertebral venous plexus.* These venous plexuses are thin walled and functionally valveless, so they communicate freely with veins in the neck, thorax, abdomen, and pelvis, as well as the occipital and basilar venous sinuses intracranially.[1,2]

Lymphatics

The deep lymphatics of the paraspinal soft tissues follow the veins and drain into the *deep cervical, posterior mediastinal, lateral aortic,* and *sacral nodes,* also referred to as glands.[1]

The deep cervical glands are large in size and number, forming a chain along the carotid sheath, where they follow the pharynx, esophagus, and trachea from the base of the skull to the root of the neck. In addition to the paraspinal musculature of the neck, they drain the scalp, pectoral, and some upper arm muscles, as well the thyroid and trachea.

The posterior mediastinal glands, which drain the thoracic paraspinal muscles, lie behind the pericardium and drape over the esophagus and descending thoracic aorta. In addition to their paraspinal afferents, they also drain the esophagus, posterior pericardium, diaphragm, and liver. Their efferents mostly drain into the thoracic duct.[2]

The lateral aortic glands drain the paraspinal muscles in the abdomen and pelvis. The right lateral aortic glands may be found in front of the inferior vena cava near the insertion of the renal vein, behind the lumbar vertebral origin of the psoas major and along the right crus of the diaphragm. The left lateral aortic glands drape between the abdominal aorta and the left psoas major, starting at the left crus of the diaphragm. Most of the efferent vessels from both chains converge to form the right and left lumbar trunks, which join the cisterna chyli.

The sacral glands are located in the concavity of the sacrum adjacent to the middle and lateral sacral arteries. In addition to draining the caudal-most paraspinal muscles, they receive efferents from the rectum and posterior wall of the pelvis.[1,2]

FUNCTIONAL DIVISIONS

The superficial muscles of the back create movement of the shoulder girdle. The *trapezius* and *levator scapulae* rotate and raise the scapula. The trapezius muscle also adducts and lowers the scapula. The *rhomboid minor and major* pull the scapula medially. The *latissimus dorsi* assists in extension, adduction, and rotation of the arm.

The deep muscles lie posterior to the vertebral column, extending and rotating the head and spine. The *splenius capitis* extends the neck and bends the head laterally. The *splenius cervicis* and *erector spinae* extend the cervical and upper thoracic spine. The *longissimus capitis* and *semispinalis* are major extensors of the head and neck. The semispinalis also rotates the head and vertebral column to its contralateral side. The *multifidus* and *rotatores* also rotate the column to the opposite side.

The suboccipital muscles extend and tilt the head. The *rectus capitis* extends and rotates the head, the *oblique capitis superior* extends and tilts the head to the same side, and the *oblique capitis inferior* turns the head to the same side.

The prevertebral muscles flex and bend the head and neck. The rectus capitis and *longus capitis* flex the head. The *longus colli* and *scalenes* flex the neck, with the longus colli also providing rotation and the scalenes providing lateral bending. The *psoas* muscles flex the thigh.[2,4]

IMAGING

Ultrasonography

Ultrasonography has the advantages of speed, portability, and low cost and is free of any risks of ionizing radiation. It is a useful modality in evaluating cystic or vascular structures, which are common manifestations of paraspinal pathology. It is also useful in evaluating pediatric patients, for whom radiation exposure is particularly undesirable and whose smaller size is more amenable to sound wave penetration. Ultrasonography is also a useful tool for followup after treatment (see Fig. 2-18B).

Muscles on ultrasound evaluation demonstrate a homogeneous, often striated appearance that is conspicuously interrupted in the presence of a pathologic process (see Fig. 2-35). These features are easily distinguishable from the echogenic surface and decreased through transmission that is characteristic of bone.

CT

A complex rope of muscles traversing the plane of view defines the CT appearance of the cervical paraspinal soft tissues (see Figs. 2-1A, 2-2A, and 2-3A). The *sternocleidomastoid* muscle dominates the lateral neck, whereas the *trapezius* forms the superficial layer posteriorly. *Longus colli* and *capitis* lie anterior to the vertebral body. Lateral to these muscles lie the internal carotid artery and jugular vein. In the superior portion of the cervical spine, the *oblique capitis inferior* and *semispinalis* are most closely applied to the spinous processes (see Fig. 2-1A). However, as we progress more inferiorly, and for the remainder of the spinal column, the *multifidi* remain deepest (see Figs. 2-2A and 2-3A). The next layer of the posterior paraspinal musculature includes the *longissimus capitis* anteriorly and the *splenius capitis* posteriorly. The *levator scapulae* run deep to the sternocleidomastoid on higher slices and inferiorly sweeps posteriorly as the sternocleidomastoid travels anteriorly. The *scalene* muscles appear anterolaterally as we approach the base of the neck (see Fig. 2-3A).

As we descend into the thorax (see Figs. 2-4A and 2-5A), the anterior muscles are replaced by lung and pleura. Anteriorly, the aorta lies to the left and the esophagus lies slightly to the right. The *interspinalis* may be seen connecting the adjacent spinous processes (see Fig. 2-4A). The *multifidus* continues to appear closely applied to either side of the spinous processes, with the *spinalis thoracis* and *longissimus* found laterally. The *trapezius* forms a cape superficially around these muscles

superiorly, whereas inferiorly the *latissimus* sweeps across to form the superficial layer (see Fig. 2-5A).

The lumbar spine gains the anterolaterally placed *psoas* muscles on either side of the vertebral column (see Figs. 2-6A, 2-7A, and 2-8A). Lower in the pelvis, the psoas muscles slide laterally toward the *iliacus* muscles, allowing the iliac vessels and fat to interpose between the psoas muscles and the spine. The *quadratus lumborum* lies posterior and lateral to the psoas muscles. Its anterior and posterior borders define the anterior and middle layers of the thoracolumbar fascia. The posterior layer of the thoracolumbar fascia envelops the posterior paraspinal muscles (see Fig. 2-6A). Again, the *multifidi* appear most medially, adhering to the spinous process. Heading laterally we see the *longissimus* and the *iliocostalis*. The *spinalis* muscles are intimately associated with the multifidi and are difficult to resolve as discrete muscle slips. The *internal* and *external oblique* muscles may be visualized on superior slices, lateral and superficial to the erector spinae (see Fig. 2-6A). Anteriorly, the aorta lies to the left and the inferior vena cava to the right.

MRI

MRI has the advantage of increased soft tissue contrast and multiplanar imaging (see Figs. 2-9 and 2-10). Individual muscle bellies are easily visualized on non–fat-saturated T1-weighted (T1W) imaging, whereas T2-weighted (T2W) imaging is useful to assess edema and fluid. However, CT surpasses MRI in the demonstration of calcium and bony detail.

Coronal MRI demonstrates the vertically oriented layers of the paraspinal musculature of the lower back (see Figs. 2-9 and 2-10). From medial to lateral, the *multifidi, rotatores, spinalis,* and *longissimus* lie in long ropes along the back. The *semispinalis thoracis* lies somewhat superficial to these muscles.

PATHOLOGY

Infection

Infection is a very common pathologic process affecting the paraspinal soft tissues; tuberculous infection is a classic etiology. The indolent nature of tuberculous spondylitis, with its initially subtle clinical and radiographic findings, contributes to the frequent incidence of paravertebral soft tissue involvement on presentation. Infection often spreads from the vertebral bodies to the anterior and posterior longitudinal spinal ligaments, leading to abscess formation in the paraspinal muscles. Paraspinal and subligamentous abscesses frequently become large and confluent.[6] The abscesses are often bilateral and caudal to the level of spondylitis, involving the psoas muscle most commonly (Fig. 2-11).[7]

CT is ideal for detecting bony destruction, as well as small calcifications within the abscess, which are highly specific for tuberculosis (see Fig. 2-11A). MRI is particularly useful for diagnosing recurrent disease, as well as defining the extent of disease and its relationship to the spinal cord (Figs. 2-12 and 2-13). Tuberculous spondylitis has several distinctive findings, which help to dis-

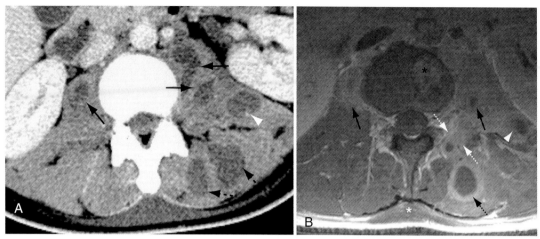

■ **FIGURE 2-11** Tuberculous vertebral osteomyelitis with paraspinal spread in a 56-year-old man. **A,** On the axial contrast-enhanced CT image, multiple abscesses are noted in the psoas (*black arrows*), quadratus lumborum, and erector spinae (*dashed black arrows*). A tiny calcification is noted adjacent to the left quadratus lumborum abscess (*white arrowhead*) highly characteristic for TB. **B,** On the MR image, a rounded focus of enhancement is noted in the vertebral body (*black asterisk*), representing one of several foci of osteomyelitis. The anterior process can be seen to violate the thoracolumbar fascia and extend posteriorly (*dashed white arrows*). Note the fluid in the posterior soft tissues, which does not have an enhancing rim (*white asterisk*).

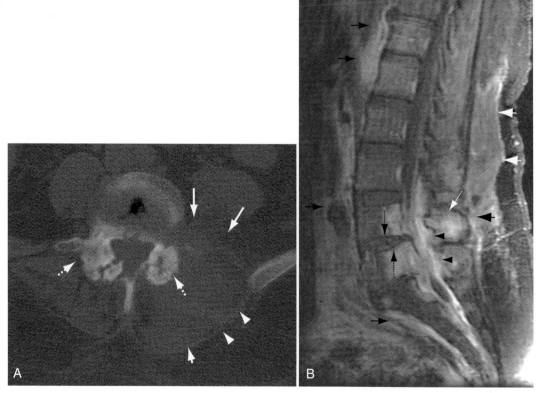

■ **FIGURE 2-12** Tuberculous spondylitis with paraspinal spread. **A,** Axial bone algorithm CT shows expansion and loss of fat planes of the left erector spinae muscles (*arrowheads*) with inflammatory tissue anterior to and destroying the left transverse process (*arrows*). The left psoas muscle is displaced anteriorly and appears ill defined and misshapen compared with the right, suggesting involvement. Note that posterior elements of this lumbar vertebral body are sclerotic (*dashed arrow*), indicating a long-standing process. **B,** Sagittal gadolinium-enhanced MR image demonstrates anterior soft tissue extension and abscess formation (*black arrows*), as well as posterior soft tissue extension (*white arrowheads*). Note how the osseous involvement spreads into the posterior elements (*white dashed arrow*) and flanks, but spares the intervertebral disc (*black dashed arrows*), as is typical of tuberculosis. The posterior ligaments enjoy no such mercy, as clear violation of the ligamentum flavum (*small black arrowheads*) and supraspinous ligament (*large black arrowhead*) is noted.

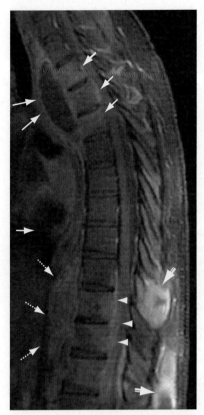

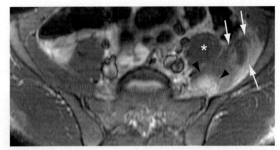

■ FIGURE 2-14 Tuberculous abscess in a 14-year-old boy. Axial T2W MR image. The left iliacus muscle is expanded and infiltrated with bright inflammatory signal (*arrows*), and a complex collection has formed medially (*arrowheads*). The psoas (*asterisk*) is anteriorly displaced but otherwise spared.

■ FIGURE 2-13 Tuberculous spondylitis with extraspinal spread. Sagittal contrast-enhanced MR image of thoracic and lumbar spine. This single image demonstrates abnormal enhancement of multiple contiguous vertebral bodies (*short arrows*) as well as extension into the prevertebral soft tissues (*dotted arrows*), epidural space (*arrowheads*), and posterior soft tissues with destruction of posterior vertebral elements (*double arrows*). A prevertebral abscess (*arrows*) lies adjacent to the enhancing vertebral bodies. The intervertebral discs are relatively spared, as is typical with tuberculous spondylitis.

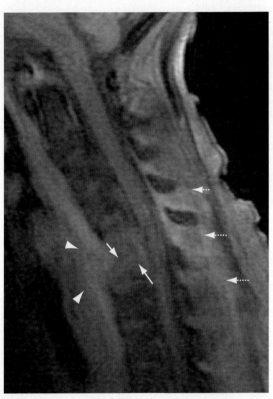

■ FIGURE 2-15 Cervical discitis and osteomyelitis with paraspinal spread. Sagittal contrast-enhanced MR image. The C5-6 space is obliterated (*arrows*), and the adjacent vertebral bodies themselves have lost height anteriorly, creating a kyphosis that narrows the spinal canal. The infectious process has spread to the prevertebral soft tissues (*arrowheads*), as well as the interspinous soft tissues (*dashed arrows*).

tinguish it from pyogenic infection. Bone destruction with relative disc preservation is the most consistent and easily noted feature of tuberculosis (see Fig. 2-12). Focal, heterogeneous enhancement (see Fig. 2-11) and well-defined abnormal signal intensity of the paraspinal areas are also suggestive of tuberculosis (Fig. 2-14). Rim-enhancing intraosseous abscesses of the vertebral body are also characteristic.[8]

In contrast, pyogenic spondylitis tends to be centered on the disc, with peridiscal bone destruction (Figs. 2-15 and 2-16). Diffuse homogeneous enhancement, particularly in the peridiscal region (see Fig. 2-15), and ill-defined signal intensity in the paraspinal regions are characteristic (see Fig. 2-16).[8] Surgical instrumentation is a common cause of pyogenic infection, with the infection centered in the surgical bed (Figs. 2-17 and 2-18) but often dissecting through the soft tissues and fascial planes (Fig. 2-19).

Neoplasm

Neoplastic involvement of the paraspinal soft tissues most frequently extends from neoplastic involvement of the vertebral column, spinal cord, and nerve roots. As a result, primary tumors tend to be neurogenic in origin. They may, however, arise from a primary osseous lesion, such as benign aneurysmal bone cysts, which have been observed to extend into the psoas.[9] Osteoid osteoma may be associated with soft tissues masses, enhancement, and swelling. Like tuberculous infection, these findings spare the intervertebral disc space.[10,11] Occasionally, primary benign or malignant tumors may arise from adjacent soft tissues, as in the case of the myelolipoma found incidentally on a metastatic workup (Fig. 2-20). Metastatic tumors of the spine are most frequently the common,

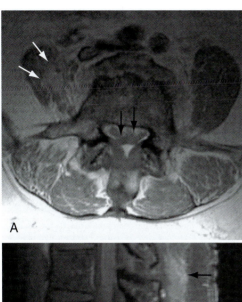

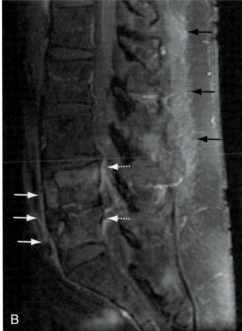

■ **FIGURE 2-16** Paraspinal extension in a patient with discitis and osteomyelitis at L4-L5. **A,** On this contrast-enhanced axial MR image, the right psoas muscle (*white arrows*), in addition to being atrophied, enhances avidly as a result of direct spread of infection. Note the epidural enhancement (*black arrows*). **B,** Sagittal contrast-enhanced MR image demonstrates flattened and enhancing disc, enhancement along the anterior longitudinal ligament (*white arrows*), epidural enhancement (*white dashed arrows*), and posterior subcutaneous enhancement (*black arrows*).

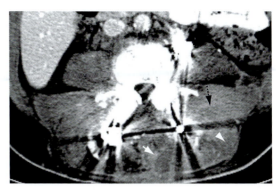

■ **FIGURE 2-17** Paraspinal abscess in a patient status post laminectomies and spinal fixation. Multiple abscesses are noted in the erector spinae (*arrowheads*) and the quadratus lumborum (*dashed black arrow*).

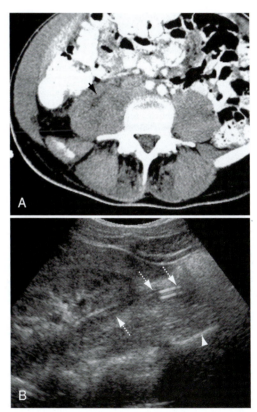

■ **FIGURE 2-18** Psoas muscle bacterial infection in an 18-year-old patient after instrumentation. **A,** Contrast-enhanced axial CT image shows the right psoas muscle is asymmetrically enlarged compared with the right and contains an elongated low-density collection (*arrowhead*). **B,** Sagittal view from an ultrasound examination performed 3 days after percutaneous drain placement demonstrates the echogenic drain (*dashed arrows*) within the psoas muscle. The collection has resolved. Superiorly we see the kidney on the left of the screen and the echogenic cortex of the iliac bone on the right (*arrowhead*).

aggressive cancers, such as lung, breast, renal cell, and gastrointestinal cancers (Figs. 2-21 and 2-22), as well as leukemia and lymphoma (Fig. 2-23). A thin-walled valveless venous plexus makes the paraspinal musculature particularly susceptible to metastatic disease. Findings include enhancement, displacement, and invasion of the paraspinal soft tissues, as well as muscle atrophy due to slowly growing tumors. Lung cancer (Figs. 2-24 and 2-25) and lymphoma (Fig. 2-26) may also extend directly into paraspinal tissues from the lung.

Neurogenic tumors may be divided into peripheral nerve sheath tumors, which are more frequent in adults, and sympathetic ganglia tumors, which are more frequent in children. They may both displace and invade the paraspinal muscles and fascia, creating edema and/or atrophy. However, the neurogenic tumors tend to remain well circumscribed without the destruction often seen in metastases or infection. Peripheral nerve sheath tumors include schwannoma and neurofibroma. Both tumors are benign, slowly growing neoplasms that present as sharply

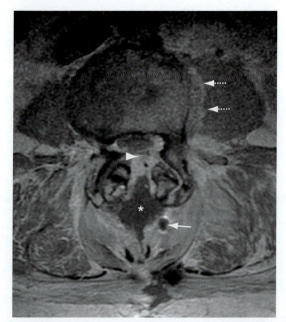

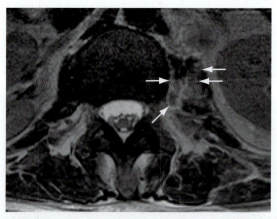

■ **FIGURE 2-21** Metastatic gastric carcinoma to the spine and psoas muscle. Axial T2W MR image demonstrates expansion, enhancement, and abnormal signal within the left psoas muscle (*arrows*). Biopsy of both the psoas lesion and a vertebral body lesion noted a couple of levels superiorly proved to be metastatic gastric adenocarcinoma.

■ **FIGURE 2-19** Surgical bed abscess in a patient after laminotomy. Contrast-enhanced axial MR image. A large abscess (*asterisk*) with extensive surrounding inflammatory change is noted extending from the laminotomy bed into the spinal canal (*arrowhead*) and into the erector spinae muscles bilaterally. Paraspinal extension is noted displacing the left psoas muscle laterally (*dashed arrows*). Note the bubble of air creating susceptibility artifact (*arrow*).

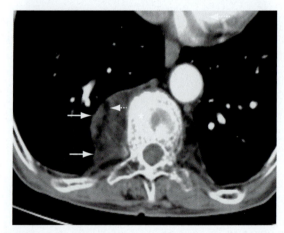

■ **FIGURE 2-20** Paraspinal mass with macroscopic fat. Contrast-enhanced CT scan. Biopsy of this incidentally found mass revealed myelolipoma, a rare benign lesion most commonly found in the adrenal glands. Note the smooth margins (*arrows*) and streaks of fat density (*dashed arrow*). Differential diagnosis includes liposarcoma and teratoma.

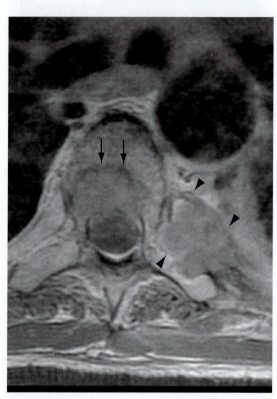

■ **FIGURE 2-22** Bony metastasis in a patient with hepatocellular carcinoma. Axial contrast-enhanced MR image. A large lesion is noted destroying the transverse process and left rib (*arrowheads*) and extending into the left apex. Note the wispy central enhancement (*arrow*).

marginated, spherical, and lobulated masses in the paraspinal region. Schwannomas tend to be solitary, may exhibit cystic degeneration, and enhance peripherally (Fig. 2-27). Neurofibromas are associated with neurofibromatosis type 1 and are frequently multiple. On T2W imaging they may demonstrate a target appearance with peripheral T2 bright signal corresponding to gelatinous zones and central intermediate signal representing solid tissue (Figs. 2-28 and 2-29). Neurofibromas tend to enhance

centrally, although diffuse enhancement may be noted. Plexiform neurofibromas are well-defined nonencapsulated tumors that infiltrate along an entire nerve trunk (Fig. 2-30).[12,13]

Sympathetic ganglia tumors include ganglioneuroma (Fig. 2-31) and neuroblastoma (Fig. 2-32), both of which present as well-marginated, oblong masses that typically span three to five vertebrae and may contain calcifications. Ganglioneuromas are benign tumors that often

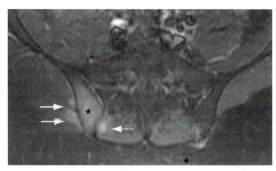

■ FIGURE 2-23 Lymphoma of the iliac bone. Axial contrast-enhanced MR image. The tumor involvement of the iliac bone enhances clearly (*asterisk*). In addition, foci of edema were seen to enhance in the adjacent gluteus maximus (*arrows*) and multifidus (*dashed arrow*). The soft tissue abnormalities were believed to be reactive edema and resolved with radiation therapy.

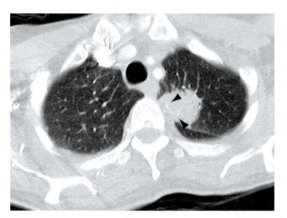

■ FIGURE 2-24 Squamous cell lung cancer in a paraspinal location. Contrast-enhanced CT scan, lung algorithm, suggests the pulmonary origins of the mass, both in its respect to the major fissure and its mildly spiculated margins. Note the calcifications with the mass (*arrowheads*), characteristic of squamous cell tumors.

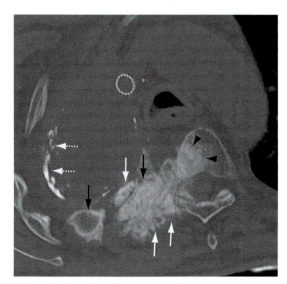

■ FIGURE 2-25 Spinal metastasis in a patient with recurrent adenocarcinoma of the lung after wedge resection. Axial CT scan shows sclerosis of the upper thoracic vertebral body (*arrowheads*), sclerosis and expansion of the ribs (*black arrows*), and surrounding neoplastic calcification (*white arrows*) in the metastatic process. Note the pleural calcifications (*dashed arrows*) peripherally. An indolent infection such as tuberculosis may also have this appearance.

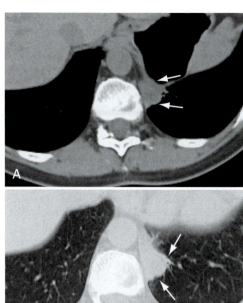
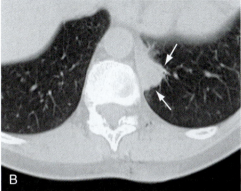

■ FIGURE 2-26 Pulmonary lymphoma. Axial CT scan, mediastinal (**A**) and pulmonary (**B**) algorithms. This heterogeneous paraspinal mass (*arrows*) presented incidentally in a 58-year-old woman with hepatitis C cirrhosis. The lung algorithm image strongly suggests its pulmonary origins.

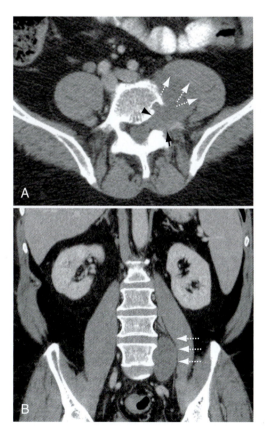

■ FIGURE 2-27 Schwannoma of the right L5 nerve root. Contrast-enhanced CT scan (**A**) and coronal (**B**) reconstructions. This well-circumscribed dumbbell-shaped lesion widens the neuroforamen through which it exits (*arrowheads*) and exerts a mass effect on the right psoas (*dashed arrows*). A clear fat plane can be visualized on the coronal plane only.

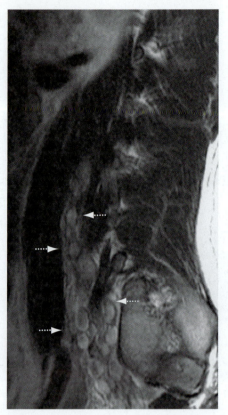

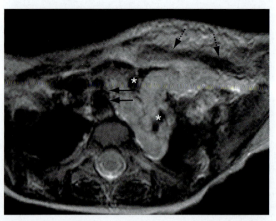

■ **FIGURE 2-30** Plexiform neurofibromas in a 34-year-old man with neurofibromatosis type 1. Axial T2W MR image through the cervical spine demonstrates the complex mass displacing the oropharynx (*black arrows*) anteriorly and to the right. Also note the atrophy and displacement of the sternocleidomastoid (*dashed arrows*) and levator scapulae (*asterisks*).

■ **FIGURE 2-28** A 22-year-old man with a family history of neurofibromatosis presented with multiple neurofibromas. Sagittal T2W MR image demonstrates the thick rope of ovoid lesions displacing the psoas muscle anteriorly (*dashed arrows*). Note the target appearance of a number of the lesions. The bright T2 signal represents the gelatinous periphery, and the dark T1 signal, the solid center.

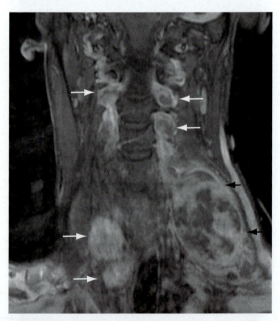

■ **FIGURE 2-29** A 36-year-old man presented with neurofibromatosis type 1. Coronal contrast-enhanced MR image. Multilevel cervical neurofibromas expand the neuroforamina (*arrows*) and extend into the lateral soft tissues of the neck (*black arrows*). Note the heterogeneous enhancement, with regions of necrotic nonenhancement, particularly in the large mass on the left. The characteristic target appearance of the neurofibromas can be noted on the left, with the bright gelatinous peripheral zone and the intermediate central solid zone.

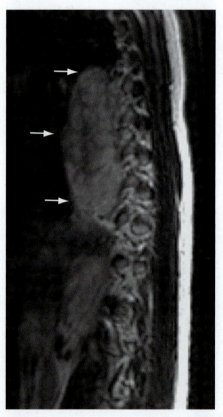

■ **FIGURE 2-31** Ganglioneuroma in a teenage boy. Sagittal T2W MR image. This benign mass spans from T4 to T9 and has neuro-foraminal and intracanalicular components. This is the classic appearance of ganglioneuroma of the spine. Note the smooth encapsulated margins (*arrows*) and heterogeneously bright T2 signal. The whorled dark signal is characteristic of ganglioneuroma.

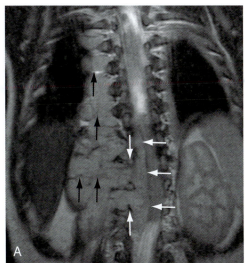

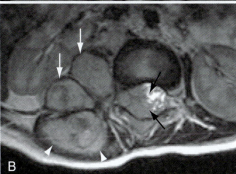

■ **FIGURE 2-32** Neuroblastoma in a 9-month-old male infant. **A,** Coronal T2W MR image shows the tumor spanning nearly the entire thoracolumbar spine, extending through neuroforamina (*vertical white arrows*), intercostal spaces (*black arrows*), and the spinal canal (*horizontal white arrows*). Note the multilobular appearance and well-circumscribed contours. **B,** Axial T2W MR image better demonstrates the multilobular appearance of the tumor (*white arrows*). Note how the posterior lobule of the mass insinuates into and expands the right longissimus and iliocostalis muscles (*arrowheads*). The mass also extends intraspinally (*black arrows*).

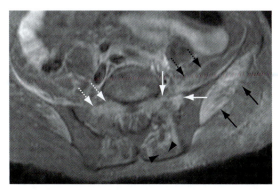

■ **FIGURE 2-33** Muscle edema in a patient with a sacral insufficiency fracture. Axial T2W MR image demonstrates the bright T2 signal of the sacral fracture, which on this image extends to the sacroiliac joint on the left (*white arrows*) but is seen only medially on the right (*white dashed arrows*). Muscle edema of the left gluteus medius (*black arrows*) and erector spinae muscles (*black arrowheads*) is noted. Edema also surrounds the left iliacus muscle (*black dashed arrows*).

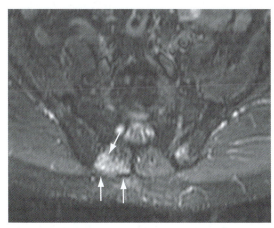

■ **FIGURE 2-34** Muscle sprain. This 45-year-old painter complained of right buttock pain. This axial STIR MRI revealed bright T2 signal in the right iliocostalis muscle (*arrows*), consistent with a muscle sprain. Note the lack of mass effect.

demonstrate a nodular or curvilinear low T1 and T2 signal, creating a somewhat whorled appearance. In contrast, neuroblastomas are nonencapsulated lesions that frequently contain hemorrhage, necrosis, and cystic degeneration. Alternatively, they may appear homogeneous on all sequences, including after contrast enhancement.[13]

Trauma

Paraspinal changes are common in the setting of trauma. Fractures, such as the sacral insufficiency fracture seen in a patient with osteopenia (Fig. 2-33), are often associated with muscle edema, both from direct contusion and altered use. Overuse or acute injury may cause muscle strain in the absence of fracture. Such injuries are characterized by edema, enlargement, and loss of fat planes (Fig. 2-34). Tendonitis, such as seen in the longus colli tendon, presents as soft tissue swelling and calcification.[3] Muscle hematoma is most commonly seen in the setting of anticoagulation therapy or bleeding diatheses, often with minimal or no history of trauma (Fig. 2-35).[14]

Degenerative Disease

Atrophy of the paraspinal muscles is a common finding in older patients, particularly those with back pain or degenerative disc disease (Fig. 2-36). In a study comparing patients with chronic low back pain to asymptomatic volunteers, MR spectroscopy demonstrated a significantly higher fat content in the lumbar multifidus muscle.[15] However, fatty infiltration and loss of muscle mass are often generalized. Paraplegia can cause marked atrophy and fatty infiltration (Fig. 2-37), and focal atrophy may be caused by neuropathy (Fig. 2-38) and radiation (Fig. 2-39).

Ligament ossification, as in diffuse idiopathic skeletal hyperostosis (DISH), may encroach on the paraspinal muscles, particularly if the ossification is robust. This most commonly affects the thoracic spine on the right, as the pulsating aorta is believed to protect the left.[16]

Synovial cysts should be considered when a paraspinal cystic lesion is seen (Fig. 2-40). Paraspinal synovial cysts are usually asymptomatic and associated with degenera-

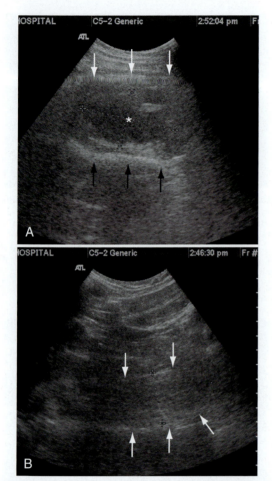

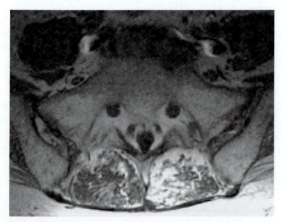

■ **FIGURE 2-35**   Left iliacus hematoma in a 15-year-old boy with sickle cell anemia. Sagittal ultrasound images of the left (**A**) and right (**B**) iliacus muscles. **A,** The left iliacus is bulging (*white arrows*) and contains a low-density collection (*asterisk and calipers*). Note the echogenic cortex of the iliac bone just deep to the muscle (*black arrows*). **B,** The normal right iliacus muscle (*arrows*), in comparison, has a concave superficial margin and a homogeneous, somewhat laminated echotexture.

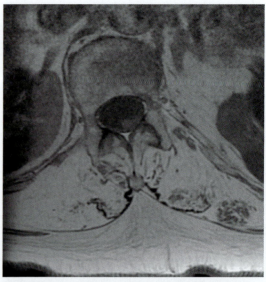

■ **FIGURE 2-37**   Near complete fatty replacement of the paraspinal muscles in a paraplegic patient. Axial T1W MR image.

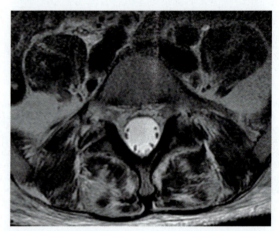

■ **FIGURE 2-38**   Diffuse paraspinal muscle atrophy in the setting of sarcoid polyneuropathy. Axial T2W MR image. Note both the decrease in muscle size and the fatty infiltration of the muscle belly.

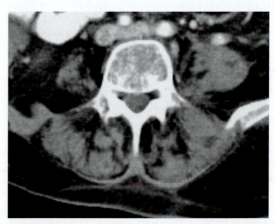

■ **FIGURE 2-36**   Asymmetric left paraspinal muscle atrophy in a patient with severe degenerative disc disease. Axial T1W MR image.

■ **FIGURE 2-39**   Psoas muscle atrophy. Axial CT scan. Note the striking asymmetry of the psoas muscles in this patient who had a remote history of radiation therapy.

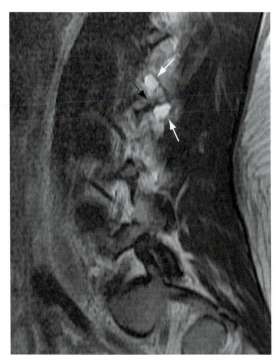

■ FIGURE 2-40   Synovial cysts. T2W MR sagittal image. These rounded fluid structures were incidentally noted at the right L3-L4 interfacet joint (*white arrows*). Note how they extend directly from the facet joint (*black arrow*).

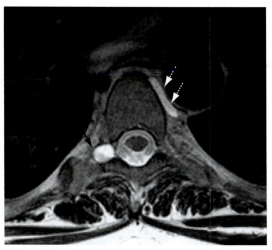

■ FIGURE 2-41   Foregut duplication cyst. Axial T2W MR image. This cylindrical fluid structure (*dashed arrows*) interposed between the descending aorta and the lower thoracic spine was found incidentally during a routine MRI for back pain. No enhancement was observed with intravenous gadolinium. Note the incidental nerve root cyst on the right (*black arrow*).

tive changes of the adjacent spine, particularly when they occur in the lumbar region. They are typically dorsally located and do not communicate with any joint cavity, supporting the theory that they represent mucinous degeneration within periarticular fibrous tissue.[17,18]

Congenital Disease

Congenital paraspinal masses tend to be mediastinal and cystic. They present as smooth, rounded masses with an enhancing wall, and they do not infiltrate adjacent structures. Included in these masses are bronchogenic cysts, which arise in the postcarinal, retrocardiac, or esophageal regions, and may occasionally calcify. They are of variable appearance on T1W imaging owing to the presence of protein or hemorrhage and may contain fluid-fluid levels. Air within the cyst suggests infection or communication with the tracheobronchial tree. Esophageal duplications cysts have an identical appearance on CT and MRI, with the occasional exception of a slightly thicker wall and closer contact with the esophagus (Fig. 2-41). Half of all esophageal foregut cysts contain ectopic gastric mucosa that may help distinguish them on nuclear medicine imaging.[12,18]

Lateral thoracic meningocele is an anomalous herniation of the leptomeninges through an intervertebral foramen or vertebral body defect (Fig. 2-42). These sharply defined paraspinal masses are often associated with neurofibromatosis and are most frequently detected in adults. They may cause bony distortion and scoliosis, widen the intervertebral foramina, and deform adjacent ribs. Other benign cystic masses may occur in the paraspinal region, including dermoid cysts and lymphangiomas. Occasion-

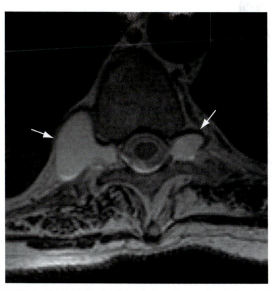

■ FIGURE 2-42   Multilevel bilateral thoracic meningoceles. T2W MR axial image. These cystic outpouchings of cerebrospinal fluid (*arrows*) widened the neuroforamina throughout the thoracic spine.

ally, primary pulmonary parenchymal disease such as congenital cystic adenomatoid malformation and sequestration may be difficult to distinguish from mediastinal disease.[12,19]

Extramedullary Hematopoiesis

Extramedullary hematopoiesis may present as unilateral or bilateral, smoothly lobulated paraspinal masses, located between T6 and T12. Unlike neurogenic tumors, they typically cause no bone erosion. Because the masses represent a compensatory response to decreased blood cell production, they are most often seen in patients with hereditary anemias, as well as malignant replacement of bone marrow.[20]

ANALYSIS

Clinical history is the most important information in interpreting a radiologic study of the paraspinal soft tissues. Unfortunately, it is frequently absent or insufficient. Whenever possible, a thorough evaluation of the patient's past trauma, surgery, medical conditions, and family history should be obtained.

Because the paraspinal soft tissues are frequently evaluated in conjunction with a spine or body study, our evaluation is usually made with knowledge of the presence of concurrent spinal, pulmonary, or visceral disease. A simple approach to differential diagnosis would be to include in our mental checklist a careful evaluation of whether the identified pathology approaches, displaces, or invades the paraspinal soft tissues.[21] This may be seen in infectious causes, such as pyogenic discitis and osteomyelitis (see Fig. 2-16), where a process centered in the vertebral column spreads to the adjacent musculature. In the setting of trauma (see Fig. 2-33), the muscles surrounding a fracture may suffer edema or hemorrhage.

If the finding is squarely centered in the paraspinal soft tissues, its borders and extent should be evaluated. Neurogenic tumors tend to be well circumscribed, causing smooth bony expansion and remodeling (see Fig. 2-29). Infection and metastasis tend to be ill defined, with extensive, messy bone destruction, and edema (see Figs. 2-19 and 2-22).

Finally, if no obvious finding leads to the paraspinal soft tissues, evaluation should be made for symmetry, enhancement, and atrophy (see Fig. 2-39). The sequela of injury may be as subtle as isolated bright T2 signal in a muscle strain (see Fig. 2-34).

A sample MRI report is presented in Box 2-1.

BOX 2-1   MRI Evaluation for Back Pain

PATIENT HISTORY

A patient presented with back pain and fever.

TECHNIQUE

The following sequences were obtained of the lumbosacral spine: axial T1W and fat-saturated T2W; sagittal T1W and fat-saturated T2W; postcontrast axial and sagittal T1W. Gadolinium chelate, 15 mL, was given intravenously.

FINDINGS

The visualized spinal cord and cauda equina are unremarkable, with the conus medullaris at the approximate level of L1.

Abnormal fluid intensity signal and heterogeneous enhancement are noted within the L1 and L2 vertebral bodies with relative sparing of the intervertebral disc. The vertebral body heights are maintained. A fluid collection measuring up to 2.3 cm is noted in the left psoas muscle at the level of L2-3, with rim enhancement and diffuse enhancement of the entire muscle at this level. A smaller rim-enhancing collection is noted in the right psoas muscle, extending into the quadratus lumborum and the erector spinae musculature. There is bulging of the anterior longitudinal ligament spanning from T12 to L3, with bright fluid signal and heterogeneous enhancement, consistent with a subligamentous abscess.

The left quadratus lumborum and erector spinae muscles are unremarkable, with preserved fat planes.

The remaining vertebral bodies and intervertebral discs are unremarkable without loss of height or abnormal enhancement. There is no evidence of abnormal extradural enhancement or collection.

The visualized kidneys and aorta are unremarkable.

IMPRESSION

This patient has spondylitis with paraspinal muscle abscess and anterior subligamentous abscess, most consistent with tuberculous infection.

KEY POINTS

■ A thin-walled, valveless venous plexus provides a pathway for metastatic and infectious disease to spread to the paraspinal soft tissues.

■ Tuberculous spondylitis spares the disc space and frequently involves the psoas muscles. Soft tissue calcifications are a specific finding for tuberculous soft tissue involvement.

■ Schwannomas are usually solitary; neurofibromas are frequently multiple and seen in the setting of neurofibromatosis type 1.

■ Extramedullary hematopoiesis does not erode the adjacent bone, unlike neurogenic tumors, which may have a similar appearance.

SUGGESTED READINGS

Donnelly LF, Frush DP, Zheng JY, Bisset GS. Differentiating normal from abnormal inferior thoracic paravertebral soft tissues on chest radiography in children. AJR Am J Roentgenol 2000; 175:477-483.

Gaisie G, Oh KS. Paraspinal interfaces in the lower thoracic area in children: evaluation by CT. Radiology 1983; 149:133-135.

Khong PL, Goh WHS, Wong VCN, Fung CW. MR Imaging of spinal tumors in children with neurofibromatosis 1. AJR Am J Roentgenol 2003; 180:413-417.

Ledermann HP, et al. MR imaging findings in spinal infections: rules or myths? Radiology 2003; 228:506-514.

Sharif HS, Clack DC, Aabed MY, et al. Granulomatous spinal infections: MR imaging. Radiology 1990; 177:101.

Silver AJ, et al. Computed tomography of the carotid space and related cervical spaces: II. Neurogenic tumors. Radiology 1984; 150:729-735.

REFERENCES

1. Snell R. Clinical Anatomy for Medical Students, 6th ed. Baltimore, Lippincott Williams & Wilkins, 2000, pp 828-830.
2. Gray H. Anatomy of the Human Body. Philadelphia, Lea & Febiger, 1918; available at Bartleby.com.
3. Harnsberger HR. Handbook of Head and Neck Imaging, 2nd ed. St. Louis, Mosby, 1995.
4. Harnsberger HR, et al. Diagnostic and Surgical Imaging: Anatomy, Brain, Head & Neck, Spine. Salt Lake City, Amirsys, 2006.
5. Osborn AG, Koehler PR. Computed tomography of the paraspinal musculature: normal and pathologic anatomy. AJR Am J Roentgenol 1982; 138:93-98.
6. Ng AHW, et al. Extensive paraspinal abscess complicating tuberculous spondylitis in an adolescent with Pott kyphosis. J Clin Imaging 2006; 29:359-361.
7. de Roos A, et al. MRI of tuberculous spondylitis. AJR Am J Roentgenol 1986; 146:79-82.
8. Chang MC, et al. Tuberculous spondylitis and pyogenic spondylitis: comparative magnetic resonance imaging features. Spine 2006; 31:782-788.
9. Turker RJ, Mardjetko S, Lubicky J. Aneurysmal bone cysts of the spine: excision and stabilization. J Pediatr Orthop 1998; 18:209-213.
10. Woods ER, Martel W, Mandell SH, Crabbe JP. Reactive soft-tissue mass associated with osteoid osteoma: correlation of MR imaging features with pathologic findings. Musculoskeletal Radiol 1993; 186:221-225.
11. Guzey FK, et al. Vertebral osteoid osteoma associated with paravertebral soft-tissue changes on magnetic resonance imaging. J Neurosurg (Pediatrics 5) 2004; 100:532-536.
12. Jeung MI, et al. Imaging of cystic masses of the mediastinum. RadioGraphics 2002; 22:S79-S93.
13. Tanaka O, et al. Neurogenic tumors of the mediastinum and chest wall: MR imaging appearance. J Thorac Imaging 2005; 20:316-320.
14. Baba Y, et al. Large paraspinal and iliopsoas muscle hematomas. Arch Neuroradiol 2005; 62:1306.
15. Mengiardi B, et al. Fat content of lumbar paraspinal muscles in patients with chronic low back pain and in asymptomatic volunteers: quantification with MR spectroscopy. Radiology 2006; 240:786-792.
16. Nakhoda K, Greene G. Diffuse idiopathic skeletal hyperostosis. emedicine 2005. Available at www.emedicine.com/RADIO/topic218.htm
17. Alguacil-Garcia A. Spinal synovial cyst (ganglion): review and report of a case presenting as a retropharyngeal mass. Am J Surg Pathol 1987; 11:732-735.
18. Choudhri HF, Perling LH. Diagnosis and management of juxtafacet cysts. Neurosurg Focus 2006; 20:E1.
19. Buckley JA, et al. CT evaluation of mediastinal masses in children: spectrum of disease with pathologic correlation. Crit Rev Diagn Imaging 1998; 39:365-392.
20. De Backer AI, et al. Extramedullary paraspinal hematopoiesis in hereditary spherocytosis. JBR-BTR 2002; 85:206-208.
21. Davis WL, Harnsberger HR. CT and MRI of the normal and diseased perivertebral space. Neuroradiology 1995; 37:388-394.

PART THREE

Normal Spinal Column and Cord

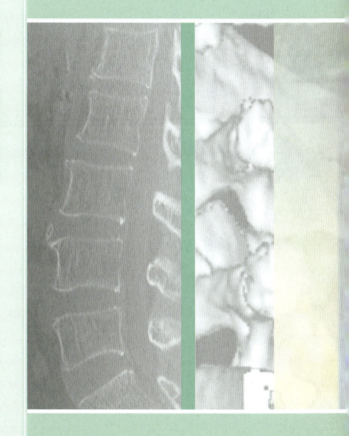

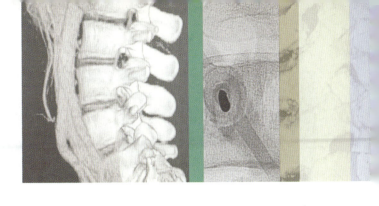

CHAPTER 3

The Normal Spinal Column: Overview and Cervical Spine

Jose Conrado Rios, Thomas Paul Naidich, David L. Daniels, Victor M. Haughton,
Cheuk Ying Tang, Joy S. Reidenberg, Patrick A. Lento, Evan G. Stein,
Girish Manohar Fatterpekar, Tanvir Fiaz Choudhri, and Irina Oyfe

The spinal column consists of multiple segmented osseous vertebrae, the intervertebral discs interposed between these segments, and the ligaments and joints that bind the segments together. The spine has 32 to 35 vertebral segments, traditionally considered as 7 cervical, 12 thoracic, 5 lumbar, 5 sacral, and 3 to 5 coccygeal segments. The relative lengths of the cervical, thoracic, lumbar, and sacral spines are in proportion as 2:5:3:2.[1-3]

The vertebrae articulate with each other by a combination of cartilaginous, synovial, and fibrous joints. The cervical spine articulates with the skull base at the craniovertebral junction and with the thoracic spine at the cervicothoracic junction. The thoracic spine articulates with the heads of the ribs at the costocapitular (costovertebral) joints, with the necks of the ribs at the costotubercular (costotransverse) joints, and with the lumbar spine at the thoracolumbar junction. The sacrum articulates with the lumbar spine at the lumbosacral junction, with the ilia at the sacroiliac joints, and with the coccyx at the sacrococcygeal junction.

The anterior surface of the spine merges into the lateral surface with no clear demarcation. The lateral surface is demarcated from the posterior surface by the articular processes in the cervical region, by the transverse processes in the thoracic region, and by the articular processes again in the lumbar region. The posterior surface is the posterior face between the articular and transverse processes of each side.[1-3]

NORMAL ANATOMY

The spinal column measures approximately 70 cm in males and 60 cm in females. Approximately 80% of that length is due to bone and 20% to the intervertebral discs.[1-3] Diurnal variation in disc hydration changes the length of the spinal column approximately 16 mm over the day. The loss of height is greatest in the first 3 hours after awakening and in adolescents and young adults.[1-3]

The spine normally displays specific dorsoventral curvatures (Figs. 3-1 and 3-2). Posteriorly directed concavity is designated *lordosis.* Posteriorly directed convexity is designated *kyphosis.* The normal cervical lordosis extends from C2 to T2, with the apex at C4-C5. The normal thoracic kyphosis extends from T2 to T11 or T12, with the apex at T6 to T9. The normal lumbar lordosis extends from T12 to the lumbosacral junction with the apex at L3.[1-3] As a result of these curvatures, a plumb line suspended from the external auditory canal of a standing adult would pass through the dens of C2, just anterior to the vertebral body of T2, through the center of the vertebral body of T12, and through the posterior portion of the vertebral body of L5, coming to hang anterior to the sacrum.[1-3] Muscle changes associated with handedness may induce slight asymmetric lateral curvatures of the upper thoracic spine to the right in right-handed persons and to the left in left-handed persons.[1-3]

The Standard Vertebra

The Osseous Vertebrae

Each osseous vertebra has a standard overall structure, composed of an anterior vertebral body and a posterior neural arch (Figs. 3-3 and 3-4). This general shape is modified secondarily at each level. Each vertebra has an outer shell of dense cortical bone and an inner core of less dense, cancellous bone. The cortical bone is thick over the neural arch, less thick along the sides of the vertebral body, and thinnest where the upper and lower surfaces of the vertebral body abut the disc. The cancellous bone contains the vertebral marrow.

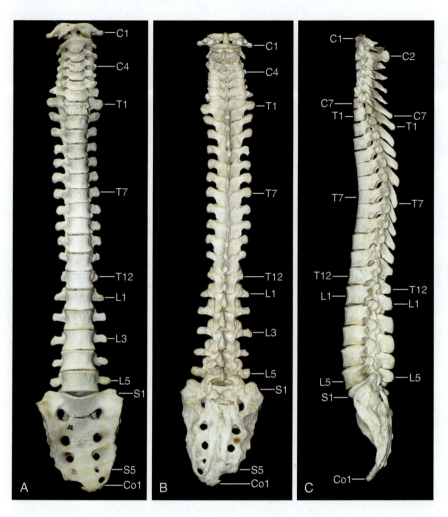

■ **FIGURE 3-1**   Full length of the spinal column. Dried osseous vertebrae. Anterior (**A**), posterior (**B**), and lateral (**C**) surfaces. This overview emphasizes the changing curvatures, proportions, and orientations of the vertebral bodies, transverse processes, neural foramina, laminae, and spinous processes over the length of the cervical (C), thoracic (T), lumbar (L), sacral (S), and coccygeal (Co) segments of the spinal column. These anatomic transitions are detailed in magnified images of each section presented sequentially through this and the following chapter.

The vertebral body forms the front of each vertebra, anterior to the spinal canal. The body is shaped like an asymmetric cylinder with concave side walls. The top and bottom of each body resembles a drum head, with a smooth, raised periphery and a roughened flat-to-scaphoid center.

The neural arch forms the lateral and posterior portions of each vertebra, lateral to and behind the spinal canal. Each neural arch is composed of paired pedicles, paired laminae, paired articular processes, and a single, posteriorly directed spinous process. The pedicles form the two sides of the spinal canal. These narrow struts arise from the upper posterolateral surface of each vertebral body and pass posteriorly to merge into the laminae. The pedicles are roughly cylindrical in coronal section. In lateral view, they show shallow curves on their upper and lower borders (the gentler superior vertebral notch and the deeper inferior vertebral notch). The laminae are flattened, obliquely oriented plates of bone that form the posterior/posterolateral walls of the spinal canal. They merge with the pedicles anteriorly and angle toward each other posteriorly to fuse with the base of the spinous process in the midline. The spinous process arises from the medial edges of the paired laminae and juts posteriorly and inferiorly in the midline behind the spinal canal.

The superior and inferior articular processes lie posterolateral to the spinal canal. They arise where the pedicles merge into the laminae. From there, the paired articular processes project superiorly and inferiorly to form synovial articulations with the articular processes of the next-higher and next-lower vertebrae (Fig. 3-5). At each articulation, the superior articular processes of the lower vertebra lie anterior to the inferior articular processes of the upper vertebra. The facets of the superior articular processes face posteriorly to fit with the anteriorly facing facets of the inferior articular processes.

The transverse processes of the vertebrae also arise where the pedicles merge into the laminae but project laterally. In the thoracic region, these processes are true transverse processes (designated *diapophyses*) that articulate with the ribs (designated *pleurapophyses, costal elements*). At other spinal levels the similar, laterally projecting bony elements are composed of *both* true transverse processes (diapophyses) and incorporated pleurapophyses (costal elements).[1-3]

The neural foramina are the soft tissue and osseous channels between vertebrae that convey the spinal nerves and blood vessels into and out of the spinal canal (Figs. 3-5 and 3-6). Superiorly and inferiorly the neural foramina are bordered by the periosteum of the concave margins

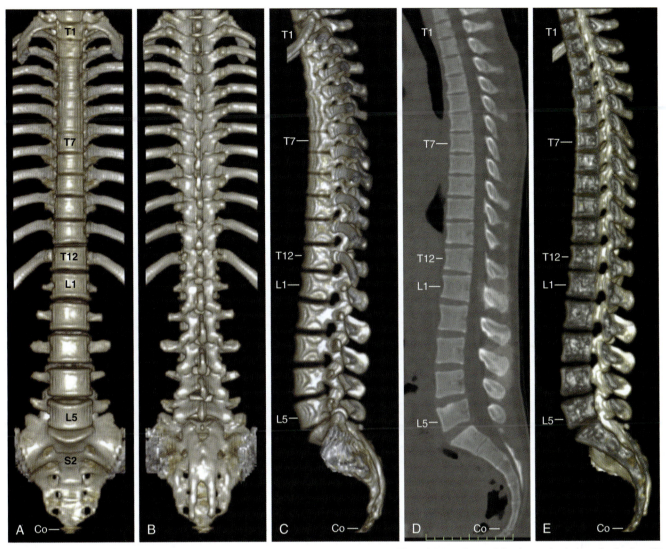

■ **FIGURE 3-2** 3D CT surface reformatted images of the anterior (**A**), posterior (**B**), and lateral (**C**) surfaces of the thoracolumbosacral spine in a 27-year-old man. **D**, Midsagittal reformatted image of the spine. **E**, 3D sagittal cut-away reformatted image to display the interior and the opposite side of the spine from the midline.

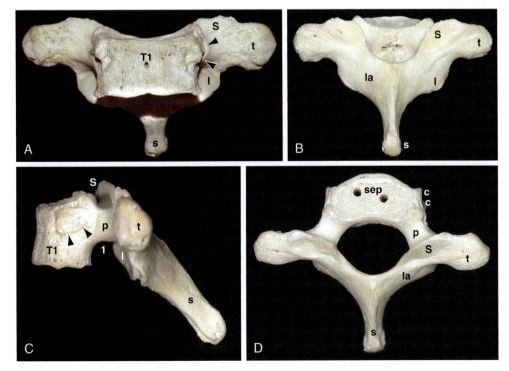

■ **FIGURE 3-3** Isolated dried T1 vertebra. Anterior (**A**), posterior (**B**), lateral (**C**), and superior (**D**) surfaces. Four views demonstrate the vertebral body (T1), pedicle (p), superior (S) and inferior (I) articular processes and facets, the transverse process (t), lamina (la), spinous process (s), and costocapitular facet (*arrowheads*). In lateral view (**C**) the gentle concavity of the upper border of the pedicle (p) is the superior vertebral notch. The deep concavity of the lower border of the pedicle is the inferior vertebral notch. The segmental T1 nerve roots (1) exit through the T1-T2 neural foramen just inferior to the T1 pedicle. The superior end plate (sep) of the vertebral body displays a rim of dense cortical bone and a central region of cancellous bone. The head of the T1 rib articulates with the side of the T1 vertebral body at the costocapitular (costovertebral) facet (*arrowheads*; cc). In this and other images, the paired "drill holes" indicate that the segmental vertebrae had been strung together to form a spinal column.

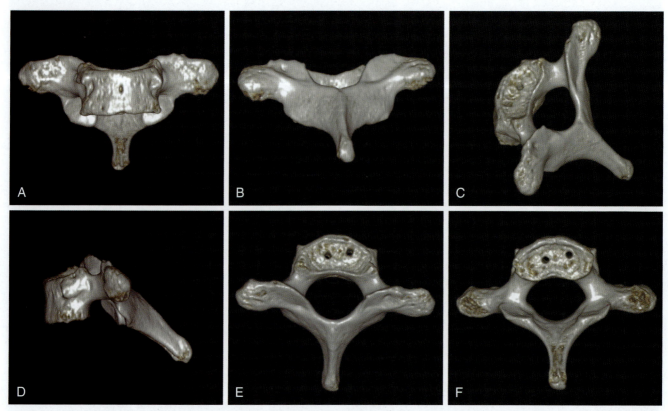

■ **FIGURE 3-4**   3D surface reformatted images of the dried T1 vertebra illustrated in Figure 3-3. Anterior (**A**), posterior (**B**), posterosuperior (**C**), lateral (**D**), superior (**E**), and inferior (**F**) surfaces. See Figure 3-3 to identify structures.

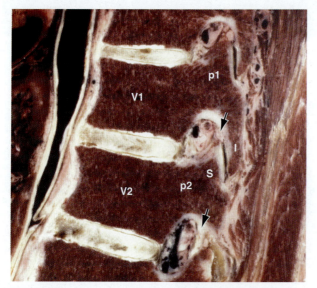

■ **FIGURE 3-5**   Parasagittal cryomicrotome section through the pedicles, neural foramina, and zygapophyseal (facet) joints of adjacent thoracic vertebrae. The outer surfaces of the vertebral bodies, pedicles, and articular surfaces of the facets show dense cortical bone. The interior surfaces show cancellous bone containing homogeneous red marrow. The facet joint (S/I) has a steep coronal orientation. The ovoid neural foramina are bounded superiorly by the deep inferior vertebral notch of the upper pedicle (p1), inferiorly by the shallow superior vertebral notch of the lower pedicle (p2), anteriorly by the posterior surfaces of the upper vertebral body (V1) and the V1-V2 disc, and posteriorly by the ligamentum flavum (*arrows*) and superior articular facet (S) of the lower vertebra (V2). The neural foramina contain epidural fat, traversing veins, segmental nerve roots, and the segmental dorsal root ganglia.

of the pedicles. The superior border of the neural foramen is the undersurface of the upper pedicle. Therefore, the deeply curved inferior vertebral notch of the upper pedicle constitutes the roof of the neural foramen. The inferior border of the neural foramen is the upper surface of the lower pedicle. Therefore, the shallower superior vertebral notch of the lower pedicle constitutes the floor of the neural foramen. On their anterior wall, from above downward, the neural foramina are bordered by the periosteum of the posterior surfaces of the upper vertebra, the syndesmosis formed by the hyaline cartilage end plates and disc, and the periosteum of the posterior surface of the lower vertebra. Posteriorly, the neural foramen is formed by the periosteum over the pars interarticularis, the ligamentum flavum, and the synovial capsule of the facet joint.[1-3] At T1 to T10 only, the anterior border of the foramen also includes the synovial capsules for the articulations of the ribs.

The marrow within the vertebra consists of both red hematopoietic marrow and yellow fatty marrow (Figs. 3-7 and 3-8). Additional small (2-4 mm) intraosseous nodules of notochordal remnants are found in 14% of spinal columns.[4] From birth to approximately age 2 years, the vertebral marrow is predominantly red hematopoietic marrow. It converts progressively, diffusely and homogeneously to yellow fatty marrow with growth and development.[4] From early middle age onward, the conversion of red to yellow marrow progresses more slowly and inhomogeneously. The fat fraction of the lumbar vertebral marrow is usually higher in men than women and may

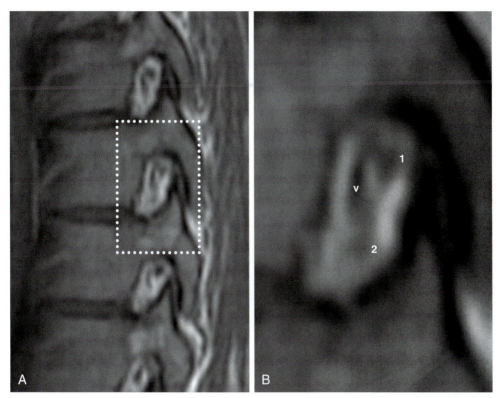

■ **FIGURE 3-6** Neural foramina in a 31-year-old woman. **A,** Sagittal T2W MR image of midthoracic foramina comparable to Figure 3-5. **B,** Magnified image of one foramen to show the radicular vein (v) anteriorly and the dorsal (1) and ventral (2) roots posteriorly.

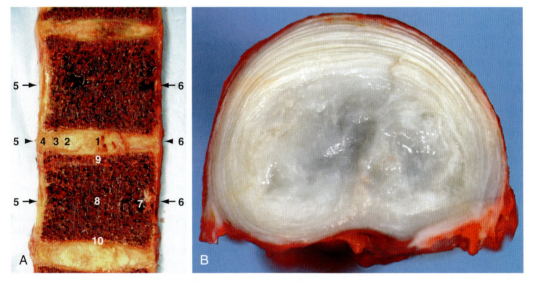

■ **FIGURE 3-7** Intervertebral junctions. Two fresh unfixed specimens. Midsagittal section (**A**) through two adjacent vertebral bodies and axial section through an intervertebral disc (**B**) show the central nucleus pulposus (1), inner annulus fibrosus (2), outer annulus fibrosus (3), Sharpey's fibers (4) inserting into the corners of the vertebral bodies, and the superior (9) and inferior (10) end plates of the vertebral bodies. The cancellous interior (8) of the vertebral body contains predominantly red, hematopoietic marrow. The anterior (5) and posterior (6) longitudinal ligaments insert very tightly (*arrowheads*) into the disc and end plates of the intervertebral symphysis but only loosely (*arrows*) into the midportions of the vertebral bodies. The basivertebral venous channel (7) drains venous blood from the vertebra into the posterior internal vertebral plexus deep to and lateral to the posterior longitudinal ligament.

increase from 27% to 70%, at a rate of approximately 7.5% per decade in adulthood.[4,5] In the adult, the fat content of the lumbar marrow usually increases from L1 to L5. However, the distribution of the fat is variable and heterogeneous. The red marrow may cluster near the anterior margin of the vertebral body and at the end plates.[4]

Because fat and hematopoietic cells both grow by expansion of cell clusters to form nodules, fatty conversion tends to create islands of juxtaposed red and yellow marrow.[4] The increase in the fat fraction with age correlates with the atherosclerotic decline in overall vascular perfusion and with reduced bone mineral density.[4,6]

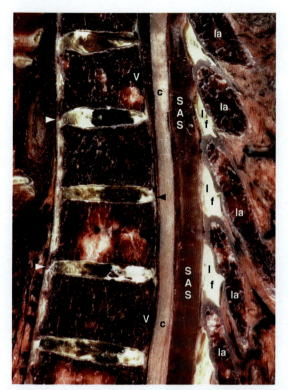

■ FIGURE 3-8   Paramedian cryomicrotome section through the midthoracic spine. The cancellous bone displays both red and yellow marrow. Superiorly and inferiorly, the vertebral bodies are joined by the intervertebral symphyses composed, in part, of the paired upper and lower vertebral margins, the hyaline cartilage end plates, and the intervening discs. Aging pigment discolors the discs in this specimen. Anteriorly and posteriorly the vertebral bodies are joined by the tough anterior longitudinal ligament (*white arrowheads*) and posterior longitudinal ligament (*black arrowhead*). Posteriorly, the laminae are joined by the segmental ligamenta flava (lf) that attach to the anterior cortical surface of the lower half of each lamina (la) and insert into the cortical surface of the upper margin and adjacent posterior face of the next-lower lamina. Because of the thoracic kyphosis, the spinal cord (c) lies in the anterior portion of the spinal canal and the subarachnoid space (SAS) appears widened behind it. The basivertebral veins (v) at the mid heights of the vertebrae drain posteriorly into the anterior internal vertebral venous plexus situated ventral to the posterior longitudinal ligament.

Craniocaudal Patterns of Osseous Anatomy (Figs. 3-1 and 3-2)

Vertebral Bodies

The heights of the vertebral bodies generally increase from the cervical to the lumbar spine. Within the thoracic spine, the T3 body is smallest. Below this, the thoracic and lumbar vertebral bodies increase in size progressively down to L4, with a slight decrease in height at L5. The width (transverse dimension) of the vertebral bodies increases progressively from C2 to L3, with variable width of L4 and L5. The width of the vertebral bodies then decreases from S1 to the lowest coccygeal vertebra.[1-3]

Vertebral Canal

The vertebral canal is large and triangular in the cervical region, small and circular in the thoracic region, and again large and triangular in the lumbar region. The lumbar canal diminishes progressively from L1 to L5. The shortest transverse distance between the most medial curvatures of the paired pedicles is the interpediculate distance. This varies systematically along the length of the spinal canal, giving a characteristic pattern that is most commonly displayed as a graph (see reference 7).[1-3,7]

Pedicles

The medial borders of the pedicles are typically convex toward the spinal canal. In the region T11 to L2, however, the medial aspects of the pedicles may be flattened or even concave as a normal variation.[8] As a result, the interpediculate distance may normally be increased at these levels.

Laminae

C1 has a posterior arch but no laminae. The C2 and C7 laminae are very thick and robust. From C3 to C6 the cervical laminae are thin and wide with narrow craniocaudal extent. The thoracic laminae are generally thicker, wider, and taller than the cervical laminae but vary along the length of the thorax. The T1 laminae are very broad. The laminae narrow from T2 to T7, broaden again from T8 to T11, and narrow again from T11 to L3. The lumbar laminae are more robust than the cervical or thoracic laminae (except C2 and C7), are narrower than most thoracic laminae, and are intermediate in their craniocaudal length.

Articular Processes and Facet Joints

The articular surfaces and synovial facet joints are relatively flat in the cervical and thoracic spines but more complex and cup shaped in the lumbar spine. The cervical facet joints are oriented in an oblique coronal plane at an angle of 30 to 50 degrees to the vertical (measuring the narrow angle from the superior facet surface to the inferior vertical). The thoracic facet joints down to about T10-T11 are oriented in a steeper oblique coronal plane, making a narrower angle of 15 to 20 degrees to the inferior vertical. From about T11-T12 to about L2-L3, the facet joints transition into a more nearly sagittal orientation. Below this, the posteroinferolateral portions of the cup-shaped facet joints are oriented in the sagittal plane whereas the anterosuperomedial portions of the same facet joints are oriented in the coronal plane.

Transverse Processes

By shape, cervical transverse processes are long and broad at C2, narrower and more delicate at C3-C6, and longer again at C7. Thoracic transverse processes are broad at T1 and decrease in breadth progressively from T1 to T12. The T12 transverse processes are nearly absent. Lumbar transverse processes become broader from L1 to L3 and usually increase at L4 and L5, so that the L5 transverse process is sturdiest and arises directly from the body and pedicle to transfer weight to the pelvis. The angulations of the transverse processes and their positions relative to the pedicles, articular facets, and neural foramina vary with the spinal level. By position, cervical transverse processes lie anterior to the articular processes, lateral to the pedicles, and vertically between the two adjacent intervertebral foramina. Thoracic transverse processes lie posterior to the pedicles and neural foramina, farther back than the transverse processes of other portions of the spine. Lumbar transverse processes lie anterior to the articular processes but posterior to the intervertebral foramina.[1-3]

Spinous Processes (Spines)

Cervical

The C1 spine is vestigial, forming only the posterior tubercle of C1. The C2 spine is large and strong, whereas the C3 spine is very short and thin. From C3 to C7 the spines gradually increase in length, so the longest cervical spine is C7. The spines are bifid at C2-C5, variably single or bifid at C6, and characteristically single and pointy at C7.

Thoracic

The T1 spine is robust and about as long as C7. From T2 to about T8 the thoracic spines are thin and long, angle far inferiorly, and overlap each other extensively. From T9 to T12 the spines shorten, thicken, and incline directly posteriorly.

Lumbar

From L1 to L3 the spines thicken, enlarge, and point directly posterior. The L4 spine is often slightly smaller than the L3 spine. The L5 spine is variable but usually smaller than the L4 spine.

Sacral

The spines of S1 to S3 (or S4) fuse together into the median sacral crest with three to four spinous tubercles marking their remnants.

Dorsal Paravertebral Grooves

Together, the spinous processes, adjoining laminae, and transverse processes form paired paraspinal gutters for the dorsal paraspinal musculature. In the cervical and lumbar regions these gutters are shallow and are composed mainly of the laminae themselves. In the thoracic region, they are deeper and broader and are formed by both the laminae and transverse processes.

Intervertebral Foramina (Neural Foramina)

The neural foramina are small in the cervical and upper thoracic regions but increase in size progressively through the mid-lower thoracic and lumbar regions. The cervical neural foramina are nearly round and face anterolaterally. The cervical transverse processes lie between the neural foramina and form trough-like semicanals that conduct the emerging roots anterolaterally and inferolaterally. The tho-racic and lumbar neural foramina are "keyhole" in shape and face laterally, with the transverse processes behind them.[1-3]

Costal Facets

The articulations of the rib heads with the vertebral bodies vary along the length of the thoracic spine. The T1 rib head articulates solely with the T1 body, so the T1 costal facet is circular and complete. From T2 to T10 each rib head articulates with the two adjoining vertebrae across the interspace. Superiorly, the rib head articulates with the inferior margin of the upper vertebral body at a small semilunar costal demifacet. Inferiorly, the same rib articulates with the superior aspect of the lower vertebral body at a large semicircular costal demifacet. At T11 and T12, the rib head again articulates solely with its own vertebral body at a complete circular costal facet. From T9 to T12 the positions of the costal facets migrate caudad from the upper lateral to the middle lateral surface of the vertebral body.

Joints between the Vertebrae

The connections between the vertebrae consist of junctions between the vertebral bodies, junctions between the posterior arches, and additional ligaments.[1-3]

Junctions between Vertebral Bodies

The junctions between the vertebral bodies consist of (1) symphyses formed by the intervertebral disc and apposing cartilaginous end plates, (2) the anterior longitudinal ligament, and (3) the posterior longitudinal ligament.

Symphyses

The intervertebral symphysis is a "sandwich" formed by the two layers of hyaline cartilage from the inferior and superior end plates and the fibrocartilaginous disc centered between them (see Figs. 3-5 and 3-7 to 3-9). At cervical, thoracic, and lumbar levels, these symphyses are tightly anchored to the anterior and posterior longitudinal ligaments (ALL and PLL). At thoracic levels, the syndesmoses are also anchored to intra-articular ligaments that are directed laterally toward the ribs at the costocapitular (costovertebral) joints. By shape, the cervical and lumbar discs are thicker anteriorly, whereas the thoracic discs are nearly uniform in thickness. By size, the intervertebral discs are thinnest in the upper thoracic region and thicker in the lumbar region. In patients with five lumbar vertebrae, the thickest disc of all is typically the L4-L5 disc.

Anterior Longitudinal Ligament (ALL)

The ALL is a smooth, thick, glistening ligament that, in aggregate, extends along the anterior surface of the whole spine from the caudal end of the clivus (basiocciput) to the upper sacrum (see Figs. 3-7 to 3-10). There are three layers. The most superficial fibers of the ALL extend over

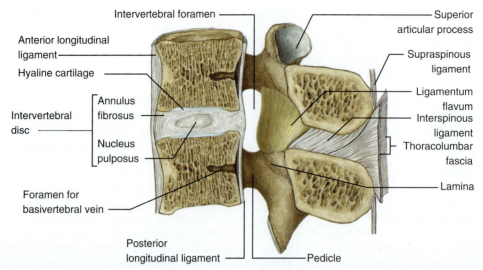

FIGURE 3-9 Intervertebral connections. Diagram of adjacent upper lumbar vertebrae showing the discs and ligaments. The posterior longitudinal ligament adheres tightly to the posterior surfaces of discs but separates from the backs of the vertebral bodies. *(From Sobotta J [ed]. Atlas of Human Anatomy, 14th ed. Volume 2: Thorax, Abdomen, Pelvis, Lower Limb. London, Churchill Livingstone, 2006.)*

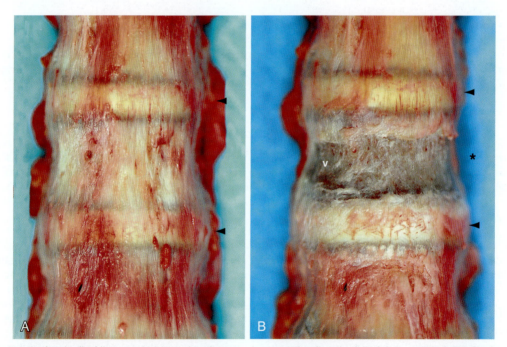

■ **FIGURE 3-10** Anterior longitudinal ligament (ALL). Fresh cadaver specimen. **A,** The glistening ALL forms a tough sheath for the anterior surface of the spinal column. The ALL is very tightly adherent (*arrowheads*) to the upper and lower margins of the bony vertebrae, to the cartilaginous end plates, and to the anterior surface of the intervertebral disc. It is loosely attached over the midvertebral bodies. **B,** Gentle scraping removes the ALL from the midvertebral body (*asterisk*), but even sharp dissection fails to separate the ALL from the intervertebral symphysis. v indicates the exposed anterior surface of the vertebral body. The dark horizontal lines above and below the discs are the margins of the adjacent bony vertebrae.

three to four segments. The next deeper fibers extend over one to three segments, whereas the deepest fibers unite only adjoining vertebrae. Overall, the ligament is broad in the cervical region, thicker and narrower in the thoracic region, and broadest in the lumbar region. The ALL attaches to the basion, the anterior tubercle of C1, the anterior surface of the body of C2, and the anterior surfaces of each intervertebral symphysis down to the upper sacrum. Specifically, the longitudinal fibers of the ALL adhere tightly to the superior and inferior margins of the vertebral bodies, the hyaline cartilage of the associated

end plates, and the anterior surfaces of the intervening discs. The ALL is very loosely attached at the concave midportions of the vertebral bodies.

Posterior Longitudinal Ligament (PLL)

The PLL is a smooth glistening ligament that extends along the posterior surfaces of the vertebral column from the body of C2 to the sacrum (see Figs. 3-7 to 3-9 and 3-11 to 3-12). Superiorly, it merges into the tectorial membrane

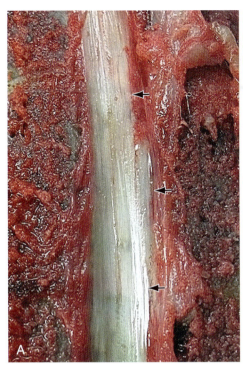
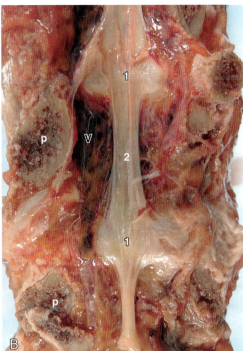

■ **FIGURE 3-11** Posterior longitudinal ligament (PLL). Fresh cadaver specimens of the anterior wall of the spinal canal, displaying the posterior surfaces of upper thoracic (**A**) and lumbar (**B**) vertebral bodies. P, pedicles. **A,** In the cervical and upper thoracic regions the PLL has uniform thickness (*arrows*) over the vertebral bodies and discs. **B,** In the lower thoracic and lumbar regions, the PLL is denticulated: wide (1) where it attaches broadly to the posterior surfaces of the discs and narrow (2) where it crosses the backs of the vertebral bodies. The anterior internal venous plexus (v) lies immediately ventral to the superficial layer of the PLL. It extends across the full transverse dimension of the vertebral body (where the narrow PLL does not adhere to the bone) but is restricted to paired lateral channels where the PLL flares laterally and adheres tightly to the disc.

(see later). Like the ALL, the PLL is a composite ligament formed by fibers that, individually, extend over shorter lengths than the ligament as a whole. Like the ALL, the PLL attaches strongly to the intervertebral symphyses along the margins of each vertebral body, the hyaline cartilage of the end plates, and the posterior surfaces of each intervertebral disc. Between the discs, the PLL is separated from the concave posterior surfaces of the vertebral bodies.[1-3] Overall, the PLL is broad and uniform in width in the cervical and upper thoracic levels, but denticulated in the lower thoracic and lumbar regions.

Surgically, the denticulated PLL is conceptualized as two layers. The deep (more ventral) layer of the PLL is an hourglass-shaped band that is narrow (2-3 mm) over the mid vertebral bodies and that fans outward widely over the annuli of the discs.[10] The superficial (more dorsal) layer of the PLL has a similar hourglass-shaped band but is wider (8-10 mm) at its narrowest extent.[10] Medially, the superficial layer is loosely adherent to the deep layer. Laterally it separates from the deep layer and extends outward bilaterally to surround the vertebral arteries, the nerve roots, and their dural sleeves within both neural foramina.[9] The lateral extension of the superficial layer of the PLL to each side forms a coronal connective tissue plane that may be termed the fascia of the PLL in the cervical region but is simply called the superficial layer of the PLL in the lumbar region.[11] This coronal fibrous layer completely divides the spinal epidural space into an anterior epidural compartment ventral to the layer and a posterior epidural compartment dorsal to it.[9,11] The anterior epidural compartment is nearly entirely filled with the veins of the anterior internal vertebral venous plexus. These rarely pass posterior to the ligament into the posterior compartment. At each disc level, metamerically, fusion of the PLL to the annulus of the disc obliterates the medial portion of the anterior compartment.

Internal Vertebral Venous Plexus

The internal vertebral venous plexus is a valveless complex of veins that extends from the clival system of veins superiorly to the sacral region inferiorly.[12] It lies along the ventral aspect of the spinal canal ventral to the superficial layer of the posterior longitudinal ligament. The anterior portion of the internal venous plexus (AIVVP) is composed of paired, interconnecting medial and lateral venous compartments. The medial compartment of the AIVVP consists of a fine plexus of veins situated in and to each side of the midline, between the superficial and the deep layers of the posterior longitudinal ligament. The AIVVP receives drainage from the vertebral body via horizontal subarticular veins from the superior and inferior endplates of the vertebra and via one or two basivertebral veins from the midportion of the vertebra.[12] The lateral compartment of the AIVVP consists of larger, better defined channels, sometimes designated the anterior longitudinal veins. These channels lie in the anterolateral epidural space ventral to the lateral extensions of the posterior longitudinal ligament. The medial and lateral portions of the AIVVP interconnect widely. The whole plexus extends laterally around the segmental nerve roots within the neural foramina to fuse with the external vertebral venous plexus lateral to the foramina.[12] Per Wiltse, the blood flow within this system is bidirectional, varying with changing intra-abdominal pressure.[10]

Junctions between Vertebral Arches

The junctions between the vertebral arches take two forms. The superior and inferior articular processes (zygapophyses) articulate to form synovial joints designated zygapophyseal joints (facet joints). The laminae, the spinous processes, and the transverse processes interconnect via fibrous syndesmoses formed by the yellow

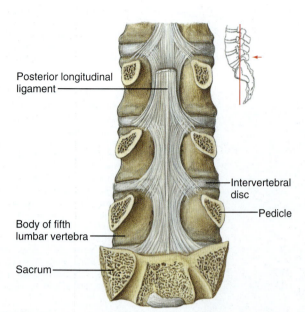

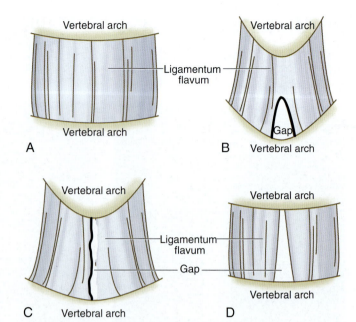

■ **FIGURE 3-12** Diagram of the denticulated posterior longitudinal ligament (PLL). The broader superficial layer of the posterior longitudinal ligament (PLL) (cut end) lies dorsal to the narrower deep layer. *(From Sobotta J [ed]. Atlas of Human Anatomy, 14th ed. Volume 2: Thorax, Abdomen, Pelvis, Lower Limb. London, Churchill Livingstone, 2006.)*

■ **FIGURE 3-14** Variable fusion of the paired ligamental flava. **A,** Complete fusion with no midline gap. **B,** Midline gap in the lower third. **C,** Nonfusion with complete gap of equal width. **D,** Nonfusion with gap wider in the inferior third. *(Modified from Lirk P, et al: Cervical and high thoracic ligamentum flavum frequently fails to fuse in the midline. Anesthesiology 2003; 99:1387-1390.)*

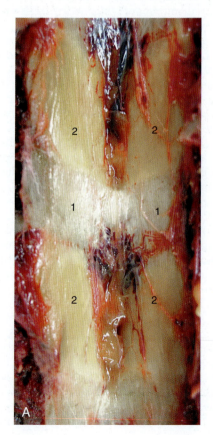

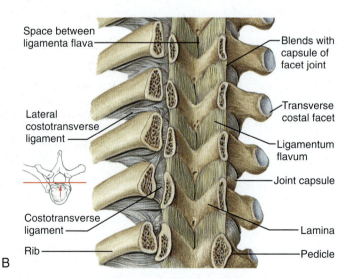

■ **FIGURE 3-13** **A,** Ligamenta flava. Fresh cadaver specimen of the posterior wall of the spinal canal displaying the anterior surfaces of lumbar vertebral laminae. The yellow elastic tissue of each ligamentum (2) arises from the anterior surface of the *lower half* of each lamina and descends across the interspace nearly vertically to insert into the upper margin and adjacent posterior surface of the next-lower lamina. The uncovered anterior surfaces of the upper laminae (1) display glistening periosteum between the segmental pairs of ligamenta flava. **B,** Diagram of the segmental origins and attachments of the paired ligamenta flava. *(B, From Sobotta J [ed]. Atlas of Human Anatomy, 14th ed. Volume 2: Thorax, Abdomen, Pelvis, Lower Limb. London, Churchill Livingstone, 2006.)*

ligaments (ligamenta flava), the interspinous ligaments, the supraspinous ligament, the intertransverse ligaments, and the ligamentum nuchae.[1-3]

Zygapophyseal Joints (Facet Joints)

The zygapophyseal joints are formed by the facets on the apposing articular processes (see Figs. 3-5 and 3-8). These are covered by a smooth layer of hyaline cartilage 2 to 4 mm thick. The articulating surfaces have a relatively simple shape in the cervical and thoracic regions but a more complex cup shape in the lumbar region. The articulations may be symmetric bilaterally or asymmetric. Facet asymmetry is designated *articular tropism.* The articulating facets are enclosed in a capsule that attaches at the periphery of the facets. In the cervical region the capsule is thin and loose. In the lumbar region, the posterior portion of the lumbar capsule is composed of elastic and fibrous tissue but the anterior wall is formed almost entirely by the ligamentum flavum.[1-3] In about 40% of adult cases, the lumbar capsule may enclose (1) fat pads at the anterosuperior, posteroinferior, or both ends of the articulation; (2) fibroadipose "meniscoids" at the upper, lower, or both poles of the articulation; and/or (3) connective tissue rims formed by reflections of the joint capsule along the upper, lower, or both margins of the facets.[1-3] The actual joint space commonly extends beyond the articular surfaces of the facet, under the ligamentum flavum and/or behind the facet joint.[13,14]

Syndesmoses of the Vertebral Arches

The paired ligamenta flava interconnect the laminae of adjacent vertebrae on each side from C1-C2 above to L5-S1 below (see Figs. 3-8, 3-9, 3-13, and 3-14). They are thickest in the lumbar region, less thick in the thoracic region, and thin, broad, and long in the cervical region.[1-3] They are made of yellow elastic fibers that attach to the lower half of the anterior surface of the upper lamina and descend vertically, ipsilaterally, to attach to the upper margin and posterior surface of the next-lower lamina. As a consequence, the upper portion of the anterior surface of each lamina remains smooth and uncovered by ligamentum. The dural sac and posterior nerve root sleeves may adhere to these smooth surfaces. The lower portion of the anterior surface of the lamina is roughened to give attachment to the overlying ligamentum flavum. On each side, the ligamentum flavum stretches across the posterior margin of the spinal canal from the capsule of the facet joint laterally to the medial margin of the lamina. The posterior edges of the paired ligamenta flava show variable, often incomplete, fusion, leaving dorsal midline gaps.[15-16] By shape, the midline gaps may be widest at the inferior third of the midline, widest at the cranial third of the midline, or complete vertical clefts of equal width along the midline (Fig. 3-14).[15] The gaps show a mean width of 1.0 ± 0.3 mm. In the cervical and high thoracic areas, up to 74% of levels show incomplete fusion of the ligamenta flava in the midline.[15] Specifically, midline gaps are found in 65% to 74% of ligamenta flava from C3-4 to T1-2, but progressively fewer caudally: T1-2: 66%; T2-3: 61%; T3-4: 41%; T4-5: 18%; and T5-6: 18%.[15] In many cases the gaps convey veins from the posterior internal venous plexus to the posterior external venous plexus. At C1-C2, fibers of the ligamentum nuchae extend through this gap to adhere to the posterior spinal dura (see Posterior Dural Attachments, later).

The supraspinous ligament is a robust cord of fibrous tissue that interconnects the tips of the spinous processes from C7 to the sacrum and merges laterally into the adjacent fascia (see Fig. 3-9). It is thickest and broadest in the lumbar region. From C7 to the external occipital protuberance it expands posteriorly to form the ligamentum nuchae. As with the ALL and PLL, the most superficial fibers of the ligament extend over three to four segments. The deeper fibers extend over two to three segments, and the deepest merge with the interspinous ligaments.

The interspinous ligaments are thin fibrous strands that interconnect the adjacent spinous processes from their base to their apex (see Fig. 3-9). In the cervical region, they merge into the ligamentum flavum anteriorly and the supraspinous ligament posteriorly. As expected from the shapes and spacing of the spinous processes in each region, the interspinous ligaments are tenuous in the cervical region, narrow and elongate in the thoracic region, and widely quadrangular in the lumbar region.

The intertransverse ligaments interconnect the transverse processes at all levels.

Segmental Osseous Morphology

Cervical Vertebrae

There are seven cervical vertebrae. Of these, C3 to C6 display a standard, archetypical cervical structure (Figs. 3-15 to 3-17). C1, C2, and C7 show special modifications.

Typical Cervical Vertebra (C3-C6)

The midcervical vertebral bodies are small, are relatively broad, and display convex anterior borders (Figs. 3-18 to 3-20). The posterior vertebral border is flat to gently concave. Basivertebral channels penetrate the midposterior surface of the body to interconnect the basivertebral veins with the anterior internal vertebral plexus.

The upper surface of the body has the shape of a saddle, with a central depression between raised lateral lips. These lips are formed by the uncinate processes (synonym: neurocentral lips). The lateral portion of the lower surface of the body shows paired demifacets that articulate with the uncinate processes of the next-lower vertebra. The anterior end of the lower surface has a prominent lip that partly overhangs the next-lower vertebra.

The cervical pedicles arise at the mid-height of the body, so the upper and lower vertebral notches are approximately equal in depth and the neural foramina are round. The laminae form thin curved plates that are slightly thicker along their inferior edges. The spinous processes are bifid and display paired posterior tubercles that are often unequal in size. The spinous processes are directed posteriorly and slightly downward. They are bifid at C3, C4, and C5 and either single or bifid at C6. The

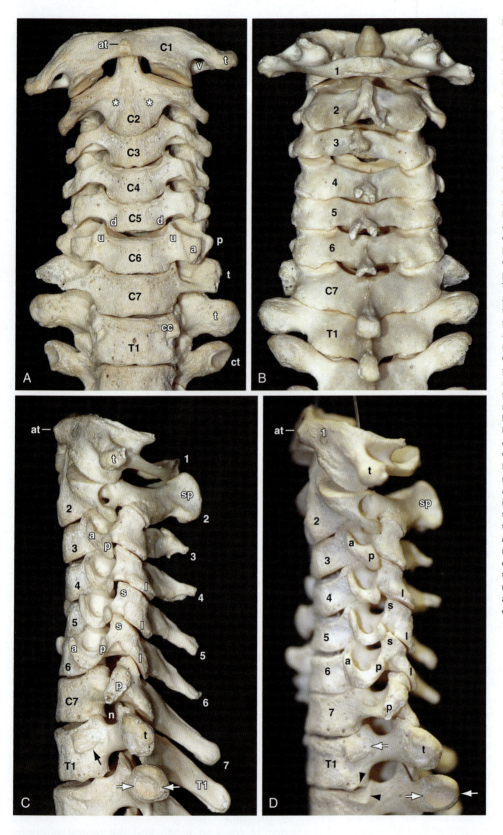

■ **FIGURE 3-15** Full cervical spine. Dried osseous vertebrae. Anterior (**A**), posterior (**B**), lateral (**C**), and anterolateral (**D**) surfaces. These images demonstrate the relative sizes of the vertebral bodies (C1-T1), transverse processes (t), and spinous processes (sp; numbers) over the length of the cervical (C) and uppermost thoracic (T) spine. The spinous processes are vestigial at C1, bifid from C2 through C6, and single again at C7. The C1 vertebral body exhibits midline anterior (at) and posterior tubercles. The uncinate processes (u) on the upper surfaces of the cervical and first thoracic vertebral bodies articulate with the demifacets (d) on the inferolateral surfaces of the next-higher vertebral bodies. The superior (s) articular processes of each vertebra articulate with the overhanging inferior articular processes (I) of the next-higher vertebra. The transverse processes (t) extend anterolaterally, forming a semicanal for the emerging roots, with the anterior tubercle of the transverse process (a) anterosuperior to the posterior tubercle (p) of the same transverse process. Cervical nerve roots (n) lie at the bottom of the foramen and are named for the nearest pedicle, so the C7 root emerges from the C6-C7 foramen, and the C8 root (8) from the C7-T1 foramen. The head (capitulum) of the first rib articulates only with lateral surface of T1 at a complete circular costocapitular (costovertebral) facet (cc) (*single white arrow*, **D**). The head of the second (and lower) rib articulates with both its own vertebra and the next-higher vertebra across the interspace, forming a small demifacet on the upper vertebra and a larger demifacet on its own vertebra (*black arrowheads*, **D**). The tubercles of all thoracic ribs articulate with the transverse processes (t) of their own vertebrae at costotubercular (costotransverse) facets (ct) (*facing white arrows*, **C, D**) on the anterolateral surfaces of the lateral ends of the transverse processes.

junction of the pedicle and lamina on each side gives rise to a large, laterally directed thickening of bone designated the *articular pillar*. The upper margin of each pillar is the superior articular process. The lower margin of each pillar is the inferior articular process. The intervening bone is the pars interarticularis. The facets of the superior articular processes are oriented posterosuperiorly. The matching facets of the inferior articular processes are directed anteriorly.[1-3]

The transverse processes lie anterior to the articular processes, lateral to the pedicles, and vertically between the two adjacent intervertebral foramina.[1-3] The cervical transverse processes have a complex origin and shape, formed from two roots. The posterior root attaches to

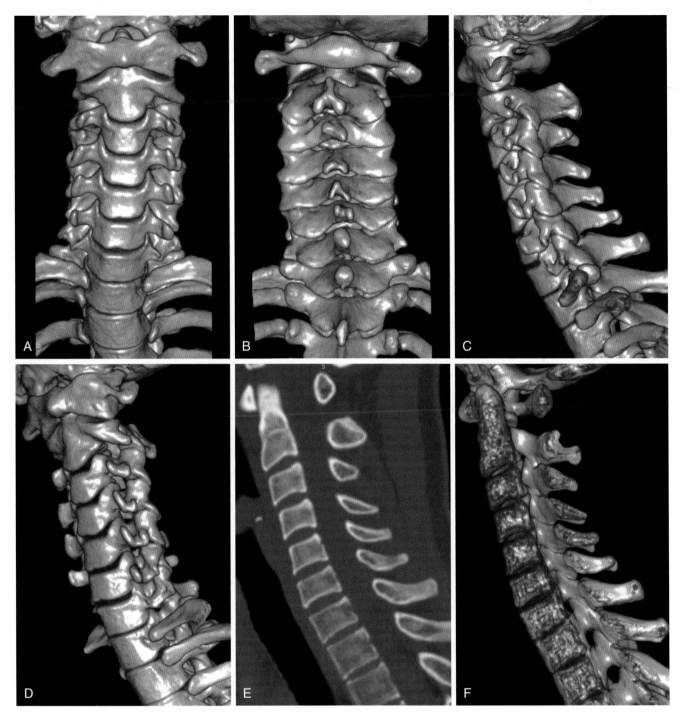

■ **FIGURE 3-16** In-vivo CT of the cervical spine of a 27-year-old woman. 3D CT surface reformatted images of the anterior (**A**), posterior (**B**), lateral (**C**), and anterolateral (**D**) surfaces of the cervical and uppermost thoracic spine. Midsagittal reformatted (**E**) and 3D cut-away (**F**) images display the interior and opposite sides of the spine from the midline.

the junction of the pedicle and lamina medially and displays a posterior tubercle laterally. This represents the true transverse process (diapophysis). The anterior root attaches to vertebral body medially and displays an anterior tubercle laterally. This root arises from costal elements and represents the pleurapophysis. An intertubercular lamella unites the two roots lateral to the foramen transversarium, enclosing the vertebral artery, vertebral veins, and vertebral nerve. The posterior tubercles lie lateral and caudad to the corresponding anterior tubercles. The resultant transverse processes form anterolater-

ally directed troughs (semicanals) leading toward the neural foramina.[11-13]

The foramen transversarium contains the vertebral artery, vertebral veins, and vertebral nerve. A ligament typically runs across the foramen, separating the vertebral artery from the veins (± nerve). Ossification of the ligament creates two parallel channels: the foramen transversarium with the vertebral artery anteromedially and the accessory foramen transversarium with the veins (± nerve) posterolaterally. The accessory foramina may form in single or multiple vertebrae, unilaterally or bilaterally.

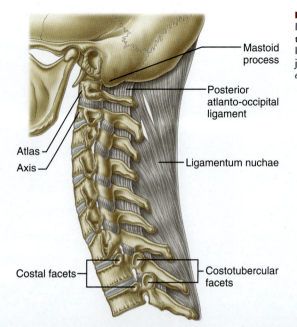

■ **FIGURE 3-17** Ligamentum nuchae and other cervical ligaments. The segmental ligamenta flava morph into the posterior atlanto-occipital membrane at C1-occiput. Capsular ligaments enclose the segmental zygapophyseal (facet) joints. *(From Kiss F, Szentagothai J. Atlas of Human Anatomy, 2nd ed. Oxford, Pergamon Press, 1964.)*

Mastoid process

Posterior atlanto-occipital ligament

Atlas

Axis

Ligamentum nuchae

Costal facets

Costotubercular facets

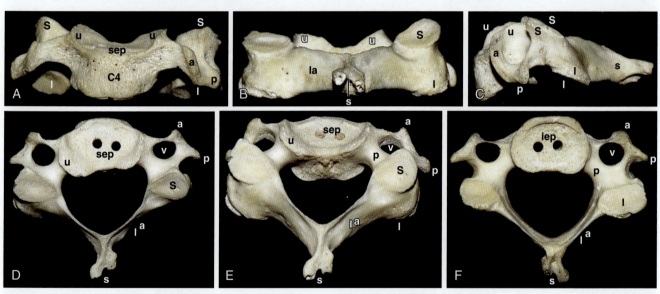

■ **FIGURE 3-18** Isolated dried C4 vertebra. Anterior (**A**), posterior (**B**), lateral (**C**), superior (**D**), posterosuperior (**E**), and inferior (**F**) surfaces. C4 displays a saddle-shaped superior surface composed of the superior end plate (sep) and uncinate processes (u), prominent articular pillar with superior (S) and inferior (I) articular processes and facets, small pedicles (*black* p), anterolaterally directed transverse processes with anterior tubercles (a), posterior tubercles (*white* p), the foramen transversarium (v) for the vertebral artery, thin laminae (la), and a small bifid spinous process (s). iep, inferior end plate.

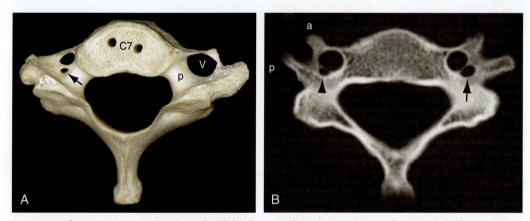

■ **FIGURE 3-19** Accessory foramen transversarium. **A,** Isolated dried C7 vertebra. Ligamentous ossification subdivides the anatomic right foramen transversarium into a true foramen transversarium (v) anterolaterally and an accessory foramen transversarium (*arrow*) posterolaterally. The pedicle (p) is designated on the left. **B,** In-vivo CT scan through C5 in a 27-year-old man. Bilateral accessory foramina transversaria are present, larger on the anatomic left (*arrow*) and smaller on the right (*arrowhead*). The transverse process displays prominent anterior (a) and posterior (b) tubercles.

They are uncommon at C1, absent at C2, and present in 19% to 45% of C3 to C7 vertebrae.[19] By level, accessory foramina transversaria are found at C7 in 15%, C6 in 23%, C5 in 17%, C4 in 5%, C3 in 5%, C2 in 0%, and C1 in 13% of cases.[19]

The cervical vertebral foramen (spinal canal) is triangular in overall shape (Figs. 3-20 to 3-23). The precise size and shape at each level of the cervical spinal canal was studied in 213 skeletons and analyzed by gender and background. Per this study, the cervical spinal canal is larger in males than females and is about 10 mm wider in transverse than sagittal dimension.[20] The anteroposterior dimension of the cervical canal averages from 13.2 to 16.8 mm and is greatest at C2. The transverse dimension averages from 22.5 to 25.5, widens progressively from C2 to C6, and is widest at C6 (Table 3-1).[20]

In sagittal cryomicrotome and CT sections, the cervical neural foramina are 8 to 9 mm high and 4 to 5 mm long. They pass anterolaterally at an angle of about 45 degrees to the coronal plane and caudad at an angle of about 10 degrees to the axial plane.[18] MRI measurements of the cervical neural foramina by MRI in 20 young adults (20-25 years of age) show that cervical neural foramen are vertical ovoids. The C2-C3 neural foramen is the largest in height, width, and cross-sectional area, whereas the C7-T1 neural foramen is the smallest (Table 3-2).[21] On average, the foramina of women measured 1% to 7% smaller than the foramina of men at each level.

C7

The spinous process of C7 is single and especially long. The transverse processes are thick and lie posterolateral to the foramina transversaria. Because the vertebral artery typically enters the foramen transversarium at C6, the C7 foramen transversarium is usually small and usually conveys vertebral veins, not the artery. However, there is substantial variation. The anterior root (pleurapophysis) of the transverse process may be small to absent at C7, leaving the foramen transversarium open anteriorly. Alternatively, the pleurapophysis (costal process) of C7 may develop into an anomalously long transverse process (~2%) or a true cervical rib (up to 3%).[15] Cervical ribs are more commonly bilateral than unilateral. Both elongated transverse processes and cervical ribs are more common in women than men.[22]

Cervical Ligaments

In addition to the ligaments common to most vertebrae the cervical spine includes the ligamentum nuchae and a complex array of ligaments restricted to the craniovertebral junction:C2-skull base.[23-29] The ligamentum nuchae is a strong intermuscular septum composed of two layers of dense fibroelastic tissue (see Fig. 3-17). These layers are separated by a thin layer of areolar tissue anteriorly but unite posteriorly to form a strong posterior free margin. The free margin of ligamentum nuchae extends downward from the external occipital protuberance and adjacent medial portions of the external occipital crest to insert into the posterior tubercle of C1, the medial aspects of the bifid spines of cervical vertebrae C2 to C6, and

the single tip of the spinous process of C7. This broad fibrous sheet gives attachment to the posterior cervical musculature.

The Atlas

The C1 vertebra is unique for lacking a defined vertebral body (Fig. 3-24). Instead, that site is occupied by the upper portion of the odontoid process of C2 (synonym: dens), which embryologically is a C1 anlage. As a result, C1 is formed of two lateral masses connected by anterior and posterior arches. The anterior arch displays a rough anterior tubercle and a concave posterior facet that articulates with the dens. The posterior arch forms the posterior wall of the spinal canal at C1 and displays a small midline posterior tubercle (abortive spinous process). The superior surface of the posterior arch has broad paired grooves for the vertebral arteries, venous plexus, and C1 root. In about 14% of individuals ossification of the posterior atlanto-occipital membrane overlying this groove creates an ossific bridge that encloses the artery, veins, and nerve, referred to as *ponticle ponticus* or *Kimerle's anomaly*.[1-3] The lateral masses of C1 are oriented obliquely, so their long axes converge anteriorly. Superiorly, the lateral masses have ovoid or reniform facets to articulate with the occipital condyles. Inferiorly, the lateral masses have nearly circular facets to articulate with the lateral masses of C2 (the axis). The medial surface of each lateral mass has a distinct tubercle that gives attachment to the transverse ligament (see later).

Special Modifications of C2 (The Axis)

The C2 vertebra is unique for having a superiorly directed odontoid process (the dens) that articulates with the anterior arch of the C1 ring (Figs. 3-25 to 3-27). In adults, the dens is formed of compact bone and is 9 to 21 mm in height. It may normally incline slightly away from the vertical, angling up to 14 degrees posteriorly and up to 10 degrees laterally.[1-3] The body of C2 is formed from the center of the embryonic C1 and C2 vertebra, so it often displays a junction (synchondrosis) within it. The superior surface of the body carries large facets for articulation with the lateral masses of C1. These extend posteriorly and laterally onto the superior surfaces of the adjacent pedicles and transverse processes. The pedicles of C2 are robust. The laminae are thick to give attachment to the ligamenta flava. The transverse processes are pointed and project inferolaterally. The foramina transversaria within them are directed laterally to conduct the vertebral arteries outward, around the large articular pillars. The spinous process is large with a very prominent bifid tip that gives attachment to the ligamentum nuchae.

The Specialized Junctions

Craniovertebral Joints

The articulations from the occipital condyles of the skull base to C1 and C2 function together as an extended joint that allows a wide range of motion. This is estimated at

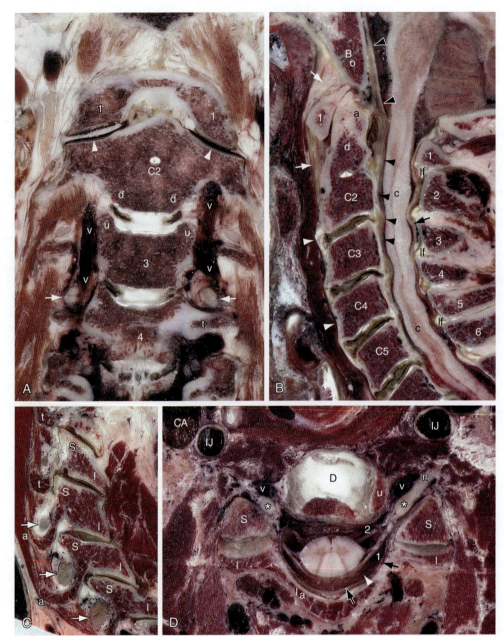

■ **FIGURE 3-20** *Cervical spine. Cryomicrotome sections in the coronal, midsagittal, parasagittal, and axial planes. Four different specimens. **A,** Coronal section through C1-C4 displays the uncovertebral joints at which the uncinate processes (u) arising from superolateral surfaces of each vertebra articulate with the demifacets (d) on the inferolateral surfaces of the next-higher vertebra. The apposing articular surfaces (arrowheads) of the lateral masses of C1 and C2 incline inferolaterally. The right C4 dorsal root ganglion (arrow) lies just above the right C4 transverse process (t). The vertebral arteries (v) ascend through the foramina transversaria bilaterally. **B,** Midsagittal section shows the cortical bone and marrow of the vertebral bodies, the anterior longitudinal ligament (ALL) (white arrowheads) and posterior longitudinal ligament (PLL) (black arrowheads), ligamentum flavum (lf), spines (1-6), and interspinous ligaments of C1-C5. From the anterior face of C2, the ALL extends superiorly as a tough narrow strap of tissue (white arrows) that crosses over the anterior tubercle of C1 to insert on the inferior surface of the basiocciput (Bo). The PLL extends upward across C2 and C1 to insert onto the posterior face of the clivus. The apical ligament extends from the apex (a) of the dens (d) to insert onto the basion (caudal edge of the basiocciput [Bo]). Offset of the vertebral bodies and infolding of ligamentum flavum in extension narrow the spinal canal and cord (c). **C,** Parasagittal section displays the oblique coronal inclination of the zygapophyseal joints, the cortical bone and facet cartilage of the superior (S) and inferior (I) articular processes, the anterior tubercles (a) of the trough-like transverse processes (t), and the relationships of the nerve roots and dorsal root ganglia (arrows) to the transverse and superior articular processes. Fat and veins surround the dorsal root ganglia within the neural foramina. **D,** Axial section through the disc (D), uncinate processes (u), and facet joints (S/I) displays the "triangular" shape of the cervical spinal canal. The dural sac (black arrows) and arachnoid mater enclose the subarachnoid space (white arrowhead) and spinal cord. The butterfly shape of the central gray matter and the peripheral columns of the white matter are well shown. The dorsal sensory root (1) and the ventral motor root (2) pass anterolaterally into the neural foramen to merge into the mixed segmental nerve root (n) distal to the dorsal root ganglion (asterisk). The ascending vertebral arteries (v) lie anterolateral to the ganglia. CA, carotid artery; IJ, internal jugular vein; la, lamina of the vertebra. Each vertebral artery is surrounded by a venous plexus.*

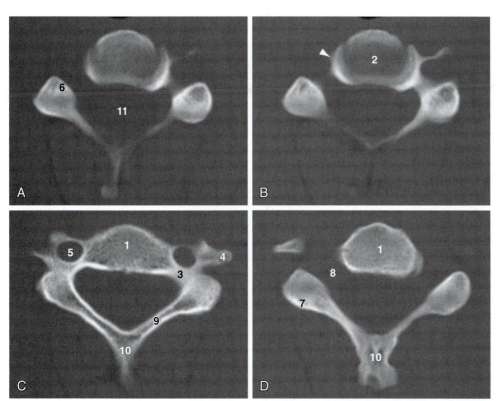

■ **FIGURE 3-21** In-vivo axial CT through C4 in a 27-year-old-man. Serial sections displayed from superior to inferior (**A** to **D**) demonstrate the C4 body (1), uncinate process of C4 (*arrowhead*), C3-C4 disc (2), C4 pedicle (3), C4 transverse process (4), foramen transversarium containing the vertebral artery (5), superior articular facet of C5 (6), inferior articular process of C4 (7), C3-C4 neural foramen containing the C4 root (8), C4 lamina (9), bifid C4 spinous process (10), and the spinal canal containing the spinal cord (11).

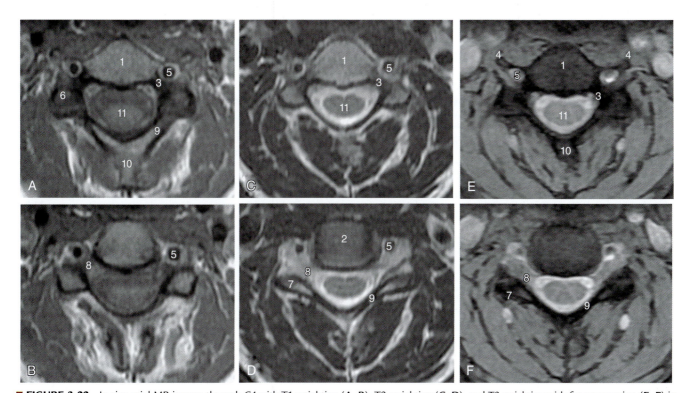

■ **FIGURE 3-22** In-vivo axial MR images through C4 with T1 weighting (**A, B**), T2 weighting (**C, D**), and T2 weighting with fat suppression (**E, F**) in a 34-year-old woman. Serial axial sections from above downward demonstrate the C4 body (1), C4-C5 disc (2), C4 pedicle (3), anterior tubercle of the C4 transverse process (4), foramen transversarium containing the vertebral artery (5), superior articular facet of C4 (6), inferior articular process of C4 (7), C4-C5 neural foramen containing the C5 root (8), C4 lamina (9), C4 spinous process (10), and the spinal cord (11).

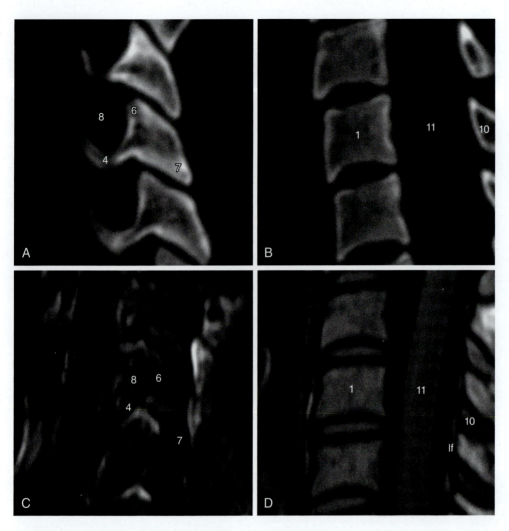

■ **FIGURE 3-23** In-vivo reformatted sagittal CT images (**A, B**) in a 27-year-old man and sagittal T1W MR images (**C, D**) in a 34-year-old woman. Sections through the articular pillars, facet joints, and midspinal canal show the C4 vertebral body (1), trough-like transverse process (4), the C3-C4 neural foramen carrying the C4 roots (8), the superior articular process (6) and inferior articular process (7) that form the facet joints, the ligamentum flavum (lf), the spinous process of C4 (10), and the spinal cord (11).

TABLE 3-1. Analysis of Cervical Spinal Canal: Sagittal and Transverse Dimensions

| | Mean Sagittal Dimension (mm)* | | | | Mean Transverse Dimension (mm)* | | | |
| | White | | African-American | | White | | African-American | |
Spinal Level	M	F	M	F	M	F	M	F
C2	16.8	16.6	16.4	15.1	23.8	22.9	23.4	**22.5**
C3	15.0	14.4	14.4	13.3	**23.4**	**22.5**	23.3	22.7
C4	14.6	13.7	**14.0**	**13.2**	24.1	23.5	24.3	23.5
C5	14.5	13.6	14.1	13.3	24.9	24.2	25.0	24.0
C6	**14.3**	**13.4**†	14.2	13.3	25.2	24.3	25.5	24.5
C7	14.3	13.4	14.4	13.6	24.3	23.4	24.5	23.5

Bold numbers indicate the narrowest dimension for each category.
*The standard deviation for each measurement listed varied from 1.0 to 1.6 mm.
†Indicates that this level measured the narrowest, before the numbers were rounded to three places for inclusion in the table.
Adapted from Tatarek NE. Technical review: variation in the human cervical neural canal. Spine J 2005; 5:623-631.

about 18 degrees of flexion and about 40 degrees of rotation.[1-3]

Occiput—C1: The atlanto-occipital junction is formed by paired synovial joints and significant supporting ligaments. The synovial atlanto-occipital joints lie between the occipital condyles above and the superior articular facets of C1 below. These are enclosed by thick fibrous capsules and may communicate with the joint cavity between the dens and the transverse ligament (see atlanto-axial junction below). The supporting ligaments include the anterior and posterior atlanto-occipital membranes.

The anterior atlanto-occipital membrane is a broad sheet of dense fibrous tissue that extends from the anterior edge of foramen magnum to the upper border of the anterior arch of C1 (Fig. 3-28). Medially it is reinforced by the ALL. Laterally, it merges with the capsular ligaments.

TABLE 3-2. Normal Cervical Neural Foramina in 20 Adults Aged 20-25 Years (10 Males, 10 Females) as Shown by In-Vivo MRI

Parameters	Vertebral Level					
	C2-C3	C3-C4	C4-C5	C5-C6	C6-C7	C7-T1
Height of foramen (mm)	12.2 ± 1.3	9.9 ± 1.2	10.5 ± 1.6	10.5 ± 1.5	10.5 ± 1.3	10.0 ± 1.4
Width of foramen (mm)	8.3 ± 1.3	7.2 ± 1.5	6.8 ± 0.9	6.9 ± 1.0	7.1 ± 1.2	6.9 ± 1.4
Cross-sectional area (mm)	64.6 ± 16.8	48.6 ± 12.2	47.7 ± 10.8	46.3 ± 9.9	48.1 ± 11.2	43.6 ± 11.6

From Lentell G, Kruse M, Chock B, et al. Dimensions of the cervical neural foramina in resting and retracted positions using magnetic resonance imaging. J Orthop Sports Phys Ther 2002; 32:380-390.

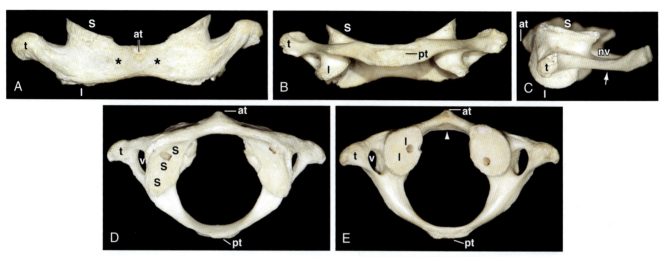

■ **FIGURE 3-24** Isolated dried C1 vertebra. Anterior (**A**), posterior (**B**), lateral (**C**), superior (**D**), and inferior (**E**) surfaces. The C1 ring displays prominent midline anterior and posterior tubercles (at, pt) and wide transverse processes (t) that enclose the foramina transversarium (v) for the vertebral artery. The superior oblique portions of longus colli attach (*asterisks*) to C1 at each side of the anterior tubercle. Paired large ovoid superior articular facets (S) and smaller, more circular inferior articular facets (I) converge toward the midline anteriorly. A cartilaginous facet (*arrowhead,* **E**) articulates with the anterior surface of the odontoid process (dens) of C2. The upper surface of the posterior arch (*arrow,* **C**) is grooved for the neurovascular bundle (nv) on each side.

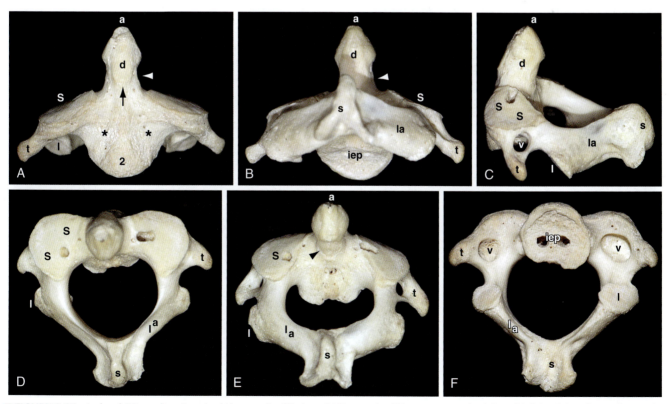

■ **FIGURE 3-25** Isolated C2 vertebra. Anterior (**A**), posterior (**B**), lateral (**C**), superior (**D**), posterosuperior (**E**), and inferior (**F**) surfaces. The anterior surface of the dens (d) displays the apex (a) that gives attachment to the apical ligament, the midline cartilaginous facet (*arrow*) for articulation with the anterior arch of C1, and the dental groove (*arrowhead*) along which the transverse ligament encloses the dens posterolaterally. Prominent depressions (*asterisks*) indicate the attachments of the vertical portions of longus colli bilaterally. iep, inferior end plate; la, lamina; s, spinous process; S and I, superior and inferior articular facets; t, transverse process; v, foramina transversaria.

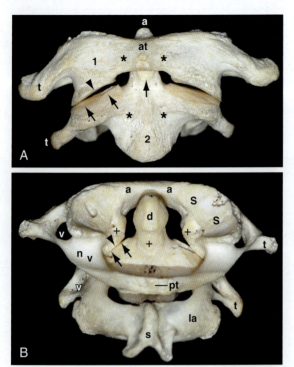

■ **FIGURE 3-26** C1-C2 articulation. Isolated dried vertebrae. Anterior (**A**) and posterosuperior (**B**) surfaces. Laterally, C1 articulates with C2 along the inferior facet of C1 (*arrowhead*) and superior facet of C2 (*paired arrows*). In the midline anteriorly, the anterior arch of C1 (a) articulates with the anterior surface of the dens along the anterior atlantodental facet of the dens (*single arrow*). In the midline posteriorly, C1 articulates with the posterior surface of the dens along the transverse ligament. The transverse ligament arches posterior to the dens (*plus sign*) to attach to prominent medial tubercles of C1 (*paired plus signs*) on each side. The vertebral artery emerges from the foramen transversarium of C2 (v), swings around the lateral masses of C2 and C1, continues superiorly through the foramen transversarium of C1 (v), and then passes over the posterior arch of C1 and along the neurovascular groove (nv) to enter the spinal canal. t, transverse process; S, superior articular facet; la, lamina; s, spinous process; at and pt, anterior and posterior tubercles. Asterisks indicate the attachments of the longus colli to C1.

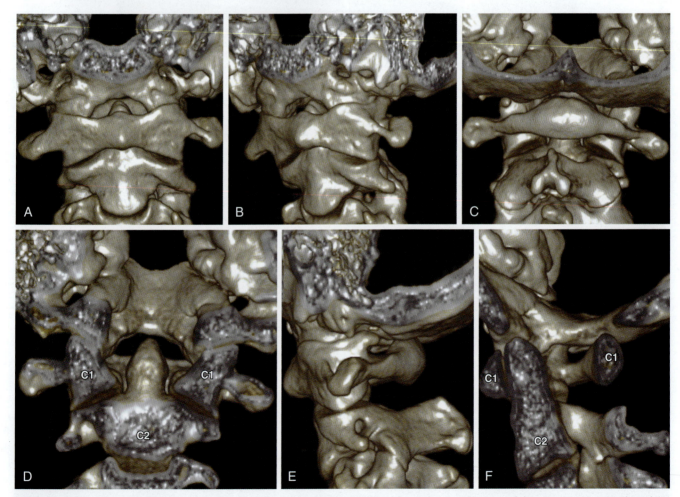

■ **FIGURE 3-27** In-vivo CT of the cervical spine in a 27-year-old woman. 3D CT surface reformatted images of the anterior (**A**), anterolateral (**B**), posterior (**C**), and lateral (**E**) surfaces of C1-C2. **D**, 3D cut-away reformatted image removing the posterior bone from **C** provides a posterior view of the relationships of the dens of C2 to the lateral masses of C1 (C1). **F**, 3D cut-away reformatted image removing the lateral bone from **E** provides a lateral view of the midline relationship of the dens to the anterior and posterior arches of C1 (C1).

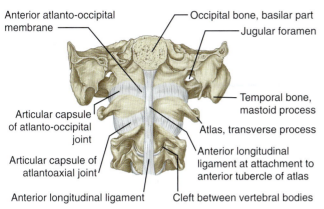

FIGURE 3-28 Diagram showing the anterior view of the atlanto-occipital and atlantoaxial joints. Small artificial clefts have been placed to mark the sites of the uncovertebral joints between the uncinate processes of C3 and the demifacets on the inferolateral surfaces of C2. *(From Standring S [ed]. Gray's Anatomy, 40th ed. Edinburgh, Elsevier Churchill Livingstone, 2009, p 733.)*

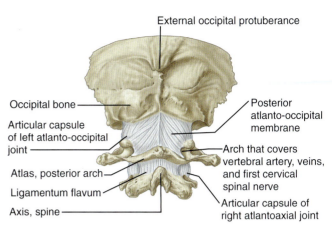

FIGURE 3-29 Diagram showing the posterior view of the atlanto-occipital and atlantoaxial joints. *(From Standring S [ed]. Gray's Anatomy, 40th ed. Edinburgh, Elsevier Churchill Livingstone, 2009, p 733.)*

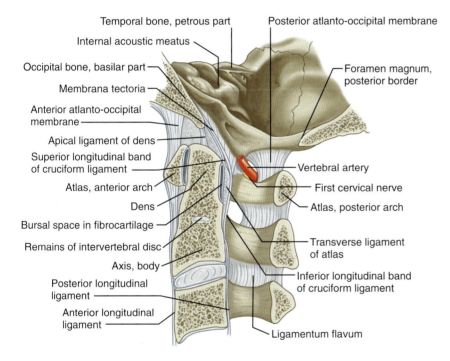

FIGURE 3-30 Diagram of midsagittal view of the atlanto-occipital, atlantoaxial, and adjacent joints. *(From Standring S [ed]. Gray's Anatomy, 40th ed. Edinburgh, Elsevier Churchill Livingstone, 2009, p 733.)*

The posterior atlanto-occipital membrane is a broad thin membrane that extends from the posterior margin of foramen magnum to the posterior arch of C1 (Fig. 3-29). It, too, merges with the capsular ligaments laterally. The posterolateral margin of this membrane arches over the vertebral artery, venous plexus, and C1 root as they cross the posterior arch of C1.

C1-C2: The atlanto-axial junction is formed by three synovial joints and significant supporting ligaments (Figs. 3-30 and 3-31).[1-3] The paired lateral synovial joints lie between the articular surfaces of the lateral masses of C1 and C2. Thin loose fibrous capsules attach to the articular margins of these paired lateral articulations. A median synovial joint lies both anterior to and posterior to the dens of C2. The anterior portion of the median joint lies

between the anterior arch of C1 and the dens. The articular surfaces of the anterior joint are formed by a cartilage-covered facet on the posterior surface of the anterior arch of C1 and an ovoid cartilage on the apposing anterior surface of the dens. The posterior portion of the median joint lies between the dens and the transverse ligament of C1 behind the dens. The articular surfaces of the posterior joint are formed by the horizontal facet that grooves the posterior surface of the dens and a cartilaginous plate on the anterior surface of the transverse ligament behind the dens. The synovial cavities of these median joints may exist as two separate noncommunicating spaces anterior and posterior to the dens or may merge into one communicating space. The capsule may be deficient superiorly. The median joints are reinforced by posteromedial acces-

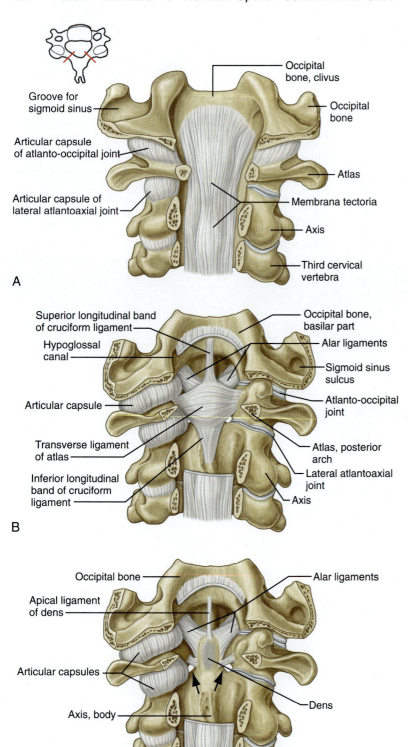

Occipital bone, clivus

Groove for sigmoid sinus

Articular capsule of atlanto-occipital joint

Articular capsule of lateral atlantoaxial joint

Occipital bone

Atlas

Membrana tectoria

Axis

Third cervical vertebra

A

Superior longitudinal band of cruciform ligament

Hypoglossal canal

Articular capsule

Transverse ligament of atlas

Inferior longitudinal band of cruciform ligament

Occipital bone, basilar part

Alar ligaments

Sigmoid sinus sulcus

Atlanto-occipital joint

Atlas, posterior arch

Lateral atlantoaxial joint

Axis

B

Occipital bone

Apical ligament of dens

Articular capsules

Axis, body

Alar ligaments

Dens

C

FIGURE 3-31 **A** to **C**, Diagrams of posterior views of the atlanto-occipital and atlantoaxial joints from within the spinal canal. The posterior portion of the occipital bone and the cervical laminae have been removed. The atlanto-occipital joint cavities have been opened. Arrows in **C** indicate the accessory ligaments. *(Adapted from Sobotta J: Atlas of Human Anatomy, 14th ed. Volume 2: Thorax, Abdomen, Pelvis, Lower Limb. London, Churchill Livingstone, 2006.)*

sory ligaments that extend from the body of C2 near the base of the dens medially to the lateral mass of the atlas near the transverse ligament.[1-3,30]

Supporting Ligaments

The atlanto-occipital and atlantoaxial joints are reinforced by a series of strong ligaments and membranes (Figs. 3-30

and 3-31).[1-3] Anteriorly, the ALL forms a tough midline cord that extends from the lower margin of the anterior tubercle of C1 onto the anterior surface of the C2 body. Posteriorly, the highest pair of ligamenta flava form thin membranes that extend from the lower margin of the C1 ring above onto the upper margins of the C2 laminae below. The paired C2 roots pierce this membrane laterally to exit from the spinal canal.

The transverse atlantal ligament is a broad strong collagenous band that sweeps across the C1 ring behind the dens. Laterally on each side the transverse atlantal ligament attaches to a small tubercle on the medial surface of the lateral mass of C1. Medially it widens into a broad band that carries a layer of cartilage on its anterior surface for articulation with the dens. Superiorly, the transverse atlantal ligament gives rise to the midline superior longitudinal ligament. The superior longitudinal ligament extends upward to insert on the basiocciput behind the apical ligament and in front of the tectorial membrane (see later). Inferiorly, the transverse atlantal ligament gives rise to a weaker, less constant inferior longitudinal ligament that extends downward to insert onto the posterior surface of C2. Together the transverse and the longitudinal ligaments form a cruciate structure, so they are designated, collectively, the cruciate ligament.

The tectorial membrane is the upward extension of the PLL and displays two layers (see Figs. 3-30 and 3-31).[1-3] The superficial (more posterior) lamina extends upward from the posterior surface of the C2 body and expands into a broad sheet that inserts onto the basiocciput, craniad to the foramen magnum. It merges into the cranial dura. The deep layer of the tectorial membrane also extends upward from the posterior surface of C2 body and forms three major bands: a strong median band that inserts onto foramen magnum and paired lateral bands that insert into and merge with capsules of the atlanto-occipital joints. Deep to the tectorial membrane, loose areolar tissue and, occasionally, a bursa separate the anterior surface of the tectorial membrane from the posterior surface of the cruciate ligament.

The alar ligaments are tough, paired fibrous cords that extend anterosuperolaterally from the posterolateral aspects of the uppermost dens to the medial aspects of both occipital condyles (see Fig. 3-31).[1-3] The alar ligaments are thought to prevent excess rotation at C1-C2, because the ligament of each side limits rotation to the opposite side.

The apical ligament of the dens extends superiorly from the apex of the dens to insert into the anterior margin of the foramen magnum between the alar ligaments.[1-3] In its course, it is separated from the anterior atlantoaxial membrane in front and the cruciform ligament behind by interposed pads of fat. The apical ligament is a remnant of the cranial notochord and its sheath.[1-3]

Together these ligaments serve to stabilize the articulations among C2, C1, and the occiput. The transverse ligament is the strongest of all. The alar ligaments are weaker. Measurement of the atlantoaxial and lateral atlantodens interval can be used to identify atlantoaxial ligamentous injuries in adults and children. Rojas and associates analyzed these parameters in 178 adult and 112 pediatric patients to establish the upper limits of normal for populations of varying ages (Table 3-3).[31] The ligamentum nuchae and the suboccipital muscles also help stabilize the head on the neck.[1-3]

Posterior Dural Attachments

At the craniovertebral junction (occiput-C2), the posterior spinal dura is thickened and anchored posteriorly by

TABLE 3-3. Atlantoaxial Interval by Patient Age

Age Group	Upper Limit of Normal Range (mm)
0-1 yr	3.6
1-2 yr	3.9
2-3 yr	4.4
3-5 yr	3.9
5-7 yr	4.1
7-9 yr	3.6
Adults (≥20 yr)	3.4

From Rojas, CA, Hayes A, Bertozzi JC, et al. Evaluation of the C1-C2 articulation on MDCT in healthy children and young adults. AJR Am J Roentgenol 2009; 193:1388-1392.

attachments to the ligamentum nuchae and the rectus capitis posterior minor (RCPM). Dissection of 30 human cadavers revealed two such attachments.[32]

In all specimens (100%) a broad ligament arose from the deep lamellar portion of the ligamentum nuchae, extended along the midline between the posterior arch of C1 and the spinous process of C2, traversed the midline gap between the left and right ligamenta flava (posterior atlanto-axial membrane), and flared out laterally to attach to the posterior spinal dura. The craniocaudal height of the ligament was 3 to 10 mm. The width of the laterally flaring attachment varied from several millimeters to 1.5 cm.[32]

In all specimens (100%) a connective tissue attachment arose from the anterior surface of the RCPM, extended along the midline between the occiput and C1, traversed a gap in the wafer-thin posterior atlanto-occipital membrane, and attached to the posterior spinal dura mater.[32]

In 27 specimens (90%), an additional connective tissue bridge arose from the posterior aspect of the RCPM, posterior and superior to the posterior arch of C1, to attach to the ligamentum nuchae. In 90% of human anatomic dissections, therefore, a connective tissue complex links the posterior spinal dura at occiput-C1 to the RCPM, the RCPM to the ligamentum nuchae, and the ligamentum nuchae back to the posterior spinal dura at C1-C2. In the dissected cadavers, traction on one of the attachments produced movement in the other attachments. These attachments may serve to prevent dural infolding and compression of the posterior spinal cord during head motion.[32]

The Neural Foramina

The neural foramina transmit the motor and sensory nerve roots that merge into a mixed spinal segmental nerve, the associated meningeal sheaths, two to four recurrent meningeal nerves, variable radiculomeningeal and radiculospinal vessels, and the plexiform venous connections between the internal and the external vertebral venous plexuses (see Figs. 3-5 and 3-6).[1-3]

The position of the neurovascular bundle is different in the cervical than the thoracolumbar region. In the cervical spine, the ventral and dorsal roots lie within the lower portion of each cervical foramen, at and inferior to the level of the cervical disc. The dorsal roots lie immediately anterior to the superior articular facets. The dorsal root

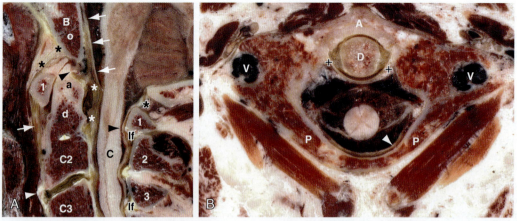

■ FIGURE 3-32 Cryomicrotome sections of the craniovertebral junction. **A,** Midsagittal section through the atlanto-occipital and atlantoaxial joints (magnified upper portion of Fig. 3-20B). A residual interspace partially separates the base of C2 from the dens (d). From anterior to posterior, five major ligaments interconnect C2 and C1 with the skull base: The anterior atlanto-occipital membrane (*double black asterisks*) interconnects the upper margin of the anterior arch of C1 with the anterior margin of foramen magnum. In the midline, this is strengthened by a tough strap (*white arrow*) of the anterior longitudinal ligament (*white arrowhead*) that crosses over the anterior surface of C2, the anterior tubercle of C1, and the anterior surface of the atlanto-occipital membrane to insert into the skull base. The apical ligament extends from a shallow concavity on the dens (*small black arrowhead*) to insert on the medical aspect of the occipital condyles. The transverse portion of the cruciate ligament (*double white asterisks*) courses posterior to the dens to form the posterior dental-transverse joint. The tectorial membrane (*three white arrows*) is the broad superior extension of the posterior longitudinal ligament that inserts onto the posterior surface of the clivus above and dorsal to the apical ligament. The posterior atlanto-occipital membrane (*black asterisk outlined in white*) extends from the upper surface of the posterior arch of C1 to the posterior rim of foramen magnum. It may be regarded, in part, as a thin counterpart to the ligamenta flava (lf) seen below. Joint spaces are seen between the posterior surface of the anterior arch of C1 (1) and the anterior surface of the dens (d) and between the posterior surface of the dens and the anterior surface of the transverse ligament (*white asterisks*). (See also Fig. 3-31.) **B,** Axial cryotome section through the atlantoaxial joint. The anterior (A) and posterior (P) arches of C1 enclose the dens, dural sac (*white arrowhead*), cerebrospinal fluid, spinal cord, and emerging nerve roots. Anteriorly, the dens (D) articulates with the posterior surface of the anterior arch (A) of C1. Posteriorly, it articulates with the anterior surface of the transverse ligament (*paired plus signs*), which inserts into a medial tubercle on the inner aspect of C1 on each side and swings posteriorly to cradle the dens. Articular cartilage can be seen just on the apposing surfaces of anterior arch, dens, and transverse ligament. The vertebral arteries (V) traverse the foramen transversarium of C1 bilaterally.

ganglion (DRG) often lies within a small concavity (fossa) at the anterior wall of the superior articular process. In axial sections, the dorsal nerve roots appear to lie just anterior to the ligamentum flavum while the anterior roots lie immediately posterior to the vertebral margin and the uncinate process.[18,33] In the thoracic and lumbar regions the nerve roots lie in the upper portion of the neural foramina, just inferior to the upper pedicle. Throughout the spine, the nerve roots are named for the pedicle they are closest to. Because the cervical roots emerge through the inferior portion of each neural foramen, closest to the inferior pedicle, the C1 root emerges between the skull base and C1, the C2 to C7 roots emerge through the C1-C2 to C6-C7 neural foramina, respectively, and the C8 root emerges at the neural foramen between C7 and T1. Conversely, because the thoracic and lumbar roots emerge through the upper portions of the neural foramina, closest to the superior pedicle, the T1 root emerges at the T1-T2 neural foramen, the T12 root emerges at the T12-L1 neural foramen, the L5 root at the L5-S1 neural foramen, and the S5 root between S5 and the first coccygeal segment.

IMAGING

CT and MRI

CT displays best the bony architecture and the many normal variants of spinal anatomy described in this chapter (Figs. 3-33 to 3-36). MRI displays the bony architecture less well than CT but shows beautifully the contained

bone marrow and often shows the ligaments and fascia better than does CT (see Figs. 3-33 to 3-36). For example, CT displays the smooth, regular dense cortical bone of the articular surfaces whereas T2-weighted (T2W) MRI imaging shows best the smooth, bright homogeneous signal of the normal 2- to 4-mm thick layer of hyaline cartilage overlying the homogeneously low signal cortical bone of the facet surfaces.[13] The imaging appearances of the normal anatomic structures presented in this chapter are illustrated within each subsection of anatomy to facilitate direct comparison of the gross anatomy with the imaging display of that anatomy.

Protocols for CT

The protocols for imaging of the cervical spine are shown in Box 3-1. A sample case report is shown in Box 3-2.

Protocols for MRI

Table 3-4 shows the present MRI protocols for the cervical spine. In any individual case, additional sequences may be indicated. Specific protocols are expected to evolve with improving technology.

Strategies for Interpreting and Reporting Cervical Spine Studies

One can interpret cross-sectional imaging of the spine in a number of ways. One format for systematic and compre-

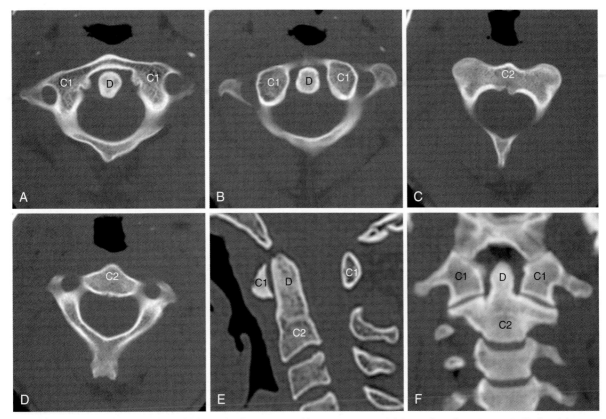

■ **FIGURE 3-33** In-vivo CT of the craniovertebral junction in a 27-year-old man. **A** to **D,** Axial CT sections from C1 to C2, displayed from superior to inferior. **E,** Reformatted mid-sagittal CT section. **F,** Reformatted coronal CT section. D, dens.

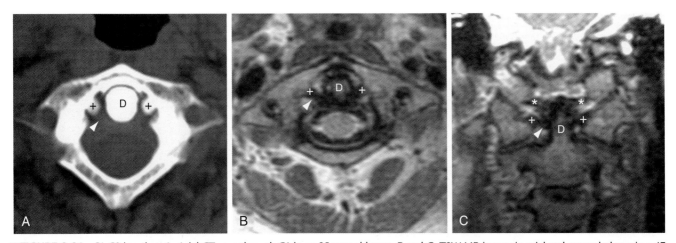

■ **FIGURE 3-34** C1-C2 junction. **A,** Axial CT scan through C1 in an 85-year-old man. **B** and **C,** T2W MR images in axial and coronal planes in a 47-year-old woman. The transverse ligament (*arrowhead*) extends from the medial tubercles (*paired plus signs*) of C1 around the posterior aspect of the dens (D) to form the posterior atlantodental joint. The alar ligaments (*paired asterisks*) arise from the lateral surfaces of the dens to insert into the medial surfaces of the occipital condyles.

hensive review of spinal images is detailed here. Other formats may also be adopted. The approach selected, however, is best followed in (nearly) identical fashion for each level of each study over the years so that the same data appear in the same order on all subsequent reports. In this way, the next radiologist and the patient's clinician can find parallel data at each site and follow the patient's status easily over time. The reporting format suggested also deliberately duplicates some data at different

points to ensure that key data in the report are readily accessible. Computer-based dictation now makes it easy to generate such standardized reports. Thus, we suggest the following:

1. On CT and MRI studies, start with the scout views, noting any gross abnormalities and all instrumentation (e.g., any indwelling catheters, drains, monitor leads, surgical hardware).

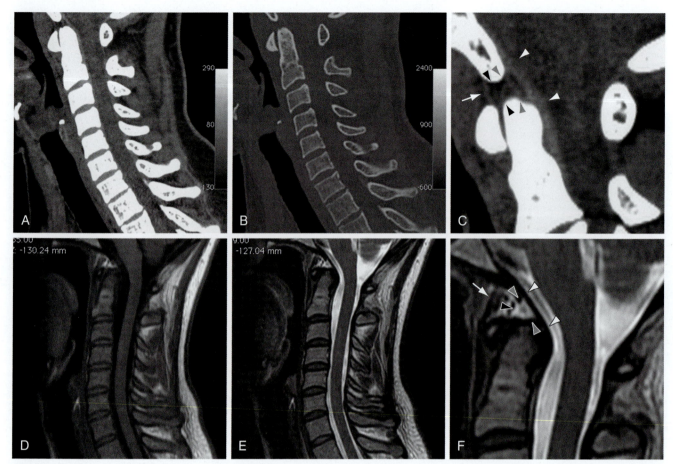

■ **FIGURE 3-35**   Craniovertebral junction. **A** to **C,** Reformatted sagittal CT sections in a 27-year-old woman. Sagittal T1W (**D**) and T2W (**E, F**) MR images in a 34-year-old woman. Images in **C** and **F** show the anterior atlanto-occipital ligament (*white arrow*) thickened in the midline by the anterior longitudinal ligament, the apical ligament (*black arrowheads*) of the dens, the posterior atlanto-occipital ligament (*gray arrowheads*), and the tectorial membrane (*white arrowheads*) that is the superior extension of the posterior longitudinal ligament.

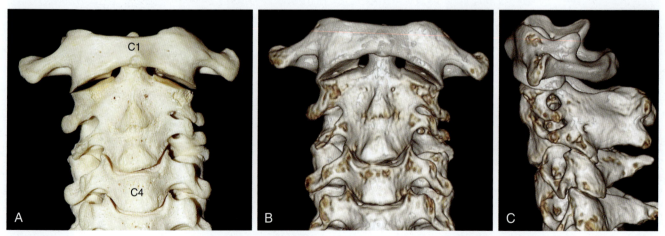

■ **FIGURE 3-36**   Malsegmentation of C2-C3. **A,** Dried osseous vertebrae. **B** and **C,** 3D CT surface reformatted images of the dried skeleton. The vertebral bodies and arches are fused, obliterating the intervertebral disc and reducing the sizes of the neural foramina.

2. Then, evaluate the sagittal (direct or reformatted) soft tissue images from the skin to skin, anteriorly to posteriorly.

3. In the cervical spine, make sure that the airway is patent without evidence of mass or stenosis. Specifically, analyze the larynx and note in the report that there is, or is not, evidence for vocal cord dysfunction.

4. Analyze the thyroid gland, the lymph nodes, the fascial planes, and other prevertebral soft tissues for evidence of inflammation, tumor, or trauma. Then, look posterior to the spinal canal for similar evidence of

---

BOX 3-1 Protocols for CT of the Cervical Spine

- Patient position: Supine
- Scan extent: Determined by radiologist
- Contrast: None
- Scan type: Helical
- Slice thickness: 0.625 mm
- Detector coverage: 20 mm
- Pitch: 0.531:1 (10.62 mm/rotation)
- Rotation time: 0.5 s
- Reconstruction: 2.5 mm
- Field of view: Sized to include entire vertebrae, including transverse and spinous processes
- Algorithm: Soft tissue and bone
- Postprocessing: 1.0 × 0.5-mm increments in coronal and sagittal multiplanar reformatted images

inflammation, tumor, or trauma affecting the retrospinal soft tissue.
5. On sagittal bone and soft tissue images, assess:
   - The overall curvature of the spine
   - The overall alignment of the vertebral bodies
   - The heights, contours, and density/signal of the bone and marrow of the individual vertebral bodies
   - The heights and density/signal of the intervertebral discs
   - The anterior and posterior longitudinal ligaments
   - The overall size of the spinal canal
   - The size, position, and configuration of the spinal cord
   - The ligamenta flava and the alignment of the spinolaminar lines at the posterior wall of the spinal canal

---

BOX 3-2 Noncontrast CT of the Cervical Spine

PATIENT HISTORY

A 40-year-old man presented with nonspecific neck pain.

TECHNIQUE

Serial thin axial sections were obtained by helical technique from the skull base to T2 and processed to generate reformatted axial, sagittal, and curved-plane "coronal" soft tissue algorithm and bone algorithm images through the length of the cervical spine. Additional oblique sagittal images were generated to display the cross sections of the neural foramina on each side. No contrast agent was administered.

FINDINGS

The paraspinal soft tissues demonstrate a patent airway with no evidence of stenosis or mass. The larynx is normal with no evidence for vocal cord dysfunction. The thyroid gland, lymph nodes, prevertebral, and retrovertebral soft tissues are within normal limits.

The spinal column shows normal cervical lordosis. There is no subluxation. The vertebral body height, contour, and density are within expected limits for patient age. The intervertebral disc spaces appear normal with no loss of height or end plate irregularity. The overall size of the spinal canal is normal. The spinal cord shows normal size, position, contour, and density. The facet joints have normal contour and alignment. The left neural foramina are normal at C2-C3 through C7-T1 inclusive. The right neural foramina are normal in size at C2-C3, minimally narrowed by uncovertebral spurs at C4-C5 and C5-C6, and normal again at C6-C7 and C7-T1. No carotid artery calcification is identified.

The visualized portions of the posterior fossa, skull base, and uppermost thoracic spine show no abnormality.

At C1-C2, the atlantodental alignment and cruciate ligaments appear normal. The anterior and posterior arches of C1 show no abnormality. The spinal canal, spinal cord, and paravertebral soft tissue are within normal limits.

At C2-C3, the spinal canal has normal contour with no impingement by disc or spur. The transverse processes, facet joints, and laminae are normal bilaterally. The neural foramina are normal in size. The C3 ganglion and emerging C3 roots are surrounded by fat bilaterally, with no compression by disc or spur. The spinal cord is normal in size, position, density, and configuration. The paravertebral soft tissues are within normal limits.

At C3-C4, the spinal canal has normal contour with no impingement by disc or spur. The transverse processes, facet joints, and laminae are normal bilaterally. The neural foramina are normal in size. The C4 ganglion and emerging C4 roots are surrounded by fat bilaterally, with no compression by disc or spur. The spinal cord is normal in size, position, density, and configuration. The paravertebral soft tissues are within normal limits.

At C4-C5, the spinal canal has normal contour with no impingement by disc or spur. The transverse processes, facet joints, and laminae are normal bilaterally. The left neural foramen, emerging left C5 roots, and ganglion are normal. The right neural foramen shows minimal narrowing by uncovertebral spurs but no impingement on the emerging right C5 roots or ganglion. The spinal cord is normal in size, position, density, and configuration. The paravertebral soft tissues are within normal limits.

(Continue serially for each level through C7-T1.)

IMPRESSION

This noncontrast CT of the cervical spine is within normal limits for stated age. There is minimal narrowing of the right C4-C5 neural foramen by uncovertebral spurs that do not impinge on the segmental C5 nerve roots or ganglion.

TABLE 3-4.   Present MRI Protocols Used in Imaging the Cervical Spine

Sequence	TE	TR	TI	Echo Train	BW	Freq	Phase	Freq Dir	NEX	FOV	ST	# Diff Dir
Precontrast												
Sagittal T1 FLAIR	22.0	2500.0	Auto	8	41.67	416	224	A/P	2.00	26.0	4.0	
Sagittal T2 FRFSE	110.0	4400.0	Auto	24	41.67	416	224	A/P	4.00	24.0	2.5	
2D MERGE	110.0	654.2	Auto	24	50.00	320	192	A/P	2.00	16.0	4.0	
3D MERGE	11.2	Minimum	Auto	24	62.50	320	160	R/L	2.00	16.0	2.0	
Axial T2 FRFSE	110.0	4617.0	Auto	1	41.67	416	224	R/L	2.00	17.0	3.0	
Axial T1 FLAIR	17.0	500.0	Auto	3	31.25	256	160	R/L	1.00	16.0	3.0	
Sagittal DTI	Minimum	1500.0	Auto	2	31.25	96	128	S/I	10.00	28.0	3.3	6
Sagittal STIR	42.0	4050.0	180	12	31.25	352	160	A/P	2.00	24.0	3.0	
Postcontrast												
Sagittal T1 FLAIR	21.0	2250.0	Auto	7	41.67	416	192	A/P	2.00	26.0	4.0	
Axial T1 FSE	17.0	2000.0	Auto	7	31.25	256	192	R/L	1.00	16.0	3.0	

TE, echo time (ms); TR, repetition time (ms); TI, inversion time (ms); FLIP, flip angle; BW, bandwidth; Freq, matrix in frequency-encoded direction; Phase, matrix in phase-encoded direction; Freq Dir, direction of frequency encoding; NEX, number of signals averaged; FOV, field of view (mm); ST, slice thickness (mm); # Diff Dir, number of diffusion directions; FLAIR, fluid-attenuated inversion recovery; FRFSE, fast recovery fast-spin echo; MERGE, multiple echo recombined gradient echo (proprietary GE sequence); DTI, diffusion tensor imaging; STIR, short tau inversion recovery; FSE, fast spin echo; A/P, anterior/posterior; R/L, right/left; S/I, superior/inferior.

- The integrity and orientation of the laminae, spinous processes, and interspinous ligaments
- The adjacent visualized portions of the posterior fossa, skull base, and upper thorax

6. Scroll side to side to assess the sagittal anatomy of the zygapophyseal (facet) joints at each level for both sides.

7. Then continue laterally on each side to see the visualized portions of the neural foramina, emerging nerve roots, brachial plexus, and musculature of the neck. Where possible also assess the carotid arteries for calcification and potential stenoses.

8. In the cervical spine, evaluate *oblique sagittal* images for the neural foramina and transverse processes, first on one side and then on the other side. Report these for each side in two separate sentences, such as "On the left, the neural foramina are normal at (list here all normal levels from superior to inferior) but show narrowing, spurring (or other pathologic processes) at (list here all abnormal levels from superior to inferior)" and "On the right, the neural foramina (*finish the sentence in parallel format*)."

9. Next turn to the axial images and assess the spinal canal level by level.

10. In the axial plane, at each level, evaluate the prevertebral soft tissues, adjoining vertebral bodies, uncinate processes, pedicles, transverse processes, foramina transversaria (for the vertebral arteries), neural foramina, facet joints, laminae, and spinous processes. Assess the anterior and posterior longitudinal ligaments, the ligamenta flava, and the cruciate and related ligaments of C1-C2.

11. Then address the cross-sectional area of the spinal canal, the contours of the vertebral bodies and intervertebral discs, and any compromise of the spinal canal or neural foramina by bulging/herniated discs or osteophytes.

12. Review the contours and density/signal of the spinal cord.

13. Check the vascularity of the spinal column and cord, and assess the integrity of the muscles, fascial planes, and other paraspinal soft tissues.

14. Report these data in the same format for each level, so each level details the same set of findings, whether the level is normal or not. To that end, one might start a new paragraph for each level: "At C1-C2 . . .", "At C2-C3 . . ." and continue, serially, to "At T1-T2. . . ." These axial data are partially redundant with the sagittal data given earlier. This deliberate duplication makes it easier, for example, to understand which of all neural foramina are most severely affected on the left or right sides (sagittal data) *and* what is the state of the two neural foramina at a specific level (axial data).

15. For the cervical spine, also specifically evaluate the sizes of the foramina transversaria of the lower cervical vertebrae to determine whether the vertebral artery enters the foramen transversarium at C6 (the most common entry) or at C7, C5, or other level (less common). Note whether loops of the vertebral artery undercut and narrow the uncinate and transverse processes thinning the bone between the disc, the neural foramen, and the vertebral artery. Report any right-sided aortic arch and any anomalous origin of the subclavian arteries from the aorta. These data may help a surgeon to avoid injury to an anomalous segment of the vertebral artery, to the segmental nerve roots in the foramina, or to an anomalous direct (rather than recurrent) laryngeal nerve.

Use of standardized computer-based reports helps to record the data in reproducible format rapidly and with little extra effort (see Box 3-2).

ACKNOWLEDGMENTS

The authors gratefully acknowledge the assistance of Edward Lugo, Steven Yuen, Nancy Hoo, Jeremy Tietjens, Aron Legler, Jalal Ahmed, Marcia Jaunoo, RTR, Artur Yadgarov, RTR, and James Stephen, RTR.

The 3D CT surface reformatted images and cut-away sections were made on a PC using Aquarius Workstation 3.7.0.12 by TeraRecon, Inc. (2995 Campus Drive #325, San Mateo, CA 94403) or Mac using OsiriX PACS Workstation DICOM Viewer v3.6.1 (64-bit). OsiriX is a freely distributed open-source software under the GNU licensing scheme and can be downloaded at http://www.osirix-viewer.com/Downloads.html.

KEY POINTS

- The sizes of the vertebral bodies, transverse processes, spinous processes, and laminae vary systematically over the length of the spine.
- The vertebral bodies are united across the interspace by symphyses made of the apposing vertebral margins, two apposing hyaline cartilage end plates, and the intervertebral disc.
- The anterior longitudinal ligament runs the length of the spine from the skull base to the first sacral vertebra. It attaches very strongly at the levels of the disc and more loosely over the midvertebral bodies.
- The posterior longitudinal ligament runs the length of the spine from the posterior surface of the clivus to the posterior surface of the first sacral vertebra. The portion from C2 to the clivus may be designated, separately, the tectorial membrane.
- The arches of the spine are united by zygapophyseal (facet) joints laterally, by the ligamenta flava posterolaterally, and by the interspinous and supraspinous ligaments posteriorly.
- The transverse processes represent a modification and (partial) fusion of the true transverse process (diapophysis) and the costal elements (pleurapophysis), accounting for the diverse shapes of the cervical, thoracic, lumbar, and sacral transverse processes and ribs.
- CT shows best the bony elements of the spine. MRI shows best the soft tissues of the muscles, ligaments, spinal cord, and nerve roots.

SUGGESTED READINGS

Atlas SW. Magnetic Resonance Imaging of the Brain and Spine, 4th ed. Volume 2, Part 4, Spine and Spinal Cord. Philadelphia. Wolters Kluwer/Lippincott Williams & Wilkins, 2009.

Bullough PG, Boachie-Adjei O. Atlas of Spinal Disorders. Philadelphia, JB Lippincott, 1988.

Castillo M. Neuroradiology Companion: Methods, Guidelines, and Imaging Fundamentals, 3rd ed. Philadelphia, Lippincott Williams & Willkins, 2006.

Daniels DL, Haughton V, Naidich TP. Cranial and Spinal Magnetic Resonance Imaging: An Atlas and Guide. New York, Raven Press, 1987.

Modic MT, Masaryk TJ, et al. Magnetic Resonance Imaging of the Spine. St. Louis, MO, Mosby–Year Book, 1994.

Newell RLM. The back. In Strandring S (ed). Gray's Anatomy: The Anatomical Basis of Clinical Practice, 39th ed. Edinburgh, Churchill Livingstone, 2009.

Ross JS, Brant-Zawadzki M, Moore KR, et al. Diagnostic Imaging Spine. Salt Lake City, UT, Amirsys, 2004.

Soames RW. Skeletal system. In Williams PL (ed). Gray's Anatomy: The Anatomical Basis of Medicine and Surgery, 38th ed. Edinburgh, Churchill Livingstone, 1995.

Van Goethem JWM, van den Hauwe L, Parizel PM (eds). Spinal Imaging: Diagnostic Imaging of the Spine and Spinal Cord (Medical Radiology/Diagnostic Imaging). Berlin, Springer, 2007.

REFERENCES

1. Williams PL (ed). Gray's Anatomy: The Anatomical Basis of Medicine and Surgery, 38th ed. New York, Churchill Livingstone, 1995.
2. Standring S (ed). Gray's Anatomy: The Anatomical Basis of Clinical Practice, 39th ed. Edinburgh, Elsevier Churchill Livingstone, 2005.
3. Standring S (ed). Gray's Anatomy: The Anatomical Basis of Clinical Practice, 40th ed. Edinburgh, Elsevier Churchill Livingstone, 2009.
4. Vande Berg BC, Lecouvet FE, Galant C, et al: Normal variants of the bone marrow at MR imaging of the spine. Semin Musculoskelet Radiol 2009; 13:87.
5. Liney GP, Bernard CP, Manton DJ, et al. Age, gender, and skeletal variation in bone marrow composition: a preliminary study at 3.0 Tesla. J Magn Reson Imaging 2007; 26:787.
6. Griffith JF, Yeung DK, Antonio GE, et al. Vertebral bone mineral density, marrow perfusion, and fat content in healthy men and men with osteoporosis: dynamic contrast-enhanced MR imaging and MR spectroscopy. Radiology 2005; 236:945.
7. Schwarz GS. The width of the spinal canal in the growing vertebra with special reference to the sacrum; maximum interpediculated distances in adults and children. Am J Roentgenol Radium Ther Nucl Med 1956; 76:476.
8. Benzian SR, Mainzer F, Gooding CA. Pediculate thinning: a normal variant at the thoracolumbar junction. Br J Radiol 1971; 44:936.
9. Hayashi K, Yabuki T, Kurokawa T, et al. The anterior and the posterior longitudinal ligaments of the lower cervical spine. J Anat 1977; 124:633-666.
10. Wiltse LL. Anatomy of the extradural compartments of the lumbar spinal canal: Peridural membrane and circumneural sheath. Radiol Clin North Am 2000; 38:1177-1206.
11. Hogan QH. Lumbar epidural anatomy: A new look by cryomicrotome section. Anesthesiology 1992; 76:866-867.
12. Crock HV, Yoshizawa H. The Blood Supply of the Vertebral Column and Spinal Cord in Man. New York, Springer Verlag, 1977.
13. Hasegawa T, An HS, Haughton VM. Imaging anatomy of the lateral lumbar spinal canal. Semin Ultrasound CT MR 1993; 14:404.
14. Xu GL, Haughton VM, Carrera GF. Lumbar facet joint capsule: appearance at MR imaging and CT. Radiology 1990; 177:415.
15. Lirk P, Kolbitsch C, Putz G, et al: Cervical and high thoracic ligamentum flavum frequently fails to fuse in the midline. Anesthesiology 2003; 99:1387-1390.
16. Lirk P, Moriggi B, Colvin J, et al. The incidence of lumbar ligamentum flavum midline gaps. Anesth Analg 2004; 98:1178-1180.
17. Lirk P, Colvin J, Steger B, et al: Incidence of lower thoracic ligamentum flavum midline gaps. Br J Anaesth 2005; 94:852-855.
18. Pech P, Daniels DL, Williams AL, et al. The cervical neural foramina: correlation of microtomy and CT anatomy. Radiology 1985; 155:143.
19. De Boeck M, Potvliege R, Roels F, et al. The accessory costotransverse foramen: a radioanatomical study. J Comput Assist Tomogr 1984; 8:117.
20. Tatarek NE. Variation in the human cervical neural canal. Spine J 2005; 5:623.
21. Lentell G, Kruse M, Chock B, et al. Dimensions of the cervical neural foramina in resting and retracted positions using magnetic resonance imaging. J Orthop Sports Phys Ther 2002; 32:380.
22. Brewin J, Hill M, Ellis H. The prevalence of cervical ribs in a London population. Clin Anat 2009; 22:331.
23. Daniels DL, Williams AL, Haughton VM. Computed tomography of the articulations and ligaments at the occipito-atlantoaxial region. Radiology 1983; 146:709.
24. Krakenes J, Kaale BR, Rorvik J, et al. MRI assessment of normal ligamentous structures in the craniovertebral junction. Neuroradiology 2001; 43:1089.
25. Menezes AH, Traynelis VC. Anatomy and biomechanics of normal craniovertebral junction (a) and biomechanics of stabilization (b). Childs Nerv Syst 2008;24:1091.

26. Mercer SR, Bogduk N. Clinical anatomy of ligamentum nuchae. Clin Anat 2003; 16:484.
27. Pfirrmann CW, Binkert CA, Zanetti M, et al. MR morphology of alar ligaments and occipitoatlantoaxial joints: study in 50 asymptomatic subjects. Radiology 2001; 218:133.
28. Schweitzer ME, Hodler J, Cervilla V, et al. Craniovertebral junction: normal anatomy with MR correlation. AJR Am J Roentgenol 1992; 158:1087.
29. Shoda N, Anamizu Y, Yonezawa N, et al. Ossification of the posterior atlantoaxial membrane and the transverse atlantal ligament. Spine 2005; 30:E248.
30. Yuksel M, Heiserman JE, Sonntag VK. Magnetic resonance imaging of the craniocervical junction at 3-T: observation of the accessory atlantoaxial ligaments. Neurosurgery 2006; 59:888.
31. Rojas CA, Hayes A, Bertozzi JC, et al. Evaluation of the C1-C2 articulation on MDCT in healthy children and young adults. AJR Am J Roentgenol 2009; 193:1388.
32. Humphreys BK, Kenin S, Hubbard BB, Cramer GD. Investigation of connective tissue attachments to the cervical spinal dura mater. Clin Anat 2003; 16:152-158.
33. Czervionke LF, Daniels DL, Ho PS, et al. Cervical neural foramina: correlative anatomic and MR imaging study. Radiology 1988; 169:753.

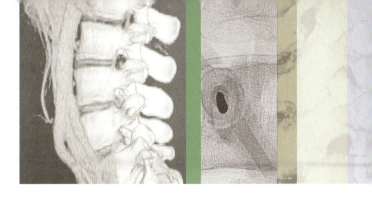

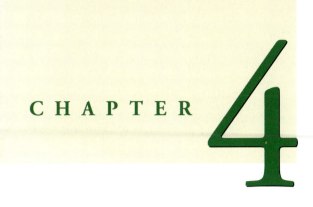

The Normal Spinal Column: Thoracic, Lumbar, Sacral, and Coccygeal Segments

Jose Conrado Rios, Thomas Paul Naidich, David L. Daniels, Victor M. Haughton, Cheuk Ying Tang, Joy S. Reidenberg, Patrick A. Lento, Evan Gary Stein, Girish Manohar Fatterpekar, Tanvir Fiaz Choudhri, and Irina Oyfe

The spinal column consists of multiple segmented osseous vertebrae, the intervertebral discs interposed between these segments, and the ligaments and joints that bind the segments together. The spine has 32 to 35 vertebral segments, traditionally considered as 7 cervical, 12 thoracic, 5 lumbar, 5 sacral, and 3 to 5 coccygeal segments. The relative lengths of the cervical, thoracic, lumbar, and sacral spines are in proportion as 2:5:3:2.[1-3] An introduction to the spinal column and a detailed anatomy of the cervical segment was presented in Chapter 3; in this chapter the thoracic, lumbar, sacral, and coccygeal segments of the spinal column are addressed and imaging of the bone marrow is discussed.

NORMAL ANATOMY

Segmental Osseous Morphology

Thoracic Vertebrae

The 12 rib-bearing thoracic vertebrae are similar to each other but show a progressive transition from more nearly cervical to more nearly lumbar shape over the length of the thorax (Figs. 4-1 and 4-2).[1-3] The vertebral bodies resemble cylinders with concave side walls and nearly equal anteroposterior and transverse dimensions. The T1 and T2 bodies show flat anterior faces. The T3 body is the smallest thoracic vertebral body and shows a convex anterior surface. From T4 downward the thoracic vertebral bodies become progressively larger to bear increasing weight. The two thoracic pedicles extend directly posteriorly from the vertebral body, nearly parallel to each other, rather than angling posterolaterally as do the cervical pedi-

cles (Figs. 4-3 and 4-4). The thoracic pedicles increase in size progressively from above downward. The articulations with the ribs extend onto the lateral surfaces of the pedicles. For that reason, the upper surfaces of thoracic pedicles (except T1) are straight or convex superiorly, with little to no superior vertebral notch. The inferior surfaces of the thoracic pedicles are markedly concave with deep inferior notches. As a consequence, the neural foramina lie predominantly behind the lower portion of the vertebral bodies. They are round, face directly laterally, and are nearly equal in size over the length of the thoracic spine.

Thoracic laminae are short, thick, and wide. From above downward they overlap each other like shingles of a roof. Thin superior articular processes arise from the junctions of the body with the pedicles, extend mostly superiorly, and display flat facets that face mostly posteriorly. The inferior articular processes project caudad from the inferior margins of the laminae and display facets that face predominantly anteriorly. The paired superior articular facets lie closer to the midline and to each other than do the paired inferior articular processes. Thoracic transverse processes arise from the pediculolaminar junctions and extend posterolaterally. The transverse processes are longest at T1 and decrease in length progressively down the spine, so the T12 transverse processes may be nearly absent (Figs. 4-5 to 4-7).

Lumbar Vertebrae

The five lumbar vertebrae are the largest of the spine (Figs. 4-8 and 4-9).[1-3] They increase in size from L1 to L3. L4 and

Text continued on p. 82

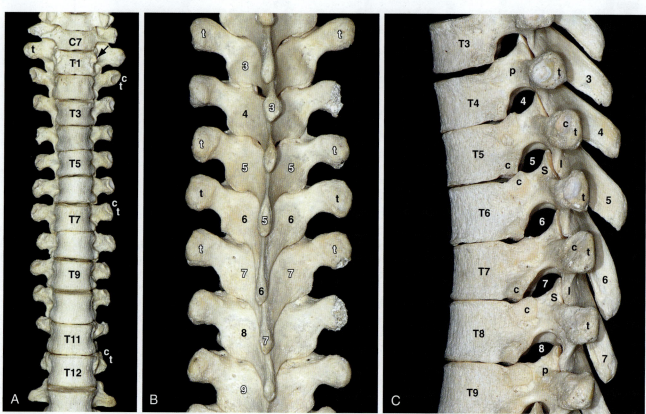

■ **FIGURE 4-1**   Thoracic spine. Dried osseous vertebrae. **A,** Full anterior surface. **B,** Midportion of posterior surface. **C,** Corresponding lateral surface. Anteriorly these images demonstrate the changing sizes and relationships of the thoracic bodies and transverse processes (t). The costotubercular (costotransverse) facets (ct) for the rib articulations change orientation progressively over the length of the thoracic spine. At T1, the prominent costocapitular (costovertebral) facet (*black arrow* in **A**) forms a circular depression and raised edges that mold the lateral contour of the T1 body. Posteriorly, the broad laminae and long spinous processes (3-9) of the vertebrae overlap extensively. The tips of the spine are single, not bifid. Laterally, the vertebral bodies form a gentle kyphosis. The costocapitular (cc) demifacets for each articulating rib mold the adjoining inferior and superior margins of the vertebrae at each interspace. The lateral ends of the transverse processes (t) bear costotubercular (costotransverse) (ct) facets that face anterolaterally to articulate with the tubercles of the ribs. The zygapophyseal (facet) joints between the superior (S) and inferior (I) articular processes show steep, near-coronal angulation superiorly. These gradually become more shallow and complex inferiorly. The neural foramina lie between the deep inferior vertebral notch of the upper pedicle (p) and the shallow or flat superior vertebral notch of the lower pedicle. In the thoracic (and lumbar) regions, the nerve roots lie within the upper portion of the neural foramina, near to the superior pedicle, so they are named for the uppermost pedicle. White numbers 4 to 8 in **C** indicate the sites at which the nerve roots exit the spinal canal beneath the T4-T8 pedicles.

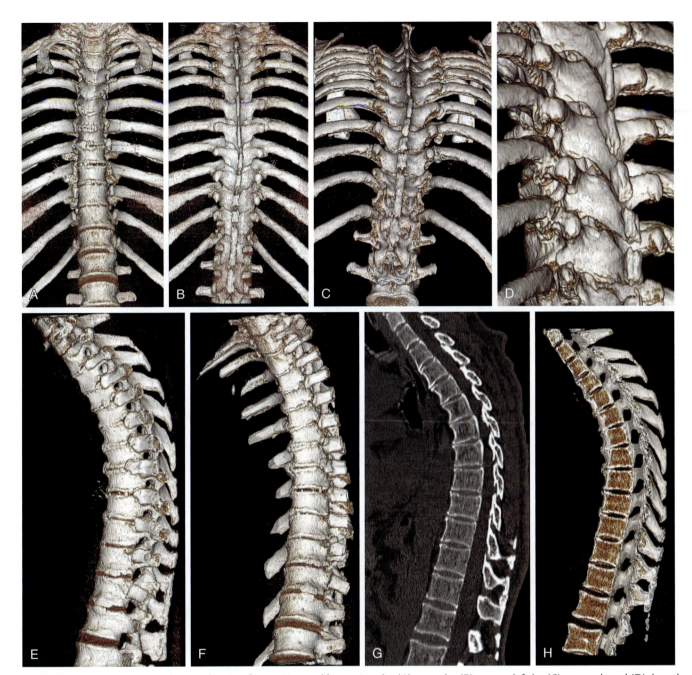

■ **FIGURE 4-2**   In-vivo 3D CT reformatted images from a 56-year-old man. Anterior (**A**), posterior (**B**), posteroinferior (**C**), posterolateral (**D**), lateral (**E**), and anterolateral (**F**) surfaces. **G,** Midsagittal CT reformatted image. **H,** 3D cut-plane removal of lateral bone from **E** reveals the surfaces of the contralateral side as viewed from the midsagittal plane.

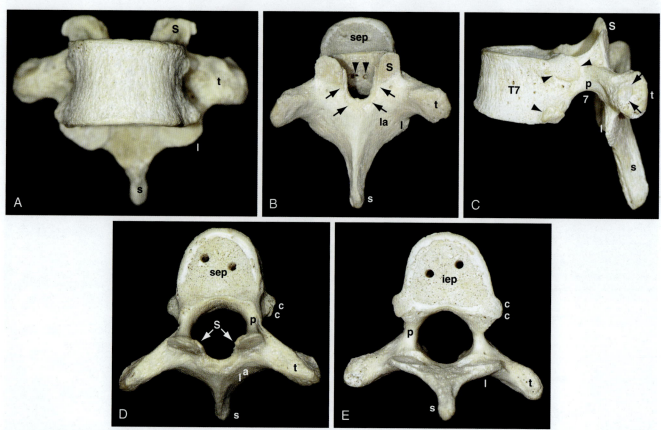

■ **FIGURE 4-3**   Isolated dried T7 vertebra. Anterior (**A**), posterior (**B**), lateral (**C**), superior (**D**), and inferior (**E**) surfaces. The sides of the vertebral body are concave. At each level the widths of the vertebral bodies are nearly equal to the widths of the laminae. The pedicles arise at the lateral edges of the bodies and run nearly parallel. The transverse processes sweep posterolaterally. The superior articular processes (s, *white arrow*) are much thinner than the inferior articular processes and point sharply superiorly. The inferior articular processes diverge inferolaterally, so the transverse distance between the superior articular processes is less than the transverse distance between the inferior articular processes. The laminae are roughened (*black arrows*, **B**) along their upper margin and upper posterior surface for the attachments of the paired ligamenta flava. The posterior surface of the vertebral body shows basivertebral venous foramina (**B**, *black arrowheads*). The superior and inferior vertebral end plates (sep; iep) show a perimeter of smooth cortical bone and a center of rougher more cancellous bone. In **C**, *arrowheads* indicate demifacets for costocapitular (costovertebral) joints and *arrows* indicate the costotubercular facet on the anterior face of the transverse process. In **D** and **E**, cc indicates costocapitular (costovertebral) facets. In this and other images, paired "drill holes" seen in the vertebral bodies indicate that the segmental vertebrae had been strung together to form a spinal column.

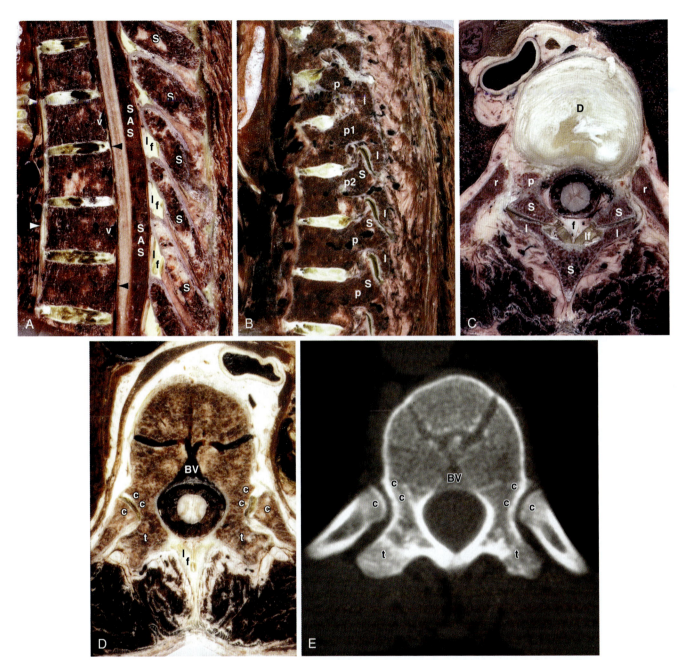

■ **FIGURE 4-4** Anatomic and CT images of the thoracic spine. Cryomicrotome sections in the midsagittal (**A**), parasagittal (**B**), and axial (**C** and **D**) planes. Four specimens. **E,** Noncontrast in vivo CT similar to **D**. Midsagittal section shows the cortical bone and marrow of the vertebral bodies, the anterior (*white arrowheads*) and posterior (*black arrowheads*) longitudinal ligaments, ligamentum flavum (lf), steep angulation and marked overlap of the spines (S), and the interspinous muscles and ligaments. The gray matter and white matter of the spinal cord are well seen. The posterior subarachnoid space (SAS) appears large, because the spinal cord lies anteriorly along the thoracic kyphosis. Parasagittal section displays the cortical bone of the superior (S) and inferior (I) articular processes, the cartilage on the facet surfaces, and the oblique coronal inclination of the zygapophyseal joints. The neural foramina are defined superiorly by the deep inferior vertebral notch of the upper pedicle (p1), inferiorly by the shallow to flat superior vertebral notch of the lower pedicle (p2), anteriorly by the posterior surfaces of the upper vertebra and disc, and posteriorly by the ligamentum flavum and the superior articular process of the lower vertebra. The emerging nerve roots and dorsal root ganglia lie within the upper portion of the neural foramina, close to the upper pedicle. **C,** The axial section through the disc (D), pedicles (p), and facet joints (S/I) displays the round shape of the thoracic spinal canal, paired ligamenta flava (lf) just deep to the base of the spinous process (S), triangular packet of dorsal epidural fat (f), dura, subarachnoid space, and spinal cord. The round shape of the thoracic spinal cord, the "butterfly" of spinal gray matter, and the surrounding columns of white matter are clearly depicted. The ribs (r) flank the disc bilaterally. **D,** The axial section at the mid height of the vertebral body demonstrates the basivertebral channel (BV) leading to the anterior internal vertebral venous plexus posteriorly and the anterolaterally directed venous channels. The paired rib heads (c) articulate with the vertebral bodies at the costocapitular (cc) joints and with the tubercles of the ribs at the costotubercular joints. lf, ligamentum flavum. Non-contrast axial CT of a different patient shows the similar appearance of the midposterior channel for the basivertebral veins (BV), the anterolaterally directed venous channels within the vertebral body, and the articulations of the rib heads (c) with the vertebral body at the costocapitular (costovertebral) (cc) facets. The angular orientation of the anterior venous channels varies greatly from level to level and from person to person.

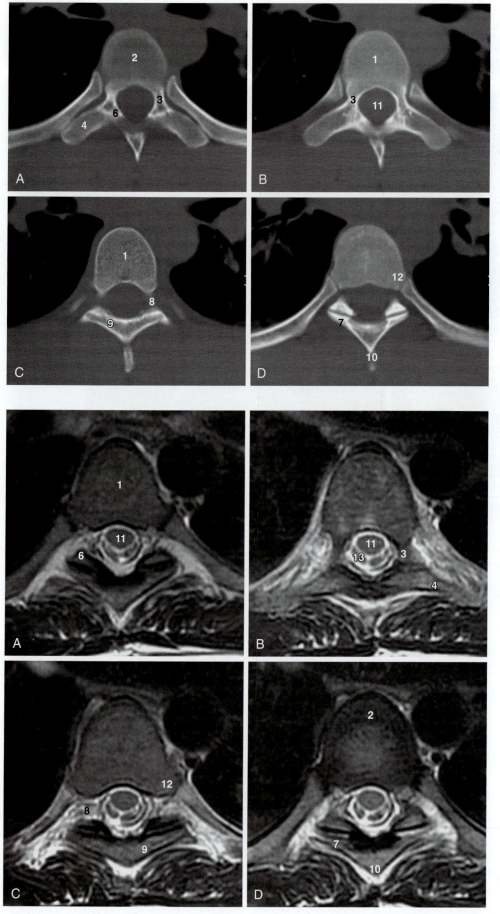

■ **FIGURE 4-5** In-vivo axial CT sections through T7 in a 27-year-old man. **A** to **D,** Serial axial images displayed from superior to inferior show the T6-T7 disc (2), T7 vertebral body (1), T7 pedicle (3), transverse process (4), base of the superior articular process (6), inferior articular process (7), neural foramen (8), transmitting the segmental T7 nerve roots, lamina (9), spinous process (10), spinal canal and cord (11), and costocapitular (costovertebral) joint (12). In **A,** the ribs are also seen to articulate with the transverse processes bilaterally at the costotubercular joints.

■ **FIGURE 4-6** In-vivo axial T2W MR images through T7 in a 31-year-old woman. **A** to **D,** Serial axial MR images displayed from superior to inferior show the T7 vertebral body (1), T7-T8 disc (2), T7 pedicle (3), superior articular process of T7 (6), inferior articular process of T7 (7), laterally directed T7-T8 neural foramen (8), transmitting the segmental T7 nerve roots, lamina of T7 (9), spinous process of T7 (10), spinal cord (11), costal facet of the T7 rib (12), and flow voids from moving cerebrospinal fluid posterolateral to the cord (13).

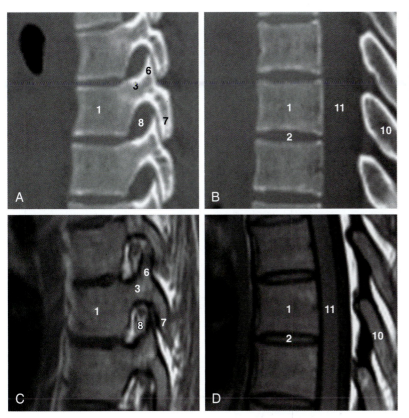

■ FIGURE 4-7 **A** and **B,** In-vivo sagittal CT images in a 27-year-old man. **C** and **D,** T1W MR images in a 31-year-old woman. These images demonstrate the T7 vertebral body (1), T7-T8 intervertebral disc (2), T7 pedicle with deep inferior vertebral notch (3), superior articular process (6), inferior articular process (7), neural foramen containing the segmental T7 roots (8), low-hanging spinous process of T7 (10), and the spinal canal and cord (11). The upper surface of the pedicles is flat to convex superiorly, so there is little to no superior vertebral notch.

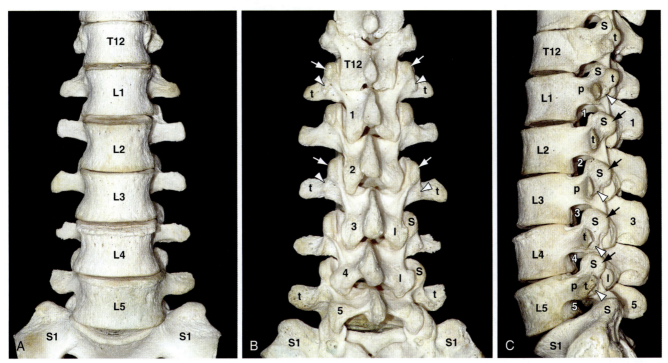

■ FIGURE 4-8 Full lumbar spine. Isolated dried vertebrae. Anterior (**A**), posterior (**B**), and lateral (**C**) surfaces. From T12 to L3 the vertebral bodies increase in height, width, and span of the transverse processes. L4 and L5 morphology is variable. The orientation of the zygapophyseal (facet) joints modulates from above downward, appearing more nearly simple and coronal superiorly and more complex inferiorly. Prominent mammillary processes (*white and black arrows*) arise from the superior lateral aspects of the superior articular processes (s). The lumbar transverse processes (t) lie posterior to the neural foramina. Prominent accessory processes (*white arrowheads*) arise from the posteroinferior aspect of the base of each transverse process. The inferior articular processes (I) appear narrower and closer together in the upper lumbar region and then widen outward caudad. The spinous processes thicken and enlarge from T12 to L3 and angle inferiorly. At L4 and L5 the spinous processes usually become smaller and angle more directly posteriorly. The nerve roots emerge through the upper portion of the neural foramina, just beneath the upper pedicle, so they are named for the nearer pedicle (*white numbers* in **C**).

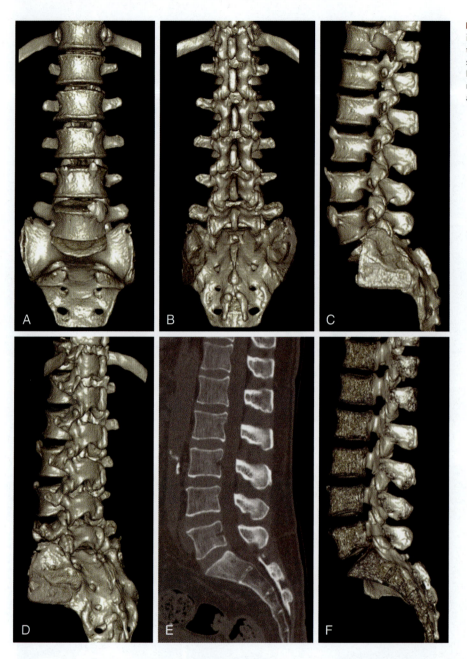

■ **FIGURE 4-9** In-vivo 3D CT reformatted images in a 49-year-old man. Anterior (**A**), posterior (**B**), lateral (**C**), and posterolateral (**D**) surfaces. **E**, Midsagittal CT reformatted image. **F**, 3D cut-plane removal of lateral bone from **C** reveals the 3D surfaces of the contralateral side as viewed from the midsagittal plane.

L5 have variable sizes. The lumbar vertebral bodies are wider transversely than sagittally and show prominent concavity of their anterior surface. Short thick pedicles arise from the posterolateral surfaces of the vertebral bodies near to their superior margins. The superior vertebral notches are shallow. The inferior vertebral notches are deep. As a consequence, the neural foramina lie predominantly posterior to the upper vertebral body but do extend inferiorly behind the next lower vertebra (Figs. 4-10 to 4-12).[1-3]

Lumbar laminae are short, broad, and overlap less than do thoracic laminae. The superior articular processes have concave articular facets that face posteromedially (Figs. 4-13 to 4-15). They exhibit prominent mammillary processes on their posterior border.[1-3] The inferior articular processes have convex articular facets that face anterolaterally. At L1 to L3 the transverse width between superior articular processes is greater than the transverse width between inferior articular processes. At L4 and L5, these widths are nearly equal.[1-3]

The lumbar transverse processes are relatively thin and increase in length from L1 to L3. The L4 transverse process remains thin and is slightly shorter than the L3 transverse process. The L5 transverse process is thicker, more robust, and variably shorter or longer than those above. It typically angles posterosuperiorly and exhibits a blunt tip. At its root, the posteroinferior surface of each lumbar transverse process displays a small accessory process.[1-3] Along its anterior surface, each lumbar transverse process displays a vertical ridge to which the anterior layer of the

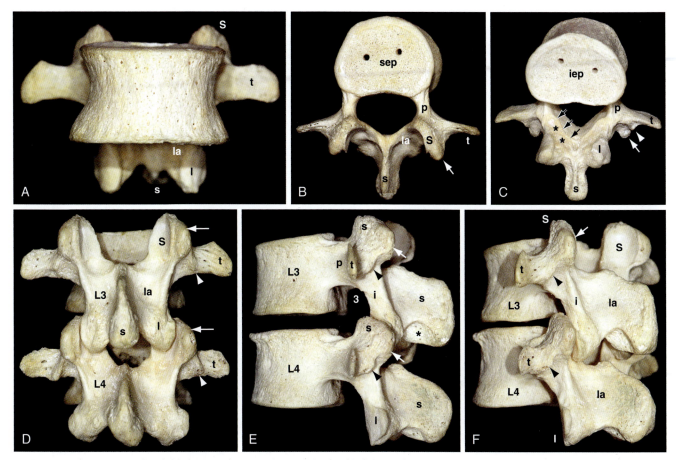

■ **FIGURE 4-10** A to C, Isolated dried L3 vertebra: anterior, superior, and inferior surfaces. D to F, L3-L4 articulations: posterior, lateral, and posterolateral surfaces. The sides of the vertebral body are deeply concave. The pedicles (p) are robust. The superior articular processes (S) are broad with prominent mammillary processes (*white arrows*) protruding posterolaterally from their surfaces. The laminae are short and squat. The inner aspect of the laminae shows a sharp demarcation (*black arrows* in **C**) between the smooth upper lamina that is free of ligamentum flavum and the roughened lower lamina (*asterisks*, **C**) to which the ligamentum flavum attaches. The inferior articular processes (I) are relatively narrow, so the transverse distance between the superior articular processes is wider than the transverse distance between the inferior articular processes. This is the reverse of their relationship in the thoracic spine. The facet surfaces are cupped, so the lateral portions of the facet joints are nearly sagittal and the medial portions nearly coronal in orientation. The bases of the transverse processes (t) show accessory processes (*black and white arrowheads* in **D**, **E**, and **F**). i, pars interarticularis. The inferior margin of the spinous process (s) shows a sharply demarcated depression (*asterisk*, **E**) for the interspinous muscles and ligaments.

thoracolumbar fascia attaches. At its tip, each transverse process gives attachment to the middle layer of thoracolumbar fascia. The spinous processes of L1-L4 are nearly horizontal with thick posteroinferior margins. The spinous process of L5 is small with a rounded downturned apex.[1-3] The tips of the lumbar spinous processes give attachment to the posterior layer of thoracolumbar fascia.

Sacrum

The sacrum is the name given to the triangular bony mass made by fusion of the five sacral vertebrae (Figs. 4-16 and 4-17).[1-5] It has a superior base that articulates with L5, an inferior apex that articulates with the coccyx, a concave ventral (deep) surface that forms the posterior superior wall of the pelvis, and a convex dorsal (superficial) surface that is palpable beneath the skin. The dorsal surface displays a series of tubercles. These tubercles mark the borders of the multiple spinal elements that fused into the single dorsal bone plate. On each side, lateral surfaces articulate with the iliac bones.

Base

The base of the sacrum is formed by the wide upper surface of the S1 vertebral body (Fig. 4-18). The prominent anterior lip of S1 forms the most anterior portion of the sacrum, designated the sacral promontory (see Fig. 4-16D). The S1 transverse processes merge with broad bone masses that arise from the body, pedicle, and superior articular process on each side. These project posterolaterally to form the upper portion of each sacral ala. The pedicles are short and diverge posterolaterally to form the narrow sacral canal. The oblique laminae converge posteromedially to form the roof of the spinal canal in the midline. The superior articular processes of S1 project upward to articulate with L5 and display cortical thickenings analogous to the lumbar mammillary processes.

Apex

The inferior surface of S5 has an oval facet that articulates with the coccyx.

Text continued on p. 90

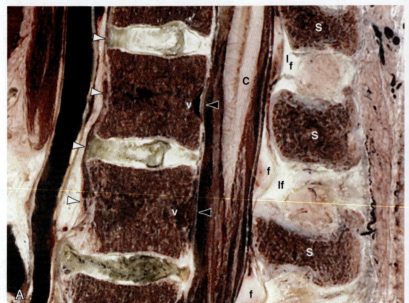
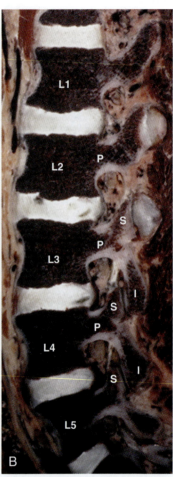

■ **FIGURE 4-11**   Sagittal cryomicrotome sections of the lumbar spine. **A,** Midsagittal section at L1-L2 displays the anterior longitudinal ligament (*white arrowheads*) and posterior longitudinal ligament (PLL) (*black arrowheads*), the dense white cortical bone at the edges of the vertebral body, mottled red and yellow marrow within the cancellous bone, the basivertebral channel (v) draining into the anterior internal vertebral venous plexus ventral to the PLL along the mid posterior vertebral body, lipofucsin aging pigment within the intervertebral discs, the dura, dorsal epidural fat (f) and ligamentum flavum (lf) along the posterior wall of the spinal canal, the spines (S), and the interspinous muscles and ligaments. The tip of the spinal cord (conus medullaris) lies at L1-L2, surrounded by the roots of the cauda equina. **B,** Parasagittal section from L1 to uppermost S1 demonstrates uniform color and height of young adult discs, homogeneous red marrow within the vertebral bodies, keyhole shape of the lumbar neural foramina, the nerve roots and dorsal root ganglia within the upper portions of the neural foramina, the angulation of the zygapophyseal (facet) joints between the superior (S) and inferior (I) articular processes of adjoining vertebrae, and the bright yellow ligamenta flava that extend from the inferior half of the anterior surface of the upper vertebra to insert into the lamina and articular processes of the next-lower vertebra. The ligamentum flavum forms the anterior surface of the lumbar facet joints.

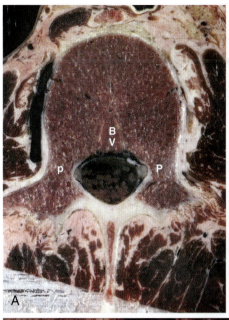
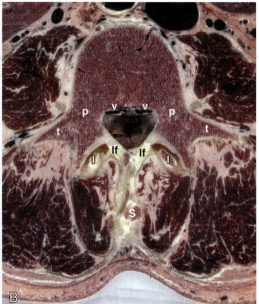
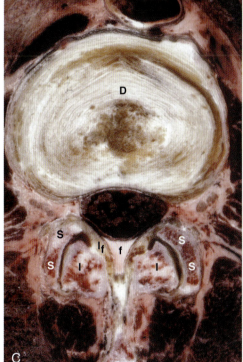
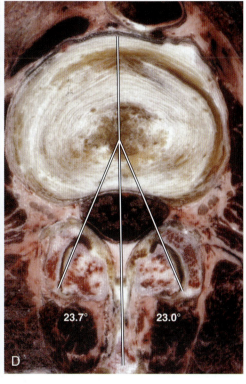

■ **FIGURE 4-12** Axial cryomicrotome sections of the lumbar spine. Upper lumbar vertebrae (**A**) show short robust, nearly parallel pedicles, while lower lumbar vertebrae (**B**) show thicker pedicles that diverge posterolaterally. The midline basivertebral venous channel (BV) leads into the prominent venous plexus of the ventral epidural space (vv). The thick dural sac contains the subarachnoid fluid and roots of the cauda equina. **C,** Section through the intervertebral disc, neural foramina, and facet joints displays the superior (S) and inferior (I) articular processes of the cup-shaped facet joint and the spinous process (s). As they sweep across the back of the spinal canal, the paired ligamenta flava form the posterior wall of the spinal canal, the anterior walls of the synovial joints, and the posterior walls of the neural foramina. The midline triangle of dorsal epidural fat (f) fits snuggly between the posteromedial margins of the ligamenta flava. **D,** Diagrammatic representation of the facet joints in C demonstrates one method to measure the articular angles and assess articular tropism. Here the right facet measures 23.7 degrees to the midline, whereas the left measures 23.0 degrees. An angular difference of less than 7 degrees is considered to be within normal limits.

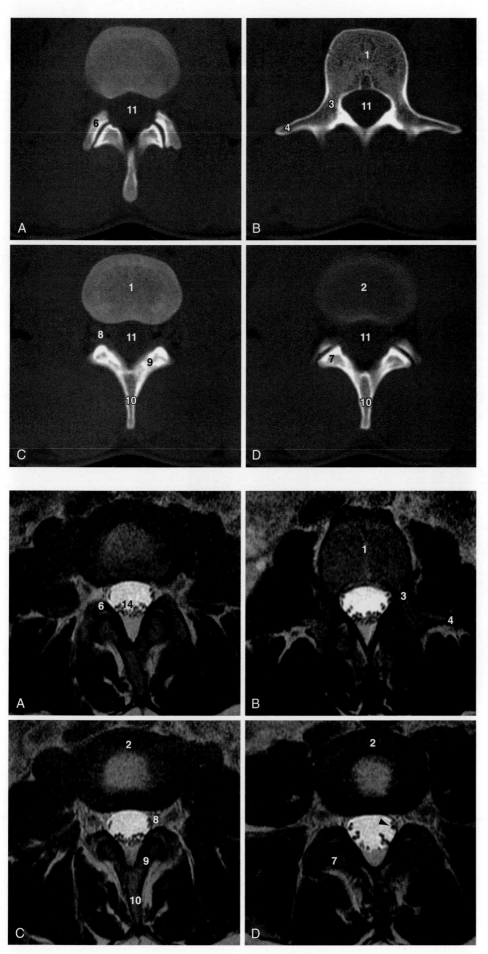

■ **FIGURE 4-13** In-vivo axial CT sections through L3 in a 27-year-old man. **A** to **D,** Serial axial images displayed from superior to inferior show the L3 vertebral body (1) with basivertebral channel in the midposterior surface, L3-L4 intervertebral disc (2), L3 pedicle (3), transverse process (4), superior articular process (6), inferior articular process (7), L3-L4 neural foramen containing the segmental L3 roots (8), L3 lamina (9), L3 spinous process (10), and spinal canal containing the cauda equina (11).

■ **FIGURE 4-14** In-vivo axial T2W MR sections through L3 in an 18-year-old woman. **A** to **D,** Serial axial images displayed from superior to inferior show the L3 vertebral body (1), L3-L4 intervertebral disc (2), L3 pedicle (3), transverse process (4), superior articular process (6), inferior articular process (7), L3-L4 neural foramen containing the segmental L3 roots (8), L3 lamina (9), L3 spinous process (10), roots of cauda equina within the spinal canal (14), and the pair of L4 nerve roots moving caudally and laterally toward the next-lower L4-L5 neural foramen (*black arrowhead,* **D**).

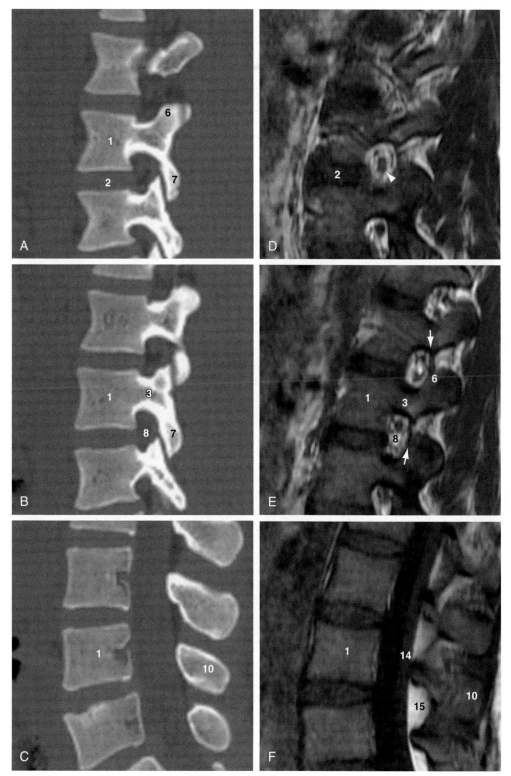

■ **FIGURE 4-15** In-vivo sagittal sections of the L2-L4 spine centered on L3. **A** to **C,** Reformatted sagittal CT sections in a 27-year-old man. **D** to **F,** T1W MR images in an 18-year-old woman. These images display the L3 vertebral body (1), L3-L4 disc (2), L3 pedicle (3), superior articular process (6), inferior articular process (7), L3-L4 neural foramen (8) containing the segmental L3 roots (*white arrowheads*), and L3 spinous process (10). The ligamentum flavum (*white arrows*) forms the posterior wall of the neural foramina. The dorsal epidural fat appears segmentally as interrupted plates.

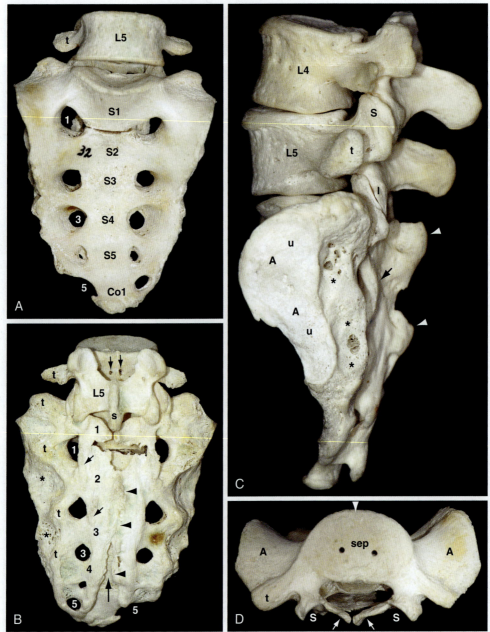

■ **FIGURE 4-16** Sacrum and lumbosacral articulation. Anterior (**A**) and posterior (**B**) surfaces of L5 plus sacrum. The sacrum is roughly triangular. The transverse processes of S1 form the widest portion of the sacral alae (wings). On the anterior surface, ridges (and occasional gaps) mark the sites of the embryonic interspaces. The upper four sacral nerve roots S1 to S4 emerge through four paired sacral foramina. The S5 root emerges just inferior to S5 (right). If the transverse process for coccygeal 1 fuses to the sacrum (left) then the S5 root emerges via its own "fifth sacral" foramen. On the posterior surface, the rudimentary spinous processes fuse into a median sacral crest (*black arrowheads*, **B**) with variably distinct spinous tubercles. At S3 or S4 the spinal canal opens onto the dorsal surface at the sacral hiatus (*large vertical black arrow*, **B**). The articular processes fuse into paired intermediate sacral crests with variably distinct articular tubercles. The transverse processes (t) fuse into the lateral sacral crest (t on sacrum) with variably distinct transverse tubercles. In this specimen, the laminae of S1 did not fuse, leaving an S1 spina bifida occulta. Far laterally, the posterior surface is roughened (*asterisk*) for attachment of the multiple sacroiliac ligaments. Two small vertical *black arrows* in **B** mark the basivertebral venous channels in the midposterior surface of L5. **C**, Lateral surface of L4, L5, and S1 (second specimen). The sacrum articulates with the ilium laterally via the ear-shaped auricular facet (Au). The roughened surface for tendinous attachments lies posterior to this facet. *White arrowheads* indicate spinous tubercles of S1 and S2. *Black arrow* in **C** shows the articular tubercle of S1-S2. **D,** Top surface of S1. The sacral promontory (*white arrowhead*) is the most anterior portion of the upper sacrum. The sacral alae (A) evolve from the transverse processes: the true transverse processes (diaphyses) posterolaterally and the pleurapophyses (costal element) anterolaterally. The laminae (*white arrows*) remain unfused in the midline. sep, Superior end plate.

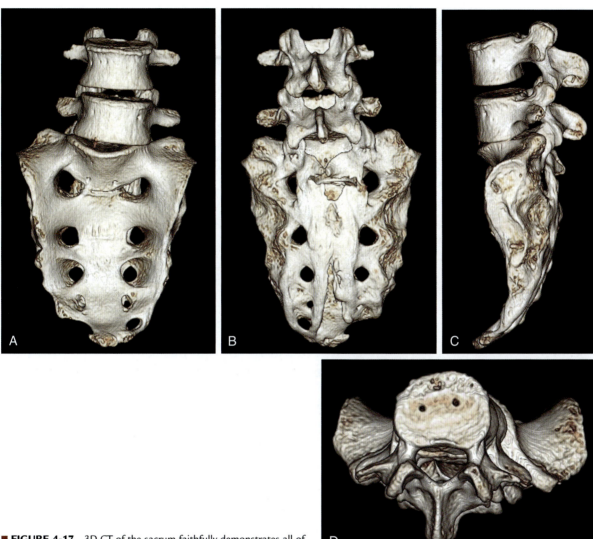

■ **FIGURE 4-17** 3D CT of the sacrum faithfully demonstrates all of the anatomic features of the sacrum, as labeled on Figure 4-16.

■ **FIGURE 4-18** Axial cryomicrotome section through the anterior portion of L5-S1 disc (D) and the sacral alae (SA) displays the laminae (la) and inferior articular processes (I) of L5 forming the facet joint with S1, and the paired ligamenta flava (yellow ligaments) (lf). The sacral spinal canal is triangular. The S1 (1) root sleeves bud off the thecal sac anterolaterally. The anterior internal venous plexus (v, v) lies ventral to the superficial layer of the posterior longitudinal ligament.

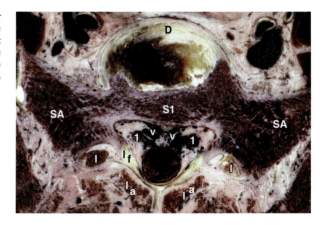

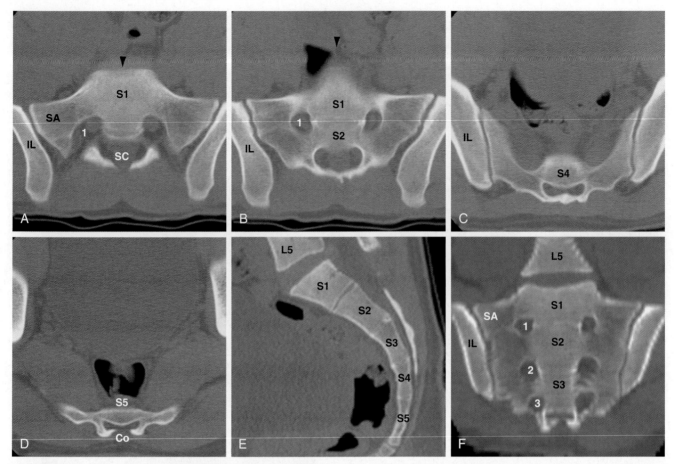

■ **FIGURE 4-19**   In-vivo CT sections through the sacrum in a 27-year-old man. **A** to **D,** Axial images. **E,** Reformatted midsagittal image. **F,** Reformatted coronal image. These studies display the sacral promontory (*black arrowhead*) and the five sacral segments from S1 downward, the neural foramina (1, 2, 3) for the sacral nerve roots, the sacral alae (SA), the sacroiliac joints formed between the sacral alae and the ilia (IL), and a portion of the coccygeal cornua (Co) that articulates with S5. Inferiorly the sacral spinal canal opens dorsally to form the sacral hiatus.

Pelvic Surface

The pelvic surface is concave ventrally, although the anterior surface of the S2 body often forms a prominent forward bulge (Figs. 4-19 and 4-20). Medially, the superior and inferior margins of the original sacral vertebral bodies form prominent transverse ridges that mark the old interspaces. Four pairs of ventral sacral foramina extend from the intervertebral foramina to the ventral surface to give exit to the ventral rami of the sacral roots. The laterally directed bony bars between the foramina are formed by costal elements (rib analogs) fused to the vertebrae. Lateral to the foramina, these costal elements fuse with each other and with the true transverse processes behind them to form the lateral portion of the sacral triangle. Superiorly, this surface enlarges into the sacral alae. Inferiorly, it curves gently medially to the inferolateral angle, then angles more sharply medially to the apex.

Dorsal Surface (From Medial to Lateral)

In the midline, the spinous processes of S1 to S3 (or S4) fuse into a median sacral crest that retains three to four spinous tubercles at the tips of the spines (see Fig. 4-16B). Just inferior to the lowest tubercle, the laminae of S5 (or S4 and S5) remain unfused, leaving an arched sacral hiatus that opens into the vertebral canal. Lateral to the median sacral crest, the sacral laminae and articular processes fuse to form the dorsal wall of the sacrum. The lateral edges of these exhibit four pairs of articular tubercles, collectively designated the intermediate sacral crests (articular crests). Just lateral to these, four pairs of dorsal sacral foramina extend from the intervertebral foramina to the dorsal surface to give exit to the dorsal rami of the sacral roots S1 to S4. Each foramen lies immediately superolateral to each articular tubercle. Caudad, the inferior articular processes of S5 morph into prominent paired ridges—the sacral cornua—that flank the sacral hiatus. The sacral cornua articulate with the paired coccygeal cornua of Co1 inferior to them. The S5 roots emerge just medial to the sacral cornua and groove the lateral surface of S5. Farther laterally, the transverse processes of S1 to S5 fuse together lateral to the dorsal sacral foramina to form the lateral sacral crest. The apices of these transverse processes form a vertical line of small transverse tubercles.

Lateral Surface

The lateral surface of the sacrum is formed by the fused costal elements (anteriorly) and the fused transverse

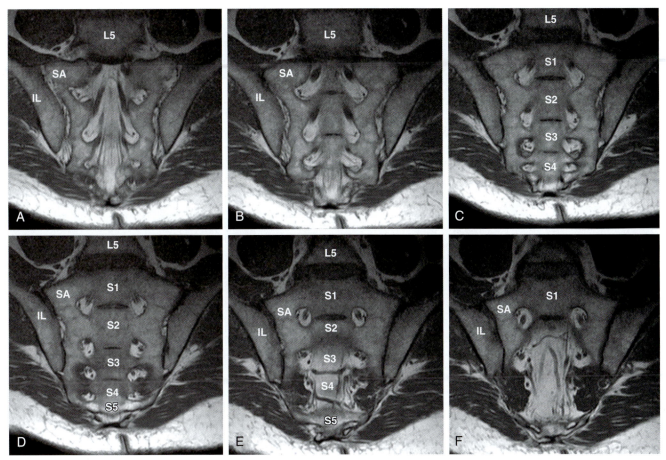

■ **FIGURE 4-20** In-vivo oblique coronal T1W MR sections (**A** to **F**) through the sacrum in a 62-year-old man. This plane demonstrates the relationships among the sacral segments S1-S5, the sacral alae (SA), the ilia (IL), the sacroiliac joints, the sacral foramina, and the emerging nerve roots.

processes (posteriorly) (see Fig. 4-16C). Anteriorly and superiorly the fused costal processes form an auricular facet that articulates with the ilia. The upper portion of the facet is formed by the costal elements of S1. The inferior portion is formed by the costal elements of S2 and part of S3. Behind the auricular facet the lateral surface is roughened for attachment of ligaments. Inferior to S3 the lateral surface of sacrum does not articulate with other bones and rapidly becomes reduced in size.

Lumbosacral Vertebral Specialization

Transitional lumbosacral vertebrae typically occur in 5% to 7% of the population, although numbers as high as 21%[6] have been reported.[7-9] These transitional vertebrae may be classified by the Castellvi criteria (Table 4-1; Fig. 4-21).[10] Overall, sacralization of L5 occurs about as often as lumbarization of S1. Among types II-IV, subtypes IIA and IIIB are most common and IIIA least common.[11]

The incidence of sacral spina bifida has been reported to range from 1.2% to 50%.[12] Fidas and associates found a 23% incidence of spina bifida occulta in 2707 Swedish adults.[13] Spina bifida occulta was twice as common in men as women. Most commonly, it affected S1 alone or S1 plus S2. Isolated defects at L5 or S2 were rare (Table 4-2).[13]

TABLE 4-1. Classification of Lumbosacral Transitional Vertebrae

Type	Description
I	Dysplastic transverse process of the vertebra with width >19 mm
IA	Unilateral
IB	Bilateral
II	Incomplete lumbarization or sacralization. Enlarged transverse process that has unilateral or bilateral pseudoarthrosis with the adjacent sacral ala.
IIA	Unilateral
IIB	Bilateral
III	Complete lumbarization or sacralization. Enlarged transverse process that has unilateral or bilateral complete fusion with the adjacent sacral ala.
IIIA	Unilateral
IIIB	Bilateral
IV	Mixed type with type IIA on one side and type IIIA on the other

From Castellvi AE, Goldstein LA, Chan DP. Lumbosacral transitional vertebrae and their relationship with lumbar extradural defects. Spine 1984; 9:493-495.

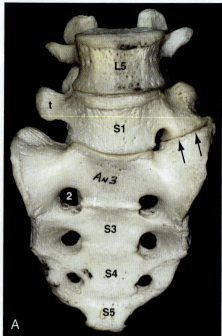
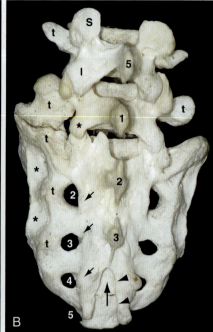
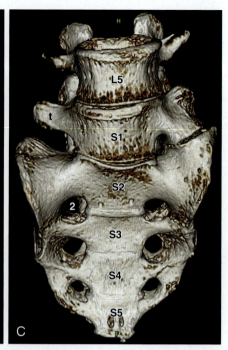

■ **FIGURE 4-21**   Transitional lumbosacral vertebra: anterior (pelvic) (**A**) surface and dorsal (**B**) surface. **C,** 3D surface reformatted image of this dried specimen. The S1 vertebra is partially lumbarized with a lumbariform right transverse process (t) and sacriform left transverse process that is incompletely united (*arrows,* **A**) with the sacral ala formed by S2. Note that the fused sacral bones enclose only three neural foramina, indicating that the fused sacrum includes only S2-S5. **B,** The left S1 inferior articular process (*upper asterisk*) is hypoplastic and articulates with an anomalous S2 superior articular process. The spinous processes of L5 (5) and S1 (1) are free, while those of S2 (2) and S3 (3) have fused into the median sacral crest. The sacral hiatus (*black arrowheads*) opens dorsally (*vertical black arrow*) at S4. The articular tubercles (*oblique black arrows*) mark the intermediate sacral crest (synonym: articular crest). The foramina for the dorsal sacral roots S2-S4 lie immediately lateral to these. Further laterally, the transverse tubercles of S2-S5 (t, t, t) mark the lateral sacral crest. The sacriform left transverse process of S1 (*upper t*) aligns with these. Further laterally, the roughened sacral surface (*lower two asterisks*) gives attachment to numerous tendons. In this case, the transverse processes of the first coccygeal segment did not fuse to the sacrum, so the S5 roots (*white 5*) exit lateral to S5 with no osseous neural foramen (see Fig. 4-16).

TABLE 4-2.   Incidence and Combinations of Spina Bifida Occulta in 2707 Adults

Type	Males (%)	Females (%)
None	70.4	83
L5 only	0.1	0.1
S1 only	17.8	11.5
S2 only	1.0	0.7
L5 + S1	0.8	0.4
L5 + S2	0.1	0.0
S1 + S2	8.5	3.7
All three	1.1	0.6
Any form	29.6	17

From Fidas A, MacDonald HL, Elton RA, et al: Prevalence and patterns of spina bifida occulta in 2707 normal adults. Clin Radiol 1987;38:537.

Coccyx

The coccyx is a small, triangular bone formed by the fusion of three to five rudimentary coccygeal vertebrae (Fig. 4-22).[1-3] It may show incomplete fusion and irregular asymmetric shape. In analogy with the sacrum, the upper surface of the coccyx (Co1) is designated the coccygeal base. The caudal portion of the lowest coccygeal segment is designated the coccygeal apex. The base has an oval facet that articulates with the apex of the sacrum. The coccyx angles forward at the sacrococcygeal joint, so the pelvic surface of the coccyx inclines superiorly and ventrally. The pedicles and superior articular processes of Co1 morph into coccygeal cornua that articulate with the sacral cornua of S5. On one or both sides, rudimentary transverse processes of Co1 may project superolaterally to articulate or fuse with the inferolateral angle(s) of the lateral sacral surfaces to form (variably) complete S5 neural foramina. Inferior to Co1, Co2 to Co4 decrease rapidly in size and may resemble fused bony nodules.

Ligaments

Ligamentum Flavum

The posterior edges of the paired ligamenta flava may fuse completely or leave dorsal midline gaps (see detailed review in Chapter 3, The Normal Spinal Column: Overview and Cervical Spine).[14-16] In the low thoracic and lumbosacral regions, the paired ligamenta flava appear to be either completely fused or completely separated, without the intermediate partial fusions seen in the cervical and upper thoracic regions.[15,16] Within the lower thoracic spine, the incidence of midline gaps is very low from T6-7 to T8-9, increases caudally to a peak of 28% to 35% at T10-11 and T11-12, and decreases again further inferiorly.[16] Within the lumbar spine, the incidence of midline gaps is generally lower than in the low thoracic region, but shows a peak incidence at L1-2.[15] Specifically, the incidences of midline gaps in the ligamentum flavum are T6-7: 4.4%; T7-8: 2.1%; T8-9: 4.4%; T9-10: 17.9%; T10-11: 35.2%; T11-12: 28.5%; T12-L1: 15.8; L1-2: 22.2%; L2-3: 11.4%; L3-4: 11.1%; L4-5: 9.3%; and L5-S1: 0%.[15]

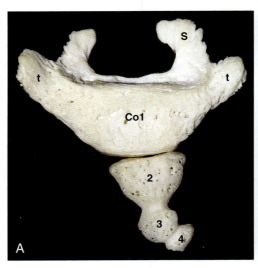
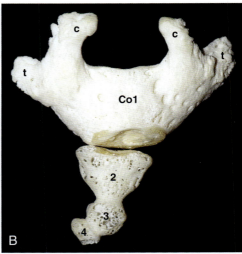

■ **FIGURE 4-22** Coccyx. Anterior (**A**) and posterior (**B**) surfaces. The first coccygeal segment (Co1) has coccygeal cornua (s) that articulate with S5. The transverse processes (t) of Co1 may articulate with the sacrum at the inferolateral angles to create osseous S5 neural foramina. The caudal coccygeal segments (c) often manifest as unequal and asymmetric nubbins.

Lumbosacral Junction

The most inferior fibers of the anterior and posterior longitudinal ligaments attach to the anterior and posterior surfaces of S1 (Figs. 4-23 and 4-24).[17] The lowest pair of ligamenta flava arise from L5 and insert onto the upper margins of the S1 laminae. The iliolumbar ligament helps to attach L5 to the ilium and sacrum. From the tip and anteroinferior margin of the L5 transverse process (± the L4 transverse process) the iliolumbar ligament radiates laterally to form upper and lower bands. The upper band extends to the iliac crest anterior to the sacroiliac joint and merges with the anterior layer of the thoracolumbar fascia above. The lower band extends from the inferior edge of the L5 transverse process and the L5 body across the anterior sacroiliac ligament to attach to the posterior margin of the iliac fossa.[1-3] A posterior portion of the iliolumbar ligament extends posterior to the quadratus lumborum to attach to the ilium.[1-3]

Sacrococcygeal Junction

The sacrococcygeal articulation is formed by the sacrococcygeal symphysis and multiple ligaments. The anterior sacrococcygeal ligament comprises irregular ligaments that attach to the anterior (pelvic) surfaces of the sacrum and coccyx. It functions like the anterior longitudinal ligament.[1-3] The deep dorsal sacrococcygeal ligament extends from the posterior aspect of the S5 body to the dorsum of the coccyx. It functions like the posterior longitudinal ligament.[1-3] The posterior superior sacrococcygeal ligament extends from the lips of the sacral hiatus to the dorsal surface of the coccyx, covering the sacral hiatus (Figs. 4-23 to 4-24).[1-3]

Spinal Epidural Space

The spinal epidural space is situated between the spinal dura mater and the walls of the vertebral canal (Fig. 4-25). Anatomically, it begins at foramen magnum and continues caudally to the sacral hiatus at approximately S4. It is delimited deeply by the spinal dura mater and peripherally by the walls of the canal. It extends laterally as far as the narrowest portion of each neural foramen.[18] The spinal epidural space contains connective tissue, fat cells, and the internal vertebral venous plexus (Fig. 4-26).[19]

Meningovertebral Ligaments

The dural sac is suspended within the spinal canal by segmental meningovertebral ligaments composed of dense connective tissue, primarily type I collagen, and elastic fibers (Fig. 4-27). The arrangement of these ligaments varies from level to level and subject to subject.[20,21] The most nearly constant and characteristic of these are the ventral meningovertebral ligaments that tether the anterior wall of the thecal sac to the dorsal (superficial) layer of the posterior longitudinal ligament and vertebral endosteum.[21,22] These ligaments are about 1 to 1.5 mm wide, are often widened or bifurcated (Y-shaped) anteriorly, and insert into the posterior longitudinal ligament (PLL) overlying both the vertebral bodies and the discs. Single ventral bands may be replaced by paired, sometimes asymmetrical, paramedian bands. Overall, the ventral ligaments become increasingly better developed caudally and are thickest at the L5-S1 levels. Taken together, they form a discontinuous ventral median or paramedian septum along the length of the spinal canal.[21]

Additional paired lateral meningovertebral ligaments extend anteriorly and caudally from the anterior surface of the dural sac to anchor the sac to the superficial layer of the PLL. These lateral ligaments may be 1 cm or more wide at L2, narrow to threadlike at L5, and are absent at S1.[23]

The sacral level has two named meningovertebral ligaments. Anteriorly, thick fibrous bands form a strong fenestrated membrane that anchors the dura to the sacrum (Trolard's anterior sacrodural ligament).[21] Posteriorly, thinner, paired ligaments arise from the lateral surfaces of the dura at the intervals between the neural foramina and pass slightly caudally to anchor the dura to the vertebral arches and ligamenta flava posteriorly (Hofmann's dorsolateral sacral-dural ligaments).[21] Other variable ligaments also extend from the outer surface of the dura to the borders of the neural foramina, the vertebral laminae, and the ligamenta flava over the full length of the dural sac.[20]

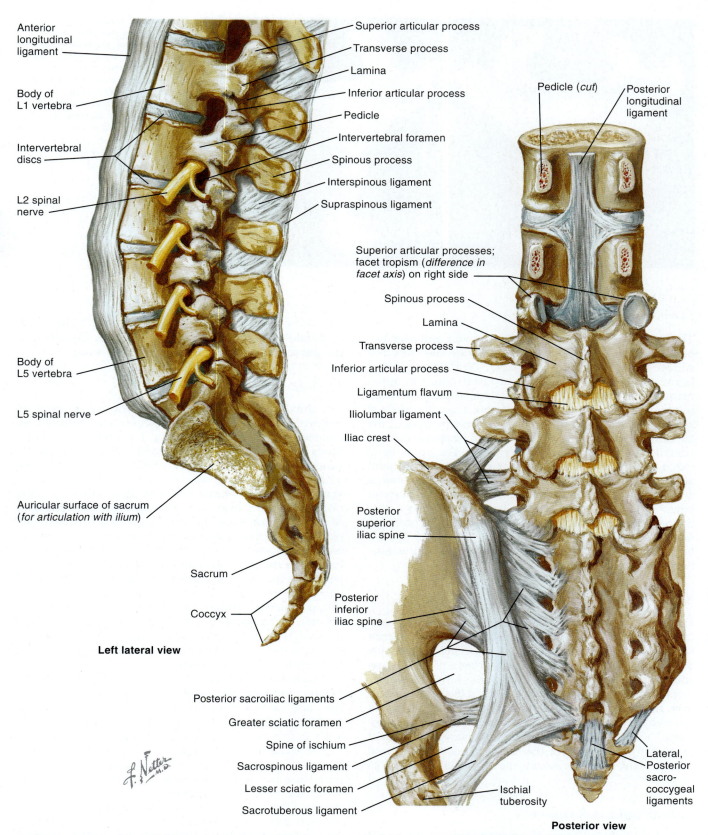

Anterior longitudinal ligament

Body of L1 vertebra

Intervertebral discs

L2 spinal nerve

Body of L5 vertebra

L5 spinal nerve

Auricular surface of sacrum (*for articulation with ilium*)

Sacrum

Coccyx

Left lateral view

Superior articular process

Transverse process

Lamina

Inferior articular process

Pedicle

Intervertebral foramen

Spinous process

Interspinous ligament

Supraspinous ligament

Pedicle (*cut*)

Posterior longitudinal ligament

Superior articular processes; facet tropism (*difference in facet axis*) on right side

Spinous process

Lamina

Transverse process

Inferior articular process

Ligamentum flavum

Iliolumbar ligament

Iliac crest

Posterior superior iliac spine

Posterior inferior iliac spine

Lateral, Posterior sacro-coccygeal ligaments

Posterior sacroiliac ligaments

Greater sciatic foramen

Spine of ischium

Sacrospinous ligament

Lesser sciatic foramen

Sacrotuberous ligament

Ischial tuberosity

Posterior view

■ **FIGURE 4-23** Ligaments of the lumbosacral and coccygeal spine. *(Reprinted from Netter FH. Atlas of Human Anatomy, 4th ed. Philadelphia, WB Saunders, 2006, plate 159. Netter Anatomy Illustration Collection. © Elsevier, Inc. All rights reserved.)*

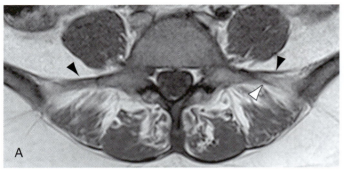
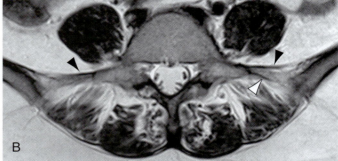

■ FIGURE 4-24 Iliolumbar ligaments. **A** and **B**, In-vivo axial T1W and T2W MR images in a 34-year-old woman. The iliolumbar ligaments comprise two bands. An upper band (*black arrowheads*) passes to the iliac crest anterior to the sacroiliac joint. A lower band (*white arrowheads*) arises from the L5 body and transverse process to reach the posterior margin of the iliac fossa.

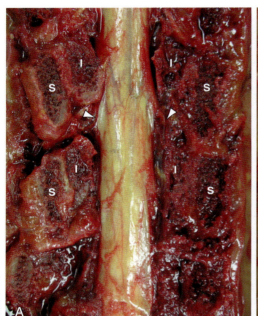
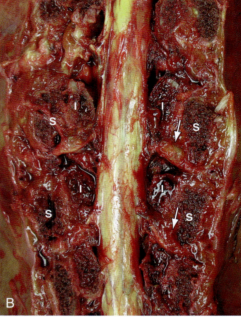

■ FIGURE 4-25 Spinal epidural space. Fresh cadaver specimen viewed from posterior after removal of the anterior spinal column and the dural sac by far posterior section through the superior (S) and inferior (I) articular processes. The epidural fat (*yellow*) and vessels (*red*) separate the bony canal from the thecal sac (just visible through the epidural tissue). In **A**, one pair of dural root sleeves (*arrowheads*) is just visible through the fat. In **B**, multiple root sleeves extend to the dorsal root ganglia (*white arrows*) lying within the posterior portions of the neural foramina.

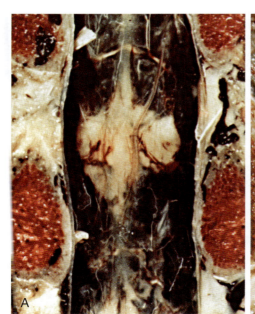
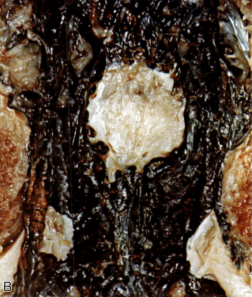

■ FIGURE 4-26 Internal vertebral venous plexus (IVVP). Two specimens. **A**, Upper lumbar spine with intact dura. India ink injected into the vertebral body traversed the basivertebral veins to fill the anterior IVVP (*black zones*). Rendering the dura transparent discloses the denticulate shape of the posterior longitudinal ligament (PLL), the wide width of the venous plexus over the vertebral bodies (where the PLL is narrow), and restriction of the venous plexus to paired narrow lateral channels over the discs (where the laterally flaring PLL adheres to the posterior surface of the annulus). **B**, Removal of the dura and the PLL discloses multiple small resin-filled channels of the anterior IVVP. (*Adapted from Crock HV, Yoshizawa H. The Blood Supply of the Vertebral Column and Spinal Cord in Man. New York, Springer-Verlag, 1977.*)

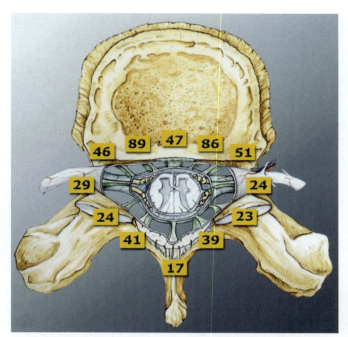

■ **FIGURE 4-27** Sites and percentage frequencies of finding ligaments at those sites in dissections of 70 adult lumbar spines. *(From Geers C, Lecouvet FE, Behets C, et al. Polygonal deformation of the dural sac in epidural lipomatosis: Anatomic explanation by the presence of meningovertebral ligaments. AJNR Am J Neuroradiol 2003; 24:1276-1282.)*

Purely dorsal meningovertebral ligaments are said to be present only in the cervical spine, and connect the dura to the ligamenta flava.[21]

Dural Relations to the Bone

The dural sac appears to be applied directly against the inner aspect of the bony canal at specific sites. At the level of each vertebral arch, segmentally, the dural sac appears to be applied directly onto the inner surfaces of the pedicles and laminae. Between the vertebral arches, the dura abuts the fat in the intervertebral foramina laterally, the ligamenta flava posterolaterally, and the epidural fat in the recess between the ligamenta flava posteriorly.[24]

Epidural Fat

The spinal epidural fat is a white-yellow adipose tissue the exact color of which depends on the carotenoids in the diet.[25] It provides a cushion for the pulsatile movements of the dural sac, protects nerve structures, facilitates the movement of the dural sac over the periosteum of the spinal column during flexion and extension, and may form a pharmacologic reservoir of lipophilic substances.[25]

The distribution of epidural fat varies along the length of the spinal canal. In the cervical spine, epidural fat is normally sparse to nonexistent anteriorly, laterally, and posteriorly. A tiny point of posterior epidural fat may be found at C7 and T1.[25] In the thoracic spine, the epidural fat is normally sparse anteriorly but abundant posteriorly (see Figs. 4-4 to 4-7). The posterior thoracic epidural fat usually forms a continuous sheet of fat from T1-T7, but separates into discontinuous, segmented packets of fat

from T8-T12.[25] In the lumbar spine, the anterior epidural fat and the posterior epidural fat show independent configurations (see Figs. 4-12C and 4-13 to 4-15). The anterior lumbar epidural fat often forms a continuous fatty sheet from approximately L4 down to about S2. The posterior epidural fat typically forms discontinuous, segmented (metameric) packets of fat, separated from each other where the dural sac abuts the inner surface of the bony canal. The volume of posterior lumbar epidural fat typically increases caudally from L1-2 to L4-5. The posterior lumbar fat volume varies with patient weight (obesity) but not with patient gender, patient height, or body habitus.[25] Younger patients show larger quantities of anterior, but not posterior, lumbar epidural fat.[25] In addition, the volume of spinal epidural fat becomes increased wherever the curvature of the spinal canal is greatest, especially in patients with kyphoscolioses.

In sagittal sections through the lumbar spine, the posterior fat packets form vertical crescents along the deep surfaces of the ligamenta flava. They pass from the middle of the lamina above along the deep surface of that lamina to the uppermost portion of the next-lower lamina (see Figs. 4-11A and 4-15). The heights of the dorsal lumbar fat packets are nearly identical from level to level, measuring ~21 mm (range, 16 to 25 mm) at each level. The fat packets are thickest at their cephalic ends. They become increasingly bulky caudally: L1-2: 6 mm; L2-3: 9 mm; L3-4: 11 mm; and L4-5: 13 mm.[18,25] In axial sections, each posterior fat packet appears triangular (tetrahedral) in shape with a concave base along the dorsal surface of the dura, concave sides along the deep surfaces of the ligamenta flava, and an apex in the dorsal midline just deep to the spinous process. A fine layer of connective tissue encapsulates each fat packet from its dural surface anteriorly toward the ligamenta flava and neural foramina laterally. Within each dorsal fat packet, sparse collagen fibers and vessels converge posteriorly to a vascular pedicle that emerges from the inferior (rarely superior) pole of the tetrahedron to pierce the dorsal midline between the paired left and right ligamenta flava. These fat packets adhere to spinal structures only at their posterior midline vascular pedicle, so the open interfaces between fat and spine facilitate free movement of the dura and other spinal structures during flexion and extension. The vascular pedicle coincides topographically with the plica mediana dorsalis described by epidurography.[26,27] The lateral margins of the tetrahedral fat packets conform to the "transverse connective tissue planes" shown in the dorsal epidural space by CT epidurography.[18,27]

Unlike the dorsal epidural fat, the lateral epidural fat is lobulated by septae.[18] The plane of septation typically extends from the lateral edge of the posterior longitudinal ligament into the dural-arachnoid sheaths of the exiting nerve roots.[18] Electron microscopy discloses fat within the epidural space around the root sleeves and layers of fat within the dura mater (interleaved with the individual laminae of the dura). Fat also surrounds and separates small fascicles of the nerve roots within the dural sleeves but no fat is interposed between the axons of the nerve roots. In the zones proximal to the dorsal root ganglia, fat may constitute one third of the thickness of the entire root sleeve.[25]

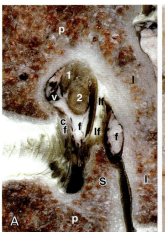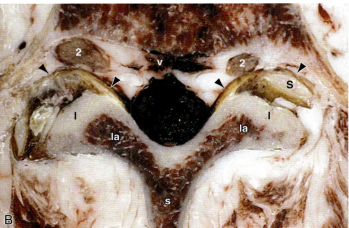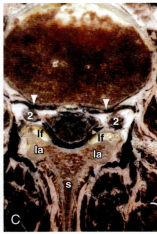

■ **FIGURE 4-28** Neural foramen. Cryomicrotome sections. **A,** Sagittal section through the neural foramen shows the keyhole shape of the foramen formed superiorly and inferiorly by the pedicles (p) above and below, anteriorly by the posterior surfaces of the upper vertebral body and disc, and posteriorly by the ligamentum flavum (lf) and superior articular process (S) of the lower vertebra. The segmental roots lie within the upper portion of the neural foramen with the ventral motor root (1) anterosuperior and the dorsal sensory root (2) posteroinferior. There is fat (f) within the upper portion of the zygapophyseal joint formed by the superior and inferior articular processes. cf, cribriform fascia. **B,** Axial section through the neural foramina and facet joints. The paired ligamenta flava (*arrowheads*) form the posterior wall of the spinal canal, the anterior portions of the capsules of the facet joints, and the posterior wall of the neural foramina. The neural foramina are filled with fat, vessels, and nerves. The dorsal root ganglia (2) lie immediately anterior to the lateral portions of the ligamenta flava within the neural foramina. The anterior internal vertebral venous plexus (IAVVP) (v) lies within the anterior compartment of the spinal epidural space. la, lamina; S, superior articular process; I, inferior articular process; s, spinous process. **C,** Axial section through the neural foramina shows the prominent radicular veins (*arrowheads*) traversing the neural foramina anterior to the dorsal root ganglia.

Neural Foramina

The neural foramina transmit the motor and sensory nerve roots that merge into a mixed spinal segmental nerve, the associated meningeal sheaths, two to four recurrent meningeal nerves, variable radiculomeningeal and radiculospinal vessels, and the plexiform venous connections between the internal and the external vertebral venous plexuses (Figs. 4-28 to 4-30).[1-3]

The position of the neurovascular bundle is different in the cervical than the thoracolumbar region. In the cervical spine, the ventral and dorsal roots lie within the lower portion of each cervical foramen, at and inferior to the level of the cervical disc. The dorsal roots lie immediately anterior to the superior articular facets. The dorsal root ganglion often lies within a small concavity (fossa) at the anterior wall of the superior articular process. In axial sections, the dorsal nerve roots appear to lie just anterior to the ligamentum flavum while the anterior roots lie immediately posterior to the vertebral margin and the uncinate process.[28] In the thoracic and lumbar regions the nerve roots lie in the upper portion of the neural foramina, just inferior to the upper pedicle.

Throughout the spine, the nerve roots are named for the pedicle to which they are closest. Because the cervical roots emerge through the inferior portion of each neural foramen, closest to the inferior pedicle, the roots are named for the lower pedicle of the foramen. Thus, the C1 root emerges between the skull base and C1, the C2 to C7 roots emerge through the C1-C2 to C6-C7 neural foramina, respectively, and the C8 root emerges at the neural foramen between C7 and T1. Because the thoracic and lumbar roots emerge through the upper portions of the neural foramina, closest to the superior pedicle, these roots are named for the lower pedicle of the foramen. Thus, the T1 root emerges at the T1-T2 neural foramen, the T12 root emerges at the T12-L1 neural foramen, the L5 root at the L5-S1 neural foramen, and the S5 root between S5 and the first coccygeal segment.

The lateral ends of the lumbar neural foramina of L1 through L4 are "closed" by a thin fibrous sheet designated the cribriform fascia (Fig. 4-31).[29] This fascia runs from the posterolateral aspect of the vertebral body and disc anteriorly to the transverse or articular processes posteriorly and is thicker superiorly than inferiorly. It separates the neural compartment from the paraspinal tissue and is detectable by both CT and MRI. This fascia is not evident at L5-S1. Other, inconstant ligaments within the neural foramina create another layer of cribiform fascia. These structures include the superior and inferior transforaminal ligaments and the superior and inferior corporotransverse ligaments (Figs. 4-28 and 4-31).[30]

The lumbar neural foramina were measured in serial sagittal cryomicrotome sections of 100 foramina from 18 cadavers and scored for each level L1-L2 through L5-S1 (Table 4-3). Normal lumbar neural foramina measure more than 15 mm in height.[31] The mean cross-sectional areas of the intraforaminal nerve roots increase caudad from L1 to L5. Those of the neural foramina do not. Therefore, the nerve roots occupy an increasingly large percentage of the area of more caudal neural foramina.[31]

IMAGING

CT

CT displays best the bony architecture and the many normal variants of spinal anatomy described earlier and in

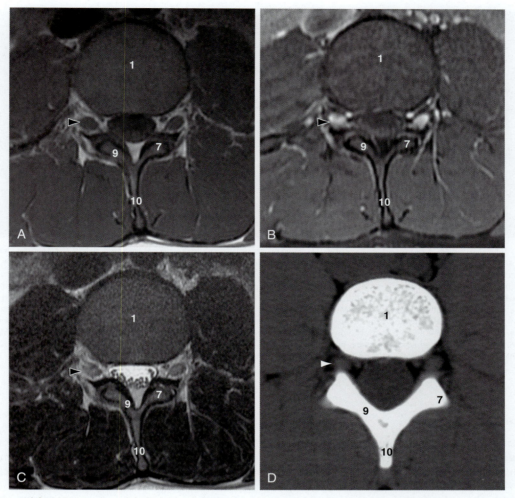

■ **FIGURE 4-29**   Neural foramina. In-vivo axial MR images in a 20-year-old man: noncontrast axial T1W (**A**), contrast-enhanced T1W (**B**), and non-contrast T2W (**C**) images. **D**, Noncontrast axial CT image in a 27-year-old man. These images show the vertebral bodies and discs (1) forming the anterior wall of the foramina, the ligamenta flava and superior articular processes forming the posterior walls of the foramina, the dorsal root ganglia (*arrowheads*) within a small concavity along the posterior wall of the foramina, and prominent enhancement of the intraforaminal venous plexus. 7, Inferior articular process; 9, lamina; 10, spinous process.

this section. MRI displays the bony architecture less well than CT but displays beautifully the contained bone marrow and often shows the ligaments and fascia better than does CT.

Articular Angles and Tropism

The symmetry or asymmetry of the facet joints is assessed by measuring the angles between the articulating surfaces of the superior articular facets and a midsagittal line drawn from the center of the disc through the center of the base of the spinous process (Figs. 4-12D and 4-32). In the lumbar spine, the individual facet joints orient at 10 to 77 degrees to the midline.[32] The mean angle of the facet joints increases at each lumbar level from T12-L1 to L4-L5 but decreases from L4-L5 to L5-S1.[32]

 Articular tropism is defined as asymmetry in the angles of the two sides on well-centered studies. In the lumbar spine, normal asymmetry is considered to be less than 7 degrees. Moderate articular tropism is taken to be asym-metry of 7 to 15 degrees, and severe tropism to be asym-metry greater than 15 degrees. CT and MRI studies in 79 vertebral levels in 88 living patients showed a mean asym-metry of 5 to 6 degrees (± 5 degrees).[33] CT study of 104 lumbar facets in cadavers disclosed no tropism (i.e., asym-metry <7 degrees) in 90%, moderate tropism in 6%, and severe tropism in 4% of specimens.[32]

Absent Articular Processes

The superior and/or inferior articular processes of one or more vertebrae may anomalously fail to develop.[34] Meta-analysis of 40 anomalies in 37 individuals shows that these can appear as *one or more* unilateral defects of the superior articular process (SAP) (12%), unilateral defect of the inferior articular process (IAP) (17%), unilateral defects of the SAP, IAP, and lamina of the same level (10%), uni-lateral absence of both the SAP and the IAP of the same facet joint (50%), or bilateral absence of the IAP of the same segment (10%).[34]

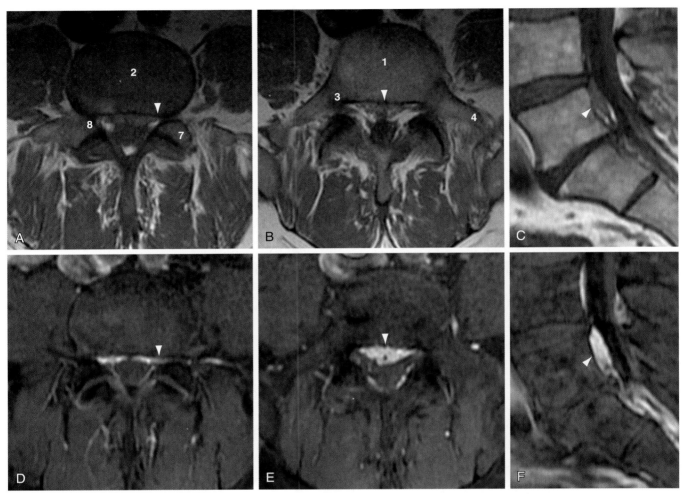

■ **FIGURE 4-30** Neural foramina: venous structures. In-vivo axial (**A, B, D, E**) and sagittal (**C and F**) T1W MR images before (**A-C**) and after (**D-F**) contrast enhancement in a 50-year-old man. There is intense enhancement of the epidural venous plexus (*white arrowheads*) at the ventral spinal canal and within the neural foramina. See also Figure 4-28. Also labeled: vertebral body (1), intervertebral disc (2), pedicle (3), transverse process (4), superior articular process (7), and neural foramen (8).

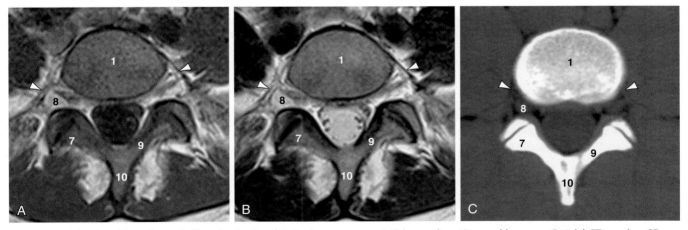

■ **FIGURE 4-31** Neural foramina: cribriform fascia. **A and B,** In-vivo noncontrast MR images in a 40-year-old woman. **C,** Axial CT scan in a 27-year-old man. Fat within and around the neural foramina outlines the tenuous bands of low signal and intermediate density. The cribriform fascia (*white arrowheads*) occupies the lateral ends of the neural foramina. Also labeled: vertebral body (1), inferior articular process (7), neural foramen (8), lamina (9), and spinous process (10).

TABLE 4-3. Normal Lumbar Neural Foramina in 18 Cadavers Aged 35-86 Years at Death

Parameter	Vertebral Level				
	L1-L2	**L2-L3**	**L3-L4**	**L4-L5**	**L5-S1**
Height of foramen (mm)	20.3 ± 2.3	21.8 ± 2.3	22.2 ± 2.5	20.5 ± 2.7	21.7 ± 2.5
Posterior disc height (mm)	6.8 ± 1.1	7.6 ± 1.5	7.3 ± 2.0	6.9 ± 1.5	6.1 ± 1.3
Cross-sectional area					
Foramen (mm)	126.7 ± 26.6	132.3 ± 26.9	141.0 ± 24.0	123.0 ± 22.6	147.3 ± 39.0
Nerve root (mm)	29.8 ± 10.7	32.5 ± 8.3	38.2 ± 12.5	34.3 ± 8.1	41.8 ± 13.5
Ratio (percent)	23.3 ± 6.7	25.1 ± 6.5	27.0 ± 6.6	28.4 ± 6.8	29.2 ± 4.3

Data from Hasegawa T, An HS, Haughton VM, et al. Lumbar foraminal stenosis: critical heights of the intervertebral discs and foramina: a cryomicrotome study in cadavera. J Bone Joint Surg Am 1995;77:32.

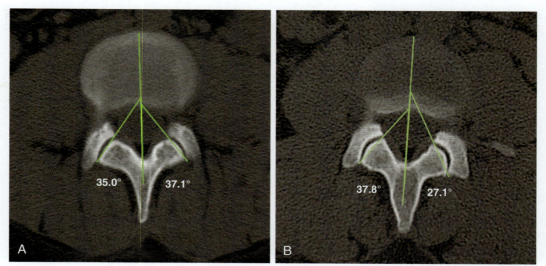

■ **FIGURE 4-32** Articular tropism. In-vivo axial CT scans at L3-L4. **A,** Normal facet angles in a 22-year-old woman. The difference between the right and left facet angles is 2.1 degrees. Angular differences less than 7 degrees are normal. **B,** Mild articular tropism in a 21-year-old woman. The difference between the right and left facet angles is 10.7 degrees. Angular differences of 7 to 15 degrees are classified as mild articular tropism. Only angular differences greater than 15 degrees are classified as severe tropism.

Unfused Ossicles at the Lumbar Facet Joints

Secondary or accessory ossification centers that fail to fuse with their parent bones may appear as accessory ossicles about the joint (Fig. 4-33).[35] Plain radiographs show these ossicles in 0.7% to 1.5% of lumbar spine studies.[35] Anatomic imaging study of 273 lumbar facet joints in 38 cadavers disclosed accessory ossicles in 5 of 38 cadavers (13%) and 7 of 273 lumbar facet joints (2.6%). The ossicles could be single or multiple and symmetric or asymmetric. They all showed smooth well-defined cortical margins, distinguishing them from fracture fragments.[35]

Lumbar Spinal Canal

Schmid and colleagues[36] used an open 0.5-T MR unit and T2-weighted (T2W) fast spin-echo sequences to measure the size of the lumbar spinal canal at L4-L5 in 12 normal patients aged 19 to 33 years in multiple body positions. At the level of the pedicles, the mean cross-sectional area of the spinal canal measured 260 to 280 mm² and did not change significantly with differing body positions. At the level of the L4-L5 disc, however, the mean cross-sectional

area varied approximately 16% from a maximum of 268 mm² in an upright flexed position to a minimum of 224 mm² in an upright extended position.[36] The ligamentum flavum showed similar change with a minimum mean thickness of 1.8 mm in an upright flexed position and a maximum mean thickness of 4.3 mm in an upright extended position.[36]

Lumbar Lateral Recesses

Normal measurements were established for the sagittal dimension of the lateral recess; a measurement of 5 mm or greater is normal. A measurement of 3 to 4 mm raises question of stenosis, whereas a measurement of 2 mm is pathologic.[37]

Neural Foramina

Changes with Body Position

Schmid and colleagues[36] also measured the changes in the neural foramina with changing body position at each level

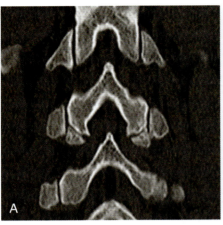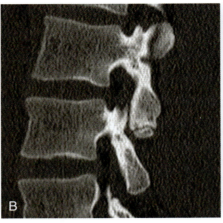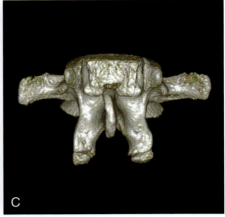

■ **FIGURE 4-33** Accessory ossification centers in a 32-year-old man. Bone algorithm CT images reformatted as coronal plane **(A)**, sagittal plane **(B)**, and 3-D rendering of the posterior surface **(C)** of the lumbar spine demonstrate symmetrical accessory ossification centers for the inferior articular processes of L2.

from L1-L2 to L5-S1. The mean cross-sectional areas of the neural foramina decreased by 30% to 40% from the upright flexion to upright extended positions. Broken down by difference from neutral position, the mean cross-sectional areas of the neural foramina increased by 5% to 20% from the upright neutral to upright flexion positions. The mean cross-sectional areas of the neural foramina decreased by 20% to 30% from the upright neutral to upright extended positions.[36]

Changes with Axial Loading

Hasegawa and associates correlated vertical measurements of the lumbar neural foramina with nerve root compression, disc disease, and axial loading.[31] Nerve root compression was present in 80% of lumbar neural foramina in which the height of the neural foramen was 15 mm or less and in 80% of the foramina in which the height of the posterior disc margin measured 4 mm or less. Therefore, a posterior disc height of 4 mm or less and a lumbar neural foramen height of 15 mm or less were taken to be critical values at and below which there was high probability of neural compression.

In cadaver studies, axial loading of the lower spine from T12 to S2, with pressure levels approaching the failure load of the motion segments, causes reduced disc height, bulging of the intervertebral disc, bulging of the ligamentum flavum, and consequent narrowing of the cross-sectional area of the neural foramina in 74% of specimens.[38] These disc and foraminal changes were significantly greater in motion segments with radial tears than in motion segments with normal discs. However, the changes induced did not cause displacement, deformity, or compression of the spinal roots or nerves, even in segments with common chronic degenerative changes such as annular tears.[38]

Protocols for CT

Present protocols for imaging of the thoracic/lumbar spine are shown in Box 4-1. A sample case report is shown in Box 4-2.

BOX 4-1   Protocols for CT of the Thoracic/ Lumbar Spine

- Patient position: Supine
- Scan extent: Determined by radiologist
- Contrast: None
- Scan type: Helical
- Slice thickness: 0.625 mm
- Detector coverage: 20 mm
- Pitch: 0.531:1 (10.62 mm/rotation)
- Rotation time: 0.5 s
- Reconstruction: 3.75 mm
- Field of view: Sized to include entire vertebrae, including transverse and spinous processes
- Algorithm: Soft tissue and bone
- Postprocessing: 1.0 × 0.5-mm increments in coronal and sagittal multiplanar reformatted images

---

MRI

MRI displays the expected features of normal anatomy detailed earlier. In addition, MRI has provided information about the bone marrow not previously available by imaging.

Bone Marrow Imaging

Standard T1-weighted (T1W) and T2W MRI displays the vertebral marrow as intermediate signal intensity secondary to mixed contributions of lower-intensity red marrow and higher-intensity yellow fatty marrow. The lower-intensity red marrow is usually distributed uniformly through the vertebral body but may be more concentrated near the vertebral end plates or at the anterior aspect of the body.[39]

In the adult lumbar spine, the high signal of marrow fat may appear nearly equal in all lumbar vertebrae or may appear progressively brighter from L1 to L5.[40] On T1W images, owing to the high fat content of their marrow, normal lumbar vertebral bodies appear just slightly

BOX 4-2   Noncontrast CT of the Lumbar Spine

PATIENT HISTORY

A 25-year-old man presented with nonspecific lower back pain.

TECHNIQUE

Serial thin axial sections were obtained by helical technique from the lower thoracic spine to upper sacrum and processed to generate reformatted axial, sagittal, and curved-plane "coronal" soft tissue algorithm and bone algorithm images through the length of the lumbar spine. No contrast agent was administered.

FINDINGS

The aorta and iliac vessels show no evidence of stenosis, aneurysm, or dissection. The paraspinal soft tissues demonstrate no organomegaly, pathologic calcification, or evidence of traumatic injury. The visualized lymph nodes and prevertebral and retrovertebral soft tissues are within normal limits.

No transitional vertebra is identified. The spinal column shows normal lumbar lordosis. There is no malalignment of the vertebral bodies. The vertebral body height, contour, and density are within expected limits for patient age. The intervertebral disc spaces appear normal with no loss of height or end plate irregularity. The overall size of the spinal canal is normal. The distal spinal cord and roots of the cauda equina are normal in size, position, contour, and density. The facet joints have normal contour and alignment. The pars interarticularis of L5 on the left is narrow and shows a linear defect with adjacent sclerosis consistent with spondylolysis. The right pars interarticularis is normal. The left neural foramina are normal at T12-L1 through L4-L5 inclusive. The left L5-S1 neural foramen is mildly narrowed in association with the spondylolysis. The right neural foramina are normal at T12-L1 through L5-S1 inclusive.

The visualized portions of the lower thoracic spine and sacrum show no abnormality.

At T12-L1, the spinal canal has normal contour with no impingement by disc or spur. The transverse processes, facet joints, and laminae are normal bilaterally. The neural foramina are normal in size. The T12 ganglion and emerging T12 roots are surrounded by fat bilaterally, with no compression by disc or spur. The spinal cord is normal in size, position, density, and configuration. The paravertebral soft tissues are within normal limits.

At L1-L2, the spinal canal has normal contour with no impingement by disc or spur. The transverse processes, facet joints, and laminae are normal bilaterally. The neural foramina are normal in size. The L1 ganglion and emerging L1 roots are surrounded by fat bilaterally, with no compression by disc or spur. The conus medullaris is normal in size, position, density, and configuration. The paravertebral soft tissues are within normal limits.

(Continue serially for each level through L4-L5.)

At L5-S1, the spinal canal has normal contour with no impingement by disc or spur. The transverse processes, facet joints, and laminae are normal bilaterally. There is narrowing and sclerosis of the left pars interarticularis with a linear defect consistent with spondylolysis. No spondylolisthesis is identified. The left neural foramen is mildly narrowed with no evidence of compression of the emerging left L5 roots and ganglion. The right pars interarticularis is normal. The right neural foramen, emerging L5 nerve roots, and L5 ganglion are normal. The roots of the cauda equina are normal in size, position, density, and configuration. No evidence of arachnoiditis is appreciated. The paravertebral soft tissues are within normal limits.

The upper sacrum is normal.

IMPRESSION

There is narrowing, sclerosis, and linear defect within the left pars interarticularis of L5, consistent with spondylolysis. Minimal narrowing of the left L5-S1 neural foramen with no impingement on the emerging L5 roots or L5 ganglion is evident. No evidence of spondylolisthesis is noted when scanning with the patient supine.

---

brighter than the adjacent skeletal muscle and *usually* appear brighter than the interposed discs.[39] In children younger than age 6 months, and even in some children younger than age 2 years, normal vertebral bodies can appear darker than the intervertebral discs owing to heavy concentrations of normal red marrow.[39] In adults, normal *thoracic* vertebrae may also show lower signal intensity than the adjacent discs.[39]

With age, the proportion of fatty marrow (fat fraction) increases and the distribution of red and yellow marrow becomes more inhomogeneous (Figs. 4-34 and 4-35).[40] Four common patterns of marrow signal are seen on T1W MR images: (1) uniformly low signal of the vertebral body with dual linear bands of high signal fat paralleling the basivertebral veins, (2) peripheral bands and triangles of high-intensity fat along the end plates and corners of the vertebrae, (3) multiple small (few millimeter) areas of high-intensity fat dispersed through the body, and (4) multiple large (5-15 mm) areas of high-intensity fat dispersed through the body.[41] In the cervical spine, most

patients with the first pattern are younger than age 40 years, whereas most with the second to fourth patterns are older than age 40 years. In the thoracic spine, a pure second pattern is rare to absent and the age distribution of those with the third pattern is relatively uniform. In the lumbar spine, the first pattern was again seen predominantly in the young (<20 years) and is not seen after age 30 years. The second and third patterns increased monotonically with age.[41] The difference in the patterns of the thoracic versus the cervical and lumbar spines may reflect reduced axial loading and torque on the thoracic vertebral body, because the ribs also bear and distribute the axial compressive forces of weight and motion.

Vande Berg and coworkers noted that the low signal intensity of red marrow may be concentrated along the anterior ends of the vertebral bodies, forming wedges of low signal intensity in multiple adjacent bodies on T1W and T2W images.[39] The zones of red and yellow marrow may both expand into nodules. Nodules of fat may impinge upon and scallop the borders of adjacent regions of red

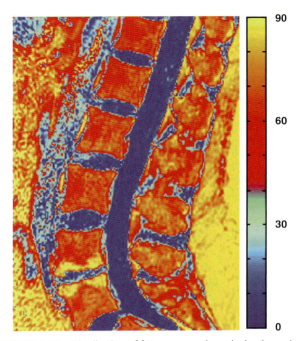

■ **FIGURE 4-34** Distribution of fatty marrow along the lumbar spine in a 57-year-old woman. Sagittal image of the lumbar spine from T12 to uppermost S1. The fat fraction (FF) increases from L1 to L5. The color scale shows a range of FF values from dark blue (0% fat) to bright yellow (90% fat). *(Reprinted from Liney GP, Bernard CP, Manton DJ, et al. Age, gender, and skeletal variation in bone marrow composition: a preliminary study at 3.0 Tesla. J Magn Reson Imaging 2007; 26:787-793.)*

marrow of low signal intensity.[39] The foci of fatty marrow may become very large. Conversely, nodules of red marrow may grow to produce single or multiple foci of low signal intensity with indistinct or defined borders.[39] Such islands of red marrow often lie along the periphery of the vertebrae. As a further complication, small (2-4 mm) islands of notochordal tissue may also be seen within the vertebral bodies as foci of slightly low T1 signal intensity and high T2 signal intensity.[39]

Proton MR spectroscopy is more effective than routine T1 spin-echo MRI for defining the extent of fatty vertebral marrow. MR spectroscopy shows definite increase in bone marrow fat in postmenopausal women with osteopenia and osteoporosis. There is greater increase in saturated fats versus unsaturated fats, and the increasing fat content correlates well with reduced bone mineralization.[42]

Contrast Enhancement

The extent of vertebral contrast enhancement varies greatly among healthy persons (range, 3%-59%) (Fig. 4-36). The mean increase in T1 signal intensity with contrast enhancement is approximately 21% and typically does not exceed 35% to 40% in individuals older than 35 years.[39,43] However, many normal subjects (up to 21%) show no perceptible enhancement of the vertebral marrow on routine T1W MR images without fat saturation.[44] The enhancement is greatest in patients older than age 30

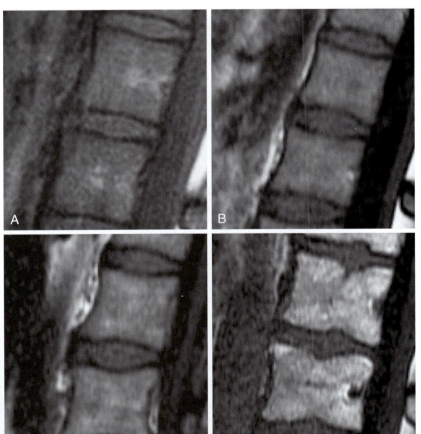

■ **FIGURE 4-35** In-vivo T1W MR images of four different patients show the high signal fatty marrow in the four general patterns.
A, 14-year-old girl. Pattern 1: high signal fatty marrow confined to linear areas along the basivertebral vein.
B, 18-year-old woman. Pattern 2: band-like and triangular areas of fatty marrow located peripherally along the vertebral margins and corners.
C, 44-year-old woman. Pattern 3: multiple small areas of high signal fatty marrow throughout the vertebra.
D, 53-year-old woman. Pattern 4: multiple large areas of high signal fatty marrow throughout the vertebra.

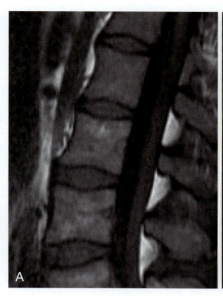
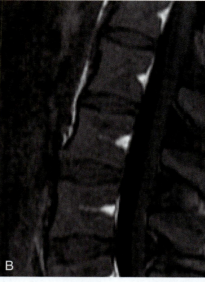

■ **FIGURE 4-36** Contrast-enhancement of the normal lumbar spine in a 44-year-old woman. Sagittal T1W MR images before (**A**) and after (**B**) administration of gadolinium chelate contrast agent (17 mL, Magnevist) in a dose of 0.1 mmol/kg. The basivertebral veins and anterior internal vertebral venous plexus show intense enhancement at each level. No other change is readily discernible. In **B**, application of a fat-saturation pulse has reduced the signal intensity of the epidural fat and other fat tissue.

years and decreases significantly with age. As a result, young healthy individuals may show much greater enhancement of the vertebral marrow than do elderly individuals with diffuse malignant infiltration of the vertebral marrow.[43]

Dynamic perfusion MRI shows that initial perfusion of the vertebrae is very rapid while washout is relatively slow. The peak of enhancement is reached within the first 40 to 60 seconds after bolus infusion (Fig. 4-37). Thereafter, progressive slow washout of contrast agent occurs at 6% per minute over the next 7 minutes.[43] Age and gender significantly influence the rate of perfusion and the extent of enhancement of vertebral marrow.[45] Men and women younger than age 50 years show a higher rate and higher peak of contrast enhancement than those older than age 50 years. Among subjects younger than 50 years, women have a higher rate and peak of enhancement than men. This declines steeply after age 50 years, when men have higher values.[45] Montazel and associates confirmed these findings in normal subjects, showing a very wide range of maximal contrast enhancement (0% to 430% at <1 minute), markedly more rapid and greater enhancement in subjects younger than age 40 years, and logarithmic decline in maximal enhancement with age after age 40 years.[44] These researchers found no gender effect.

The extent of vertebral marrow perfusion also correlates with bone mineral density. In older male patients, subjects with normal bone density show significantly greater marrow perfusion than those with osteopenia, and those with osteopenia show significantly greater marrow perfusion than those with osteoporosis.[46]

Protocols for MRI

Table 4-4 shows the present MR protocols for the thoracic spine, the lumbar spine, and the sacrum. In any individual case, additional sequences may be indicated. Specific protocols are expected to evolve with improving technology.

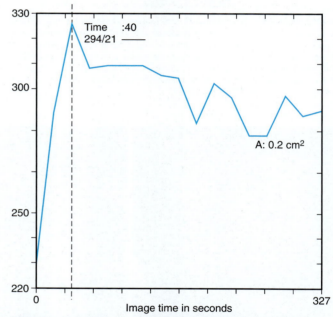

■ **FIGURE 4-37** Time course of MRI contrast enhancement of the vertebral bone marrow. The x-axis is image time in seconds. The y-axis is signal intensity. After intravenous administration of gadopentetate dimeglumine (Gd-DTPA) at a dose of 0.1 mmol/kg, healthy normal adults show a steep increase in the T1 signal intensity of the bone marrow within the first milliseconds and a slow decrease in signal intensity over the next 7 minutes. (TR/TE = 572/15 ms). A: 0.2 cm² indicates the area measured. *(Reprinted from Baur A, Stäbler A, Bartl R, et al. MRI gadolinium enhancement of bone marrow: age-related changes in normals and in diffuse neoplastic infiltration. Skeletal Radiol 1997; 26:414-418.)*

Strategies for Interpreting Thoracic and Lumbar Spine Studies

One can interpret cross-sectional imaging of the spine in a number of ways. One format for systematic and comprehensive review of spinal images is detailed here. Other formats may also be adopted. The approach selected,

TABLE 4-4. Present MRI Protocols in Imaging the Thoracolumbosacral Spine

The Thoracic Spine

Sequence	TE	TR	TI	Echo Train	BW	Freq	Phase	Freq Dir	NEX	FOV	ST
Precontrast											
Sagittal T1 FLAIR	22.0	1550.0	Auto	8	41.67	512	256	A/P	2.00	35.0	4.0
Sagittal T2 FRFSE	110.0	4450.0	Auto	24	31.25	512	256	A/P	4.00	35.0	2.0
2D MERGE Disc	111.0	300.0	Auto	24	62.50	320	192	A/P	2.00	18.0	7.0
Axial T2 FRFSE	110.0	5300.0	Auto	1	41.67	320	224	R/L	2.00	17.0	5.0
Sagittal STIR	42.0	4050.0	180	12	31.25	352	160	A/P	2.00	35.0	4.0
Postcontrast											
Sagittal T1 FLAIR	22.0	2500.0	Auto	8	41.67	512	256	A/P	2.00	35.0	4.0
Axial T1 FSE	20.0	425.0	Auto	4	31.25	288	160	R/L	2.00	22.0	4.0

The Lumbar Spine

Sequence	TE	TR	TI	Echo Train	BW	Freq	Phase	Freq Dir	NEX	FOV	ST
Precontrast											
Sagittal T1 FLAIR	20.0	2500.0	Auto	8	41.67	448	224	A/P	2.00	26.0	4.0
Sagittal T2 FRFSE	102.0	4300.0	Auto	24	41.67	416	288	A/P	4.00	26.0	3.0
Axial T2 FRFSE	110.0	5717.0	Auto	32	41.67	288	256	R/L	4.00	16.0	4.0
Axial PD	32.0	3200.0	Auto	10	50.00	320	192	R/L	2.00	16.0	4.0
Sagittal STIR	42.0	4050.0	180	12	31.25	352	160	A/P	2.00	26.0	4.0
Postcontrast											
Sagittal T1 FLAIR	20.0	2000.0	Auto	8	41.67	448	224	A/P	2.00	26.0	4.0
Axial T1 FSE	20.0	825.0	Auto	4	31.25	256	192	R/L	2.00	22.0	4.0

The Sacrum

Sequence	TE	TR	TI	Echo Train	BW	Freq	Phase	Freq Dir	NEX	FOV	ST
Precontrast											
Sagittal T1 FLAIR	15.0	3000.0	Auto	7	62.50	448	224	A/P	1.00	26.0	4.0
Sagittal T2 FRFSE	102.0	4300.0	Auto	24	41.67	448	224	A/P	2.00	26.0	3.0
Sagittal IR	38.0	2900.0	180	8	62.50	448	192	A/P	1.00	26.0	4.0
Coronal T1 FLAIR	15.0	2975.0	Auto	7	62.50	448	224	S/I	1.00	26.0	4.0
Coronal IR	42.0	2875.0	180	8	62.50	448	160	S/I	1.00	30.0	5.0
Postcontrast											
Sagittal T1 FLAIR	20.0	2250.0	Auto	8	41.67	448	224	A/P	2.00	26.0	4.0
Axial T1 FSE	20.0	825.0	Auto	4	31.25	256	192	R/L	2.00	36.0	4.0
Coronal T1 FLAIR	15.0	2725.0	Auto	7	41.67	448	224	S/I	1.00	26.0	4.0

TE, echo time (ms); TR, repetition time (ms); TI, inversion time (ms); BW, bandwidth; Freq, matrix in frequency-encoded direction; Phase, matrix in phase-encoded direction; Freq Dir, direction of frequency encoding; NEX, number of signals averaged; FOV, field of view (mm); ST, slice thickness (mm); FLAIR, fluid-attenuated inversion recovery; FRFSE, fast recovery fast-spin echo; MERGE Disc, multiple echo recombine gradient echo (proprietary GE sequence) at the level of each disc; STIR, short tau inversion recovery; FSE, fast spin echo; PD, proton density; IR, inversion recovery; A/P, anterior/posterior; R/L, right/left; S/I, superior/inferior.

however, should be followed in (nearly) identical fashion for each level of each study over the years so that the same data appear in the same order on all subsequent reports. In this way, the next radiologist and the patient's clinician can find parallel data at each site to follow serial changes in the patient over time. The reporting format suggested also deliberately duplicates some data at different points to ensure that key data in the report are readily accessible. Computer-based dictation now makes it easy to generate such standardized reports. Thus, we suggest the following (see Box 4-2):

1. On CT and MRI studies, start with the scout views, noting any gross abnormalities and all instrumentation including any indwelling catheters, drains, monitor leads, surgical hardware, and so on.
2. Then, evaluate the sagittal (direct or reformatted) soft tissue images from the skin to skin, anteriorly to pos-teriorly. Specifically, evaluate the aorta and its major branches to report any stenosis, aneurysm, or dissection. Also report concurrent masses, fluid collections, or free air.
3. In the lower thoracic and lumbar spine, evaluate the liver, spleen, pancreas, kidneys/ureters, aorta, bowel, and gynecologic structures for pathologic processes that may mimic the symptoms of spinal disease. Note the presence of masses, calculi, organ lacerations, hemorrhages, fluid collections, and/or aortic lesions, among other emergent findings. Analyze the paravertebral soft tissues for evidence of inflammation or tumor.
4. After this overview, begin to evaluate the spine itself.
5. On sagittal bone and soft tissue images, assess:
   - The overall curvature of the spine
   - The overall alignment of the vertebral bodies
   - The heights, contours, and density/signal of the bone and marrow of the individual vertebral bodies

- The heights and density/signal of the intervertebral discs
- The anterior and posterior longitudinal ligaments
- The overall size of the spinal canal
- The size, position, and configuration of the spinal cord
- The ligamenta flava and the alignment of the spinolaminar lines at the posterior wall of the spinal canal
- The integrity and orientation of the laminae, spinous processes, and interspinous ligaments
- The visualized portions of the adjacent spine

6. Then scroll side to side to assess the sagittal anatomy of the zygapophyseal (facet) joints at each level for both sides.

7. Continue laterally on each side to see the visualized portions of the neural foramina, emerging nerve roots, lumbosacral plexus, and musculature of the back.

8. Next turn to the axial images and assess the spinal canal level by level.
   - Evaluate the prevertebral soft tissues, adjoining vertebral bodies, pedicles, transverse processes, neural foramina, facet joints, laminae, and spinous processes.
   - Assess the anterior and posterior longitudinal ligaments, ligamenta flava, and iliolumbar ligaments.
   - Then address the cross-sectional area of the spinal canal, the contours of the vertebral bodies and intervertebral discs, and any compromise of the spinal canal or neural foramina by bulging/herniated discs or osteophytes.
   - Review the contours and density/signal of the spinal cord and cauda equina.
   - Check the vascularity of the spinal column and cord, and assess the integrity of the muscles, fascial planes, and other paraspinal soft tissues.

- Report these—often redundant—data in the same format for each level, so each level details the same set of findings, whether the level is normal or not.

9. In the thoracic region, the great number of interspaces precludes description of axial findings level by level. Instead, it is usual to have three paragraphs beginning: (1) "In the upper thoracic region, . . ." (2) "In the midthoracic region, . . ." and (3) "In the lower thoracic region,. . . ." Any local findings should be described specifically by level within these broad paragraphs.

10. In the lumbar region, first describe any transitional lumbosacral vertebrae. Since the segmental nerve roots are named by the vertebrae, variations in numbering transitional vertebrae may lead to misidentification of specific nerve roots. Clinicians attempting to correlate clinical findings might then discount the radiologic features, because the levels reported do not correlate with the level of their patient's signs and symptoms. Reporting of transitional vertebrae may also clarify apparent discordances in the sites of pathology reported by different physicians and help to avoid wrong-level surgery. Thereafter, describe the positive and negative imaging findings, level by level, from the lower thoracic region into the sacrum, as outlined earlier.

ACKNOWLEDGMENTS

The authors gratefully acknowledge the assistance of Edward Lugo, Steven Yuen, Nancy Hoo, Jeremy Tietjens, Aron Legler, Jalal Ahmed, Marcia Jaunoo, RTR, Artur Yadgarov, RTR, and James Stephen, RTR.

The 3-D CT surface reformatted images and cut-away sections were generated on a PC using Aquarius Workstation 3.7.0.12 by TeraRecon, Inc. (2995 Campus Drive #325, San Mateo, CA 94403) or Mac using OsiriX PACS Workstation DICOM Viewer v3.6.1 (64-bit). OsiriX is a freely distributed open-source software under the GNU licensing scheme and can be downloaded at http://www.osirix-viewer.com/Downloads.html.

SUGGESTED READINGS

Atlas SW. Magnetic Resonance Imaging of the Brain and Spine, 4th ed. Volume 2, Part 4, Spine and Spinal Cord. Philadelphia, Wolters Kluwer/Lippincott Williams & Wilkins, 2009.

Bullough PG, Boachie-Adjei O. Atlas of Spinal Disorders. Philadelphia, JB Lippincott, 1988.

Castillo M. Neuroradiology Companion: Methods, Guidelines, and Imaging Fundamentals, 3rd ed. Philadelphia, Lippincott Williams & Wilkins, 2006.

Daniels DL, Haughton V, Naidich TP. Cranial and Spinal Magnetic Resonance Imaging: An Atlas and Guide. New York, Raven Press, 1987.

Modic MT, Masaryk TJ, et al. Magnetic Resonance Imaging of the Spine. St. Louis, Mosby–Year Book, 1994.

Newell RLM. The back. In Standring S (ed). Gray's Anatomy: The Anatomical Basis of Clinical Practice, 39th ed. Edinburgh, Churchill Livingstone, 2009.

Ross JS, Brant-Zawadzki M, Moore KR, et al. Diagnostic Imaging Spine. Salt Lake City, UT, Amirsys, 2004.

Soames RW. Skeletal system. In Williams PL (ed). Gray's Anatomy: The Anatomical Basis of Medicine and Surgery, 38th ed. Edinburgh, Churchill Livingstone, 1995.

Van Goethem JWM, van den Hauwe L, Parizel PM (eds). Spinal Imaging: Diagnostic Imaging of the Spine and Spinal Cord (Medical Radiology/Diagnostic Imaging). Berlin, Springer, 2007.

REFERENCES

1. Williams PL (ed). Gray's Anatomy: The Anatomical Basis of Medicine and Surgery, 38th ed. Edinburgh, Churchill Livingstone, 1995.

2. Standring S (ed). Gray's Anatomy: The Anatomical Basis of Clinical Practice, 39th ed. Edinburgh, Elsevier Churchill Livingstone, 2005.

3. Standring S (ed). Gray's Anatomy: The Anatomical Basis of Clinical Practice, 40th ed. Edinburgh, Elsevier Churchill Livingstone, 2008.

4. Marty C, Boisaubert B, Descamps H, et al. The sagittal anatomy of the sacrum among young adults, infants, and spondylolisthesis patients. Eur Spine J 2002; 11:119.

5. Puhakka KB, Melsen F, Jurik AG, et al. MR imaging of the normal sacroiliac joint with correlation to histology. Skeletal Radiol 2004; 33:15.

6. Hughes RJ, Saifuddin A. Numbering of lumbosacral transitional vertebrae on MRI: role of the iliolumbar ligaments. AJR Am J Roentgenol 2006; 187:W59.

7. Tini PG, Wieser C, Zinn WM. The transitional vertebra of the lumbosacral spine: its radiological classification, incidence, prevalence, and clinical significance. Rheumatol Rehabil 1977; 16:180.

8. Kim YH, Lee PB, Lee CJ, et al. Dermatome variation of lumbosacral nerve roots in patients with transitional lumbosacral vertebrae. Anesth Analg 2008; 106:1279.

9. Lee CH, Park CM, Kim KA, et al. Identification and prediction of transitional vertebrae on imaging studies: anatomical significance of paraspinal structures. Clin Anat 2007; 20:905.

10. Castellvi AE, Goldstein LA, Chan DP. Lumbosacral transitional vertebrae and their relationship with lumbar extradural defects. Spine 1984; 9:493.

11. Hsieh CY, Vanderford JD, Moreau SR, et al. Lumbosacral transitional segments: classification, prevalence, and effect on disk height. J Manipulative Physiol Ther 2000; 23:483.

12. Eubanks JD, Cheruvu VK. Prevalence of sacral spina bifida occulta and its relationship to age, sex, race, and the sacral table angle: an anatomic, osteologic study of three thousand one hundred specimens. Spine 2009; 34:1539.

13. Fidas A, MacDonald HL, Elton RA, et al. Prevalence and patterns of spina bifida occulta in 2707 normal adults. Clin Radiol 1987; 38:537.

14. Lirk P, Kolbitsch C, Putz G, et al. Cervical and high thoracic ligamentum flavum frequently fails to fuse in the midline. Anesthesiology 2003; 99:1387-1390.

15. Lirk P, Moriggi B, Colvin J, et al. The incidence of lumbar ligamentum flavum midline gaps. Anesth Analg 2004; 98:1178-1180.

16. Lirk P, Colvin J, Steger B, et al. Incidence of lower thoracic ligamentum flavum midline gaps. Br J Anaesth 2005; 94:852-855.

17. Netter FH. Atlas of Human Anatomy, 4th ed. Philadelphia, Elsevier Saunders, 2006.

18. Hogan QH. Lumbar epidural anatomy. A new look by cryomicrotome sections. Anesthesiology 1991; 75:767-775.

19. Hamid M, Fallet-Bianco C, Delmas V, Plaisant O. The human lumbar anterior epidural space: morphological comparison in adult and fetal specimens. Surg Radiol Anat 2002; 24:194-200.

20. Geers C, Lecouvet FE, Behets C, et al. Polygonal deformation of the dural sac in lumbar epidural lipomatosis: anatomic explanation by the presence of meningovertebral ligaments. AJNR Am J Neuroradiol 2003; 24:1276-1282.

21. Scapinelli R. Anatomical and radiologic studies on the lumbosacral meningovertebral ligaments of humans. J Spinal Disord 1990; 3:6-15.

22. Schellinger D, Manz HJ, Vidic B, et al. Disk fragment migration. Radiology 1990; 175:831-836.

23. Wiltse LL. Anatomy of the extradural compartments of the lumbar spinal canal. Peridural membrane and circumneural sheath. Radiol Clin North Am 2000; 38:1177-1206.

24. Parkin IG, Harrison GR. The topographical anatomy of the lumbar epidural space. J Anat 1985; 141:211-217.

25. Reina MA, Pulido P, Castedo J, et al. Characteristics and distribution of normal human epidural fat. Rev Esp Anestesiol Reanim 2006; 53:363-372.

26. Luyendijk W. The plica mediana dorsalis of the dura mater and its relation to lumbar peridurography (canalography). Neuroradiology 1976; 11:147-149.

27. Savolaine ER, Pandya JB, Greenblatt SH, Conover SR. Anatomy of the human lumbar epidural space: New insights using CT-epidurography. Anesthesiology 1988; 68:217-220.

28. Pech P, Daniels DL, Williams AL, et al. The cervical neural foramina: correlation of microtomy and CT anatomy. Radiology 1985; 155:143.

29. Paz-Fumagalli R, Haughton VM. Lumbar cribriform fascia: appearance at freezing microtomy and MR imaging. Radiology 1993; 187:241.

30. Nowicki BH, Haughton VM. Neural foraminal ligaments of the lumbar spine: appearance at CT and MR imaging. Radiology 1992; 183:257-264.

31. Hasegawa T, An HS, Haughton VM, et al. Lumbar foraminal stenosis: critical heights of the intervertebral discs and foramina: a cryomicrotome study in cadavera. J Bone Joint Surg Am 1995; 77:32.

32. Grogan J, Nowicki BH, Schmidt TA, et al. Lumbar facet joint tropism does not accelerate degeneration of the facet joints. AJNR Am J Neuroradiol 1997; 18:1325.

33. Lee DY, Lee SH. Effects of facet tropism and disk degeneration on far lateral lumbar disk herniation: comparison with posterolateral lumbar disk herniation. Neurol Med Chir 2009; 49:57.

34. Ikeda K, Nakayama Y, Ishii S. Congenital absence of lumbosacral articular process: report of three cases. J Spinal Disord 1992; 5:232.

35. Wang ZL, Yu S, Sether LA, et al. Incidence of unfused ossicles in the lumbar facet joints: CT, MR, and cryomicrotomy study. J Comput Assist Tomogr 1989; 13:594.

36. Schmid MR, Stucki G, Duewell S, et al. Changes in cross-sectional measurements of the spinal canal and intervertebral foramina as a function of body position: in vivo studies on an open-configuration MR system. AJR Am J Roentgenol 1999; 172:1095.

37. Hasegawa T, An HS, Haughton VM. Imaging anatomy of the lateral lumbar spinal canal. Semin Ultrasound CT MR 1993; 14:404.

38. Nowicki BH, Yu S, Reinartz J, et al. Effect of axial loading on neural foramina and nerve roots in the lumbar spine. Radiology 1990; 176:433.

39. Vande Berg BC, Lecouvet FE, Galant C, et al. Normal variants of the bone marrow at MR imaging of the spine. Semin Musculoskelet Radiol 2009; 13:87.

40. Liney GP, Bernard CP, Manton DJ, et al. Age, gender, and skeletal variation in bone marrow composition: a preliminary study at 3.0 Tesla. J Magn Reson Imaging 2007; 26:787-793.

41. Ricci C, Cova M, Kang YS, et al. Normal age-related patterns of cellular and fatty bone marrow distribution in the axial skeleton: MR imaging study. Radiology 1990; 177:83.

42. Yeung DK, Griffith JF, Antonio GE, et al. Osteoporosis is associated with increased marrow fat content and decreased marrow fat unsaturation: a proton MR spectroscopy study. J Magn Reson Imaging 2005; 22:279.

43. Baur A, Stabler A, Bartl R, et al. MRI gadolinium enhancement of bone marrow: age-related changes in normals and in diffuse neoplastic infiltration. Skeletal Radiol 1997; 26:414.

44. Montazel JL, Divine M, Lepage E, et al. Normal spinal bone marrow in adults: dynamic gadolinium-enhanced MR imaging. Radiology 2003; 229:703.

45. Chen WT, Shih TT, Chen RC, et al. Vertebral bone marrow perfusion evaluated with dynamic contrast-enhanced MR imaging: significance of aging and sex. Radiology 2001; 220:213.

46. Griffith JF, Yeung DK, Antonio GE, et al. Vertebral bone mineral density, marrow perfusion, and fat content in healthy men and men with osteoporosis: dynamic contrast-enhanced MR imaging and MR spectroscopy. Radiology 2005; 236:945.

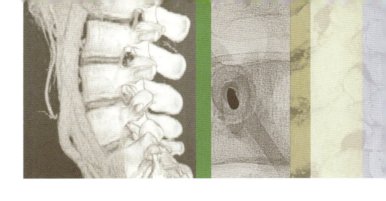

The Normal Spinal Cord and Meninges

Thomas P. Naidich, Bradley N. Delman, Cheuk Y. Tang, Mary Elizabeth Fowkes, Girish M. Fatterpekar, Jose C. Rios, Evan G. Stein, Victor M. Haughton, and David L. Daniels

I. THE SPINAL CORD

The spinal cord is the segment of the central nervous system that lies within the spinal canal caudal to the foramen magnum (Figs. 5-1 to 5-3).[1-24] The top of the spinal cord is taken to be the plane immediately rostral to the emergence of the C1 nerve roots.[11] The bottom of the spinal cord merges into the filum terminale at approximately the L1-L2 vertebral level. The spinal cord is subdivided into 31 segments: 8 cervical, 12 thoracic, 5 lumbar, 5 sacral, and 1 coccygeal.[11]

Grossly, the spinal cord is a tubular neural structure situated with the cranial two-thirds of the spinal canal.[21,24] It is approximately 45 cm long and weighs about 30 g.[21,24] In cross section, the spinal cord is narrow anteroposteriorly and wide transversely, especially where the cervical and lumbar segments enlarge to innervate the shoulder and pelvic girdles. The cervical enlargement lies at C5-T1, with a maximum circumference at the C6 level (38 cm).[21,24] The lumbar enlargement occurs at the L2-S3 neural levels, with a maximum circumference at the T12 vertebral level (35 cm).[21,24] The portion of the spinal cord caudal to the lumbar enlargement tapers to a point, so that the caudal portion is designated the conus medullaris. In the average adult, the caudal tip of the conus medullaris lies at approximately the L1-L2 vertebral level. However, the specific level of termination varies widely (see Imaging, MRI, later in this chapter).[15]

A connective tissue filament, the filum terminale, extends caudad from the conus.[21,24] The filum terminale is approximately 20 cm long and has two portions. The proximal intradural portion of the filum (15 cm) arises at the precise tip of the conus medullaris and descends through the subarachnoid space to penetrate the precise tip of the arachnoid sac at approximately S2.[21,24] The distal extradural portion of the filum (5 cm) fuses with the dura and continues through the sacral canal to insert into the dorsum of the first coccygeal segment.[21,24] As with the conus, the precise level of termination of the dural sac varies widely (see Imaging, MRI, later in this chapter).[15]

Internal Organization

Grossly, the spinal cord is organized as a series of hollow cylinders arrayed concentrically along the length of the cord. From deep to superficial these are the central canal of the cord, the deep gray matter of the cord, and the surrounding white matter. The ratio of gray matter to white matter within each spinal segment varies systematically along the length of the cord (Fig. 5-4). Upper spinal segments show larger proportions of white matter, because they carry the white matter tracts to and from the entire distal cord. Lower spinal segments carry only the white matter for the few segments distal to them.[6] The spinal gray matter is usually sharply delimited from the white matter, except in the cervical cord where strands of gray matter extend into the lateral white matter as the reticular formation.[21,24]

The central canal extends downward from the caudal end of the fourth ventricle into the proximal filum terminale (see Fig. 5-4). It is lined by ciliated ependyma and surrounded by neuroglia and a network of fine nerve fibers constituting the substantia gelatinosa centralis.[21,24] The central canal typically measures less than 1 mm in diameter in youth, partially closes in adulthood, and is mostly obliterated by age 40 years. Within the distal cord and/or proximal filum terminale, the caudal end of the central canal widens into a fusiform "terminal ventricle," 8 to 10 mm long, that contains less than 1 mL of cerebrospinal fluid.[21,24] There may be ependymal rests and lumina of abortive accessory canals within the conus medullaris and proximal filum.

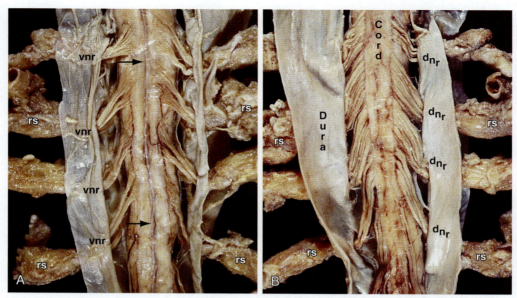

■ **FIGURE 5-1**   Gross anatomy of the cervicothoracic spinal cord seen through the opened dura and arachnoid at postmortem examination. **A,** Anterior surface. The ventral (motor) roots (vnr) arise from the spinal cord segmentally. They form relatively narrow bundles of rootlets that cross the subarachnoid space anterior to the denticulate ligament toward the segmental root sleeves (rs). **B,** Posterior surface. The dorsal (sensory) rootlets (dnr) arise laterally from the segmental dorsal root ganglia and cross the subarachnoid space dorsal to the denticulate ligament. The dorsal rootlets form relatively broad "brushes" of fibers that enter the spinal cord at the dorsal root entry zone over the full length of each segment. The anterior spinal artery (*arrow,* **A**) appears as a single vessel that courses longitudinally in the midline. The paired dorsal spinal arteries (unlabeled) appear as more tenuous, incomplete vessels that course longitudinally just medial to the dorsal root entry zone.

Just external to the central canal, and surrounding it, the longitudinal column of spinal gray matter forms a "fluted gray column" that appears H-shaped in cross section (Figs. 5-4 and 5-5). The ventral arms of the H are the symmetric ventral horns containing motor neurons. The dorsal arms of the H are the symmetric dorsal horns receiving the central fibers of sensory neurons that reside in the dorsal root ganglia. The crossbar of the H is the central gray matter. In the thoracic region, paired additional lateral horns project into the lateral white matter and contain the preganglionic sympathetic neurons. Considered vertically over the length of the spinal cord, the ventral, dorsal, and lateral horns form ventral, dorsal, and lateral columns of gray matter.

External to the gray matter, the white matter of the spinal cord is subdivided into paired dorsal, lateral, and ventral columns (funiculi) by fissures, septa, sulci, and nerve roots (see Figs. 5-4 and 5-5). In the ventral midline, the deep ventral median fissure extends nearly to the central canal, dividing the white matter of the ventral cord into paired ventral columns (anterior columns, anterior funiculi). Anterolaterally, the paired ventrolateral sulci mark the line of exit of the ventral motor nerve roots. The ventral columns are the paired white matter tracts situated to each side of the ventral median sulcus as far laterally as the ventrolateral sulci (including the emerging ventral roots). In the dorsal midline, the shallow dorsal median sulcus and subjacent posterior median glial septum extend nearly to the central canal, dividing the dorsal white matter into paired dorsal columns (posterior columns, dorsal funiculi).[11] Posterolaterally, the paired dorsolateral sulci mark the line of entry of the dorsal nerve roots. The dorsal columns are the paired white matter tracts situated

to each side of the dorsal median sulcus and septum as far laterally as the dorsolateral sulci (but not including the entering dorsal roots). At cervical and thoracic levels above T6, a posterointermediate sulcus and septum further divide each dorsal column into a medial fasciculus gracilis and a lateral fasciculus cuneatus. The lateral columns are the white matter tracts situated between the ventrolateral and dorsolateral sulci.

The fibers coursing within the longitudinal columns may cross the midline close to the central canal of the cord via the gray and white commissures. The dorsal and ventral gray commissures are tracts of crossing unmyelinated (hence "gray") fibers situated just dorsal and ventral to the central canal. The ventral white commissure is a tract of crossing myelinated (hence "white") fibers situated ventral to the ventral gray commissure and dorsal to the depth of the ventral median fissure (Fig. 5-6A).[21,24]

The ventral motor roots arise from cell bodies situated within the ventral horns of the spinal gray matter. The cell bodies are organized longitudinally into medial, central, and lateral longitudinal cell columns, which supply different groups of muscles. The motor roots emerge into the subarachnoid space through the ventrolateral sulci and course ventrolaterally toward the exiting segmental root sleeves.

At each level the dorsal (sensory) roots arise from cell bodies situated within the dorsal root ganglia in the neural foramina. Each dorsal root ganglion cell gives rise to one short fiber that quickly divides into a central and a peripheral process. The central process (central axon) of the dorsal root ganglion cell passes centrally through the subarachnoid space toward the spinal cord. Multiple central processes arise from each segmental ganglion. These fan

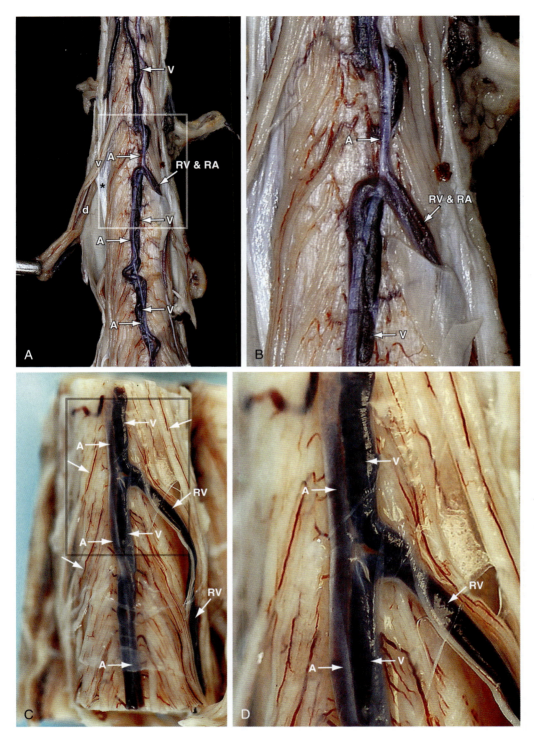

■ **FIGURE 5-2** Anterior surfaces of the formalin-fixed thoracolumbar spinal cord. Short segments of two specimens (**A, C**) with magnified views (**B, D**) of the anterior vessels. **A,** The ventral (motor) rootlets (v) pass anterior to the denticulate ligament (*asterisk,* **A**) to enter the root sleeves with the dorsal nerve roots (d). Radiculomedullary arteries (RA) and veins (RV) course along the nerve roots of either side to supply the thinner, more superficial anterior spinal axis (A) and drain the larger, deeper midline anterior spinal vein (V). Note the fine radicular vessels (*arrows,* **C**) that supply each rootlet.

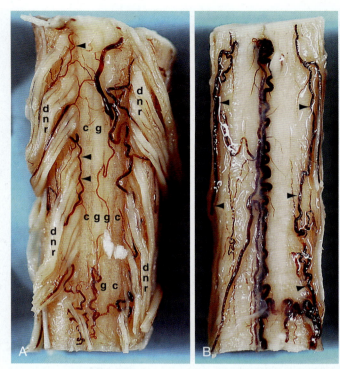

■ **FIGURE 5-3**   Posterior surfaces of the formalin-fixed cervicothoracic spinal cord. Short segments of two specimens. The dorsal nerve roots (dnr) fan out into multiple rootlets that enter the cord at the dorsolateral sulci. The paired gracile (g) and cuneate (c) fasciculi are faintly outlined by the shallow midline dorsal median sulcus, the paired dorsal intermediate sulci between them, and the dorsal root entry zones at the dorsolateral sulci lateral to them. Multiple radiculomedullary arteries feed the paired dorsal spinal arteries (*arrowheads*), which form incomplete longitudinal channels just medial to the dorsal root entry zones. These channels feed into a pial arterial plexus (designated the "vasocorona") that supplies the dorsal portion of the spinal cord. The posterior median vein may form a dorsal midline "hairpin turn" as it drains peripherally via radiculomedullary veins. These may mimic the hairpin turn of the radiculomedullary arteries to the anterior spinal axis. The dorsal midline veins are often serpiginous.

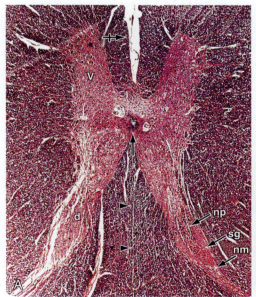
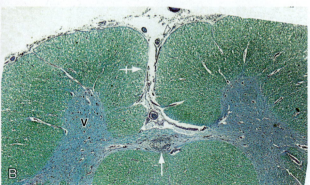

■ **FIGURE 5-4**   Axial histologic specimens. **A,** Central spinal cord (H & E stain). **B,** Ventral spinal cord (Luxol Fast Blue stain for myelin). The central canal of the spinal cord (*vertical midline arrows*) is lined by ependyma. The surrounding cylinder of gray matter appears H-shaped in axial sections with paired ventral horns (v) and dorsal horns (d). The crossbar of the H is formed by the gray matter that surrounds the central canal. Differing concentrations of cells within the gray matter correspond to named histologic laminae and named spinal nuclei, such as the cellular nucleus proprius (np), more myxoid substantia gelatinosa (sg), and apical cap of the nucleus marginalis (nm). The ventral midline shows the deep open ventral median sulcus (*crossed horizontal arrows*) containing the sulcomarginal vessels. The dorsal midline shows the glial dorsal median septum (*black arrowheads*). The vessels within the white matter show a radial distribution.

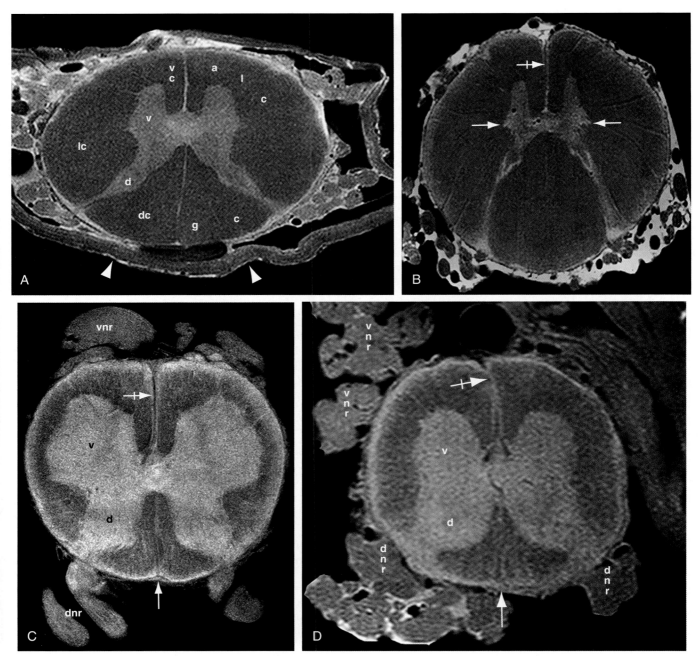

■ **FIGURE 5-5** Normal spinal cord at the cervical (**A**), thoracic (**B**), lumbar (**C**), and sacral (**D**) cord levels shown on axial postmortem 9.4-T MR images. The sagittal dimension of the cord is relatively constant from cervical to lumbar levels and then tapers distally. The transverse dimension shows cervical and lumbar expansions for the shoulder and pelvic girdles. The volume of white matter is greatest in the cervical cord and diminishes progressively caudad. In cross section, the central gray matter forms an H or "butterfly" shape with paired ventral (v) and dorsal horns (d) united by a transverse band of gray matter that encloses the central canal. The thoracic cord displays additional paired lateral horns (*horizontal arrows,* **B**). The cord surface is demarcated by a deep ventral median sulcus (*crossed horizontal arrows*), a shallow dorsal median groove with subjacent deep dorsal median septum (*vertical white arrow,* **C**), paired ventrolateral sulci at which the ventral nerve roots (vnr) emerge from the ventral horns, and paired dorsolateral sulci at which the dorsal roots (dnr) enter the dorsal horns. The dorsolateral fasciculus of Lissauer (Lissauer's tract) manifests as high signal intensity at the dorsal root entry zone (**B**). Superficial to the gray matter, the white matter of the spinal cord is arrayed in longitudinal tracts designated columns (funiculi). The paired ventral columns (vc) extend between the ventral median sulcus and the lateral margins of the emerging ventral roots, including the ventral roots. The paired dorsal columns (dc) lie between the dorsal median septum and the entry of the dorsal roots at the dorsolateral sulci. The lateral columns (lc) lie between the ventral and dorsal columns. The term *anterolateral column* (alc) is useful to designate the adjoining portions of the anterior and lateral columns that surround the emerging ventral nerve roots. In the upper thoracic and cervical cords (from T6 upward), a dorsal intermediate septum subdivides the dorsal columns into paired fasciculi graciles (g) medially and paired fasciculi cuneati (c) laterally. Note the low signal intensity of the fibrous dura (*arrowheads,* **A**) surrounding the nerve roots and cord and the intermediate signal intensity of nerve roots versus the low signal intensity of vessels in the subarachnoid space (**B**).

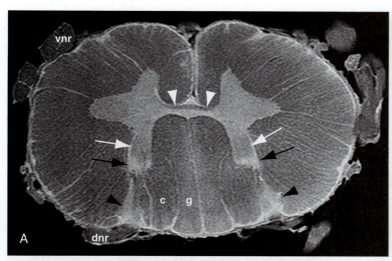

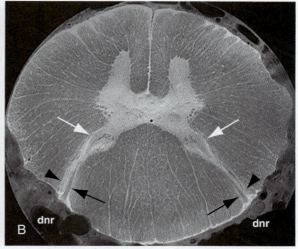

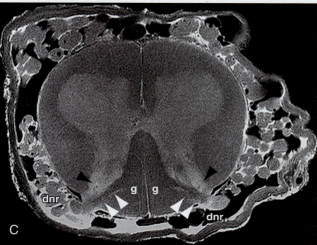

■ **FIGURE 5-6** Axial postmortem 9.4-T MR images of the spinal cord. **A** and **B**, Cervical levels in two specimens. Myelinated fibers crossing the midline form the ventral white commissure (*white arrowheads*, **A**) just dorsal to the ventral median sulcus and just ventral to the ventral gray commissure. As they approach the dorsal root entry zone (DREZ) dorsal nerve rootlets (dnr) sort out into more heavily myelinated fibers (*black arrows*, **B**) that enter the medial portion of the DREZ and thinly myelinated or unmyelinated fibers that enter the lateral portion of the DREZ. The dorsal tract of Lissauer (*black arrowheads*) surrounds the entering dorsal nerve roots and appears bright owing to the limited myelination of its fibers. **C**, Lumbar level. The dorsal root fibers with thick myelination (*white arrowheads*) enter the medial aspect of the DREZ. The dorsal tract of Lissauer (*black arrowheads*) appears bright. The dorsal columns contain only the fasciculus gracilis (g) at the lumbar level but fasciculi graciles (g) and cuneati (c) at the cervical level. Also labeled: nucleus proprius (*thick white arrows*, **A**, **B**), substantia gelatinosa (*black arrows*, **A**), ventral nerve roots (vnr), and dorsal nerve roots (dnr).

out to form six to eight dorsal rootlets that enter the corresponding segment of the spinal cord at the dorsolateral sulcus.[21,24] As the central processes approach the cord, they become sorted by size and degree of myelination.[3] Larger, more heavily myelinated fibers pass medially to enter the dorsal root entry zone as a medial bundle of central fibers (see Fig. 5-6B,C). Lightly myelinated and unmyelinated fibers pass laterally to enter the dorsal root entry zone as a lateral bundle of central fibers. Each entering central process bifurcates into ascending and descending branches.[3] Long ascending branches of the medial fibers enter the dorsal columns directly or pass through the medial portion of the dorsal horn to deeper layers of gray matter. Thin lightly myelinated or unmyelinated branches of the lateral fibers enter the dorsolateral tract (fasciculus) of Lissauer (see later).

The peripheral process of the dorsal root ganglion cell courses laterally through the root sleeve toward the sensory receptor. Within each segmental neural foramen, the ventral motor rootlets that arise from the spinal cord unite with the peripheral sensory processes that arise from the dorsal root ganglion distal to (on the far side of) the dorsal root ganglion to form the spinal nerve. Thus, the term *nerve* signifies the united motor and sensory roots of a segment starting distal to the dorsal root gan-

glion. In humans, there are 8 cervical nerve roots, 12 thoracic roots, 5 lumbar roots, 5 sacral roots, and 1 coccygeal root.[21,24] The C1 nerve exits the spinal canal between the foramen magnum and C1, superior to the bony C1 ring. The C8 nerve exits the spinal canal between C7 and T1, superior to the T1 vertebra. All of the subsequent thoracic, lumbar, and sacral roots exit the spinal canal immediately inferior to the pedicles of the same-named vertebrae. That is, the T7 nerve exits the canal immediately under the T7 pedicle via the T7-T8 neural foramen and the L4 nerve exits the spinal canal immediately under the L4 pedicle via the L4-L5 neural foramen. In the upper cervical spine, some nerve roots also emerge directly through the lateral surface of the lateral columns of white matter to form the spinal accessory nerves (cranial nerve XI) that course superiorly through the subarachnoid space and foramen magnum to join the medullary portion of the spinal accessory nerve within the posterior fossa.[21,24]

Vascularization of the Spinal Cord

Arterial Supply

The spinal cord receives its arterial supply from a single anterior spinal axis and paired dorsal and/or dorsolateral

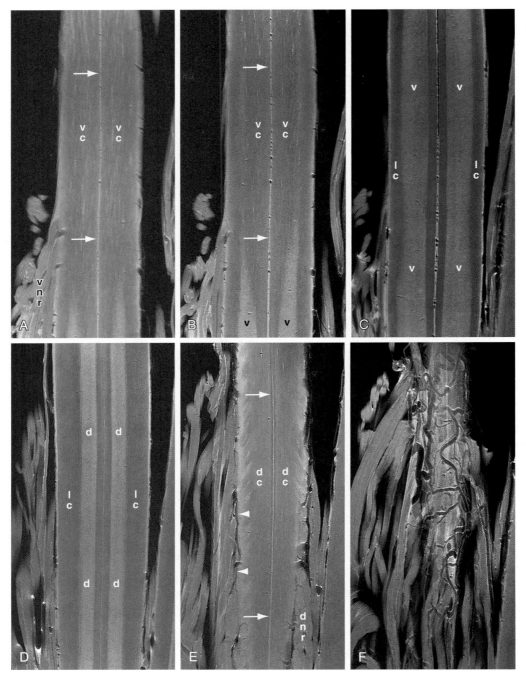

■ **FIGURE 5-7** Normal thoracolumbar spinal cord. Coronal postmortem 9.4-T MR images displayed from ventral (**A**) to dorsal (**F**). **A** and **B,** Coronal sections through the ventral columns (vc) display the ventral median sulcus (*white arrows*) in the midline and motor roots (vnr) exiting at the ventrolateral sulcus. The sulcomarginal vessels enter the ventral median sulcus singly, not in pairs, and pass dorsally toward the depth of the sulcus. **C,** Further dorsally, coronal MR sections display the deep portion of the ventral median sulcus and the vessels within it, the deep portions of the ventral white columns just to each side of the sulcus, the broad ventral horns (v) that flank them, and anterior portions of the lateral columns superficially. **D,** Within the dorsal half of the cord, coronal MR sections display the dorsal median septum, the deep portions of the dorsal columns, the thin dorsal horns (d), and the dorsal portion of the lateral columns. **E,** Coronal section through the dorsal columns shows the dorsal median septum (*white arrows*), the emerging dorsal nerve roots (dnr), and the dorsal spinal arteries that form an incomplete longitudinal plexus just medial to the dorsal nerve roots. **F,** The dorsal surface of the cord shows the dorsal venous plexus that drains into radiculomedullary veins.

arteries (Figs. 5-1 to 5-3 and 5-7 to 5-9). Ventrally, the anterior spinal axis is a long, usually continuous midline trunk that is 0.2 to 0.8 mm in diameter.[22] It arises near the foramen magnum by union of the paired anterior spinal branches of the vertebral arteries and courses caudad

within the anterior median fissure. It varies in caliber along its length, being relatively narrow in the thoracic region and widest inferior to the anastomosis with the artery of Adamkiewicz (0.5-1.0 mm).[1] The anterior spinal axis receives supplemental feeders at multiple, irregularly

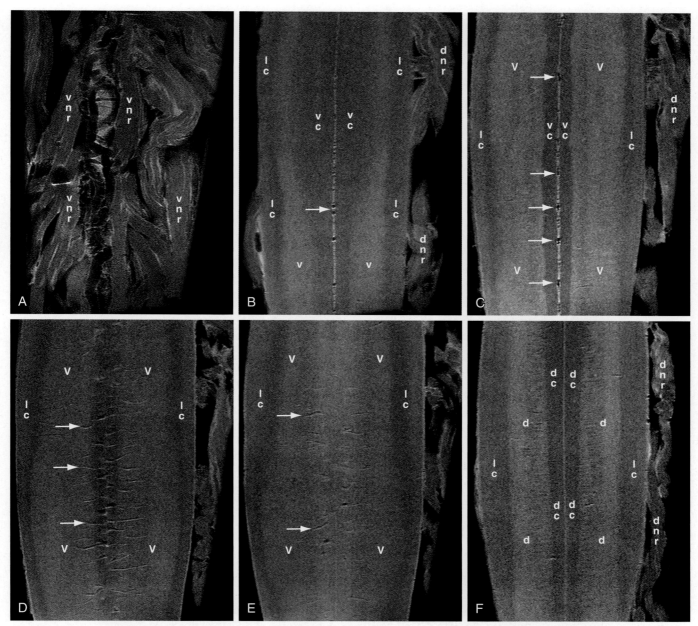

■ **FIGURE 5-8** Normal thoracolumbar spinal cord. Coronal postmortem 9.4-T MR images displayed from ventral (**A**) to dorsal (**K**). **A,** Vasculature of the ventral surface of the cord and the ventral nerve roots (vnr). **B** and **C,** The sulcomarginal vessels (*horizontal white arrows*) course dorsally through the ventromedian sulcus flanked, from medial to lateral, by the deep portions of the ventral white columns (vc), the gray matter of the ventral horns (v), and the anterior portions of the lateral columns (lc). Behind the ventralmost end of the ventral horn, the nerve roots seen about the cord are the dorsal nerve roots (dnr) passing ventrally toward their root sleeves. **D** and **E,** In these sections the deep extent of white matter of the ventral columns gives way to the gray matter that surrounds the central canal. The dorsal ends of the sulcomarginal arteries (*arrows*) ramify dorsolaterally into the ventral horns (v) and into the central gray matter (**E**). **F** and **G,** Dorsal to the central canal, the midline is formed by the glial dorsal median septum (*horizontal white arrows*). The dorsal horns (d) diverge dorsolaterally from near to the midline (in **E**) into the lateral portions of the dorsal cord (in **F**) to give rise to the dorsal nerve roots (dnr). They are flanked by the deep portions of the dorsal columns (dc) medially and the dorsal portions of the lateral columns (lc) laterally.

spaced intervals. These typically join the main arterial axis with a hairpin turn. One large feeder entering between C4 and C8 may be designated the artery of the cervical enlargement.[22] The largest supplementary feeder (arteria radicularis magna) typically arises between T9 and T12 and passes to the thoracolumbar enlargement. It may be designated the artery of the lumbar enlargement (i.e., the artery of Adamkiewicz).[22] Within the anterior median

fissure, the anterior spinal axis gives rise to numerous sulcomarginal branches that supply the anterior two thirds of the spinal cord, including most of the gray matter and much of the white matter.

At each feeder, the blood entering the anterior spinal axis is directed both craniad and caudad. This creates multiple less well-vascularized "watersheds" at the junctions of the feeder territories. At these watersheds, there-

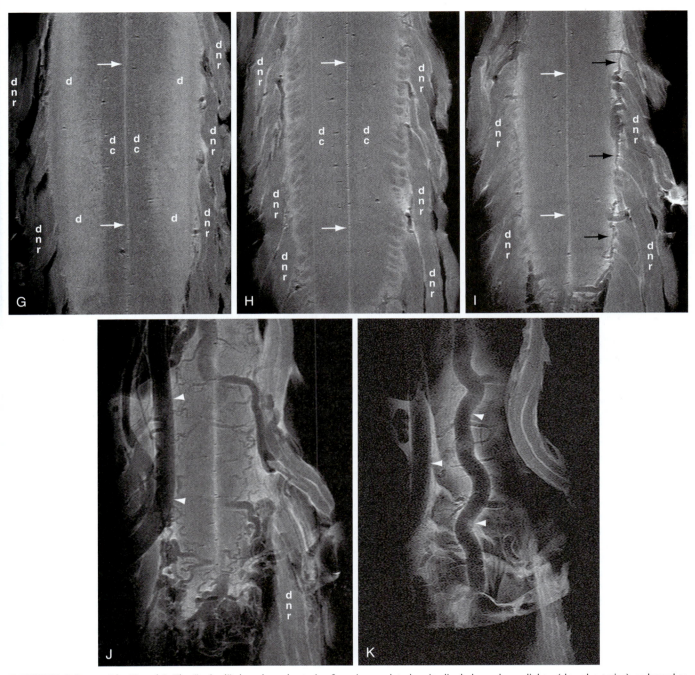

■ **FIGURE 5-8, cont'd** H and I, The "paired" dorsolateral arteries form incomplete longitudinal channels medial to (dorsal arteries) or lateral to (dorsolateral arteries) the dorsal root entry zones. The dorsal median septum (*white arrows*) separates the paired fasciculi graciles of the dorsal columns. J and K, The dorsal surface of the cord also displays a prominent dorsal vein (*arrowheads*) that exhibits a hairpin turn similar to that formed by the anterior spinal artery on the opposite side of the cord.

fore, flow within the anterior axis may be markedly reduced or nearly absent.

Dorsally, the paired arterial trunks form a variably complete plexus of longitudinal vessels (<0.5 mm in diameter) that course along the dorsal surface of the cord, either medial to (dorsal spinal arteries) and/or lateral to (dorsolateral spinal arteries) the entry of the dorsal nerve roots at the dorsolateral sulci.[22] The paired dorsal/dorsolateral trunks do not supply the spinal cord directly. Instead they feed into a circumferential pial vascular plexus called the vasocorona. The vasocorona then gives rise to multiple small arterial branches that enter each segment of the cord radially, perpendicular to the circumference of the cord, to supply the posterior one third of the spinal cord.[22]

Venous Drainage

The venous drainage of the spinal cord is more variable than the arterial supply and shows no real parallelism to

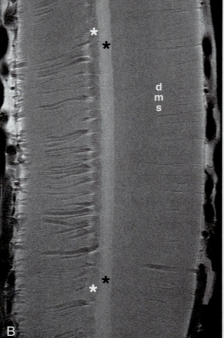
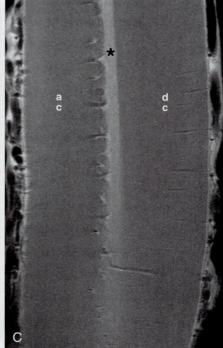

■ **FIGURE 5-9** Sulcomarginal arteries. Sagittal postmortem 9.4-T MR images. Midline (**B**) and flanking paramedian (**A**, **C**) sections oriented with ventral to the reader's left. Each sulcomarginal artery ascends dorsally into the ventral median sulcus, reaches the depth of the sulcus just anterior to the ventral white commissure (*white asterisks*), and branches outward, unilaterally, to the ipsilateral gray and white matter. Just dorsal to the ventral white commissure, the central gray matter (*black asterisks*) and gray commissures form the "horizontal" of the H. The anterior (ac) and dorsal (dc) columns of white matter and the dorsal median septum (dms) are also labeled.

the arterial tree (Figs. 5-2, 5-3, and 5-7 to 5-11).[22] On the ventral surface, a continuous anterior median spinal vein (0.4-1.0 mm) is located within the ventral median fissure, deep to the anterior spinal axis. This vein is largest in the lumbosacral region and, in 60% to 70% of cases, continues along the filum terminale as a very large terminal vein.[22] The anterior median spinal vein is typically larger than the corresponding anterior spinal axis.[1] The largest vein draining the anterior thoracolumbar cord is designated the great anterior radiculomedullary vein (see Fig. 5-2). This is easily mistaken for the artery of Adamkieciwz.[1]

On the dorsal surface, the most nearly constant vein is a large posterior median spinal vein. This is largest rostral to the thoracolumbar enlargement and continues into the cervical region.[22] It is easily recognized because it has a tortuous course at the dorsal aspect of the lumbar enlargement and because there is no posterior midline artery.[1,22]

A secondary system of short, smaller-caliber veins also courses along the surface of the spinal cord. The most nearly continuous of these are the anterolateral veins, which may replace the median veins wherever the median veins are interrupted.[22] An additional plexus of superficial transverse veins interconnects the longitudinal channels. The intrinsic veins of each segment drain outward, radially, to the superficial venous plexus. Within the spinal cord, true transmedullary anteroposterior venous anastomoses may arise from the ventral median vein, course through the ventral median fissure into the spinal cord, zigzag craniocaudad as they circle around the central canal, and then pass directly outward along

the dorsal median septum to enter the dorsal median vein (see Fig. 5-10). Such transmedullary venous anastomoses typically ascend rostrally as they pass from ventral to dorsal. They receive few, if any, veins draining from the spinal cord.

Gray Matter of the Spinal Cord

The gray matter of the spinal cord is composed of neurons, their terminal axons and dendrites (collectively designated neurites), and the neuroglial support cells.[21,24] The neurons may be designated intrasegmental if their processes remain within the same spinal segment, intersegmental if their processes extend over adjacent segments, and suprasegmental if their processes extend beyond the spinal cord into the brain. The neurons and neurites of the spinal cord interconnect widely across the midline commissures, so the paired halves of the spinal gray matter form one functional system (see Figs. 5-4 and 5-6A).[21,24]

In cross section, the spinal gray matter resembles an H or a "butterfly" with dorsal horns, ventral horns, and lateral horns (at T2-L1 levels only) (see Figs. 5-4 to 5-6). The volume of gray matter varies with the spinal level (see Fig. 5-5). The gray matter is most extensive at lumbosacral levels, where it supplies the lower extremities, perineum, and pelvis. It is thinnest in the thoracic region, where it supplies only the axial musculature, and second most prominent in the cervical region, where it supplies the shoulder girdle. The broad ventral horns are considered to have a base oriented toward the central canal and a

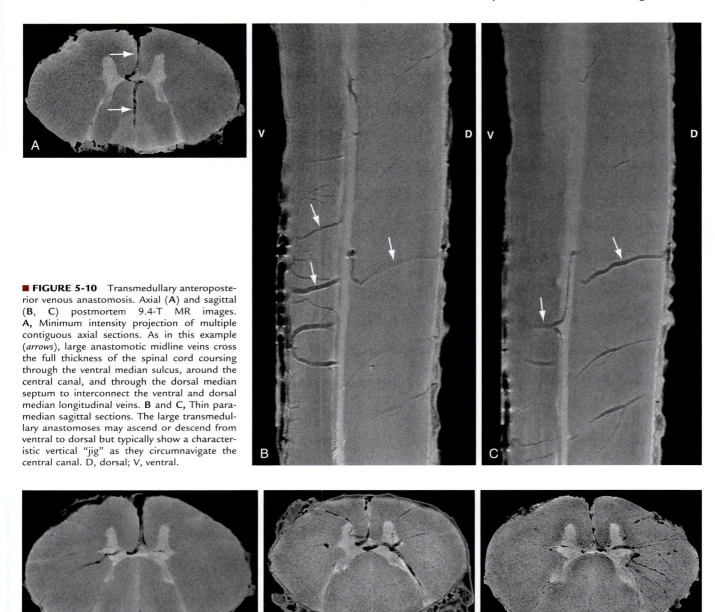

■ **FIGURE 5-10** Transmedullary anteroposterior venous anastomosis. Axial (**A**) and sagittal (**B, C**) postmortem 9.4-T MR images. **A**, Minimum intensity projection of multiple contiguous axial sections. As in this example (*arrows*), large anastomotic midline veins cross the full thickness of the spinal cord coursing through the ventral median sulcus, around the central canal, and through the dorsal median septum to interconnect the ventral and dorsal median longitudinal veins. **B** and **C**, Thin paramedian sagittal sections. The large transmedullary anastomoses may ascend or descend from ventral to dorsal but typically show a characteristic vertical "jig" as they circumnavigate the central canal. D, dorsal; V, ventral.

■ **FIGURE 5-11** Intrinsic vasculature of the cervical spinal cord seen on axial postmortem 9.4-T MR images. **A** to **C**, Composite minimum intensity projections of multiple contiguous axial sections emphasize the ventral supply via the ventral median sulcus, the presence of vessels oriented along the dorsal horns, and the radial array of the vasculature within the white matter.

large head that projects ventrolaterally. The narrow dorsal horns have a similar base near to the central canal, a constricted neck, an oval to fusiform head, and an apex that projects dorsolaterally (see Figs. 5-4 to 5-6). The junction of the dorsal and ventral horns centrally is designated the intermediate gray matter.

The spinal gray matter contains multiple specific nuclei. The most important of these are discussed below.

Dorsal Spinal Nuclei

Three major cell groups may be identified within the dorsal horns.[21,24]

- The nucleus marginalis (posteromarginal nucleus, marginal zone) is a thin superficial layer of neurons at the apex of the dorsal horn, projecting into the dorsolateral tract of Lissauer (see later). It is present at all levels and has prominent input from cutaneous nociceptors (Figs. 5-4, 5-12, and 5-13; see later discussion of Rexed lamina I).
- The substantia gelatinosa (of Rolando) lies just deep to the marginal nucleus. It is present at all levels. It receives afferents for pain and temperature from the entering dorsal nerve roots and connects with the spinothalamic tract to convey pain and temperature data onward to the brain (see Figs. 5-4, 5-6C, 5-12, and 5-13; see later discussion of Rexed laminae II and III).

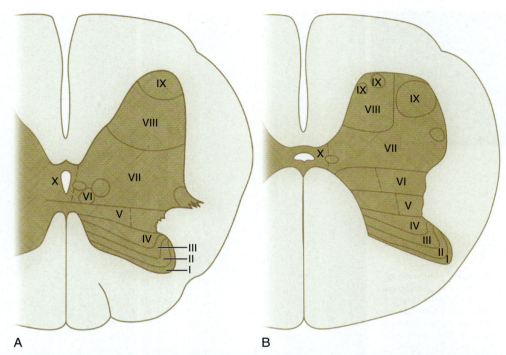

A   B

■ **FIGURE 5-12**   Rexed laminae of the thoracic (**A**) and lumbar (**B**) spinal cord. Diagrammatic representation. Roman numbers designate the approximate sites of the Rexed laminae of the gray matter in the cat. See text and the legend for Figure 5-13. *(Redrawn from Williams PL [ed]. Gray's Anatomy: The Anatomical Basis of Clinical Practice, 38th ed. Edinburgh, Churchill Livingstone, 1999.)*

● The nucleus proprius (proper sensory nucleus) is a prominent nucleus situated just deep to the substantia gelatinosa within the dorsal horn. It is present at all levels. It receives sensory impulses for light touch, among other modalities and corticospinal fibers for motor control (see Figs. 5-4, 5-6, 5-12, and 5-13; see later discussion of Rexed lamina IV).[3]

Intermediate Spinal Nuclei

Four major cell groups may be identified within the intermediate gray matter.

● The nucleus dorsalis of Clarke (nucleus thoracicus, Clarke's column) is found in the gray matter at the base of the dorsal horn, medially, along the length from C8 to L2[6] or even L3-L4.[21,24] It is largest in the lower thoracic and upper lumbar levels, where it may bulge medially into the dorsal funiculus (see Figs. 5-12 and 5-13). The nucleus dorsalis gives rise to the dorsal spinocerebellar tract (see later discussion of Rexed lamina VII).[3]

● The intermediolateral spinal nuclei occupy the lateral horn (column of Terni) that extends from approximately T1 to L2-L3. Neurons in this column send axons into the ventral spinal roots and, via white rami communicantes, to the sympathetic trunk.[21,24]

● An intermediate column of neurons in similar location at S2-S4 gives rise to the sacral preganglionic parasympathetic outflow. However, at this level, the cell column does not project laterally to form a lateral horn.[6,21,24]

● The intermediomedial column of neurons from T1-L2 receives pain afferents from the viscera.[6]

Ventral Spinal Nuclei

Three major groups of motor nuclei, designated the medial, central, and lateral longitudinal cell columns, may be identified within the ventral gray matter. These columns extend over multiple segments, either as long columns that are continuous throughout the cord or as island-like aggregations of cells in specific spinal locations.[21,24]

● The medial cell column extends along the length of the spinal cord, except at L5 and S1. The medial motor group innervates the axial musculature of the trunk, including the erector spinae dorsally and the flexors of the trunk ventrally.[21,24]

● The central cell column is found in limited cervical and lumbosacral segments. From C1 to C5-C6, neurons in the central column form the spinal accessory nucleus. At C3-C7, central neurons constitute the phrenic nucleus that innervates the diaphragm.[21,24]

● The lateral cell column is most prominent at the cervical and lumbar enlargements. It innervates the musculature of the upper and lower extremities.[21,24]

Rexed Laminae

The Swedish neuroscientist Bror Rexed classified the spinal gray matter into 10 cytoarchitectonic zones.[12-14] These Rexed laminae (RLs) I to X are organized from dorsal to ventral as successive strata of gray matter that extend along most of the length of the cord (see Figs. 5-12 and 5-13). RL I forms the most dorsal portion of the dorsal horn. RL IX forms the most ventral portion of the ventral horn, and RL X forms the central gray matter that

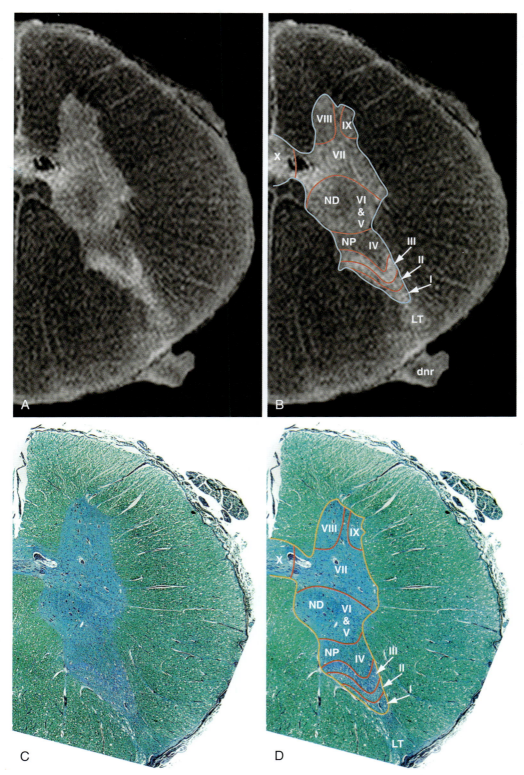

■ **FIGURE 5-13** Rexed laminae. **A,** Axial postmortem 9.4-T MR image of the thoracic hemicord. **B,** Luxol Fast Blue stain of the same specimen. **C** and **D,** Rexed laminae delineated on **A** and **B**. RLs I to X extend across the full thickness of the gray matter, as shown in Figure 5-12. RL I corresponds to the nucleus marginalis. RLs II and III correspond to the substantia gelatinosa. RL IV contains the nucleus proprius (NP). RLs V and VI are not distinguishable in humans. The full extent of RL VII is better depicted in Figure 5-12. At spinal levels C8 to L2, the nucleus dorsalis (ND) (of Clarke, Clarke's column) lies at the base of RL VII medially. In the distal cord, RL VIII lies medially and RL IX laterally within the ventral horn, interspersed within the broad RL VII. RL X corresponds to the gray matter about the central canal. The dorsolateral fasciculus (tract) of Lissauer (LT) lies at the entry of the dorsal nerve roots (see also Figs. 5-5B and 5-6).

surrounds the central canal.[6] Integrated over the length of the spinal cord, these laminae may be regarded as 10 long columns of gray matter, layered sequentially, each one cradling the next.

Anatomic Organization

- RLs I to VI lie within the dorsal horns. The neurons in these layers receive sensory information entering via the dorsal (sensory) nerve roots and transmit it onward.[6] RL I is a thin layer of marginal cells sometimes designated the marginal nucleus.[6] RLs II and III correspond to the substantia gelatinosa. RL IV contains the nucleus proprius.[11] RLs V and VI give rise to many propriospinal neurons and cannot be distinguished from each other in humans.[11]
- RL VII is in the intermediate gray matter and adjoining ventral horn. It contains the nucleus dorsalis of Clarke and the intermediomedial and intermediolateral cell columns.[6]
- RL VIII lies within the ventromedial portion of the ventral horn. Many of its neurons send commissural axons to the opposite side of the spinal cord.
- RL IX lies within the ventral horn. It contains motor cell columns from which alpha, beta, and gamma motor neurons send their axons into the ventral motor roots to innervate skeletal muscle.[6]
- RL X surrounds the central canal.

Functional Organization

- RLs I to IV are the major reception zones for cutaneous primary afferent nerves and their collateral branches. In turn, these give rise to long afferent tracts that ascend to higher levels and to complex polysynaptic intrasegmental and intersegmental pathways that course ipsilaterally or contralaterally.[21,24]
- RLs V to VI are major reception zones for both primary proprioceptive afferent fibers and corticospinal projections to the spinal cord from the motor and sensory cortices. This anatomic conjunction indicates that these laminae play a substantial role in controlling motor function.[21,24]
- RL VII (lateral portion) has extensive ascending and descending connections with the midbrain and cerebellum for regulating posture and movement. RL VII (medial portion) has numerous propriospinal connections with gray matter segments concerned with movement and autonomic function.[21,24]
- RL VIII is largely composed of propriospinal interneurons that receive ipsilateral fibers from adjacent laminae, commissural fibers from the contralateral RL VIII, and descending fibers from the reticulospinal tract, vestibulospinal tract, and the medial longitudinal fasciculus. It appears to influence and coordinate motor neurons of both the left and right sides.[21,24]
- RL IX contains alpha and gamma motor neurons and many interneurons involved with activity and control of the motor units of striated muscles.[21,24]
- RL X is the gray matter surrounding the central canal plus the dorsal and ventral gray commissures and the substantia gelatinosa centralis.[21,24]

White Matter of the Spinal Cord

The spinal white matter contains nerve fibers, neuroglia, and blood vessels.[21,24] Those nerve fibers that are well myelinated appear white. Nonmyelinated and lightly myelinated nerve fibers appear gray, hence the terms *white commissure* and *gray commissure* to indicate different groups of fibers crossing the midline near to the central canal.

The white matter tracts are typically considered in three groups: propriospinal tracts, long ascending tracts, and long descending tracts (Fig. 5-14).[21,24] The major propriospinal tracts lie immediately external to the gray matter of the spinal cord within each of the ventral, lateral, and dorsal columns. The major ascending tracts include the fasciculi gracilis and cuneatus in the dorsal columns, the spinocerebellar tracts in the lateral columns, and the spinothalamic tracts in adjoining portions of the ventral and lateral columns ("anterolateral" columns). The major descending tracts include the corticospinal and vestibulospinal tracts in the ventral and lateral funiculi, and possibly a minor contribution from the rubrospinal tract in the dorsal portion of the lateral funiculus.[21,24]

Propriospinal Tracts

Propriospinal tracts (fasciculi proprii) are intersegmental tracts that arise from neurons in the dorsal and ventral horns, travel in the white matter immediately external to the gray matter, and link nearby and distal segments of the spinal cord to integrate local reflexes into coordinated body movement and visceral function.[6,21,24] Most spinal neurons are actually propriospinal neurons and are found predominantly within RLs V through VIII. By definition, the axons of propriospinal neurons remain confined to the spinal cord. Among other roles, the propriospinal system is responsible for the automatic functions that continue after the spinal cord is transected (e.g., sudomotor and vasomotor activities, bowel and bladder function). Many axonal projections of neurons in the substantia gelatinosa (RL II) and in RL VIII stay within the gray matter of their own laminae, so they do not contribute to the propriospinal pathways.[6]

The propriospinal fibers of humans are considered in three groups: ground bundles, the dorsolateral tract (of Lissauer), and the ventral white commissure of the spinal cord.[21,24]

Ground Bundles

Ground bundles are fasciculi proprii that descend or ascend within their own fasciculus. The ventral, lateral, and dorsal ground bundles, therefore, lie solely within the ventral, lateral, and dorsal columns, respectively.

The ventral ground bundle extends the length of the cord and is the first spinal tract to myelinate.[21,24] Within it, individual fibers vary in length from one segment to the full extent of the cord. The shortest fibers lie immediately adjacent to the gray matter. Longer fibers lie more peripherally. All the fibers of the ventral ground bundle terminate in the ventral gray matter throughout the cord.

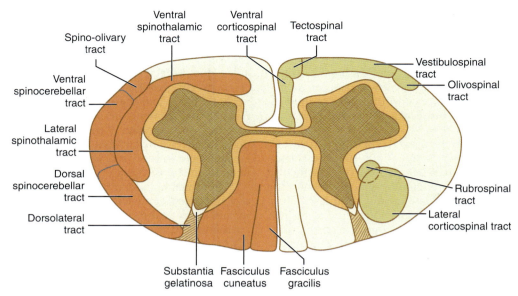

■ **FIGURE 5-14** Overview of the white matter tracts of the spinal cord. The propriospinal fibers (*pale orange*) hug the external surface of the gray matter. They include the ventral, lateral, and dorsal ground bundles (*no hatching*) that course solely within their own funiculi, the dorsolateral tract (fasciculus) of Lissauer (*cross hatched*) that courses intersegmentally at the dorsal root entry zone, and the ventral white commissure in the midline. The ascending fiber tracts (*dark orange*) include the fasciculi gracilis and cuneatus in the dorsal columns, the dorsal spinocerebellar tract, ventral spinocerebellar tract, and spino-olivary tract that form the lateral surface of the lateral columns, and the ventral and lateral spinothalamic tracts that lie between the ground bundles and these superficial tracts in the lateral and ventral columns. The descending fiber tracts (*yellow-green*) include the ventral and lateral corticospinal tracts, the vestibulospinal tracts, and the rubrospinal tracts, as well as other smaller bundles. (*Modified from Williams PL [ed]. Gray's Anatomy: The Anatomical Basis of Clinical Practice, 38th ed. Edinburgh, Churchill Livingstone, 1999.*)

The lateral ground bundle also extends the length of the cord, but it is particularly well developed in the cervical and lumbar enlargements.[21,24] The individual fibers arise mainly from the intermediate gray and dorsal gray matter of the cord. The fibers have variable length, course craniad or caudad, pass ipsilateral or contralateral to their cells of origin, and have many collaterals throughout the gray matter.

The dorsal ground bundle comprises only the fine unmyelinated fibers of the fasciculi proprii, which ascend and descend through the posterior white columns.[21,24] They probably arise from cells of the posterior gray columns and are distributed to the gray matter of the medial part of the posterior gray column.

Dorsolateral Tract

The dorsolateral tract (of Lissauer) consists of fine myelinated (white) and unmyelinated (hence gray) fibers that surround the entering fibers of the dorsal nerve roots. The tract runs the length of the cord in the dorsolateral zone between the dorsolateral sulcus on the cord surface and the apex of the posterior gray horn.[6,11,21,24] It is best developed in the upper cervical region. The small, less well-myelinated and unmyelinated dorsal root fibers that enter through the lateral portion of the dorsal root entry zone bifurcate into ascending and descending branches that enter the dorsolateral tract. These send collaterals to multiple dorsal horn cells. In addition, the dorsolateral tract contains many propriospinal fibers, including short axons of small neurons of the substantia gelatinosa, which then re-enter the posterior gray column.

The White and "Gray" Commissures

Myelinated fibers that cross the midline ventral to the central canal are designated the ventral white commissure.[11] Short and long spinal fibers in this pathway include fibers of the ascending spinothalamic tract and the descending anterior corticospinal tract.[6] Unmyelinated (hence gray) fibers cross the midline dorsal and ventral to the central canal in the anterior and posterior gray commissures.[11] In this sense, the term *gray* signifies unmyelinated white matter, not gray matter.

Ascending Fiber Tracts

The ascending fiber tracts of humans are grouped by location into those of the dorsal columns, ventral columns, and combined portions of the anterior and lateral columns, designated the anterolateral columns.[21,24]

Dorsal Columns

The fasciculus gracilis begins at the caudal end of the spinal cord. It is composed of long ascending fibers arising from the dorsal spinal roots of coccygeal, sacral, lumbar, and lower thoracic segments.[21,24] These fibers ascend topographically, with fibers from the most caudal roots situated most medially, directly against the median septum, and fibers from sequentially higher roots applied successively along the lateral border of those fibers that entered more caudad. A significant contingent of ascending gracile fibers from the lower limb exits the fasciculus gracilis at L2-L3 to synapse in the caudal end of the dorsal nucleus of Clarke (Clarke's column, nucleus thoracicus) at approximately L2. From there, secondary fibers form the dorsal spinocerebellar tracts that convey proprioception to the cerebellum via the inferior cerebellar peduncle. The gracile fibers that continue past Clarke's column terminate at the cranial end of the fasciculus gracilis by synapsing within the nucleus gracilis in the lowermost medulla. From there, secondary fibers ascend through the medial lemniscus to the ventral posterolateral nucleus of the thalamus.

The fasciculus cuneatus begins at the midthoracic level. From approximately T6 superiorly, a posterointermediate septum demarcates the lateral border of the fasciculus gracilis and separates the fasciculus gracilis from the medial border of the fasciculus cuneatus. The fasciculus cuneatus is composed of long ascending fibers arising from the dorsal spinal roots of upper thoracic (above T6) and cervical segments. The cuneate fibers also array themselves somatotopically, with caudal fibers situated medial to those fibers entering more cephalically.[21,24] Some cuneate fibers end by synapsing within the nucleus cuneatus at the cranial end of the fasciculus cuneatus in the lower medulla. From there, secondary fibers ascend through the medial lemniscus to the ventral posterolateral nucleus of the thalamus. Other cuneate fibers terminate by synapsing within the lateral (external, accessory) cuneate nucleus situated just superolateral to the cuneate nucleus within the medulla. Secondary fibers from the lateral cuneate nucleus ascend through the cuneocerebellar tract to the cerebellum.

The gracile and cuneate fasciculi mediate proprioception (position and kinesthesia) and exteroception (touch pressure) as well as vibration.[6] Within the caudal portions of the fasciculi gracilis and cuneatus, the ascending afferent fibers are organized by dermatome. As they ascend, the fibers re-sort into a somatotopic pattern that is preserved through all sequential synapses into the primary sensory cortex of the brain. The fibers of fasciculi gracilis and cuneatus show no, or minimal, overlap, so each fasciculus should be regarded as a separate anatomic entity.[6,21,24]

Lateral Columns (Dorsal and Ventral Spinocerebellar Tracts; Spinothalamic Tracts)

Dorsal Spinocerebellar Tract

The dorsal spinocerebellar tract begins at approximately L2-L3, ascends through the spinal cord to the medulla, and extends to the cerebellum via the inferior cerebellar peduncle (Figs. 5-14 and 5-15).[6,11,21,24] It consists of axons arising from large neurons of the dorsal nucleus of Clarke (Clarke's column, nucleus thoracicus) situated within RL VII of spinal segments T1-L2 (or perhaps as low as L3-4).[21,24] Two different components of fibers relay through Clarke's nucleus to pass into the dorsal spinocerebellar tract. Ascending fibers of the dorsal roots of segments caudal to L2 first pass superiorly within the fasciculus gracilis, exit the gracilis at approximately L2-3, and enter the caudal end of Clarke's column at approximately L2. Additional dorsal root fibers from the more cephalic segments L2 to T1 enter Clarke's column directly, segmentally, at sequentially higher levels. Both sets of fibers relay within Clarke's column.[6,11,21,24]

The dorsal spinocerebellar tract ascends through the peripheral part of the lateral funiculus, lateral to the corticospinal tract and ventral to the dorsolateral fasciculus (of Lissauer) (see Figs. 5-14 and 5-15). Because new fibers are added at each level, the dorsal spinocerebellar tract thickens progressively as it ascends. The new, more cephalic fibers join the deep aspect of the tract, so fibers from lower segments lie superficial to fibers from more rostral segments (Fig. 5-16).[6,11,21,24] At the medulla, the dorsal spinocerebellar tract traverses the inferior cerebellar peduncle to reach the cerebellum and terminates ipsilaterally in the rostral and caudal vermis.

The dorsal spinocerebellar tract conveys proprioceptive and exteroceptive information from the lower extremity and trunk to the cerebellum. Similar data for the upper extremity and neck pass to the cerebellum via the fasciculus cuneatus and the cuneocerebellar tract. Proprioceptive and exteroceptive information from the upper limb travels in primary afferent fibers of the fasciculus cuneatus. These fibers end somatotopically in the accessory cuneate nucleus and the adjoining cuneate nucleus. Cells of these nuclei give rise to the cuneocerebellar tract that enters the cerebellum via the inferior cerebellar peduncle. The accessory cuneate nucleus and the lateral part of the cuneate nucleus are considered to be homologous to the dorsal nucleus of Clarke, so the cuneocerebellar tract is functionally allied to the posterior spinocerebellar tract (but for the upper extremity).[11]

Ventral Spinocerebellar Tract

The ventral spinocerebellar tract begins in the sacral region. Primary afferent fibers for proprioception and exteroception pass from the dorsal roots of the lumbosacral segments into fasciculus gracilis. They then exit gracilis and enter the ipsilateral spinal gray matter to synapse on cells in RLs V to VII of the lumbosacral cord. These cells give rise to secondary fibers that (mostly) decussate through the ventral commissures to enter the ventral spinocerebellar tract (although a few fibers remain ipsilateral). The ventral spinocerebellar tract ascends through the peripheral portion of the lateral funiculus, ventral to the dorsal spinocerebellar tract. Within the ventral spinocerebellar tract new fibers joining the tract are applied somatotopically to the deep aspect of the tract, so fibers from upper segments lie deep to fibers from more caudal segments (see Figs. 5-14 and 5-16). At high cervical levels, the fibers of the ventral spinocerebellar tract shift dorsally to intermingle with those of the dorsal tract. Therefore, most ventral spinocerebellar fibers enter the inferior cerebellar peduncle to reach the cerebellum. Only a small medial component of the anterior tract ascends through the brain stem and passes around the superior cerebellar peduncle to reach the cerebellum. This component terminates mainly contralaterally in the anterior cerebellar vermis.[6,11,21,24]

Rostral Spinocerebellar Tract

The rostral spinocerebellar tract begins in the cervical enlargement from cells in the intermediate zone of the spinal gray matter. It ascends in the dorsal portion of

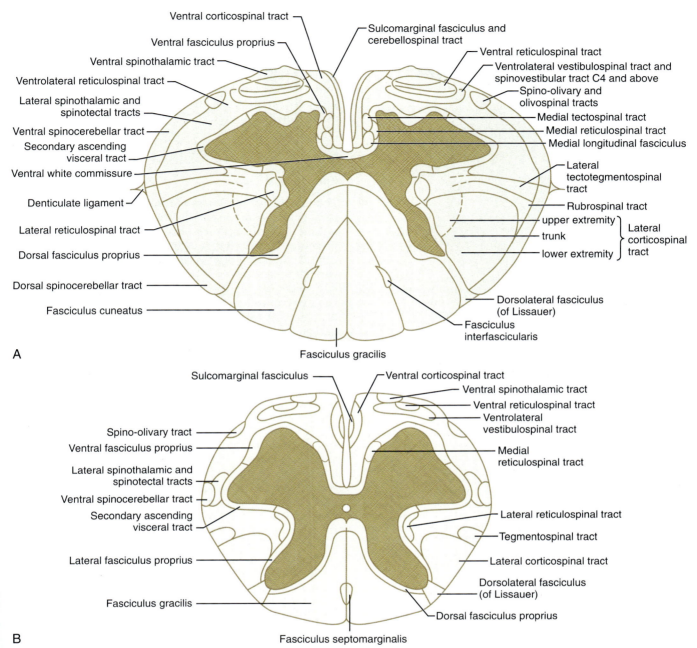

A

B

■ **FIGURE 5-15** More detailed presentation of the white matter tracts. This figure presents the distribution and relative sizes of the major and minor white matter tracts at the midcervical (**A**) and lumbar (**B**) spinal neural segments. *(Adapted from Crosby EC, Humphrey R, Lauer EW. Correlative Anatomy of the Nervous System. New York, Macmillan, 1962.)*

the lateral funiculus and terminates with the fibers of the ventral spinocerebellar tract.[6,11,21,24] It is the upper extremity counterpart of the ventral spinocerebellar tract.

The dorsal, ventral, and rostral spinocerebellar tracts and the cuneocerebellar tract all end in the midline vermis and the intermediate zone of the cerebellum, especially the anterior lobe and the caudal portion of the posterior lobe.[5]

Although the ventral and dorsal spinocerebellar tracts both convey proprioceptive and exteroceptive information to the cerebellum, they serve different functions.[6,11,21,24] In the dorsal spinocerebellar tract, the proprioceptive signals often arise from one muscle or a few synergistic

muscles acting at one joint. Thus, the dorsal spinocerebellar tract transmits modality-specific and space-specific information that is used in fine coordination of posture and movement of individual limb muscles. The ventral spinocerebellar tract does not differentiate among modalities or segments of a limb, so the ventral spinocerebellar tract conveys signals for the coordinated movement and posture of the entire lower limb.

Spinothalamic Tracts

The anterior and lateral spinothalamic tracts lie within the anterior and lateral funiculi along both sides of the ventral

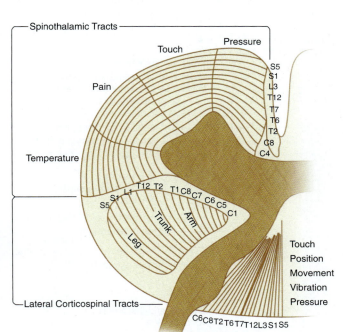

■ **FIGURE 5-16**   Overall somatotopy of the white matter tracts. In the dorsal columns, the fibers of fasciculi gracilis and cuneatus are arrayed with the most caudal fibers situated medial to more cranial fibers. In the dorsal portion of the lateral columns, the fibers of the crossed lateral corticospinal tract are arrayed with the most caudal (longest) fibers situated superficial to more cranial (shorter) fibers. In the anterolateral fasciculus, the fibers of the spinothalamic tracts are arrayed with the most caudal fibers situated superficial to more cranial fibers. These arrangements can be understood as follows. In the dorsal columns, the entering ascending fibers are first layered against the median septum. Therefore, all fibers entering at higher levels are just layered onto the lateral surface of those already there. In the crossed lateral corticospinal tract, the descending fibers traveling the greatest distance course superficial to those traveling a shorter distance. In the anterolateral fasciculus, the ascending spinothalamic fibers first arise on the contralateral side and then cross through the ventral white commissure to reach the opposite side. Therefore, all new fibers must enter deep to those already there, so they layer onto the deep aspect of the existing fibers. (*Adapted from Foerster O. Motorische Felder und Bahnen. In Bumpke O, Foerster O [eds]. Handbuch der Neurologie. Berlin, Springer-Verlag, 1936, vol 6, pp 1-357.*)

nerve roots.[6,11,21,24] Thin dorsal root fibers for pain and temperature enter the spinal cord through the lateral portion of the dorsal root entry zone. These divide into ascending and descending fibers that course in the dorsolateral tract of Lissauer and then pass to RL I (marginal nucleus), RL II (substantia gelatinosa), and RLs III to V. Axons from RLs I and V cross the midline via the anterior white commissure within one segment of their origin and then ascend through the anterolateral quadrant of the spinal white matter to reach the thalamus. The spinothalamic fibers are organized topographically. Fibers crossing at any level join the deep aspect of the tract formed by those that already crossed, so fibers of upper segments lie deep to those of more caudal segments. Because of a slight spiral twist, the superficial fibers become progressively more dorsal as they ascend. Somatotopy is maintained within the brain stem, as the fibers of the anterior spinothalamic tract join the medial lemniscus to reach the thalamus, while the fibers of the laterall tract ascend through the spinal lemniscus to the thalamus.[6,11,21,24] Within the thalamus, fibers conveying pain and temperature sensa-

tion from the lower limb extend dorsally, whereas those for the trunk and upper limb lie more ventrally. Classically, the anterior spinothalamic tract carries impulses for crude tactile and pressure modalities, whereas the lateral spinothalamic tract carries fibers for pain and temperature. However, the positions of the fibers are not known precisely, so the "two" tracts are best considered together as one functional unit.[11,21,24]

Descending Fiber Tracts

Corticospinal Tracts

The majority of the fibers of the corticospinal tracts arise from cells situated in the upper two thirds of the precentral motor cortex (Brodmann area [BA] 4) and from the premotor cortex (BA 6). A small contribution arises from cells of the postcentral gyrus (BA 3, 1, 2) and the adjacent parietal cortex (BA 5). These pass caudad into the medullary pyramids on the anterior surface of the medulla. Each pyramid contains about a million fibers of varying diameter. At the level of the pyramidal decussation, the descending corticospinal fibers follow one of three separate paths.[3,21,24]

Seventy-five to 90 percent of the descending pyramidal fibers do decussate and cross to the contralateral side to form the crossed lateral corticospinal tract. This tract lies within the dorsolateral portion of the lateral funiculus. It runs caudad for the length of the spinal cord and decreases in size progressively to end at about the S4 neural segment. In the cervical and thoracic regions, the crossed lateral corticospinal tract lies medial to the posterior spinocerebellar tract. In the lumbar and sacral regions (where there is no posterior spinocerebellar tract), the crossed lateral corticospinal tract reaches the surface of the cord. These crossed lateral corticospinal fibers terminate on cells in the lateral portions of RLs IV to VI, VII, and IX on the same side as the tract.

Ten to 25 percent of the corticospinal fibers do not decussate and descend ipsilaterally within the anterior funiculi as the uncrossed anterior corticospinal tracts to the cervical and upper thoracic levels. The anterior corticospinal tracts are stated to lie immediately to each side of the ventromedian fissure, medial to the medial longitudinal fasciculus (see Figs. 5-15 and 5-16).[11] However, in the 38th edition of *Gray's Anatomy*, the ventral corticospinal tract is shown to be separated from the ventral median fissure by the intervening sulcomarginal fasciculus.[24] At each spinal level, the fibers for that level exit the anterior corticospinal tract, mostly cross the midline through the anterior white commissure, and synapse with spinal neurons on the contralateral side. As a result, both the crossed lateral and the uncrossed anterior corticospinal tracts innervate neurons on the side opposite their side of cortical origin, even though these fibers decussate at different levels (pyramidal decussation vs. segmental spinal decussation).

A third portion of the corticospinal system descends through the corticomedullary junction without decussating and passes inferiorly in the anterior portion of the lateral funiculus as the uncrossed lateral corticospinal tract.[3] These remain uncrossed to innervate ipsilateral spinal neurons.

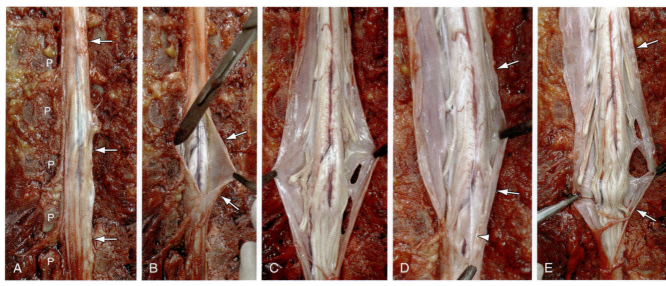

■ **FIGURE 5-17** Spinal meninges of an unfixed adult human cadaver. **A,** Removal of the lumbar vertebral bodies exposes the ventral aspect of the dura mater (*white arrows*) and the dural root sleeves exiting beneath the pedicles (P). The spinal cord and anterior spinal axis are seen faintly through the dura. **B,** Sharp incision (*scalpel*) of the dura (*white arrows*) exposes the ventral surface of the intact arachnoid mater and the contained spinal cord. The artery of Adamkiewicz executes a characteristic hairpin turn as it supplies the anterior spinal axis. **C,** Opening the dura widely exposes the glistening inner aspect of the dura mater, the sheen reflecting from the intact ventral arachnoid, the arachnoid sheaths for the nerve roots, the multiple radiculomedullary vessels passing along the roots to and from the spinal cord, and the proximal cauda equina. **D,** Delicately raising the ventral arachnoid (*tip of forceps* and *white arrowhead*) demonstrates the thin, separate, nearly transparent quality of the arachnoid mater. **E,** Incising and reflecting the arachnoid mater opens the subarachnoid space and exposes the pial-lined ventral surface of the distal spinal cord, conus medullarris, and proximal cauda equina. The nerve root bundles are now seen passing to the nerve root sleeves. Remnants of the arachnoid are still evident in some places.

The descending corticospinal fibers are arranged in lamellae, with longer fibers situated at the periphery of the tract and shorter fibers placed more medially. Overall, approximately 55% of all pyramidal fibers supply the cervical cord, 20% supply the thoracic cord, and 25% supply the lumbosacral cord.[3]

Vestibulospinal Tracts

The vestibular nuclei give rise to the descending lateral and medial vestibulospinal tracts.[21,24]

Individual portions of the lateral vestibular nucleus of the brain stem give rise to fibers that descend somatotopically to each of the cervical, thoracic, and lumbar segments of the cord. The lateral vestibulospinal fibers descend ipsilaterally, first in the periphery of the anterolateral funiculus and then in the medial portion of the anterior funiculus, to terminate in the medial ventral horn, RL VII, and medial RL VIII.[21,24]

Neurons within the medial vestibular nucleus (and some within the inferior and lateral vestibular nuclei) of the brain stem send fibers into both the ipsilateral and contralateral medial longitudinal fasciculi. These crossed and uncrossed fibers descend into the cervical and upper thoracic cord, where they lie ventrolateral to the uncrossed anterior corticospinal tracts. The medial vestibulospinal tracts project mainly to the cervical cord segments, ending in the posterior portion of RL VII and in the adjoining RL VIII.[21,24]

Functionally, the medial and lateral vestibulospinal tracts participate in posture and motor control.[21,24] Lateral vestibulospinal fibers excite motor neurons of the extensor muscles of the neck, back, and limbs and inhibit motor neurons of the flexor limb muscles. Medial vestibulospinal fibers mainly inhibit motor neurons innervating the axial muscles of the neck and upper back.[21,24]

Rubrospinal Tracts

In primates, neurons of the magnocellular layer of the red nucleus of the midbrain give rise to rubrospinal fibers that cross the midline in the ventral tegmental decussation of the brain stem and descend into the lateral funiculus of the upper three segments of the cervical spinal cord.[21,24] Within the cord, these fibers lie anterior to and intermingle with fibers of the lateral corticospinal tract. The rubrospinal tract is important in other mammals but appears to regress with development of the corticospinal system in humans.[21,24]

The positions of other smaller white matter tracts are illustrated in Figures 5-14 and 5-16 for completeness, although their discussion is beyond the scope of this chapter.

II. THE SPINAL MENINGES

Grossly, the spinal meninges consist of four meningeal sleeves concentrically arrayed around the spinal cord. From superficial to deep these are (1) the thick external dura mater; (2) the thin, subjacent arachnoid mater; (3) a highly fenestrated, incomplete "intermediated layer" situated along the deep aspect of the arachnoid, between the arachnoid and the pia; and (4) the deep pia mater that invests the spinal cord (Figs. 5-17 to 5-21).[25-40] The spinal dural sleeve is a thick, vascularized connective tissue layer that extends from the foramen magnum to the filum

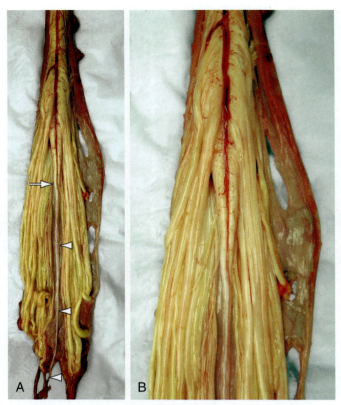

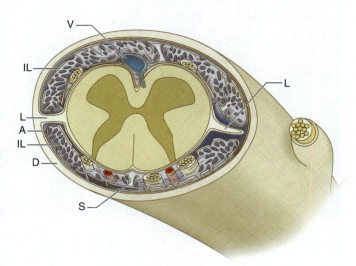

■ **FIGURE 5-18** Conus medullaris, cauda equina, and filum terminale. **A,** Distal cord and cauda equina. **B,** Magnified portion of **A**. Same specimen as in Figure 5-17 (but different lighting conditions). Opening the arachnoid and gently brushing the roots of the cauda equina to each side exposes the conus medullaris tapering down to the midline filum terminale (*arrowheads*). The termination of the conus (*arrow*) and transition to filum terminale show substantial individual variation but typically occur at the L1 vertebral level (see below). The roots of the cauda equina are arrayed symmetrically with those roots exiting more proximally situated lateral to those extending further caudally. In vivo, the descending roots of the cauda lie far closer to the midline, enclose the tip of the conus and the proximal filum terminale, and sometimes obscure their location.

■ **FIGURE 5-19** Diagrammatic representation of the human spinal cord with surrounding meninges. The arachnoid mater (A) is closely applied to the thick outer dura (D). An intermediate leptomeningeal layer (IL) lies between the arachnoid mater and the pia mater. This layer is fenestrated and is attached to the inner aspect of the arachnoid mater. It is reflected to form the dorsal septum (S). The intermediate layer spreads over the surface of the cord and is connected to blood vessels, nerve roots, and pia mater by fine trabeculae. Dentate ligaments (L) are present on either side of the cord and are covered by a layer of pia arachnoid. The collagenous core of the dentate ligament fuses with the subpial collagen medially and (at intervals) with the dural collagen laterally, as shown on the left side of the diagram. Blood vessels (V) within the subarachnoid space are coated by a leptomeningeal sheath continuous with the pia mater. (*Reproduced from Nicholas DS, Weller RO. The fine anatomy of the human spinal meninges. A light and scanning electron microscopy study. J Neurosurg 1988; 69:276-282. This image and its labels have been inverted from the original to place ventral anatomy toward the top in accord with the other images in this chapter.*)

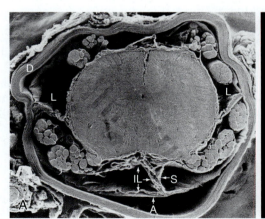

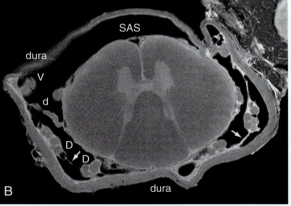

■ **FIGURE 5-20** Spinal meninges and cord. Two fixed cadaveric specimens. **A,** Scanning electron micrograph of the lumbar spinal cord of a 15-month-old child. The intermediate leptomeningeal layer (IL) is closely applied to the inner aspect of the arachnoid (A). It reflects to form the dorsal septum (S) and arborizes over the dorsal surface of the cord. The dentate ligaments (L) are seen on each side of the cord; that on the left of the image merges with the dura (D). On the other side the free margin of the dentate ligament abuts upon the arachnoid mater. **B,** Intermediate-weighted postmortem axial MR image at 9.4 T shows many of the same features: the thick dura (dura), subarachnoid space (SAS), encapsulated bundles of dorsal (D) and ventral (V) roots to each side of the denticulate ligament (d), and a membrane (*white arrows*) that stretches across the subarachnoid space to link the root bundles. (*A, Reproduced from Nicholas DS, Weller RO. The fine anatomy of the human spinal meninges. A light and scanning electron microscopy study. J Neurosurg 1988; 69:276-282. This image and its labels have been inverted from the original to place ventral anatomy toward the top in accord with the other images in this chapter.*)

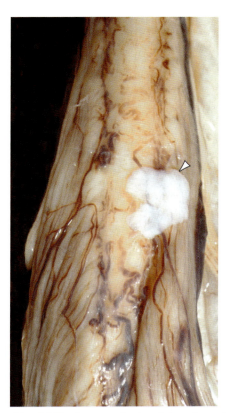

■ **FIGURE 5-21** Calcific plaque on the dorsal thoracic arachnoid. Fixed postmortem specimen. Opening the dura discloses the thin plate of calcification loosely adherent to the surface of the arachnoid. The spinal cord, roots, and vasculature are normal.

cranial arachnoid. The intermediate layer of the spinal meninges does not appear to be present in the cranial meninges, and the spinal pia mater is thicker, firmer, and less vascular than the cranial pia.[25,27]

The spinal dura mater is formed by (1) *a thin, outer dural border cell layer* composed of fibroblasts, loose collagen, and elastic fibers oriented mostly parallel with the flat surface of the dura; (2) *a middle highly vascularized fibrous layer* of interwoven lamellae of extracellular collagen and elastic fibers oriented at diverse angles; and (3) *an inner dural border cell layer* composed of flat cells oriented mostly parallel with the inner surface of the dura.[27,28] The inner dural border cells (DBC) interdigitate with each other but are not connected to each other by cell junctions. There is sparse extracellular collagen and multiple large extracellular spaces between the inner dural border cells. The inner DBC layer is easily disrupted, so shearing between inner dural border cells is thought to "create" the artifactual subdural space seen in disease.[27,28] In the dura, the extracellular collagen is organized into interwoven lamellae that are wrapped spirally around the spinal axis to provide tensile strength.[27]

The arachnoid mater is formed by *an outer layer of arachnoid barrier cells* and *an inner, more collagenous layer* of loosely arranged arachnoid reticular cells. The arachnoid barrier cell (ABC) layer has no extracellular collagen.[27] It displays tightly packed cells interconnected by numerous desmosomes and gap junctions, varying numbers of intermediate filaments, and a distinct continuous basal lamina that separates its deep surface from the underlying collagenous arachnoid reticular cell layer.[27] The ABC layer is believed to be the effective morphologic and physiologic barrier between the blood circulating within the dura mater and the cerebrospinal fluid within the subarachnoid space.[27]

The pia mater is formed by a "continuous" layer of flat pial cells, 3 to 6 cells thick, joined together by desmosomes and other specialized junctions. The pia invests the outer surface of the spinal cord, the ventral median sulcus, the conus medullaris, the filum, and the nerve roots.[29] The pial surface exhibits variable numbers of fenestrations along the conus medullaris and the nerve roots, with fewer fenestrations at the thoracolumbar junction and none in the upper thoracic cord.[29] The presence and number of pial fenestrations vary considerably. Pial cells are absent within the fenestrations, so the basal membrane is the only continuous structure interposed between the cerebrospinal fluid and the neural cells.[29] The pia is separated from the neuroglia of the spinal cord by a subpial layer of collagen, sparse elastic fibers, and amorphous material. This subpial layer is thickest at the thoracic and lumbar cord and thinner at the conus medullaris, proximal cauda equina, and nerve roots.[29]

The arachnoid trabeculae that interconnect the pia-arachnoid across the subarachnoid space (SAS) show mixed features. The core of each trabecula is formed by collagen and amorphous intercellular substance that merge directly into the collagenous subpial layer of the spinal cord. These cores are covered by leptomeningeal cells, which may be conceptualized in two ways. In one view, the deep layer of the arachnoid is considered to be covered by a layer of flattened branching arachnoid

terminale, invests the filum terminale, and continues along the filum to the coccyx, where it merges into the periosteum of the coccyx. Laterally the dura continues outward around the nerve roots as the dural root sleeves. The spinal arachnoid sleeve is a thin avascular layer that is intimately related to—and in direct contact with—the deep aspect of the dura mater. There is no anatomic subdural space between the dura mater and the arachnoid. The arachnoid mater encloses the spinal subarachnoid space and extends trabeculae across the subarachnoid space toward the pia mater. Thin isolated plaques of arachnoid calcification are found on the arachnoid in 43% to 73% of routine autopsies (see Figs. 5-19 and 5-21).[26] The intermediate layer of leptomeninges forms a fenestrated, lace-like layer that lines the deep aspect of the arachnoid and extends inward across the subarachnoid space.[25] The intermediate layer thickens focally to form dorsal, dorsolateral, and ventral ligaments that anchor the spinal cord to the arachnoid.[25] The spinal pia mater is a dual-layered membrane composed of an inner (deep) *pia intima* that is adherent to the nervous tissue and an outer (more superficial) *epipial layer* that is continuous with the arachnoid trabeculae. The blood vessels of the spinal cord lie within the epipial layer.[25]

Histologically, the spinal meninges closely resemble the cranial meninges.[27] However, the dorsal spinal dura lacks the rich innervation present in the cranial dura. The spinal arachnoid shows a richer collagen content than the border cells.[27] These arachnoid border cells may be considered to extend from the deep layer of the arachnoid onto the arachnoid trabeculae. Alternatively, where the arachnoid trabeculae merge into the subpial layer of the spinal cord, pial cells can be seen to overlap arachnoid cells and are not differentiable from arachnoid cells histologically.[29] Thus, it is not clear whether leptomeningeal "trabecular" cells are arachnoid cells, pial cells, or both at different sites.[27]

The intermediate leptomeningeal layer is loosely attached to the inner aspect of the arachnoid (see Fig. 5-20). From there, it reflects inward to form a series of dorsal and ventral septae that reach the surface of the spinal cord. These then arborize bilaterally to envelop the surface of the spinal cord, surround the nerve roots, and enclose the blood vessels.[25] The intermediate layer is a highly fenestrated, discontinuous sheet of cells, especially laterally over the nerve roots and blood vessels. The series of broad discontinuous dorsal leaflets formed by the intermediate layer appear to account for the "septum posticum" demonstrated myelographically and for the freely communicating "arachnoid pouches" in the dorsal thoracic spine.[25,30]

Denticulate Ligaments

The denticulate ligaments are symmetric pairs of lateral ligaments that suspend the spinal cord from the dura mater (Figs. 5-22 and 5-23). They usually number 21 pairs, but range from 18 to 24 pairs. Histologically, the denticulate ligaments consist of a collagenous core that is thinner where it connects to the subpial collagenenous layer of the spinal cord medially and thicker where it connects to the dura mater laterally.[21-25] The collagen core is covered by pia-arachnoid that is continuous with the spinal cord medially and the arachnoid laterally. The highest denticulate ligament is cord-like and inserts into the lateral border of the foramen magnum between the vertebral artery anteriorly and the hypoglossal nerve posteriorly. The spinal portion of the spinal accessory nerve passes posterior to it. The other denticulate ligaments are triangular in shape and are spaced evenly along the length of the spinal cord. Each triangle has its base aligned vertically along the equator of the spinal cord, between the exit/entry sites of the ventral and dorsal roots, and has its apex directed laterally to attach to the dura about 2 mm dorsal and 3 mm cephalic to the neural foramen. Over the length of the spinal canal, sequentially, each denticulate attachment lies slightly closer to the neural foramen inferior to it than does the ligament just cephalic to it. The most inferior denticulate ligament ends at the level of the conus medullaris, between the emerging fibers of the T12 and L1 segmental roots. The pia of the lowest denticulate ligament fuses with the filum terminale at this level.[21-24]

The denticulate ligaments influence the effect of masses on the spinal cord. Masses expanding anterior to the cord first press against the anterior columns of the cord and then deflect the cord posteriorly.[31] The posterior deflection pulls taut the attachments of the denticulate ligaments to the lateral spinal cord, exerting pressure on the lateral columns. In such cases, the posterior columns

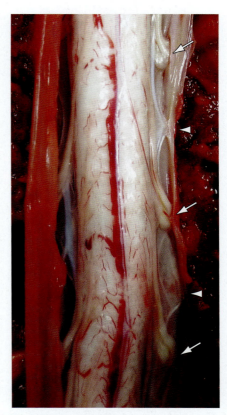

■ **FIGURE 5-22** Ventral view of the denticulate ligaments. Unfixed cadaveric specimen. The triangular denticulate ligaments have their bases aligned vertically along the equator of the cord and extend laterally to insert their apices (*white arrowheads*) into the inner aspect of the dura at spaced intervals between the meningeal sleeves of the nerve roots (*white arrows*). Proximally, the dorsal and ventral roots course laterally, each to its own side of the denticulate ligament. Distally, the nerve roots cross over the narrower free margins of the ligaments to enter the root sleeves.

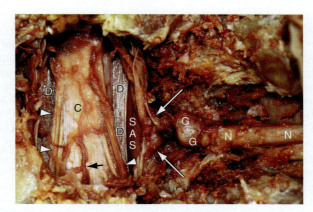

■ **FIGURE 5-23** Dorsal view of the denticulate ligament in situ. Fixed cadaveric specimen. Dissection of the back and entry into the dorsal subarachnoid space (SAS) discloses the denticulate ligaments (D) passing from the lateral margin of the spinal cord (C) toward the lateral dura, where they attach posterosuperior to the dural root sleeve. The dorsal nerve roots (*white arrowheads*) traverse the subarachnoid space dorsal to the denticulate ligaments and cross the free lateral edge of the ligament, inferior to its lateral attachment, en route toward the next lower root sleeve. At this level, dissection of the root sleeve (*white arrows*) shows the bilobed dorsal root ganglion (G) and the segmental intercostal nerve (n) distal to it. The posterior median vein (*black arrow*) makes a hairpin turn on the dorsal surface of the spinal cord.

CHAPTER 5 ● *The Normal Spinal Cord and Meninges* **131**

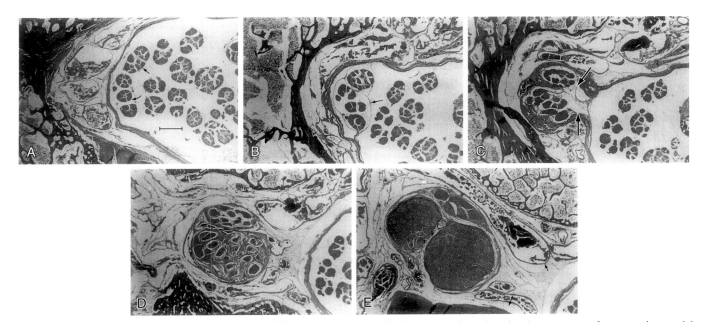

■ **FIGURE 5-24** Exiting nerve roots. Photomicrograph of dura and nerve roots of the human cauda equina, showing a sequence from rostral to caudal as the spinal nerve roots leave the dural sac (H and E stain). **A,** The enclosing membranes of the three exiting dorsal root bundles have fused (*curved arrow*). The membrane of the single ventral root bundle is clearly evident (*arrow*). Large veins fill the spinal canal just outside the dura (scale bar = 1 mm). **B,** More distally, the ventral and dorsal root membranes (*arrow*) have fused and attached to the dura. **C,** The roots leave the dural sac through a single evagination dragging along a subarachnoid pocket (*arrows*). The root bundles are dissociating into their component fascicles. **D,** The nerve roots are fully separated from the dural sac and enclosed in a sheath. The individual fascicles are no longer grouped as bundles and are each surrounded by a tubular extension of the subarachnoid space. **E,** The dorsal root ganglion forms in two masses, with the ventral root adjacent and ventral to it. A large vein (*arrows*) passes through the intervertebral foramen ventral to the neural structures. (*Reproduced from Hogan Q, Toth J. Anatomy of soft tissues of the spinal canal. Reg Anesth Pain Med 1999; 24:303-310. Please note that each figure part (A-E) has been inverted from the original image to display ventral and dorsal in the standard imaging orientation.*)

suffer least stress. Posteriorly situated masses cause the inverse effect. However, the denticulate ligaments are thickest in the cervical spine and less thick caudally, so, inferior to T8, posterior masses may displace the spinal cord against the anterior wall of the spinal canal before the denticulate ligaments become taut. Denticulate ligaments also limit cord motion from side to side. Lateral displacement of the cord tightens the denticulate ligaments before there is tension on the segmental ventral or dorsal nerve roots.

The denticulate ligaments absorb caudally directed forces better than cranially directed forces.[31] Superior masses cause detectable caudal shift of the cord for only 6 to 7 segments below the mass, whereas inferior masses cause detectable cranial shift of the cord for 10 to 11 segments above the mass. In postmortem studies, the upper cervical denticulate ligaments allow a maximum of 1 cm of inferior displacement of the cord from extreme upward to extreme downward position.

Nerve Roots

Within the subarachnoid space (SAS), the nerve roots of the cauda equina are composed of minor elements (fascicles) that are grouped into gross structures (bundles) (see Figs. 5-17, 5-18, 5-24, and 5-25). From 1 to 10 fascicles are joined together into a bundle by encircling pia-arachnoid that appears as a fine membrane. The dorsal

roots contain 1 to 5 principal bundles, usually 2 to 3 bundles.[32] In most cases the ventral roots are composed of 1 bundle and are smaller than the corresponding dorsal roots.[32] As the exiting root bundles extend laterally, the limiting pia-arachnoid membranes of the individual dorsal and the ventral bundles fuse together to form a common, distended sheath that loosely surrounds all of the fascicles of all the exiting dorsal and ventral roots. These almost always pass into a single trough of dura that surrounds the roots as they exit the sac. Rarely the dorsal and ventral roots pierce the dura through two separate sleeves.[32] Within the dural sleeve, the root bundles dissociate into their component fascicles, each surrounded by a tubular extension of the subarachnoid space and each separated from the others by connective tissue. The extent to which the dorsal roots separate into individual fascicles proximal to the dorsal root ganglion varies among individuals. The dorsal root ganglia are almost always bilobed, even when more than two bundles emerge from them.[32] The ventral motor root passes adjacent and ventral to the ganglion. Lateral to the ganglion, multiple peripheral fascicles of the dorsal root ganglion fuse with the ventral root to form the segmental mixed nerve at each level.[32] As the roots extend further outward, ventrally and laterally, the dura closes around the root bundles to constitute the dural sleeve.[32] Electron microscopy discloses fat within the epidural space around the root sleeves, fat interwoven within the layers of the dura mater of the sheath, fat within and around small fascicles of nerve roots within the dural

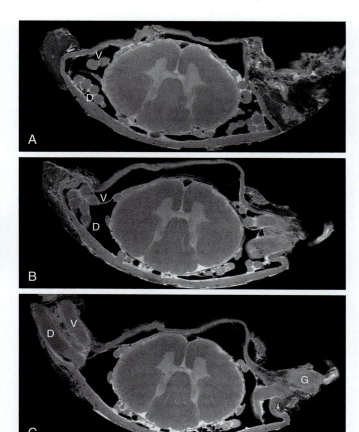

■ **FIGURE 5-25** Exiting nerve roots. A-C, Serial axial MR images of the thoracic spinal cord and exiting nerve roots displayed from cranial (A) toward caudal (C). A, Four bundles of dorsal roots (D) and two bundles of ventral roots (V) lie within the thecal sac dorsal and ventral to the denticulate ligament. B, The ventral and dorsal root bundles enter a common sheath lateral to the free edge of the denticulate ligament. C, The root bundles coalesce into two nerve roots within the sheath. The dorsal root ganglion (G) is shown on the contralateral side.

sleeves, but no fat actually interposed between the axons of the nerve roots.[33]

Variant Nerve Roots

Conjoined Nerve Roots

Conjoined nerve roots are adjacent nerve roots that share a common dural sleeve at some point during their exit from the thecal sac.[34] According to Neidre and MacNab, variant roots may be classified into four types (Fig. 5-26, A to G).

Type 1 anomalies have two adjacent roots that arise from a common dural sheath, with each root ultimately exiting through its expected neural foramen.

Type 2 anomalies have two adjacent nerve roots that arise either separately or together from the thecal sac, with both roots exiting together through the same neural foramen. The adjacent foramen may be empty (type 2a) or may also contain a nerve root (type 2b).

Type 3 anomalies show plexiform anastomoses with adjacent roots linked by a connecting root.

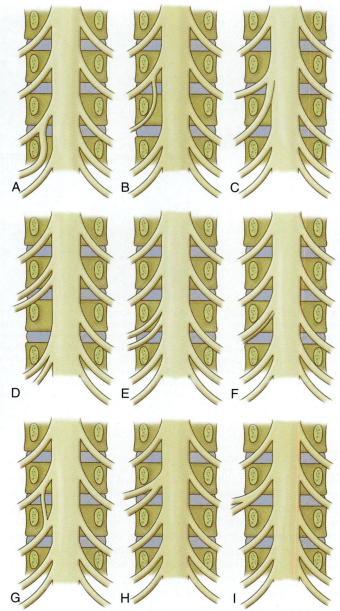

■ **FIGURE 5-26** Anomalous nerve roots. Diagrammatic representations. A-G, Conjoined nerve roots. Conjoined roots are nerve roots that form plexiform arrays with neighboring roots and/or that exit the spinal canal anomalously in conjunction with neighboring roots. They may be classified as types 1 to 4. A to C, Type 1 anomalies have two adjacent roots that arise from a common dural sheath, with each root ultimately exiting through its expected neural foramen. Conjoined roots arising at usual angles are type 1A, while upper roots arising at nearly right angles are type 1B. Per Neidre and MacNab, A and B would be classified as type 1A, whereas C would be classified as type 1B. D to F, Type 2 anomalies have two adjacent nerve roots exiting through the same neural foramen. D would be classified as type 2A, whereas E and F would be classified as type 2B. G, Type 3 anomalies show plexiform anastomoses between adjacent roots. G would be classified as type 3. Type 4 anomalies are those combining features of both type 2 and type 3. H and I, Furcal roots. Furcal roots are single roots that have split or forked into two portions. They are subclassified as intraforaminal (H) or extraforaminal (I) by the point of bifurcation. (*Parts A to G are compiled from Figures 1 to 3, pages 294 to 295 from Neidre A, MacNab I. Anomalies of the lumbosacral nerve roots. Review of 16 cases and classification. Spine 1983; 8:294-299. H and I, reproduced from Figure 13 page 92 of Scuderi GJ, Vaccaro AR, Brusovanik GV, et al. Conjoined lumbar nerve roots. A frequently underappreciated congenital anomaly. J Spinal Disord Tech 2004; 17:83-93.*)

Type 4 anomalies exhibit any combination of the first three types.

Conjoined roots are found in approximately 0.5% to 4% of imaging studies and have been reported in up to 14% of one postmortem study.[34-37] The roots most frequently conjoined are L5 with S1 (50% of cases) and S1 with S2 (33% of cases).[34,36] In one MR study of 12 cases with conjoined roots, the roots affected were S1-S2 (75%), L5-S1 (16.7%), and L3-L4 (8.3%).[37] Other levels are affected rarely. Conjoined roots occur equally frequently on the left and the right sides and in males and females.[34] Spinal anomalies such as retroisthmic clefts and hypoplastic/absent pedicles concur infrequently.[34]

Imaging features suggesting conjoint roots include a wide lateral recess of the bony canal, asymmetric contour of the anterolateral corner of the thecal sac (corner sign), a curvilinear layer of fat interposed between the dural sac and the anomalous root sleeve (the fat crescent), and an anomalously long, horizontal course of one nerve root extending far laterally, within and lateral to the neural foramen on a single axial section (parallel root).[37] Less frequently one may see both nerve roots and/or dorsal root ganglia within a single widened neural foramen and dual, not single, concavities for the ganglia along the posterior bony wall of the neural foramen.[38] In sagittal images through the neural foramen, conjoined roots compressed by herniated disc may show a band of neural tissue connecting adjacent roots immediately dorsal to the disc (shoulder sign).[39]

Bifurcation Anomalies

Bifurcation anomalies are splitting or forking of single nerve roots, either medial to the lateral edge of the pedicle (intraforaminal form) or lateral to the pedicle (extraforaminal form) (see Fig. 5-26, H and I). Bifurcation anomalies are most common at L3 and L4 levels, are commonly bilateral, and are often multiple.[34,40]

IMAGING

CT

There is very little role for routine CT in the display of the spinal cord unless MRI is contraindicated. CT angiography has real utility for assessing the vascularity and perfusion of the spinal cord (see Special Procedures).

MRI

MRI is the primary modality for imaging the spinal cord. At present, clinical MRI at 1.5 and 3.0 T does not yet achieve the fine resolution and anatomic detail of the postmortem 9.4-T images shown earlier in this chapter (see Figs. 5-5 to 5-10 and 5-13). Standard sagittal images at 1.5 T display the length and width of the spinal cord at each level (Fig. 5-27). A 3D (volumetric) gradient-recalled-echo series depicts finer detail of the gray matter and the white matter of the normal cervical spinal cord (Fig. 5-28). Standard axial T1-weighted and T2-weighted (T1W, T2W) images display the normal relationships within the neural foramina (Fig. 5-29). Fast imaging employing steady-state

acquisition (FIESTA) and constructive interference in steady state (CISS) sequences demonstrate finer detail of the nerve roots within the subarachnoid space in relationship to surrounding structures, including the denticulate ligament, nerve roots, and root sleeves (Figs. 5-30 and 5-31).

Terminations of the Conus Medullaris and Thecal Sac

The terminations of the spinal cord and the thecal sac are classified by the vertebral and disc levels at which they lie (Fig. 5-32). These terminations show a wide range of normal variation and some gender variation (Figs. 5-33 and 5-34).[41-45]

Conus Medullaris

In 300 consecutive spinal MR images from 150 males and 150 females aged 1 to 89 years Righi and Naidich showed that the modal termination for the conus medullaris was L1 for both males and females (63%).[41] The range of normal variation was from T11-T12 to L2-L3 and was wider in females (see Fig. 5-33). The study showed that 84% of cords ended between the T12-L1 disc level and the L1-L2 disc level, inclusive. Only 5.5% ended at the L1-L2 disc level itself. In a later study of 136 MR images from 47 males and 89 females McDonald and associates similarly found a modal termination at L1 (57%), and a range of variation from mid T11 to mid L3.[42]

The tip of the conus shifts slightly with patient position. As patients change from supine to lateral decubitus position, the tip of the conus shifts anteriorly in all patients and to the dependent side in 77% of patients.[43] The mean anterior shift is 6.3 mm (standard deviation (SD) 2.2 mm), and the mean lateral shift is 1.63 mm (SD 1.2 mm).[43] The emerging roots of the cauda equina shift with the conus as patients change position.

Thecal Sac

Righi and Naidich found that the modal termination of the thecal sac was S2 (63%), with 85% of sacs terminating between upper S1 and lower S2.[41] The range of variation was from above S1 to lower S3 and was wider in females (see Fig. 5-34).[41] McDonald and coworkers similarly found a modal termination at S2 (60%) and a range of variation from upper S1 to upper S4.[42] The terminal thecal sac usually displays a long and tapering shape (78% in males, 72% in females) but can normally appear short and rounded (17% in males, 23% in females) or bullet shaped (5% in males, 5% in females).[41] In pediatric patients, bending the spine from neutral to flexion may raise the tip of the thecal sac one-third of a vertebral height, from a mean of termination at mid S2 to a mean termination at upper S2.[44] In an anatomic study of 27 cadavers dissected specifically to assess the level of termination of the thecal sac, Hansasuta and associates found that most fila fused with the dura in the midline at S2 (range: lower L5 to upper S3).[45] Four fila (15%) fused above S1. Three fila (11%) fused approximately 1 cm off midline.[45]

Text continued on p. 138

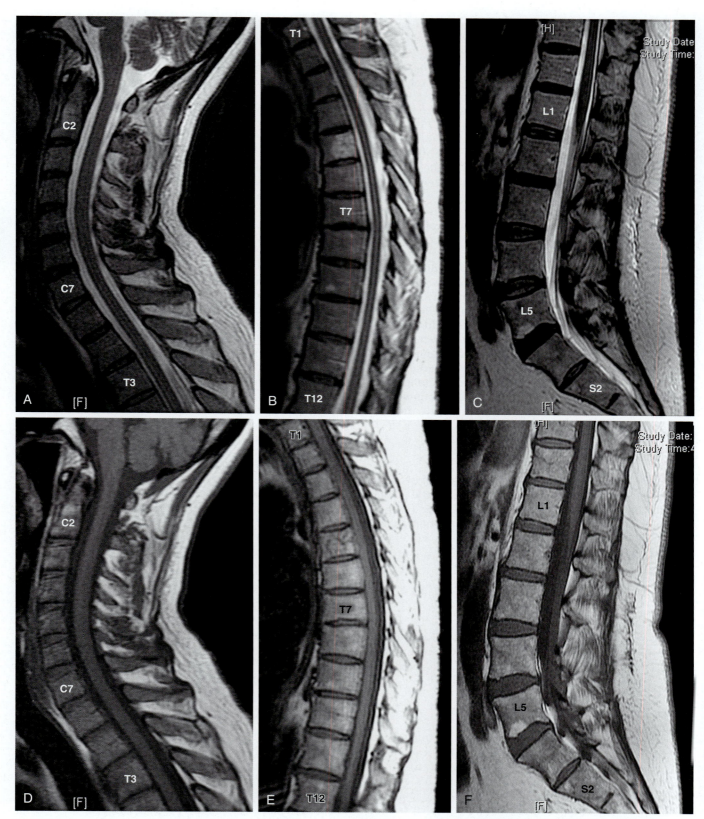

■ **FIGURE 5-27**   Sagittal 1.5-T MR images of the spinal cord. **A** to **C**, T2W images of the cervical (**A**), thoracic (**B**), and lumbar (**C**) spine. **D** to **F**, Corresponding T1W images. The specific vertebral levels are indicated on the images. A hemangioma is present within the T5 vertebral body. A rudimentary disc is present at S1-S2.

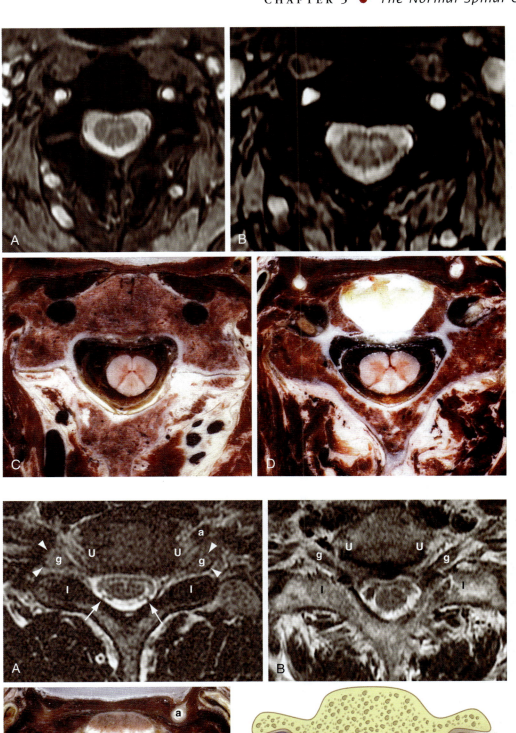

■ **FIGURE 5-28** Cervical spinal cord. **A** and **B**, Axial 1.5-T clinical MR images at C3 and C4. 3D Multiple-echo-recalled gradient-echo (MERGE) technique. **C** and **D**, Axial cryomicrotome specimens matched to **A** and **B**. The MR images display the "butterfly" contour of the ventral and dorsal horns of the spinal gray matter in relation to the ventral, lateral, and dorsal columns of white matter.

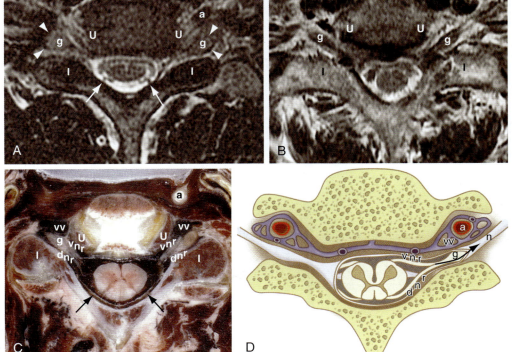

■ **FIGURE 5-29** Cervical spinal cord, nerve roots, and dorsal root ganglia. **A** and **B**, Axial T2W MR images at C6-C7 and C7-T1. **C**, Cryomicrotome image matched to **A**. **D**, Diagrammatic representation of the anatomy. Note the spinal cord within the subarachnoid space, the ventral median sulcus (compare with Fig. 5-17A, D), the dural sheath of the thecal sac (*black arrows*), the dorsal (d) and ventral (v) nerve roots (nr), and the dorsal nerve root ganglion (g) and veins (vv) within the neural foramina. The neural foramina lie between the uncinate processes (U) of the cervical vertebrae and the inferior articular processes of the facet (zygapophyseal) joints. a, the vertebral artery within the foramen transversarium. *White arrows* indicate the dorsal nerve roots within the subarachnoid space. (*D, modified from Daniels DL, Haughton EM, Naidich TP (eds). Cranial and Spinal Magnetic Resonance Imaging: An Atlas and Guide. New York, Raven Press, 1987.*)

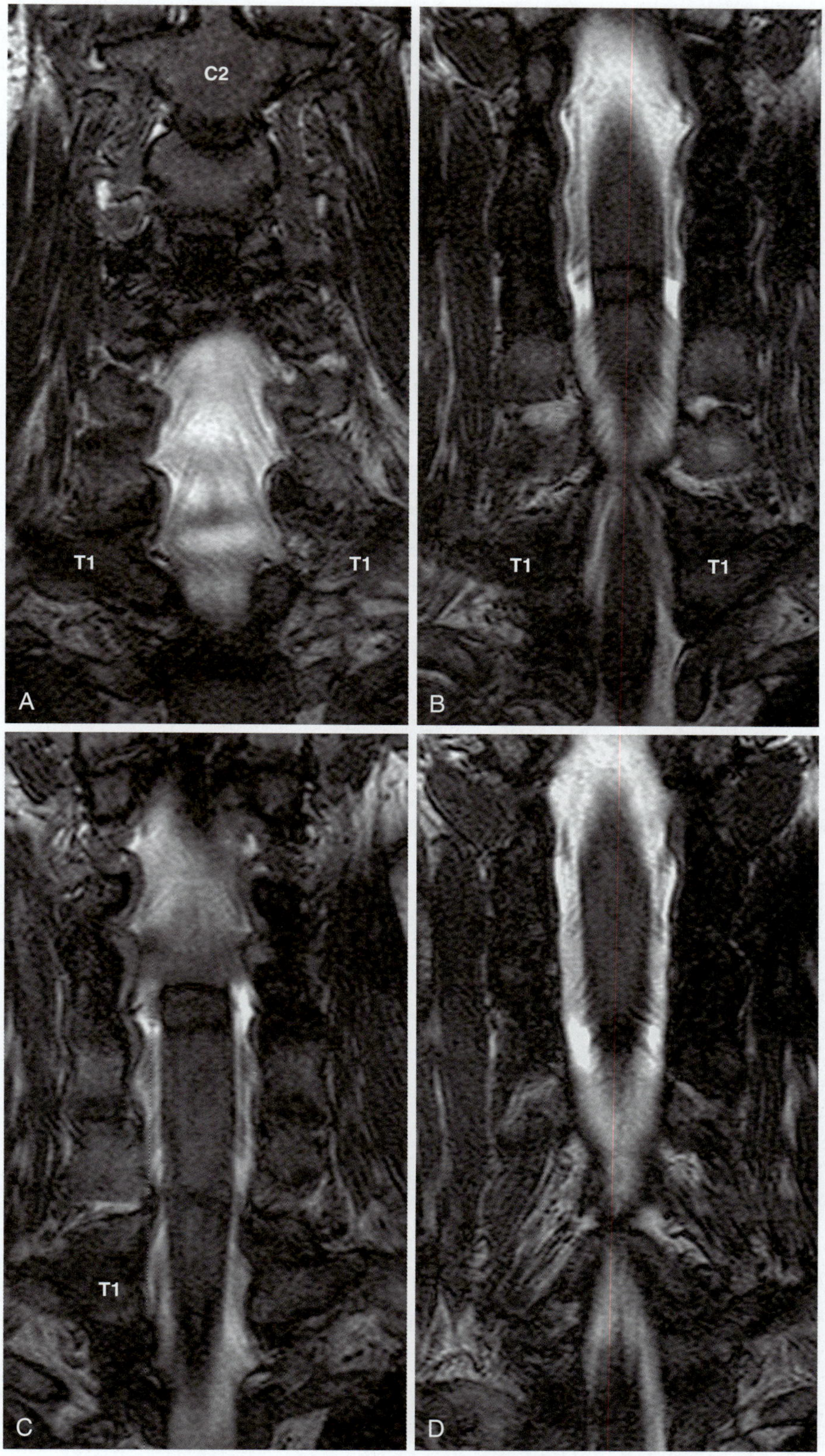

■ **FIGURE 5-30** *Cervical spinal cord. Coronal high resolution T2W MR images displayed from ventral (**A**) to dorsal (**D**). The cervical enlargement at C4-C7 and the emerging segmental ventral and dorsal nerve roots are well displayed.*

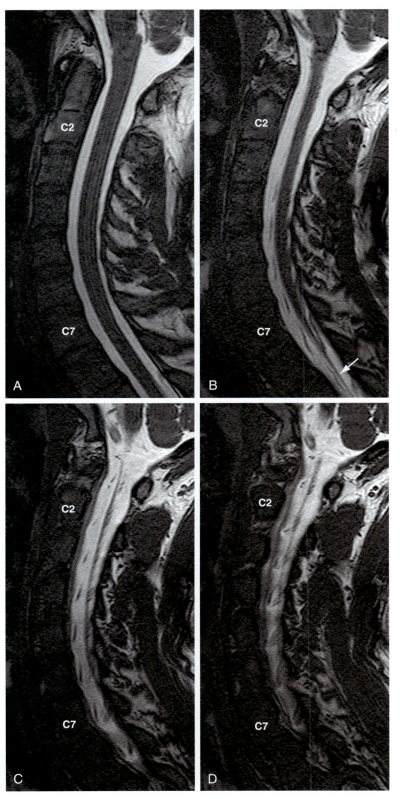

■ **FIGURE 5-31** Cervical spinal cord. Sagittal high-resolution T2W MR images displayed from medial (**A**) to lateral (**D**). The pial denticulate membrane (*arrow,* **B**) extends from the equator of the cord to the lateral wall of the arachnoid mater. It forms an *incomplete* transverse band that partially divides the arachnoid sac into ventral and dorsal compartments. The thinner motor roots arise from the ventrolateral surface of the cord and extend laterally, entirely ventral to the denticulate ligament. The broader, brush-like sensory roots arise from the dorsal root ganglia and extend medially, entirely dorsal to the denticulate ligament to reach their entry zone along the dorsolateral surface of the cord.

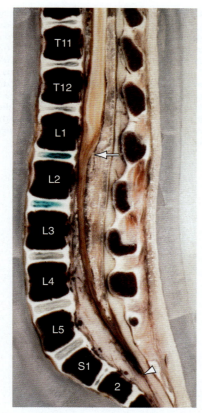

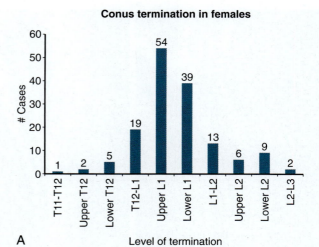

Conus termination in females

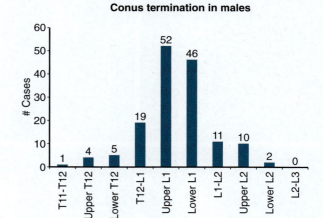

Conus termination in males

■ **FIGURE 5-32** Terminations of the conus medullaris (*arrow*) and thecal sac (*arrowhead*). Sagittal cryomicrotome specimen. To identify the positions of these landmarks, the spine is first analyzed to detect and characterize transitional vertebrae that might require especially careful use of nomenclature. The level at which the conus medullaris transitions into the filum and the level at which the thecal sac terminates are then given in terms of the nearest disc level or the nearest portion of vertebra at which they lie. In this example, the tip of the conus medullaris lies at lower L1 and the tip of the thecal sac lies at lower S2. The conal-dural interval is 6 vertebrae.

■ **FIGURE 5-33** Termination of the conus medullaris. Distribution of the termination of the conus medullaris by vertebral level in 150 females **(A)** and 150 males **(B)** of all ages. *(Reprinted from Righi A, Naidich TP. The normal termination of the thecal sac. Internat J Neuroradiol 1996; 2:188-195.)*

Conal-dural Interval

In most cases (77%) the tip of the dural sac at its junction with the filum lies six segments lower than the caudal end of the spinal cord.[41] The conal-dural interval varies very narrowly from 5 segments (8.5%) to 6 segments (77%) to 7 segments (8.8%), but not more. Thus the terminations of both the cord and the thecal sac shift together, systematically and concordantly, with both ending high, or low, together.

T1 and T2 Relaxation Times, Magnetization Transfer Ratios, Myelin, and Water Content

T1

In-vivo measurements of the T1 relaxation times of the human cervical spinal cord at 3.0 T by both inversion recovery (IR) techniques and B₁-corrected double flip-angle gradient-recalled-echo (GRE) techniques show a significant difference between the T1 values of gray matter and white matter.[19] IR techniques show T1 values of 973

± 33 ms in gray matter versus 876 ± 27 ms in white matter. GRE techniques show T1 values of 994 ± 54 ms in gray matter versus 838 ± 54 ms in white matter. IR techniques also show a significant difference in the T1 relaxation time of the lateral column white matter (863 ± 23 ms) versus the dorsal column white matter (899 ± 18 ms), but that difference is not confirmed by GRE techniques.[19]

T2

In-vivo measurements of the T2 relaxation times of the human cervical spinal cord at 3.0 T show a T2 relaxation time of 73 to 76 ms, with no significant difference in the T2 values of spinal gray matter versus dorsal column white matter or lateral column white matter.[19] The T2 of spinal white matter is very similar to the T2 of densely packed cerebral white matter tracts like the corpus callosum.[19] The T2 value of spinal gray matter is very similar to the T2 of the deep gray matter of the basal ganglia and brain

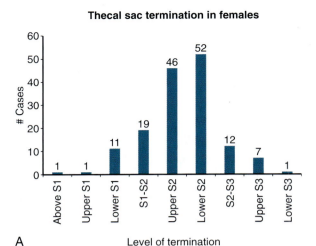

Thecal sac termination in females

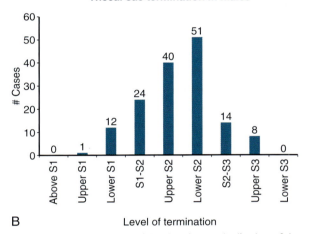

Thecal sac termination in males

■ **FIGURE 5-34** Termination of the thecal sac. Distribution of the termination of the thecal sac by vertebral level in 150 females **(A)** and 150 males **(B)** of all ages. *(Reprinted from Righi A, Naidich TP. The normal termination of the thecal sac. Internat J Neuroradiol 1996; 2:188-195.)*

stem, although not to the T2 of the lamellar gray matter of the neocortex.[19]

There are three distinct water compartments within the spinal cord, leading to three distinct T2 relaxation compartments. These three correspond to water *within* the myelin bilayers with T2 relaxation time less than 20 ms, intracellular/extracellular water with T2 relaxation time between 30 and 100 ms, and cerebrospinal fluid (CSF) with T2 relaxation time greater than 1000 ms.[8] The component of water trapped within the myelin bilayers may be designated the myelin water fraction (MWF). In rats, the average myelin water fractions in the cervical spinal cord are 5% in gray matter and 24% in white matter. These data accord well with the approximately five times greater myelin content in rat spinal cord white matter versus gray matter.[8]

Quantitative in-vivo measurements of the magnetization transfer (MT) ratio (qMTR) of the human cervical spinal cord at 1.5 T show that the mean rate (R) of MT exchange is just slightly higher in gray matter (67 ± 12 Hz)

than white matter (56 ± 11 Hz averaged over both the dorsal and lateral columns).[20] There is no significant difference in the mean rate (R) of MT exchange of dorsal versus lateral column white matter.[20] The mean macromolecular fraction (M_{ob}) is significantly higher in white than gray matter: $14 \pm 2\%$ in white matter versus $8 \pm 2\%$ in gray matter.[20] The dorsal and lateral column white matter show equal mean macromolecular fractions.[20] The mean macromolecular relaxation time (T_{2b}) across all columns is measured as 9 ± 2 μs for both gray and white matter.[20]

Vascularity and Perfusion

In the human cervical spinal cord, CT studies estimate the blood flow at 6 to 9 mL/min/100 g tissue, the blood volume at 1 to 4.3 mL/100 g tissue, the mean transit time at 16 to 17 seconds, and the permeability at 0.7 to 2 mL/100 g tissue/min.[2] At present, however, these estimates are not very reproducible and depend, in part, on technical factors. These include the software packages used, the placement of the region of interest cursor in the largest internal carotid artery versus the largest vertebral artery to assess the arterial input function, and specifics regarding timing the bolus.[2]

Diffusion Weighted Imaging

Diffusion-weighted imaging provides a measure of the number, size, and orientation of the fiber tracts of the spinal cord. Within the cord, the membranes and myelin sheaths of the axons restrict the diffusion of water, both in vivo and ex vivo, causing anisotropic diffusion of water (Fig. 5-35). As a result, water diffusion occurs principally longitudinally, in both white matter and gray matter, and mainly follows the longitudinal fiber tracts. A second component of diffusion occurs in the transverse direction, following the collateral nerve fibers that course radially as they pass into and out of the spinal gray matter over a limited number of segments.[10] Specific correlation of histologic features with diffusion-weighted imaging shows that transverse and longitudinal diffusion correlate with differing histologic factors.

Transverse diffusion across the spinal cord, orthogonal to the long axis of the cord, correlates closely with axonal spacing and the fraction of tissue composed of extracellular water (extracellular volume fraction).[18] Transverse diffusion shows significant inverse correlation with axonal count (expressed as $\log_{10}$ [axon count]) and with the fraction of tissue composed of myelin (myelin volume fraction).[18] These factors may reflect the tortuosity of the extracellular space. The transverse diffusion does not appear to correlate with axon diameter or the thickness of the myelin sheaths.[18]

Longitudinal diffusion along the long axis of the spinal cord correlates closely with the axon diameter, measured both with and without the myelin sheath. Longitudinal diffusion shows very strong inverse correlation with axon count (expressed as $\log_{10}$ [axon count]) and less strong correlation with axon diameter exclusive of the myelin sheath.[18] This correlation with the diameter of the axon itself suggests that intracellular diffusion may be the

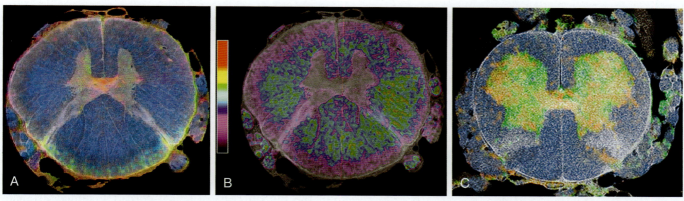

■ **FIGURE 5-35** Diffusion tensor imaging. **A** and **B**, Thoracic spinal cord depicting the color-coded directional diffusion map (**A**) and the fractional anisotropy map (**B**). Compare with Figures 5-5B and 5-6B. **C**, Lumbar spinal cord. Color-encoded directional diffusion map. Compare with Figures 5-5C and 5-6C. In **A** and **C**, the colors indicate the tissue vectors directed superoinferior (*blue*), ventrodorsal (*green*), and transversely (left-right) (*red*). Fibers coursing oblique to the three orthogonal directions are represented by intermediate colors directly proportional to the components of their vectors that are directed along each of the three orthogonal directions. The predominantly blue color of the white matter bundles and the nerve roots around the cord emphasizes the craniocaudal direction of the fibers of the funiculi and the nerves. The reddish color of the entering dorsal nerve roots and ventral white commissure indicates their predominantly transverse course. The multicolored appearance of the gray matter nuclei likely reflects the fibers entering and exiting from them in all directions. The light blue area of the dorsal horns in C likely reflects the substantia gelatinosa (Rexed laminae II and III).

predominant factor in longitudinal diffusivity. It may be that in larger axons the neurofilaments and cytoskeleton proteins have lower physical concentration and present fewer barriers to longitudinal diffusion within the axon.[18]

Fractional anisotropy (FA) varies with developmental and chronologic age. In vivo, the diffusion values of the spinal cord are highest in infants, lowest in mature adults ages 30 to 50 years, and begin to increase again after age 50.[9] In adult males, the diffusivity is reported as $0.87 \pm 0.04 \, \mu m^2/ms$ in the spinal white matter and $0.81 \pm 0.02 \, \mu m^2/ms$ in the spinal gray matter.[9] The FA (averaged over 20 signals) is reported as 0.65 ± 0.04 in the spinal white matter and 0.34 ± 0.05 in the spinal gray matter.[9]

Performing diffusion-weighted imaging in vivo at 1.5 T using echoplanar sequences and a b-value of 700 s/mm², Rossi and associates found that the FA of gray matter was significantly lower than the FA of all white matter.[16] Furthermore, the FA of the lateral column white matter was lower than the FA of the dorsal column white matter.[16] Specifically, Rossi and associates found FA values of 0.45 ± 0.06 for spinal gray matter, 0.69 ± 0.08 for lateral column white matter, and 0.79 ± 0.07 for dorsal column white matter.[16] Expressed as a percentage of the dorsal column FA (taken as 100%), the FA of the gray matter was 57% and the FA of the lateral column white matter was 87%.[16] These values partly reflect the differing sizes and packing of the axons within the dorsal and lateral columns. The ascending sensory tracts of the dorsal white matter contain both thinner (fasciculus gracilis) and thicker (fasciculus cuneatus) myelinated fibers with a mean diameter of 13 to 20 μm.[16] The lateral columns contain both descending motor (crossed corticospinal) tracts that have myelinated fibers with a mean diameter of 1 to 4 μm and ascending sensory (lateral spinothalamic) tracts that have only thinly myelinated or unmyelinated fibers.[16]

Fixation does not affect the relative anisotropy or the radial diffusivity of the spinal cord but does significantly decrease the longitudinal diffusivity.[7] Once specimens are well fixed, however, the diffusivity parameters do not change over time. Fixatives that combine glutaraldehyde with formalin preserve axonal ultrastructure more completely and permit detection of greater relative anisotropy, especially in longitudinally oriented fiber tracts.[18] Therefore, postmortem diffusion MR of formalin-fixed specimens (see Fig. 5-35) remains useful for the analysis of the anatomic bases of the fractional anisotropies seen in vivo.

Special Procedures

CT myelography does display the contours of the spinal cord and the relationships of the spinal cord to surrounding structures but carries the risk of performing the spinal tap and instilling the water-soluble contrast agent (Figs. 5-36 and 5-37).

CT and MR angiography may both be used to display the artery of Adamkiewicz. Contrast-enhanced CT and contrast-enhanced MRI are reported to have comparable success for detecting the artery of Adamkiewicz (CT: 68%-90% vs. MRI: 67%-93%).[23] Performing the CT angiogram after intra-arterial injection into the proximal descending aorta achieves a substantially greater success (94.1%) than does performing the CT angiogram after intravenous injection at the antecubital vein (60.0%).[23] Important factors determining the success rate for MR angiography include a sufficiently large craniocaudal field of view (≤50 cm including vertebral levels T8-L5), the administration of at least 0.2 mmol of gadolinium per kilogram of body weight, accurate timing of the contrast administration to acquire the center of K space at peak bolus concentration, and skill in postprocessing.[1]

ACKNOWLEDGEMENTS

The authors would like to thank Mr. Calvin Keys for his help in preparing the fresh cadaver specimens. His work is much appreciated.

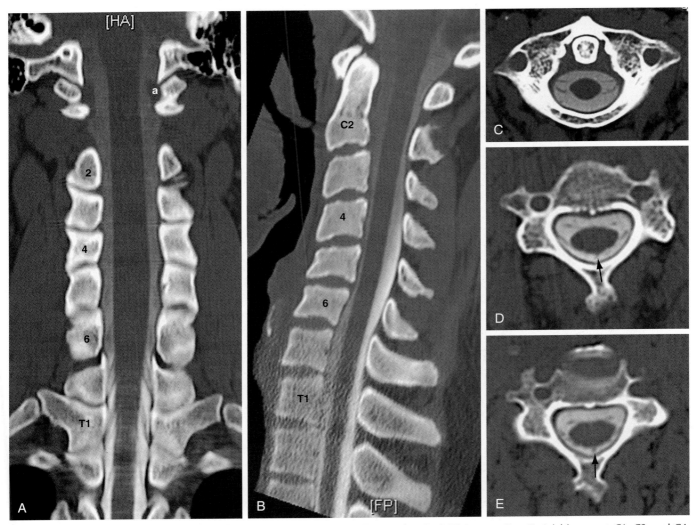

■ **FIGURE 5-36** CT myelography of the cervical spine. Reformatted coronal (**A**) and sagittal (**B**) images. **C** to **E**, Axial images at C1, C3, and C4, respectively. The water-soluble subarachnoid contrast agent outlines the spinal cord and nerve roots to depict their contours and their relationships to the surrounding structures. The vertebral artery (a) characteristically protrudes into the spinal canal at C1. *Black arrows* on **D** and **E** indicate the dorsal median vein that courses longitudinally along the spinal cord.

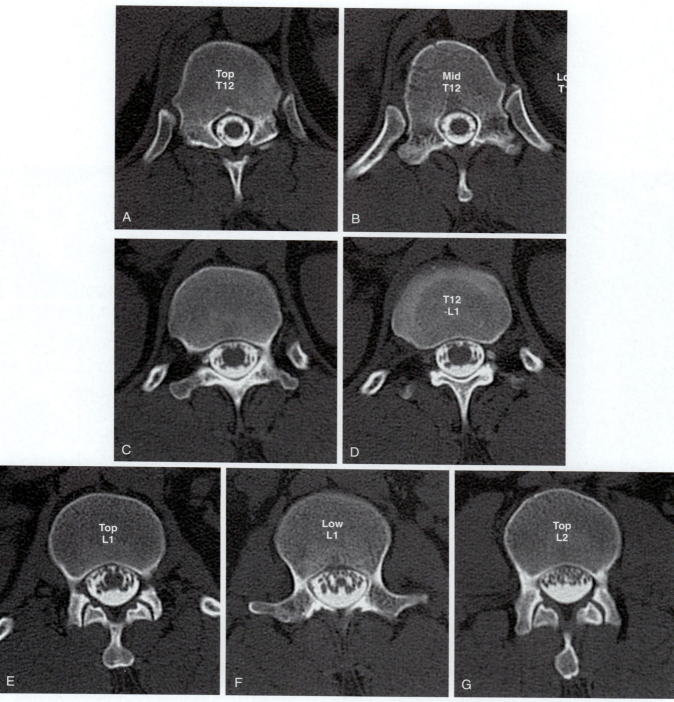

■ **FIGURE 5-37** CT myelography, thoracolumbar transition. **A to G,** Serial axial CT sections from the top of T12 to the bottom of L2 outline the changing contour of the spinal cord from the distal thoracic cord through the lumbar enlargement to the tapering conus medullaris. The ventral and dorsal nerve roots emerge segmentally and then course caudad, inferior to the tip of the conus medullaris.

KEY POINTS

- There are 31 spinal segments: 8 cervical, 12 thoracic, 5 lumbar, 5 sacral, and 1 coccygeal.
- The proportions of gray matter and white matter vary systematically over the length of the spinal cord. The white matter is greatest superiorly and decreases progressively inferiorly. The gray matter is most prominent at the lumbar enlargement, second most prominent at the cervical enlargement, and least in the thoracic cord.
- The gray matter of the spinal cord is arrayed as a fluted column, which, in cross section, displays ventral horns, dorsal horns, and (at thoracic levels) lateral horns. The gray matter is organized from dorsal to ventral in 10 cytoarchitectonic zones, designated Rexed laminae (RLs). RL I is most dorsal, RL IX is most ventral, and RL X is most central (surrounding the central canal of the spinal cord).
- The cell bodies for the ventral (motor) roots reside in the ventral horns and exit the spinal cord via the ventrolateral sulci to form the ventral nerve rootlets. The cell bodies for the dorsal (sensory) nerve roots reside within the segmental dorsal root ganglia in the neural foramina lateral to the spinal cord. Central processes of these dorsal root ganglion cells pass medially into the spinal cord via the posterolateral sulci (dorsal root entry zone) to synapse within the dorsal horns or pass through the dorsal columns to other spinal levels.
- The white matter is organized into longitudinal columns that conduct variably myelinated fiber bundles from caudad to craniad (ascending tracts) and from craniad to caudad (descending tracts). The dorsal columns convey the ascending gracile and cuneate fasciculi, which carry information regarding vibration, light touch, tactile discrimination, and joint position sense to the cerebellum and thalamus. The lateral columns convey the ascending dorsal and ventral spinocerebellar tracts that carry proprioceptive information to the cerebellum, the ascending spinothalamic tracts that carry pain and temperature information to the thalamus, and the descending crossed lateral corticospinal tracts that carry impulses to the spinal cord for cerebral control of motor function. The ventral columns convey the descending ventral uncrossed corticospinal tracts and the descending medial and lateral vestibulospinal tracts, which function in motor control, posture, and postural tone.[6]
- The arterial supply to the spinal cord is typically organized as a single anterior spinal axis and paired dorsal (or dorsolateral) arteries. The anterior spinal axis typically courses the full length of the spinal cord, giving rise to multiple segmental sulcomarginal arteries. These traverse the ventral median sulcus to supply the ventral two thirds of the spinal cord. The dorsal (dorsolateral) arteries are incomplete longitudinal feeders that supply a pial vascular plexus designated the vasocorona. In turn, the vasocorona gives rise to myriad radially oriented arteries that perforate the cord at all levels to supply the posterior one third of the spinal cord.

SUGGESTED READINGS

Carpenter MB, Sutin J. Human Neuroanatomy, 8th ed. Baltimore, Williams & Wilkins, 1983, pp 232-264.

Daniels DL, Haughton VM, Naidich TP. Cranial and Spinal Magnetic Resonance Imaging: An Atlas and Guide. New York, Raven Press, 1987.

Gilman S, Newman SW. Manter and Gatz's Essentials of Clinical Neuroanatomy and Neurophysiology, 10th ed. Philadelphia, FA Davis, 1996.

Miller RA, Burack E. Atlas of the Central Nervous System in Man, 2nd ed. Baltimore, Williams & Wilkins, 1977.

Nieuwenhuys R, Voogd J, van Huijzen C (eds). Topography of spinal cord, brain stem and cerebellum. In The Human Central Nervous System, 4th ed. Berlin, Springer-Verlag, 2008, pp 177-246.

Standring S: Gray's Anatomy: The Anatomical Basis of Clinical Practice, 39th ed. Edinburgh, Churchill Livingstone, 2005.

Thron AJ: Vascular Anatomy of the Spinal Cord: Neuroradiological Investigations and Clinical Syndromes. New York, Springer-Verlag, 1988.

REFERENCES

1. Backes WH, Nijenhuis RJ. Advances in spinal cord MR angiography. AJNR Am J Neuroradiol 2008; 29:619-631.
2. Bisdas S, Rumboldt Z, Surlan K, et al. Perfusion CT measurements in healthy cervical spinal cord: feasibility and repeatability of the study as interchangeability of the perfusion estimates using two commercially available software packages. Eur Radiol 2008; 18:2321-2328.
3. Carpenter MB, Sutin J. Human Neuroanatomy, 8th ed. Baltimore, Williams & Wilkins, 1983, pp 232-264.
4. Crosby EC, Humphrey R, Lauer EW. Correlative Anatomy of the Nervous System. New York, Macmillan, 1962.
5. Foerster O. Motorische Felder und Bahnen. In Bumpke O, Foerster O (eds). Handbuch der Neurologie. Berlin, Springer-Verlag, 1936, vol 6, pp 1-357.
6. Gilman S, Newman SW (eds). Manter and Gatz's Essentials of Clinical Neuroanatomy and Neurophysiology, 10th ed. Philadelphia, FA Davis, 1996.
7. Kim TH, Zollinger L, Shi XF, Jeong EK. Diffusion tensor imaging of ex vivo cervical spinal cord specimens: the immediate and long-term effect of fixation on diffusivity. Anat Rec 2009; 292:234-241.
8. Kozlowski P, Liu J, Yung AC, Tetzlaff W. High-resolution myelin water measurements in rat spinal cord. Magn Reson Med 2008; 59:796-802.
9. Maier SE. Examination of spinal cord tissue architecture with magnetic resonance diffusion tensor imaging. Neurotherapeutics 2007; 4:453-459.
10. Mamata H, De Grolami U, Hoge WS, et al. Collateral nerve fibers in human spinal cord: visualization with magnetic resonance diffusion tensor imaging. NeuroImage 2006; 31:24-30.
11. Nieuwenhuys R, Voogd J, van Huijzen C (eds). Topography of spinal cord, brain stem and cerebellum. In The Human Central Nervous System, 4th ed. Berlin, Springer-Verlag, 2008, pp 177-246.
12. Rexed B. The cytoarchitectonic organization of the spinal cord in the cat. J Comp Neurol 1952; 96:415-495.

13. Rexed B. A cytoarchitectonic atlas of the spinal cord in the cat. J Comp Neurol 1954; 100:297-379.

14. Rexed B. Some aspects of the cytoarchitectonics and synaptology of the spinal cord. Progr Brain Res 1964; 11:58-92.

15. Righi A, Naidich TP. The normal termination of the thecal sac. Int J Neuroradiol 1996; 2:188-195.

16. Rossi C, Boss A, Steidle G, et al. Water diffusion anisotropy in white and gray matter of the human spinal cord. J Magn Reson Imaging 2008; 27:476-482.

17. Schwartz ED, Cooper ET, Chin C-L, et al. Ex vivo evaluation of ADC values within spinal cord white matter tracts. AJNR Am J Neuroradiol 2005; 26:390-397.

18. Schwartz ED, Cooper ET, Fan Y, et al. MRI diffusion coefficients in spinal cord correlate with axon morphometry. NeuroReport 2005; 16:73-76.

19. Smith SA, Edden RAE, Farrell JAD, et al. Measurement of T1 and T2 in the cervical spinal cord at 3 T. Magn Reson Med 2008; 60:213-219.

20. Smith SA, Golay X, Fatemi A, et al. Quantitative magnetization transfer characteristics of the human cervical spinal cord in vivo: application to adrenomyeloneuropathy. Magn Reson Med 2009; 61:22-27.

21. Standring S (ed-in-chief). Gray's Anatomy: The Anatomical Basis of Clinical Practice, 39th ed. Edinburgh, Elsevier Churchill Livingstone, 2005.

22. Thron AJ. Vascular Anatomy of the Spinal Cord: Neuroradiological Investigations and Clinical Syndromes. New York, Springer-Verlag, 1988.

23. Uotani K, Yamada N, Kono AK, et al. Preoperative artery of Adamkiewicz by intra-arterial CT angiography. AJNR Am J Neuroradiol 2008; 29:314-318.

24. Williams PL (ed-in-chief). Gray's Anatomy: The Anatomical Basis of Medicine and Surgery, 38th ed. Edinburgh, Churchill Livingstone, 1995.

25. Nicholas DS, Weller RO. The fine anatomy of the human spinal meninges: A light and scanning electron microscopy study. J Neurosurg 1988; 69:276-282.

26. Wijdicks CA, Williams JM. Spinal arachnoid calcifications. Clin Anat 2007; 20:521-523.

27. Vandenabeele F, Creemers J, Lambrichts I. Ultrastructure of the human spinal arachnoid mater and dura mater. J Anat 1996; 189:417-430.

28. Orlin JR, Osen KK, Hovig T. Subdural compartment in pig: A morphological study with blood and horseradish peroxidase infused subdurally. Anat Rec 1991; 230:22-37.

29. Reina MA, De León Casasola O, Villanueva MC, et al. Ultrastructural findings in human spinal pia mater in relation to spinal anesthesia. Anesth Analg 2004; 98:1479-1485.

30. Di Chiro G, Timins EL. Supine myelography and the septum posticum. Radiology 1974; 111:319-327.

31. Tubbs RS, Salter G, Grabb PA, Oakes WJ. The denticulate ligament: Anatomy and functional significance. J Neurosurg 2001; 94:271-275.

32. Hogan Q, Toth J. Anatomy of the soft tissues of the spinal canal. Regional Anesth Pain Med 1999; 24:303-310.

33. Reina MA, Villanueva MC, López A, De Andrés JA. Grasa dentro de los mangitos durales de las raíces nerviosas de la columna lumbar humana. [English title: Fat within the nerve root sleeves of the human lumbar spinal column]. Rev Esp Anestesiol Reanim 2007; 54:297-301.

34. Scuderi GJ, Vaccaro AR, Brusovanik GV, et al. Conjoined lumbar nerve roots. A frequently underappreciated congenital anomaly. J Spinal Disord Tech 2004; 17:83-93.

35. Neidre A, MacNab I. Anomalies of the lumbosacral nerve roots. Review of 16 cases and classification. Spine 1983; 8:294-299.

36. Kadish LJ, Simmons EH. Anomalies of the lumbosacral nerve roots. An anatomical investigation and myelographic study. J Bone Joint Surg [Br] 1984; 66:411-416.

37. Song SJ, Lee JW, Choi J-Y, et al. Imaging features suggestive of a conjoined nerve root on routine axial MRI. Skeletal Radiol 2008; 37:113-138.

38. Artico M, Carloia S, Piacentini M, et al. Conjoined lumbosacral nerve roots: Observations on three cases and review of the literature. Neurocirugia 2006; 17:54-59.

39. Kang CH, Shin MJ, Kim SM, et al. Conjoined lumbosacral nerve roots compromised by disk herniation: Sagittal shoulder sign for the preoperative diagnosis. Skeletal Radiol 2008; 37:225-231.

40. Haijiao W, Koti M, Smith FW, Wardlaw D. Diagnosis of lumbosacral nerve root anomalies by magnetic resonance imaging. J Spinal Disord 2001; 14:143-149.

41. Righi A, Naidich TP. The normal termination of the thecal sac. Int J Neuroradiol 1996; 2:188-195.

42. McDonald A, Chatrath P, Spector T, Ellis H. Level of termination of the spinal cord and the dural sac. A magnetic resonance study. Clin Anat 1999; 12:149-152.

43. Ranger MRB, Irwin GJ, Bunbury KM, Peutrell JM. Changing body position alters the location of the spinal cord within the vertebral canal: A magnetic resonance imaging study. Br J Anaesth 2008; 101:804-809.

44. Koo B-N, Hong J-Y, Kim JE, Kil HK. The effect of flexion on the level of termination of the dural sac in paediatric patients. Anaesthesia 2009; 64:1072-1076.

45. Hansasuta A, Tubbs RS, Oakes WJ. Filum terminale fusion and dural sac termination: Study in 27 cadavers. Pediatr Neurosurg 1999; 30:176-179.

PART FOUR

Normal Spinal Aging and Degeneration

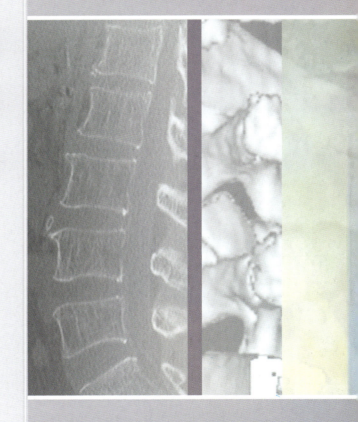

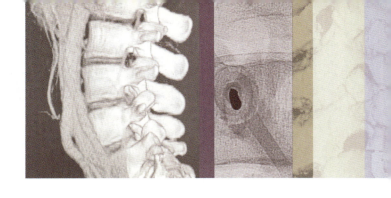

CHAPTER 6

Age-Related Changes in the Spine

Victor M. Haughton

The spines of older individuals have both the changes of normal aging and the changes of "degeneration." In the absence of accepted criteria to distinguish aging and degeneration, the features that characterize the majority of individuals at a specified age can be taken to represent normal aging rather than degeneration. The anatomic, chemical, and imaging features of the aging spine are discussed here, and the degenerative changes of the spine are reviewed elsewhere (see Chapter 7).

ANATOMY AND FUNCTIONAL ANATOMY OF THE INTERVERTEBRAL DISC

Specialized connective tissues give the intervertebral disc its biomechanical properties. For the purposes of description, the intervertebral disc can be divided into three components: outer annulus fibrosus, inner annulus fibrosus, and nucleus pulposus (Fig. 6-1). The outer annulus fibrosus has thick lamellae of dense connective tissue, containing predominantly collagen. The inner annulus has cartilaginous matrix associated with the collagenous fibers. The nucleus pulposus has predominantly cartilagenous matrix with less structure than the annulus fibrosus.

The outer annulus consists of multiple layers (lamellae), each containing dense collagenous fibers. Histologically it resembles tendinous structures such as the Achilles tendon. In each layer (lamella) of the annulus fibrosus, the fibers run parallel to each other at an angle of 60 degrees with respect to the vertebral end plate. These fibers originate and insert in bone, as do Sharpey's fibers in the anterior longitudinal ligament. The high concentration of collagen in the outer annulus fibrosus results in its low signal intensity on T1- and T2-weighted images (Fig. 6-2). In successive lamellae the fibers alternate directions (Fig. 6-3). These inelastic fibers running obliquely in the periphery of the disc resist axial rotatory torques but permit flexion and extension and lateral bending. The predominant cell type in the outer annulus fibrosus is the fibroblast, as its predominant constituent is collagen.

The inner annulus contains less well defined lamellae, together with collagenous matrix. Like the lamellae in the outer annulus, those in the inner annulus run obliquely. They insert and originate not in bone but in the thin layer of hyaline cartilage that covers the entire surface of each vertebral end plate except the ring apophysis. The transitions from outer annulus to inner annulus and from inner annulus to nucleus pulposus are indistinct. The glycosaminoglycans and water in the matrix give the inner annulus a higher T2 signal intensity than the outer annulus. The inner annulus contains fibroblasts and chondrocytes.

The nucleus pulposus also contains glycosaminoglycans, collagen, and chondrocytes, like the inner annulus fibrosus, but the structure of the nucleus pulposus is more amorphous and the fiber structure is less plentiful. The nucleus fibrosus has high signal intensity on T2-weighted images, reflecting the glycosaminoglycans and water content. A central region in the nucleus pulposus contains collagen, elastin, and reticulin fibers oriented horizontally (Fig. 6-4). The fiber content of this region results in a lower signal intensity, visible on sagittal MR images of the lumbar and thoracic spine.

The anterior longitudinal ligament and posterior longitudinal ligament have close anatomic relationships to the disc. The anterior longitudinal ligament, containing predominantly collagen and contacting the anterior and lateral surfaces of the disc, cannot be distinguished in MR images from the outer annulus fibrosus (Fig. 6-5). The posterior longitudinal ligament, which fuses to the posterior intervertebral disc margin, cannot be distinguished from the disc although it is a distinct structure posterior to the epidural venous plexus between intervertebral discs (Fig. 6-6). Containing predominantly collagen, it is not distinguished from the disc on MR.

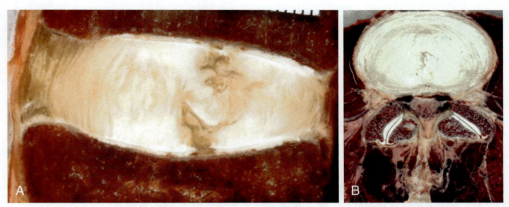

■ **FIGURE 6-1** Sagittal (**A**) and axial (**B**) anatomic sections of a lumbar intervertebral disc. In the sagittal section, notice the well-defined, faintly colored lamellae in the peripheral annulus, especially in the anterior portion of the disc (to reader's left). The lamellae become less and less well defined toward the interior of the disc where the inner annulus fibrosus is located. The central portion of the disc has an amorphous tissue, the nucleus pulposus. In the central portion of the nucleus pulposus, some fibrous structure is evident. The pigments that give the nucleus pulposus a darker color are aging changes.

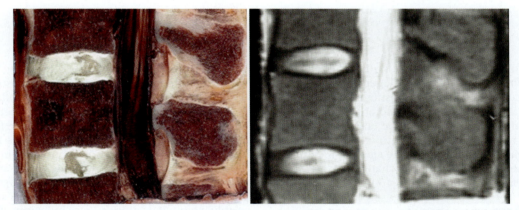

■ **FIGURE 6-2** Sagittal anatomic and T2-weighted MR images of a cadaveric lumbar spine to illustrate the MR appearance of outer annulus, inner annulus, and nucleus pulposus. The most anterior portion of the disc, consisting of inner annulus fibrosus and nucleus pulposus, has a lamellated structure, which has low signal intensity on the MR image. The region in the nucleus with higher fiber content appears also as a horizontal band of low signal intensity, the central low signal intensity region of the disc.

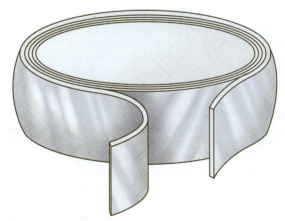

■ **FIGURE 6-3** Sketch showing the orientation of collagen fibers in the lamellae in the outer annulus fibrosus. In the most superficial layer the fibers are oriented at 60 degrees with respect to the adjacent end plate. This lamella has been delaminated from the disc to show the next adjacent lamella, which has fibers running also oriented 60 degrees with respect to the end plate, but alternating in direction with the outer lamella.

The intervertebral disc has several thousand cells in each cubic milliliter (Fig. 6-7). These cells produce collagen and glycosaminoglycan precursors. Due to the slow degradation of collagen and glycosaminoglycans in the disc, collagen and glycosaminoglycans are renewed approximately every 180 days by molecules synthesized within the disc.

The cells in the intervertebral disc receive their nutrition via diffusion because the intervertebral disc has no arteries or capillaries, except in the fetus. Oxygen, glucose, sulfates, and other nutrients diffuse into the disc through the vertebral end plates and to a lesser extent through the outer annulus fibrosus, and carbon dioxide and other waste products diffuse out. Diffusion into the intervertebral disc can be measured as an increase in signal intensity in the disc after the intravenous administration of a paramagnetic contrast medium. Reduced diffusion into the intervertebral disc may contribute to disc degeneration by impeding the normal synthetic processes in the cell population of the disc.

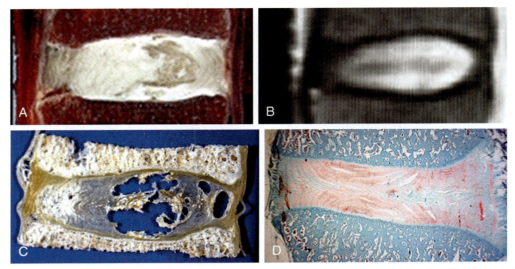

■ **FIGURE 6-4** Sagittal anatomic (**A**), MR (**B**), desiccated slice (**C**), and H&E-stained section (**D**) of a lumbar disc. The desiccated section shows the fibrous content of the disc, which is most apparent in the peripheral annulus, but also in the central nucleus pulposus. The stained section shows fibrous tissue (*staining blue*) prominent in the annulus fibrosus and the central nucleus pulposus. Matrix in the nucleus pulposus and inner annulus fibrosus stains pink.

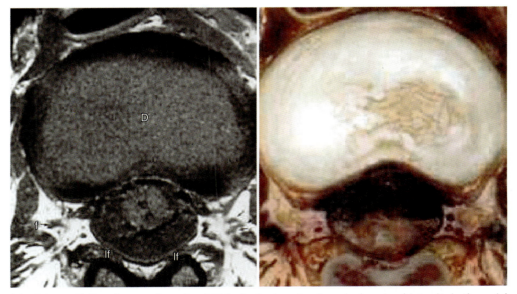

■ **FIGURE 6-5** Axial MR image (*left*) and anatomic section (*right*) of a lumbar disc show the low signal intensity in the periphery of the disc (D). The anterior longitudinal ligament along the anterior and lateral surfaces of the disc cannot be distinguished.

The intervertebral disc is normally classified as nonenhancing. Disc fragments herniated into the spinal canal are usually observed to have no enhancement, in contrast to scar tissue, which does enhance. However, increase in signal intensity in normal discs can be detected after administration of contrast medium. Images obtained 40 minutes after intravenous contrast administration may have visible contrast enhancement, especially near the periphery (Fig. 6-8).

The intervertebral discs convey flexibility to the spine. Flexion and extension and lateral bending of the spine are possible mainly because of the flexibility of discs. In response to axial rotatory torques, the spine permits little rotation because of the oblique fibers in the annulus fibrosus. Properties of the disc also explain the diurnal variation in the height of the spinal column. When the human body is in the recumbent position, axial forces on the disc are minimized and as a result the disc absorbs additional water. With the body in upright position, the water is forced out of the disc, resulting in a loss of up to an inch of height in the spine.

The intervertebral disc does not have innervation. The anterior longitudinal ligament contains nerve endings. Nerve endings may be identified in the disc tissue immediately adjacent to the ligament but not more deeply in the disc. Therefore, the disc does not normally give rise to painful stimuli.

Disc morphology varies between the cervical, thoracic, and lumbar segments of the spine. The discs between the C2 through C7 vertebrae extend laterally between

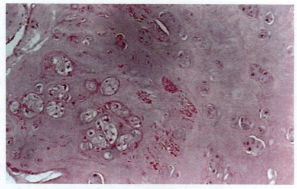

the uncinate process on the vertebra below and the demi-facet or echancrure on the vertebra above (Fig. 6-9). This region is called the "uncovertebral joint" although it contains fibrocartilage typical of the disc, without synovium. With age, a bursa or cleft may develop in this region of the disc, suggesting a joint space. In the cervical region the uncinate process lies between the disc tissue and the exiting spinal nerve root. In the thoracic region, the discs are relatively rounded and thin (Fig. 6-10). The

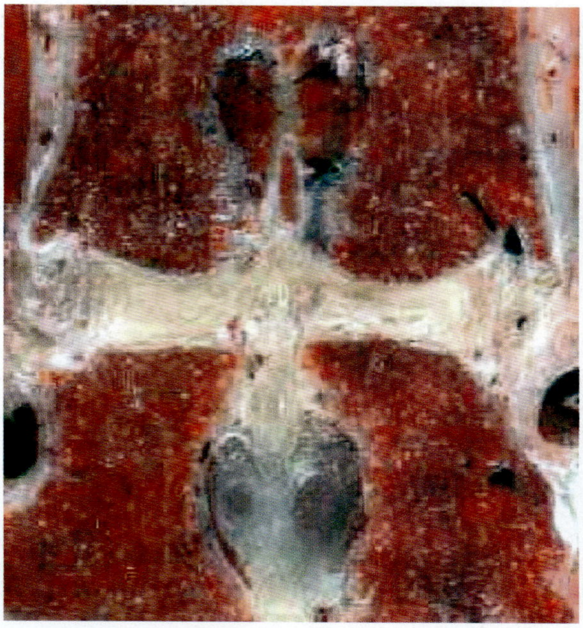

■ **FIGURE 6-6**   Anatomic section in coronal plane through the spine along the posterior margin of the intervertebral disc. The section shows fibers in the posterior longitudinal ligament running horizontally along the posterior margin of the disc. The posterior longitudinal ligament runs superiorly and inferiorly out of the plane of section, where it lies posterior to the basivertebral veins, visible as the blood-containing structures above and below the disc.

■ **FIGURE 6-7**   Histologic section through the nucleus pulposus illustrating the plentiful chondroid matrix (*staining pink*) containing numerous chondrocytes, which appear as elliptical structures containing dark dots.

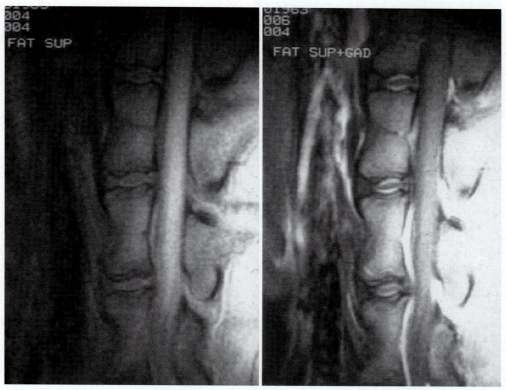

■ **FIGURE 6-8**   Sagittal MR images of a dog spine before (*left*) and 40 minutes after (*right*) intravenous contrast medium injection, illustrating enhancement in normal intervertebral discs.

outer annulus is distinguished on MR images. The lumbar discs, the thickest and largest in the spine, have a close relationship to the neural foramen.

AGE-RELATED CHANGES OF THE INTERVERTEBRAL DISC

Neonate

The neonatal disc lies between partially ossified vertebral bodies (Fig. 6-11A).[1] In anatomic sections, the nucleus pulposus and inner annulus fibrosus appear together as a colorless, translucent structure. The peripheral (outer) annulus fibrosus displays a darker color due to its collagen

content. Thin streaks that contain remnants of the primitive notochord stretch across the equator (center) of the disc from anterior to posterior. In anatomic sections, the unossified cartilage of the vertebral end plates resembles the cartilage of the disc itself. In the neonate, large blood vessels are present in the unossified vertebral cartilage. The neonatal disc is graded as stage I in the Thompson system for staging intervertebral disc degeneration.[2]

In T2-weighted (T2W) MR images, the neonatal intervertebral disc shows uniformly high signal intensity in the

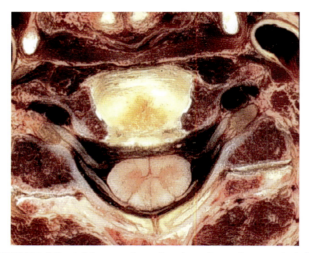

■ **FIGURE 6-9** Axial anatomic section through a cadaver cervical disc to illustrate the relationship of the disc centrally and the uncinate processes posterolaterally. The processes appear to buttress the lateral aspect of the disc. In the neural foramen, the ventral root and the dorsal root ganglion are evident.

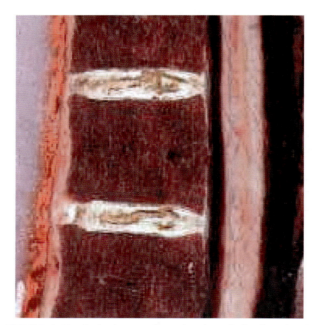

■ **FIGURE 6-10** Sagittal anatomic section through the thoracic spine. The intervertebral discs have a dense fibrous outer annulus fibrosus, as do the lumbar discs. The inner annulus fibrosus and nucleus pulposus contain cartilagenous matrix. The pigments in the inner disc represent aging changes.

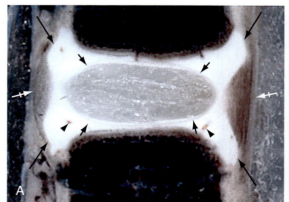
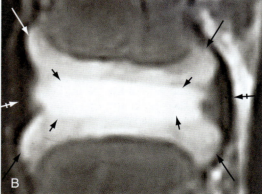

■ **FIGURE 6-11** Normal newborn lumbar intervertebral disc. **A,** Sagittal anatomic section. The newborn nucleus pulposus (*short arrows*) appears as a light gray translucent ovoid within the center of the interspace. Hyaline cartilage of the inner annulus fibrosus and the unossified portions of the adjacent vertebral bodies (*long arrows*) form a ring around the nucleus pulposus. Anteriorly and posteriorly the peripheral annulus fibrosus (*crossed arrows*) shows as a brown color and laminar structure. Small blood vessels are evident within the hyaline cartilage of the vertebral end plate (*arrowheads*). **B,** Sagittal T2W MR image of the specimen illustrated in **A**. The nucleus pulposus (*short arrows*) has high signal intensity. The hyaline cartilage in the inner annulus fibrosus and the unossified portions of the vertebral body (*long arrows*) have slightly lower signal intensity. The peripheral annulus fibrosus (*crossed arrows*) shows appreciably lower signal intensity.

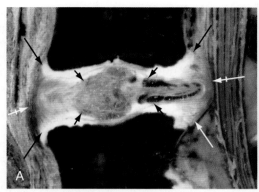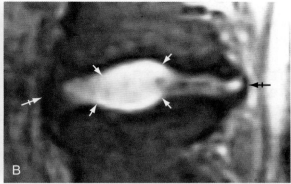

■ **FIGURE 6-12** Normal lumbar intervertebral disc of a 12-year-old. **A,** Sagittal anatomic section. The nucleus pulposus (*short arrows*) now appears inhomogeneous and semi-opaque with slightly reddish tissue and small foci of translucent material. Hyaline cartilage persists in the unossified end plates of the adjacent vertebrae (*long arrows*). The boundary between the inner annulus fibrosus and nucleus pulposus is indistinct. The peripheral annulus fibrosus (*crossed arrows*) has greater thickness and a more lamellar structure than in the newborn. No blood vessels are evident in the hyaline cartilage. **B,** Sagittal T2W MR image of the specimen illustrated in **A**. The nucleus pulposus and inner annulus fibrosus (*short arrows*) show nearly the same high signal intensity. The peripheral portion of the annulus fibrosus (*crossed arrows*) exhibits very low signal intensity.

nucleus pulposus and inner annulus fibrosus and low signal intensity in the more collagenous outer annulus fibrosus (see Fig. 6-11B). No boundary is perceptible between the nucleus pulposus and the inner annulus. However, a sharp boundary is present between the inner annulus fibrosus and the outer annulus, which contains collagen. Unossified cartilage in the adjacent vertebra has the same signal intensity as the cartilage in the disc. These MRI characteristics are considered stage I in the Pfirrmann system for classifying intervertebral disc degeneration.[3]

Second Decade

In anatomic sections, the intervertebral disc in the second decade of life appears white and opaque (Fig. 6-12A),[4] owing in part to an increase in collagen content. During this decade, the disc appears less and less homogeneous. The nucleus pulposus now has a greater concentration of collagen and elastin fibers, especially in the equator, where the syncytial notochordal cells have disappeared. The fibers of the annulus fibrosus are more distinct than in the first decade of life. The outer annulus fibrosus contains as many as 80 lamellae and has greater width than in the first decade of life.[5] The collagenous fibers of the lamellae course in parallel within each lamella, but their orientation differs by about 60 degrees from lamella to lamella. The vertebral end plates adjacent to the disc ossify by the end of the second decade of life. No blood vessels are now present in the disc or in the end plate. Water content in the disc does not decrease between the first and second decades of life.[4,6] Intervertebral discs in the second decade of life usually meet criteria for stage II by the Thompson grading system.

T2W MR images of lumbar discs now show increased thickness of the peripheral region of low signal intensity (see Fig. 6-12B). The central region of the disc maintains a relatively uniform high signal intensity. The boundary between the low and high signal intensity regions is less distinct than in the neonate. Between the ages of 4 and 20 years, the T2 relaxation time of the disc lengthens,[4] suggesting an increase in free water content. Because the

boundary between the low and high signal intensity regions is less distinct than in the neonate, the adolescent disc is graded as stage II in the Pfirrmann scale.

Third Decade

By age 20, the intervertebral disc has completed the transition to adult morphology. The nucleus pulposus appears opaque and may show reddish discoloration from the pigment lipofuscin (Fig. 6-13A). The fibers in the annulus fibrosus are now coarser. The fibers of the inner annulus fibrosus are associated with cartilage matrix. The fibers of the outer annulus, without cartilage matrix, are organized into multiple layers. Within each layer, the fibers course obliquely at about a 35-degree angle to the end plate. The collagen fibers alternate in direction between adjacent lamellae. These nonelastic fibers limit the amount of rotation between adjacent vertebrae. Conspicuous collagen and reticulin fibers form an equatorial band across the disc, about halfway between the apposing end plates.[7]

T2W MR images of intervertebral discs now show low signal intensity in the peripheral annulus fibrosus, where the collagen content is greatest (see Fig. 6-13B). The inner annulus and the nucleus pulposus display a higher T2 signal intensity, owing to their cartilage matrix. The demarcation between the high and low signal intensity regions is not sharp. A central band of greater fiber content crosses the equator of the disc, producing a band of lower signal intensity.[7] This band, called the "intranuclear cleft" or, more correctly, the central region of low signal intensity, is a typical feature of the normal adult disc.

Decade by decade, the morphology of the disc changes.[4,8] With aging, the disc cartilage appears progressively less homogeneous (Fig. 6-14). Calcium salts and pigment appear. Defects or fissures develop in the disc with aging. These defects include concentric and transverse tears of the annulus fibrosus. Concentric tears, also called crescentic tears, represent delamination of the disc between two adjacent lamellae (Fig. 6-15). The lamellar structure is otherwise intact with no signs of disc degeneration. Transverse tears, also called "rim" or "corner"

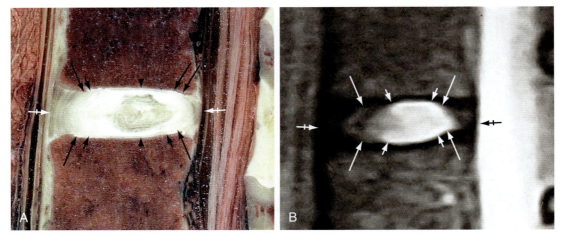

■ **FIGURE 6-13** Normal lumbar disc of a 36-year-old. **A,** Sagittal anatomic section. The nucleus pulposus (*short arrows*) and the inner annulus fibrosus (*long arrows*) are difficult to distinguish from each other. The peripheral annulus fibrosus (*crossed arrows*) has a darker color and more obvious lamellar structure. Portions of the nucleus pulposus contain lipofuscin pigment (*arrowheads*) that darkens the tissue. **B,** Sagittal T2W MR image of the specimen illustrated in **A.** The nucleus pulposus and inner annulus fibrosus (*short arrows*) both show high signal intensity with no distinct boundary between them. The peripheral annulus fibrosus (*crossed arrows*) has low signal intensity.

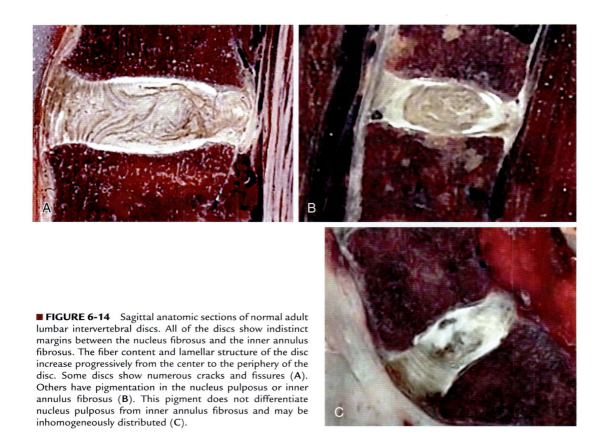

■ **FIGURE 6-14** Sagittal anatomic sections of normal adult lumbar intervertebral discs. All of the discs show indistinct margins between the nucleus fibrosus and the inner annulus fibrosus. The fiber content and lamellar structure of the disc increase progressively from the center to the periphery of the disc. Some discs show numerous cracks and fissures (**A**). Others have pigmentation in the nucleus pulposus or inner annulus fibrosus (**B**). This pigment does not differentiate nucleus pulposus from inner annulus fibrosus and may be inhomogeneously distributed (**C**).

lesions, are defects in one or more layers of the annulus fibrosus where the annular fibers insert into the ring apophysis (Fig. 6-16). Some transverse tears contain gas (Fig. 16-17). The majority of intervertebral discs in individuals older than the age of 50 have transverse and/or concentric tears in the annulus fibrosus.[9] They do not cause pain because they occur in regions of the disc

without innervation. Nerve endings have been identified only in the most peripheral layers of the disc.

On MR images, discs can be classified as normal aging discs if the height of the disc and the T2 signal intensity in the inner annulus and nucleus are retained (see Fig. 6-14).[10] Signal intensity in T2W images depends on the sequence chosen, the parameters used, and the water

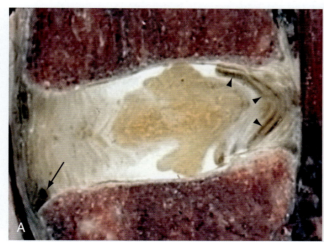

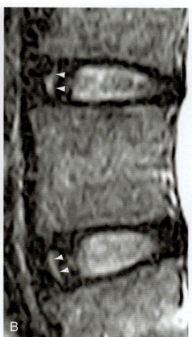

■ **FIGURE 6-15**   Concentric tear in the annulus fibrosus. **A,** Sagittal anatomic section through an adult lumbar disc. The concentric tear (*arrowheads*) in the *posterior* annulus fibrosus contains mucoid material. In this specimen transverse tears are also evident in the *anterior* annulus fibrosus (*arrow*). **B,** Sagittal T2W MR image. The concentric tear (*arrowheads*) appears as a crescentic region of high signal intensity between adjacent lamellae of the annulus fibrosus, with no signs of disc degeneration.

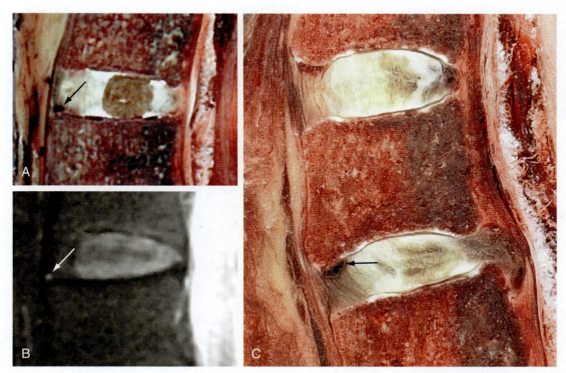

■ **FIGURE 6-16**   Transverse tears ("corner tears," "rim lesions") in the adult annulus fibrosus. **A,** Sagittal anatomic section of an adult lumbar spine. Transverse tears appear as small foci of fiber disruption and discoloration in the peripheral annulus fibrosus (*arrow*) very close to the ring apophysis. They may have less color or more color than the adjacent fibrous tissue, and they may be present without other signs of disc degeneration. Lipofuscin pigmentation is evident in the disc. **B,** Sagittal T2W MR image of the specimen illustrated in **A**. The transverse tears manifest as a region of high signal intensity in the peripheral annulus fibrosus (*arrow*). The pigmentation does not alter the signal intensity of the disc. **C,** Sagittal anatomic section of the adult cervical spine demonstrates that transverse tears in the cervical spine (*arrow*) have a similar appearance to those in the lumbar spine.

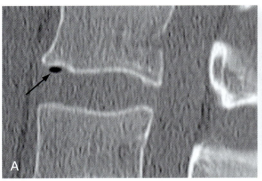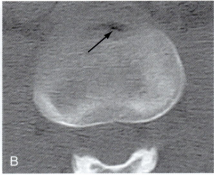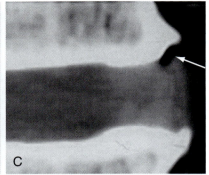

■ **FIGURE 6-17** Sagittal reformatted (**A**), axial (**B**), and coronal reformatted (**C**) CT images illustrating gas within a transverse tear. When gas accumulates within the transverse tear, CT displays it as a region of low density (*arrows*).

content of the disc. The signal intensity of the nucleus pulposus is greater in T2W spin-echo images than in T2W fast spin-echo or T1-weighted (T1W) spin-echo images. Signal intensity can be assessed more precisely by measuring T2 relaxation times than by evaluating signal intensity.[6] The boundary between the peripheral annulus and the remainder of the disc becomes less distinct with age. A central region of low signal intensity characterizes normal aging discs. MRI may show concentric (crescentic) tears or transverse (rim, corner) tears in normally aging discs. Concentric tears appear as curved regions of high signal intensity in the peripheral annulus fibrosus (Fig. 6-15). By Pfirrmann or Thompson criteria, these discs meet criteria for stage II. On sagittal T2W MR images, transverse (rim, corner) tears appear as regions of high signal intensity in the peripheral annulus fibrosus near the end plates (Fig. 6-16).

The chemistry as well as the histology of the disc changes with age. In the nucleus pulposus, the water content decreases progressively with age. In the annulus fibrosus, the water content appears to decrease in the first 3 decades of life and then stabilize (Fig. 6-18).[11] The concentration of viable cells declines to several thousand cells per cubic millimeter. The proportion of aggregating proteoglycans in the disc and the size of their aggregates both diminish with age. Collagen and noncollagen proteins increase in concentration in the nucleus pulposus and inner annulus fibrosus.[12] The aging disc loses sulfated glycosaminoglycans, specifically chondroitin sulfate, and gains collagen and noncollagenous proteins.[13] Together, these changes cause a gradual, slow decrease in T2 relaxation times and a corresponding decrease in T2 signal intensity.[10]

AGE-RELATED CHANGES OF THE VERTEBRAE AND LIGAMENTS

Age-related changes of the osseous spine have been extensively studied anatomically and biochemically.

Bone Marrow

In imaging studies, the most conspicuous age-related changes are seen in the bone marrow. The age-related

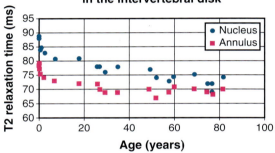

■ **FIGURE 6-18** Age-related changes in the water content of human cadaver discs. After age 20 the nucleus pulposus loses water with age. The annulus fibrosus shows little decrease with age. (From Puschel J. Der Wassergehalt normaler und degenerierter Zwischenwirbelscheiben. Beitr Path Anat 1930; 84:123-130.)

conversion of cellular to fatty bone marrow causes a grossly inhomogeneous pattern of signal within the bone marrow (Fig. 6-19).[14] This pattern may simulate a diffuse invasive metastatic process.[14]

Osteophytes

Osteophytes are found with increasing frequency and increasing size from the second decade of life onward in both men and women and in nearly all ethnic groups. Small osteophytes are universal after the age of 40 years (Fig. 6-20). Large osteophytes are essentially universal after age 80 years.[15] The osteophytes that characterize aging tend to have characteristic locations. They are more common on the anterior aspect than on the posterior aspect of the vertebral body. In the thoracic spine they are more common on the right side of the vertebral column than on the left. Anterior osteophytes occur at any level in the spine but predominate in the lower cervical levels, the lower thoracic levels, and the lumbar levels. Posterior osteophytes predominate in the lower cervical spine. These characteristic locations of anterior and posterior osteophytes may be related to the normal lordosis and kyphosis in the spine. In most cases they occur without evidence of disc degeneration.

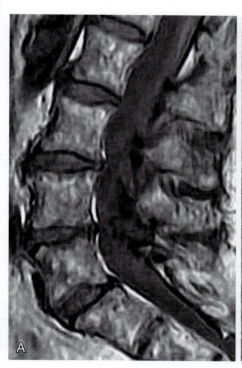
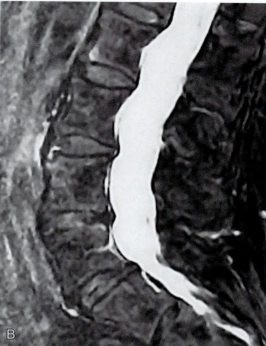

■ **FIGURE 6-19** Bone marrow. T1-weighted (**A**) and T2-weighted (**B**) MR images show inhomogeneous signal intensity in the marrow of the lumbar vertebrae in this 82-year-old man.

The osteophytes that occur in association with intervertebral disc pathology and with spinal deformity such as scoliosis or kyphosis may be considered degenerative rather than age-related changes, especially when they are larger or more numerous than other osteophytes. They may be more conspicuous in patients with vertebral infections, rickets, osteoporosis, trauma, and spinal deformities. A causal relationship between transverse tears of the annulus and development of osteophytes has been suggested.

Osteophytes begin as endochondral ossification in the outer attachment region of the annulus[16] and may enlarge progressively with age. The smallest osteophytes are isolated regions of bone formation along the ventral wall of the vertebra near the end plate. Large osteophytes appear as horizontal projections of bone extending outward from the vertebral body. As they enlarge, they involve the anterior longitudinal ligament and peripheral annulus fibrosus, producing an appearance of a "parrot's beak." With continued development they form a bridge of dense compact bone between adjacent vertebrae (see Fig. 6-20). The anatomic relationship of osteophytes to the anterior spinal ligament has suggested that the structure of collagen in the ligaments controls bone formation.

Ligamentum Flavum

In anatomic studies the ligamentum flavum (yellow ligament) is seen to lose its homogeneous appearance with age. Small cysts, collections of fat, and calcifications are common in the ligamentum flavum of older individuals. These are not demonstrated effectively on MRI.[17] The ligament does not hypertrophy or widen conspicuously with

age. The age-related changes in the anterior longitudinal ligament and the interspinous ligament have not been well characterized.

AGE-ASSOCIATED CHANGES OF THE ZYGAPOPHYSEAL AND UNCOVERTEBRAL JOINTS

Zygapophyseal (Facet) Joints

The architecture of the facet joints changes with age. In subjects younger than 20 years of age, the facets show uniform layers of cartilage and subarticular cortical bone. In older adults, the cervical facet joints have lost most of their cartilage and retain only a thin layer of discolored cartilage superimposed on irregularly thickened subarticular bone (Fig. 6-21).[18] The meniscus that characterizes zygapophyseal joints in children younger than the age of 10 years disappears in most adults. These facet changes are nearly universal, so they can be characterized as normal age-related changes.

Standard MRI sequences do not effectively demonstrate the age-associated changes in the cervical facet joint cartilage. However, high-resolution MR images obtained in planes perpendicular to the joint plane may display this pathology (Fig. 6-22). Lumbar facet joints also lose cartilage with aging.[19,20]

Uncovertebral Joints

The uncovertebral joints change with age (Fig. 6-23). In infancy, these joints consist of the uncinate process,

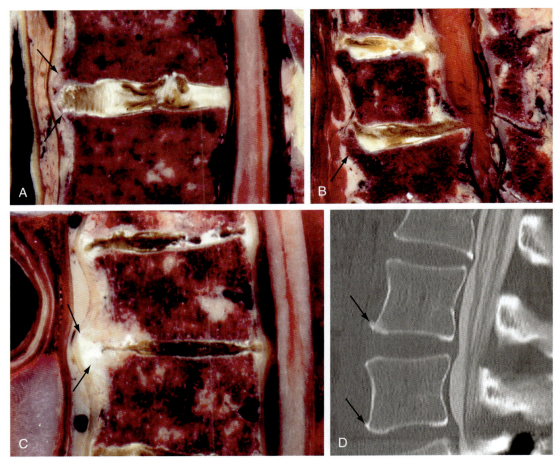

■ **FIGURE 6-20** Vertebral osteophytes. Sagittal anatomic sections show a small (**A**) osteophyte (*arrow*) extending anteriorly from a lumbar disc, a larger (**B**) osteophyte (*arrow*) at a level with disc degeneration, prominent (**C**) osteophytes (*arrow*) extending anteriorly in association with sclerotic changes in the vertebral end plates, and small (**D**) projections of bone (*arrows*) representing early osteophytes arising at intervertebral disc levels in which the disc height remains normal (sagittal reconstruction from a CT myelogram).

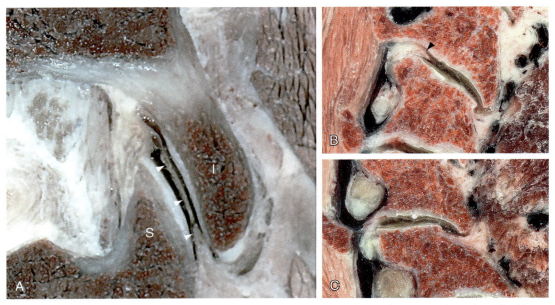

■ **FIGURE 6-21** Cervical zygapophyseal (facet) joints. Sagittal anatomic sections. **A,** In the newborn, a meniscus (*arrowheads*) occupies the space between the cartilage on the superior (S) and inferior (I) articular processes. **B,** In the young adult the meniscus is shortened (*arrowhead*) or completely absent. **C,** The articular cartilage shows thinning with age.

the slightly narrowed portion of the supra-adjacent verte-bra (enchancure), and the intervening fibrocartilage, which resembles fibrocartilage in the remainder of the disc.[21] With aging, a cleft (bursa) develops in the fibrocar-tilage between the uncinate process and enchancure. This cleft gives the impression of a joint adjacent to the unci-nate process, designated the "uncovertebral joint." Unlike diarthrodial joints, however, the uncovertebral "joint" has

no synovium and no hyaline cartilage. Because this cleft develops at each uncinate process in the cervical spine as the cervical spine matures, it is properly classified as an age-related change. In absence of degenerative changes in the intervertebral disc, the uncinate process and enchanc-ure do not display hypertrophy or erosions.

MR images of the cervical spine show the osseous unci-nate process less well than do CT images. MR images obtained in the coronal plane show the fibrocartilage between the uncinate process and enchancure as a tissue with relatively high signal intensity, as in normal disc car-tilage (see Fig. 6-23). The cleft, depending on its size and the amount of fluid in it, may or may not appear in MR images. If it is demonstrated, the cleft has high signal intensity, close to that of clear fluid.

■ **FIGURE 6-22** Oblique sagittal anatomic section through the unco-vertebral joints, neural foramina, and zygapophyseal (facet) joints of the cervical spine. Intervertebral disc cartilage occupies the space between the uncinate processes (*arrows*) and the enchancure of the adjacent vertebra. The uncovertebral joints show no evidence of joint cartilage or synovium.

KEY POINTS

- Age-related changes in the spine are those changes char-acteristic of the majority of individuals of a certain age.
- The intervertebral disc in the aging process increases in opacity, pigmentation, and collagen and decreases slowly in water content and T2 signal intensity.
- During the aging process, intervertebral discs develop concentric and transverse tears that have little effect on disc function.
- Small osteophytes that form nearly universally at all spinal levels can be classified as age-related changes.
- The zygapophyseal (facet) joints of all adults show progressive loss of cartilage and subchondral bone with age.
- Clefts that develop universally in cartilage within the uncovertebral "joint" can be classified as age related.

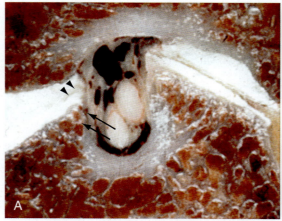
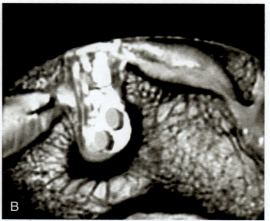

■ **FIGURE 6-23** Age-related changes in the uncovertebral joint. The anatomic section (**A**) and corresponding T1W MR image (**B**) show that tissue is present between the uncinate process (*arrows*) and adjacent vertebral disc. A small cleft or bursa (*arrowheads*) is evident in both the anatomic section and the image. This cleft, which normally develops in the second or third decade of life, represents the structure that is designated the "uncovertebral joint."

SUGGESTED READINGS

Ho PS, Yu SW, Sether LA, et al. Ligamentum flavum: Appearance on sagittal and coronal MR images. Radiology 1988; 168:469-472.

Ho PS, Yu SW, Sether LA, et al. Progressive and regressive changes in the nucleus pulposus: I. The neonate. Radiology 1988; 169:87-91.

Nowicki BH, Haughton VM, Yu S, An H. Radial tears of the intervertebral disc: Anatomic appearance, biomechanics, and clinical effects. Int J Neuroradiol 1997; 3:270-284.

Yu SW, Haughton VM, Ho PS, et al. Progressive and regressive changes in the nucleus pulposus: II. The adult. Radiology 1988; 169:93-97.

Yu SW, Haughton VM, Lynch KL, et al. Fibrous structure in the intervertebral disk: Correlation of MR appearance with anatomic sections. AJNR Am J Neuroradiol 1989; 10:1105-1110.

Yu S, Sether L, Wagner M, Haughton V. Tears of the anulus fibrosus: Correlation between MR and pathologic findings in cadavers. AJR Am J Roentgenol 1988; 9:367-370.

REFERENCES

1. Ho PS, Yu SW, Sether LA, et al. Progressive and regressive changes in the nucleus pulposus: I. The neonate. Radiology 1988; 169: 87-91.

2. Pfirrmann CW, Metzdorf A, Zanetti M, et al. Magnetic resonance classification of lumbar intervertebral disc degeneration. Spine 2001; 26:1873-1878.

3. Thompson JP, Pearce RH, Schechter MT, et al. Preliminary evaluation of a scheme for grading the gross morphology of the human intervertebral disc. Spine 1990; 15:411-415.

4. Coventry MB, Ghormley RK, Kernohan JW. The intervertebral disk: Its microscopic anatomy and pathology: II. Changes in the intervertebral disk concomitant with age. J Bone Joint Surg Am 1945; 27:233-247.

5. Andersson GB. What are the age-related changes in the spine? Bailliere's Clin Rheumatol 1998; 12:161-173.

6. Krueger EC, Perry JO, Wu Y, Haughton V. Changes in T2 relaxation times associated with maturation of the human intervertebral disk. AJNR Am J Neuroradiol 2007; 28:1237-1241.

7. Yu SW, Haughton VM, Lynch KL, et al. Fibrous structure in the intervertebral disk: Correlation of MR appearance with anatomic sections. AJNR Am J Neuroradiol 1989; 10:1105-1110.

8. Yu SW, Haughton VM, Ho PS, et al. Progressive and regressive changes in the nucleus pulposus: II. The adult. Radiology 1988; 169:93-97.

9. Yu S, Sether L, Wagner M, Haughton V. Tears of the anulus fibrosus: Correlation between MR and pathologic findings in cadavers. AJR Am J Roentgenol 1988; 9:367-370.

10. Sether LA, Yu S, Haughton VM, Fischer ME. Intervertebral disk: Normal age-related changes in MR signal intensity. Radiology 1990; 177:385-388.

11. Puschel J. Der Wassergehalt normaler und degenerierter Zwischenwirbelscheiben. Beitr Path Anat 1930; 84:123-130.

12. Eyre DR. Biochemistry of the intervertebral disk. Int Rev Connect Tissue Res 1979; 8:227-291.

13. Pritzker KP. Aging and degeneration in the lumbar intervertebral disc. Orthop Clin North Am 1977; 8:66-77.

14. Ricci C, Cova M, Kang YS, et al. Normal age-related patterns of cellular and fatty bone marrow distribution in the axial skeleton: MR imaging study. Radiology 1990; 177:83-88.

15. Hilel N. Osteophytes of the vertebral column: An anatomical study of their development according to age, race, and sex with considerations as to their etiology and significance. J Bone Joint Surg Am 1962; 44:243-268.

16. Vernon-Roberts B, Pirie CJ. Degenerative changes in the intervertebral discs of the lumbar spine and their sequelae. Rheumatol Rehabil 1977; 16:13-21.

17. Ho PS, Yu SW, Sether LA, et al. Ligamentum flavum: Appearance on sagittal and coronal MR images. Radiology 1988; 168:469-472.

18. Yu SW, Sether L, Haughton VM. Facet joint menisci of the cervical spine: correlative MR imaging and cryomicrotomy study. Radiology 1987; 164:79-82.

19. Monson NL, Haughton VM, Modl JM, et al. Normal and degenerating articular cartilage: In vitro correlation of MR imaging and histologic findings. J Magn Reson Imaging 1992; 2:41-45.

20. Ziv I, Maroudas C, Robin G, Maroudas A. Human facet cartilage: Swelling and some physicochemical characteristics as a function of age: II. Age changes in some biophysical parameters of human facet joint cartilage. Spine 1993; 18:136-146.

21. Fletcher G, Haughton VM, Ho KC, Yu SW. Age-related changes in the cervical facet joints: Studies with cryomicrotomy, MR, and CT. AJR Am J Roentgenol 1990; 154:817-820.

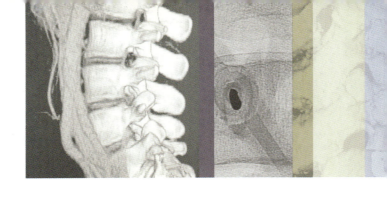

CHAPTER 7

Degenerative Disorders of the Spine

Victor M. Haughton

Degeneration of the spine should be distinguished from normal aging of the spine. Normal aging retains the biomechanical and biochemical functions of the spine, whereas degeneration does not. The claim that disc degeneration begins in the first decade of life and affects many children suggests misconceptions in the use of the term *degeneration*.[1,2] In this chapter a description is provided of the biochemical and biomechanical changes that characterize spinal degeneration and distinguish degeneration from normal aging. The multiple mechanisms by which disc degeneration may lead to back pain are emphasized, and some of the newer MRI techniques used to detect and distinguish degeneration from normal aging are illustrated.

In patients with back, neck, or radicular pain, imaging often focuses on the detection of disc herniation and nerve root compression. In most patients, however, pain results from the degeneration itself and not from direct nerve root compression. Disc degeneration affects the biochemistry of the disc, the anatomic relationships among the spinal elements, and the biomechanical integrity of the motion segments formed by the disc and adjacent vertebrae. Novel biologic and surgical therapies under development target these biochemical and biomechanical causes of degenerative back pain. As studies on novel therapies progress, knowledge of the biochemical and biomechanical changes in aging and degeneration will become increasingly important.

TECHNICAL ASPECTS

MRI Techniques Applicable to Evaluating Spinal Degenerative Changes

The anatomy of the spine can be shown by high-resolution spin-echo (SE) or gradient-recalled-echo (GRE) MR images.

SE images provide qualitative information about the integrity of the intervertebral disc. GRE images provide similar data and diminish the artifacts arising from the motion of cerebrospinal fluid (CSF). Fluid-attenuated inversion recovery (FLAIR) T1-weighted (T1W) images of the spine provide improved contrast between soft tissue and CSF. When an inversion pulse is applied a short time interval (tau) before the excitation and refocusing pulse, short tau inversion recovery (STIR) images are created. STIR images reduce the signal intensity from fat and thereby increase the contrast between tissues with differing water content. Contrast agents often help to demonstrate granulation tissue, to differentiate scar tissue from herniated intervertebral disc tissue, to measure diffusion of solutes in the intervertebral disc, and to detect disruption of the blood/tissue barrier in the spinal cord, nerve roots, and neoplasms.

SE and GRE MRI techniques provide images with differing combinations of T1, proton density, and T2 weighting. In degenerated discs, T2-weighted (T2W) images demonstrate low disc signal, due to loss of water and glycosaminoglycans within the disc (Fig. 7-1). For the purpose of MR reports, this loss of disc signal has been characterized as *dehydration*. However, the signal intensity in MR images is not due solely to water content.

Other MRI techniques useful for analyzing spine function include the measurement of the T2 relaxation times of the discs, dynamic imaging of spinal motion, MR spectroscopy (MRS), diffusion-weighted MRI (DWI), diffusion tensor imaging (DTI), and ultrashort echo time (TE) imaging (UTE). Functional MRI (fMRI) can be used to evaluate neuronal activity within the spinal cord.[3] Phase-contrast MRI helps to evaluate CSF kinetics.[4] Motion-sensitive MR angiographic images (MRA) help to evaluate the spinal vasculature. The techniques most useful for assessing spinal degeneration are summarized briefly below.

■ **FIGURE 7-1** Lumbar intervertebral discs with radial tear of the annulus fibrosus. **A,** Postmortem sagittal T2W MR image shows decreased signal intensity of the L4-L5 intervertebral disc versus the adjacent normal discs. The radial tear of the annulus fibrosus is poorly seen. **B,** The corresponding sagittal anatomic section shows the radial tear (*arrow*).

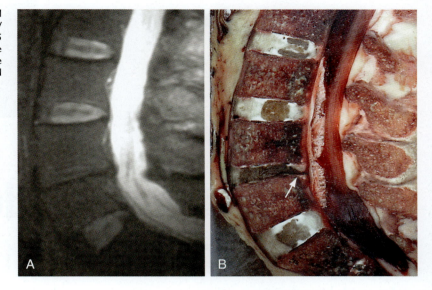

- *T2 relaxation time.* Measuring the T2 relaxation time of the intervertebral disc provides a useful, reproducible technique to assess the effects of disc aging and degeneration (Fig. 7-2).[5-7] T2 relaxation times correlate with the free water content of the disc, so they are affected by aging and degeneration. The T2 relaxation time may provide a sensitive means of detecting the slow progressive loss of disc water seen with normal aging and the more rapid, premature loss of water seen in intervertebral disc degeneration.

- *MRS.* MRS can measure metabolites within the disc (e.g., lactate) and biochemical constituents of the vertebral body (e.g., fat).[8] Degenerating intervertebral discs show increased levels of lactic acid, which may contribute to inflammation and fibrosis in the neighboring arachnoid mater.[9,10] In some storage diseases, MRS may demonstrate abnormal concentrations of lipid within the spine.[11]

- *DWI.* The diffusion of water within the disc reflects both the water content of the disc and the composition

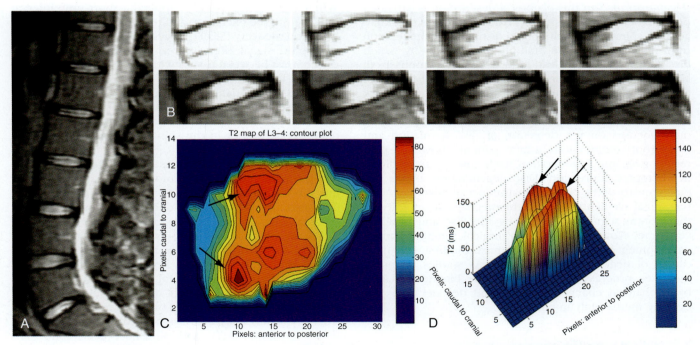

■ **FIGURE 7-2** Calculation of the T2 relaxation times from multiecho MR images. **A,** Sagittal T2W MR image of the lumbar spine at echo time (TE) = 90 ms shows normal lumbar intervertebral discs. **B,** Multiple sagittal images obtained at progressively longer TEs (*displayed from upper left to lower right*) illustrate the decrease of signal within the disc as a function of increasing TE. For each voxel the signal loss is fit to a decay model to calculate the actual T2 relaxation times. The color map (**C**) and the color contour map (**D**) depict the calculated T2 relaxation times for a sagittal slice through the L5/S1 disc shown in **A.** Superior, inferior, anterior, and posterior are marked. The highest T2 values are found in the superior and inferior portions of the nucleus pulposus (*arrows*) with a region of shorter T2 near the center of the disc. Vertebrae have short T2 relaxation times, and CSF has long relaxation times.

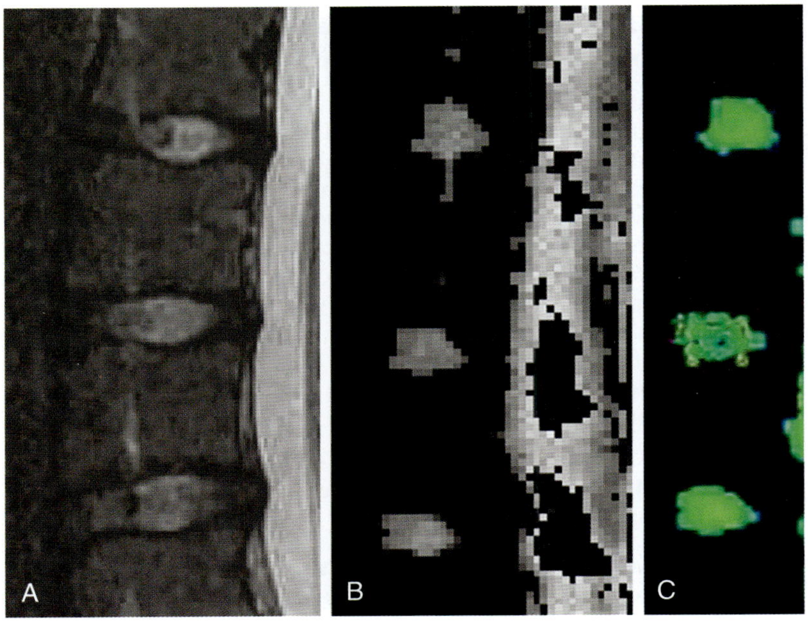

■ **FIGURE 7-3** Sagittal T2W (**A**) diffusion-weighted (**B**) MR images of the spine showing the L2-L3, L3-L4, and L4-L5 discs and adjacent lumbar spine in a 22-year-old woman. The apparent diffusion coefficient (ADC) can be calculated (**C**), and the ADC for specific voxels in the spine can be displayed for a region of interest (marked at L3-L4) in the intervertebral disc.

of the disc matrix. Therefore, measurements of water diffusion within the disc and measurements of the rate at which contrast medium diffuses from the bloodstream into the disc (contrast medium kinetics) can help to evaluate the disc matrix (Fig. 7-3).[12,13]

- **DTI.** DTI measures the magnitude and anisotropy of water diffusion within the disc. Therefore, DTI can be used to demonstrate the orientation of fibers in the annulus fibrosus[14] as a guide to disc integrity, aging, and degeneration.[15,16]
- **UTE.** Ultrashort TE imaging depicts the osseous tissues in the spine. Unlike most MRI techniques, this technique detects MR signal and contrast enhancement within the bone itself.[17] It is likely to be useful in orthopedic research and eventually in clinical evaluations.
- **MRA.** Spinal MRA may be used to identify the artery of Adamkiewicz and related spinal vessels (Fig. 7-4).[18,19] The present resolution of MRA is limited but sufficient to demonstrate some of the normal radiculomedullary arteries and the abnormal vessels associated with vascular malformations of the spinal cord.
- **Dynamic MRI.** New MRI methods attempt to measure the changes in spinal column alignment caused by axial loading and rotation. One method compares the MR images of the spine acquired before and after an axial compressive force is applied to the patient within the scanner.[20,21] Another method assesses the changes in spinal alignment as the patient assumes a variety of sitting or standing positions within an "upright" MR scanner.[22] A third technique assesses the mobility of one spinal motion segment versus adjacent segments as the patient rotates within the scanner.[23] Motion segments containing a normal disc permit rotations of up to 1 degree. Degenerated discs allow greater rotation. Rotation is significantly greater in discs that evoke "concordant pain" at discography than in discs that do not.[24] These dynamic imaging techniques may prove useful

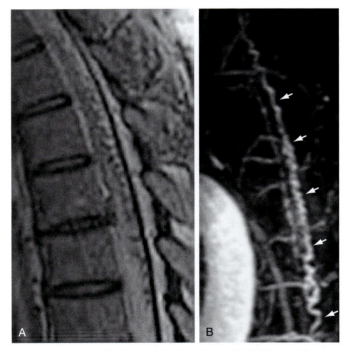

■ **FIGURE 7-4** Sagittal T2W (**A**) MR angiographic (**B**) images illustrate abnormally large and tortuous blood vessels posterior to the spinal cord in a patient with a dural arteriovenous fistula.

for detecting (1) occult spinal stenoses that become evident only when the spine is subjected to a load or force, (2) instability due to ligamentous injury, and (3) nonunion after attempted fusion procedures. The detection and measurement of hypermobility with dynamic imaging may provide objective measures of spinal instability and lead to improved selection criteria for determining when spinal fusions are indicated.[25]

Spinal instability has been defined clinically as the failure of the spine to maintain normal patterns of deformation and resistance under physiologic loading.[26,27] At present, instability is diagnosed clinically by the character of the patient's pain and is (poorly) confirmed by detecting spinal movements on flexion-extension radiographs.[28] In the future, MRI should provide a better measure of spinal of instability. Degeneration of the disc changes the resistance of the motion segment to torque, especially to axial rotatory torque.[29] Normal intervertebral discs resist axial rotation, because the radially orientated, nonelastic collagen fibers in the annulus fibrosus oppose that motion. Radial tears of the annulus fibrosus disrupt the collagen fibers of the disc, so torn discs resist axial rotation less effectively than normal discs. An old, invasive procedure called roentgen stereophotogrammetric analysis was devised to measure spinal rotations in vivo.[30] Newer, non-invasive CT and MRI techniques now measure rotations resulting from axial torque as accurately as roentgen stereophotogrammetric analysis. Imaging of the spine with applied axial rotatory torques may prove to be useful for determining the effect of disc degeneration on motion of the spinal segments in vivo.

Until now, CT and MRI have been used primarily as replacements for myelography—to detect herniated discs and degenerated facet joints that cause nerve root compression. As a result, imaging now has near-perfect accuracy for the identification of disc herniations and nerve root compression.[31] However, at present CT and MRI have limited utility for detecting the causes of back and radicular pain without nerve root compression.[32,33] CT and MRI may show highly similar degenerative changes of the spinal column in patients with and without back pain.[32] In the future, therefore, MRI and CT techniques must evolve into clinically effective tools for assessing noncompressive pain caused by functional abnormalities of the spine.

BIOCHEMISTRY AND BIOMECHANICS IN DEGENERATIVE INTERVERTEBRAL DISCS

Biochemical Changes in Intervertebral Disc Degeneration

Aging and degeneration of the intervertebral disc are both associated with decreased water content, decreased glycosaminoglycans content, and increased collagen content within the disc. However, the *rates* at which water and glycosaminoglycans are lost from the disc differ in aging and disc degeneration. Aging is associated with slow progressive changes in the chemical constituents of the disc. Degeneration manifests much more rapid change. Aging reduces the water content of the disc, primarily in the nucleus pulposus, by a few percent between the third and ninth decades of life.[34] Degeneration causes greater loss of more water over a shorter span of time.[35] Quantitative MRI measures of T2 relation times of the intervertebral disc provide precise, continuous, and reproducible measures that correlate with the free water content of the disc.[5,6] Therefore, the measured T2 relaxation times can be applied to the longitudinal study of disc aging and degeneration.[5]

Biomechanical Changes in Aging and Degeneration of the Disc

Aging and degeneration have different biomechanical effects on the intervertebral disc. Aging discs have an intact annulus fibrosus throughout life that confers normal resistance to applied forces such as axial rotatory torque. Degenerating discs exhibit mechanical failure of the disc. For that reason, biomechanical testing shows that degenerating discs with radial tears of the annulus permit greater rotation between adjacent vertebrae as axial rotatory toque is applied to the spine.[36] Dynamic MRI or CT measures the relative rotation occurring at each lumbar motion segment in response to physiologic rotations of the torso.[37]

MORPHOLOGIC CHARACTERIZATION OF INTERVERTEBRAL DISC DEGENERATION

Gross Morphologic Changes in Degenerated Intervertebral Discs

For radiologic interpretation, the gross anatomic changes in the degenerated intervertebral disc are traditionally described in terms of bulging, herniation, sequestration, and so on. Nomenclature for characterizing disc degeneration by CT and MRI has been standardized to improve agreement and consistency between readers.[38] However the gross anatomic terms used for characterizing degenerating discs do not predict symptomatology and do not correlate well with clinical findings in patients. Furthermore, the terms fail to identify the fundamental changes that cause the disc to fail or to produce pain. The next sections describe, first, the radial tear fundamental to disc degeneration and then the gross morphologic classification for disc degeneration.

Radial Tear of the Annulus Fibrosus

Radial tears of the annulus fibrosus are characteristic of all *degenerating* intervertebral discs but are not found in normally aging discs with preserved height and signal intensity.[39] By definition, a radial tear is a defect that extends through all layers of the annulus fibrosus, from its interior margin to the periphery of the disc (Fig. 7-5). The radial tear may affect the anterior annulus only, the posterior annulus only, or the full diameter of the disc with disruption of both the anterior and the posterior annulus fibrosus. Radial tears can be considered fatigue failures of the disc, because application of repetitive axial loading or axial torsion in the biomechanical laboratory produces radial tears in the annulus fibrosus.[40] Radial tears are found most commonly in the lumbar spine and are most prevalent at the L4-5 and L5-S1 disc levels. Radial tears differ significantly from those tears that involve only a few lamellae of the annulus fibrosus (transverse tears) or that result from delamination between adjacent lamellae of the annulus fibrosus (concentric tears).

Radial tears, a necessary precondition to herniation of the nucleus pulposus, accompany all disc herniations. However, they actually occur more commonly without disc herniations, even in patients with clinical findings

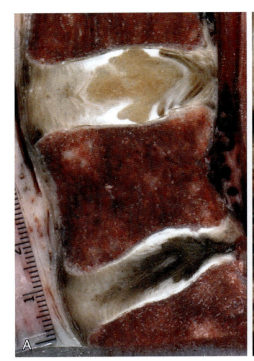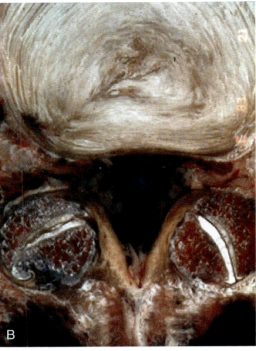

■ **FIGURE 7-5** Radial tears through the annulus fibrosus of L5-S1 illustrated in a sagittal anatomic section (**A**) and in an axial anatomic section (**B**). The radial tear extends through the entire annulus fibrosus.

typical of a herniated disc.[41] Radial tears of the annulus fibrosus may cause pain by several mechanisms, discussed next.

Granulation tissue containing nerve fibers may penetrate into the disc along the radial tear, thereby innervating the disc. Anatomic sections of degenerating intervertebral discs show granulation tissue with both blood vessels and small spinal nerve branches in many radial tears of the annulus fibrosus (Fig. 7-6).[42] Hypothetically, noxious stimulation of nerve fibers within the disc may produce pain referred to the distribution of the spinal nerve supplying the ingrowing fibers. In the lumbar region, this may result in pain referred to a lower extremity. The referred pain may be difficult to distinguish clinically from radiculopathy of a herniated nucleus pulposus compressing a spinal nerve.[41]

Fluids and tissues leaking outward from the nucleus pulposus through the radial tear may cause inflammation of the adjacent meninges. Experimental studies have shown that glycosaminoglycans or lactic acid from an intervertebral disc may initiate inflammation and fibrosus in the dura and the epidural space.[9,10] Disc contents that leak into the epidural space may initiate an immunologic reaction that produces inflammation.[43] The inflammatory process resulting from the irritating fluids escaping from the disc may cause pain.

The disruption of annulus fibers by a radial tear increases motion of the spine at the level of the affected disc.[36] Tears in the strong, obliquely oriented, inelastic collagenous fibers in the annulus fibrosus diminish the stiffness of the disc. Torques or forces, especially axial rotatory torques, produce greater rotation in the motion segment when the radial fibers are disrupted. Therefore, the spinal motion segment that has a radial tear moves nonphysiologically and excessively in the presence of a torque or force.

Hypothetically, the greater spinal motion permitted by a radial tear may cause pain by putting increased strain on other connective tissues that extend across the degenerating disc. This hypothesis has not yet been adequately tested.

A radial tear may cause occult spinal stenosis, that is, stenosis evident only when a load is applied to the spine. In patients with radial tears, normal activities may cause larger than normal changes in the diameter of the lateral spinal canal at the level of the tear.[44] Changes in posture and physiologic loading of the spine may then produce intermittent nerve root compression at spinal levels containing a radial tear of the annulus fibrosus. Changes in the neural foramina sufficient to cause nerve root compression occur when physiologic forces are applied to a disc with a radial tear.[45] When a patient is positioned comfortably in an MR or CT imager, there may be no evidence of central or lateral spinal stenosis. When the same patient is studied in a standing or weight-bearing position or while the patient is rotating his or her torso, the study may show compression of spinal nerves in the neural foramen or central spinal canal.

Radial tears create the conditions necessary for disc herniation. Disc material herniated through the annulus fibrosus may compress spinal nerves in the neural foramen or central spinal canal, causing pain. The identification of a herniated disc, even one compressing a spinal nerve, does not exclude the presence of other pain mechanisms.[46,47]

How the radial tear causes back pain or radicular pain in a specific patient may be difficult to determine. In some subjects a radial tear is asymptomatic. In other patients with back pain, the radial tear may be the cause of back pain. Especially when radial tears are present at multiple levels, the symptomatic radial tear(s) may be difficult to

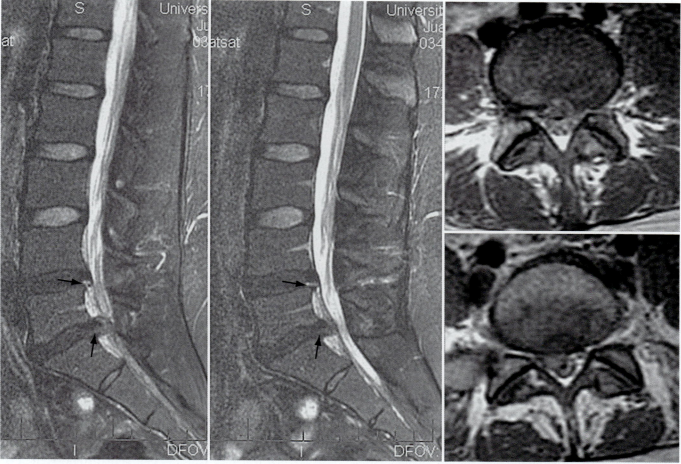

■ **FIGURE 7-6**   Axial T2W MR images illustrate decreased signal intensity and radial tears (*arrows*) in the L4-L5 and L5-S1 intervertebral discs. Axial images demonstrate a small midline protrusion of the disc at L4-L5 and an extrusion posterolaterally in the L5-S1 disc.

identify. Functional tests such as discography may provide some clues to the cause of pain. "Concordant pain," pain provoked by injecting an intervertebral disc with contrast medium at discography, may signify a symptomatic radial tear. Some clinicians perform discography to identify the specific spinal level(s) causing pain in the patient. Production of "concordant pain" by injection of a specific disc has been reported to indicate that the injected disc is the one responsible for the patient's back and radicular pain.[48,49] The value of discography for predicting the outcome from spinal fusion has been debated.

MRI Features of the Radial Tear

The most characteristic finding in a radial tear is the presence of a linear or irregular region of high signal intensity within the annulus on sagittal T2W images (Fig. 7-7).[39] This "high intensity zone" results from mucoid material within the tear. In one cadaver study, about 30% of radial tears lacked mucoid material and showed no high T2 signal intensity in the tear.[51] Because mucoid material may be present in only portions of the tear, the high intensity zone shown on MRI may not indicate the full extent of the tear. On axial MR images radial tears may appear as pie-shaped regions of high signal intensity in the posterior annulus

fibrosus (Fig. 7-8). Radial tears have a high predictive value for positive "concordant pain production" on discography.[48-50] When granulation tissue invades the radial tear, contrast-enhanced sequences may display the tear as a zone of linear enhancement within the disc (Fig. 7-9).[52]

Diminished signal intensity throughout a disc, that is, a "dark disc" on T2W images, indicates the presence of a radial tear of the annulus fibrosus. These discs are referred to popularly as "dehydrated discs," although they have diminished content of proteoglycans and increased content of collagen as well as decreased water content. At discography, "dark discs" invariably show leakage of contrast medium from the disc through the radial tear (Fig. 7-10).[53]

A herniated disc and a bulging disc also indicate the presence of a radial tear. Herniation of the nucleus pulposus requires the presence of a radial tear of the annulus fibrosus, which may or may not be demonstrated by MR (Fig. 7-11). Bulging discs also result from disruption of the annulus fibrosus, as anatomic studies show.[39] Decreased disc height and collapse of the disc indicate more chronic presence of a radial tear (Fig. 7-12).

The linear high intensity zone of the radial tear must be differentiated from concentric (crescentic) and transverse (rim, corner) tears of the annulus fibrosus, which are age-related rather than degenerative changes. Concentric tears of the annulus fibrosus represent focal delamination of the concentric lamellae of the annulus fibrosus. Concentric tears may appear as foci of high signal intensity in the shape of a parenthesis and conform in their orientation to the shape of the lamellae in the annulus fibrosus. They are not necessarily associated with diminished signal intensity or mechanical failure of the disc. Transverse tears of the annulus fibrosus occur near the ring apophysis. They may appear as small hemorrhagic or

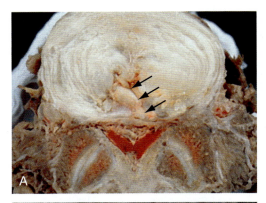

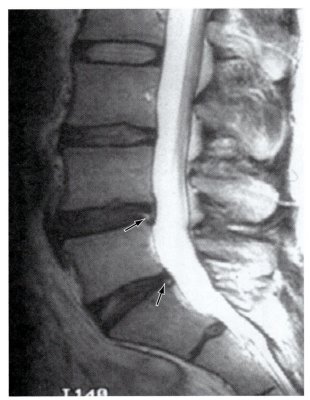

■ **FIGURE 7-7** Sagittal T2W MR image shows small high intensity zones (*arrows*) in the posterior annulus of the L4-L5 and L5-S1 discs. These high signal intensities and the loss of normal signal intensity in the central part of the disc indicate radial tears.

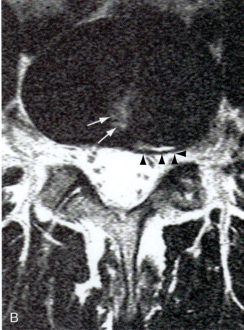

■ **FIGURE 7-8** Radial tear of the annulus fibrosus. **A,** In the axial anatomic section note the amorphous material, nucleus pulposus (*arrows*), in the radial tear. **B,** The MR image shows a region of high signal intensity in the annulus fibrosus (*arrow*), probably displaying mucoid material in a radial tear. A herniated disc shows as high signal intensity (*arrowheads*) between the disc margin and the posterior longitudinal ligament.

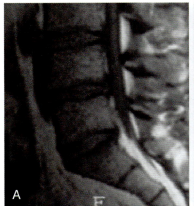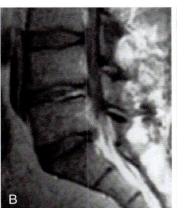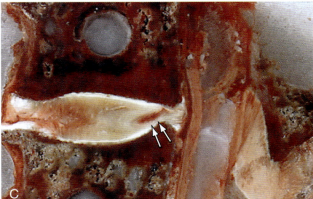

■ **FIGURE 7-9** Sagittal T1W MR images before (**A**) and after (**B**) administration of a contrast agent illustrate linear enhancement (*arrows*) of granulation tissue within a radial tear. **C,** A sagittal section through a lumbar cadaver disc shows a tear in the annulus fibrosus (*arrows*) in which granulation tissue is present. The opposite side of the disc also has a radial tear and evidence of more diffuse granulation tissue.

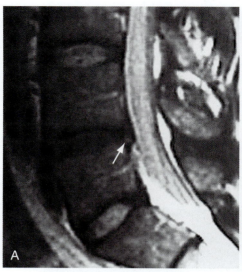
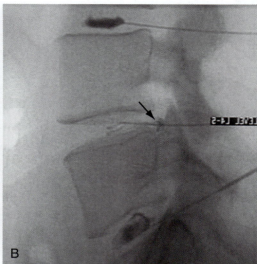

■ **FIGURE 7-10** Discography performed in a disc with a radial tear of the annulus fibrosus. **A,** Sagittal T2W MR image obtained before discography demonstrates reduced signal intensity in the L4-L5 disc and a faint posterior high intensity zone (*arrow*). **B,** The lateral radiograph from the discogram demonstrates cannulas in the L3-L4, L4-L5, and L5-S1 intervertebral discs. Leakage (*arrows*) of contrast medium from the nucleus pulposus at L4-L5 confirms the radial tear, which was barely detectable as a high intensity zone. Needles are present. The contrast medium injected into the L3-L4 and L5-S1 discs is retained in the central region.

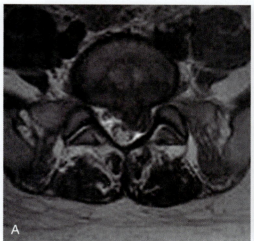
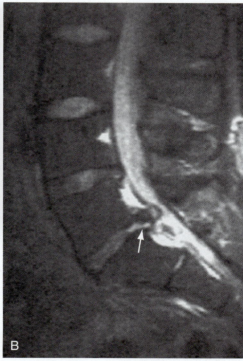

■ **FIGURE 7-11** Sagittal T2W (**A**) and axial T1W (**B**) MR images demonstrate a large herniated disc at L5-S1. The disc fragment displaces and obscures the left S1 nerve root but does not contact the L5 nerve roots. The radial tear through which the disc fragment herniated is evident as a region of increased T2 signal intensity in the posterior annulus fibrosus in the sagittal image (*arrow*).

nonhemorrhagic cleft-like foci of altered T2 signal intensity. They are not necessarily associated with diminished signal intensity or mechanical failure of the disc. Concentric and transverse tears are described in Chapter 6 and illustrated in Figures 6-5 and 6-6.

Gross Morphologic Classifications of Disc Degeneration

The gross morphologic changes in the disc have been used to define stages of disc degeneration.[54] In the staging systems, disc height, signal intensity, and morphology are

evaluated to assign the appropriate stage. The classification of a disc into one of the stages does not suggest the mechanism by which pain is produced. On the basis of gross morphologic changes, degenerating discs can be classified as herniated, bulging annulus, or disc collapse.

Staging Intervertebral Disc Degeneration

One strategy to classify intervertebral disc degeneration is the Pfirrmann staging system.[54] This system distinguishes five stages of disc degeneration (Fig. 7-13). On T2W images *stage I* is characterized by sharp demarcation between the

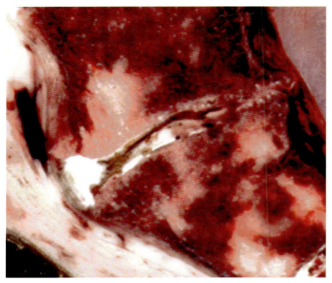

■ **FIGURE 7-12** Sagittal anatomic section illustrates complete collapse of the L5-S1 intervertebral disc with essentially no disc cartilage remaining.

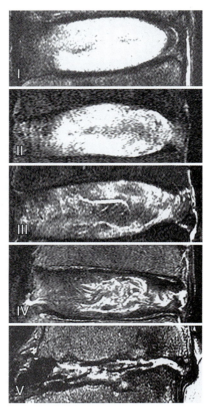

■ **FIGURE 7-13** MR images selected to illustrate the five stages of the Pfirrmann classification for disc degeneration. *From top to bottom:* Type I, a uniform high signal intensity in the central disc that is sharply demarcated from the peripheral lower signal intensity portion of the disc; type II, a less uniform central high signal intensity region and less sharp demarcation from the peripheral lower signal intensity region; type III, diminished signal intensity in the central region; type IV, loss of disc height and fissuring in the disc; and type V, collapse of the intervertebral disc.

dark outer annulus and the higher intensity combined nucleus pulposus plus inner annulus and is typical of normal juvenile intervertebral discs. *Stage II* is characterized by less sharp demarcation between the high and low signal intensity regions of the disc and is typical of normal adolescent and young adult discs. *Stage III* and *stage IV* discs are characterized by fissures and cracks within the disc, diminished signal intensity of the disc, and some reduction in disc height. *Stage V* is characterized by disc collapse. Stages III and IV indicate degenerating intervertebral discs. The precise classification assigned to individual discs in stages III and IV has shown variability among readers.

Classifying the Gross Morphologic Changes of Disc Degeneration

Disc degeneration can be classified by the appearance of the disc margin.[38] This classification system distinguishes normal disc margins, bulging of the annulus fibrosus, and herniation of the disc (subclassified as disc protrusions, disc extrusion, extrusions with subligamentous extension, and sequestrations (free fragments). These classifications have practical value but are not anatomically accurate. Disc *bulging* is defined as centrifugal displacement of 50% or more of the disc margin outside the boundary (perimeter) of the adjacent vertebral body (Fig. 7-14A). The displacement can be symmetric or asymmetric. Disc *herniation* is defined as displacement of less than 50% of

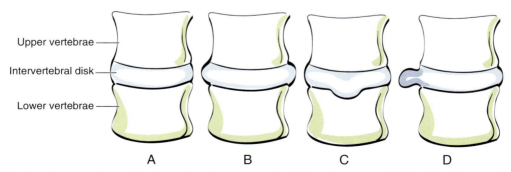

Upper vertebrae

Intervertebral disk

Lower vertebrae

A   B   C   D

■ **FIGURE 7-14** Sketches of two vertebrae and the intervening disc seen posteriorly illustrating a normal (**A**), bulging (**B**), protruded (**C**), and extruded (**D**) intervertebral disc. Note that the normal disc conforms in cross section approximately to the adjacent vertebrae whereas the bulging disc extends beyond the adjacent vertebrae completely around the circumference of the disc or at least halfway around. The protruded disc appears as a focal displacement of the disc margin. The extruded disc appears as a mass of tissue, with a connection to the intervertebral disc that is smaller in dimension than the extrusion itself.

the disc margin outside the perimeter of the adjacent vertebra (see Fig. 7-14B). The term *protrusion* applies when the broadest diameter of the herniation is located at the margin of the disc itself (see Fig. 7-14C). Disc protrusions have a greater diameter at their base than at any other region. The terms *protrusion* and *contained herniation* are also used to indicate that the nucleus pulposus has not herniated outside the posterior longitudinal ligament, although the term *contained herniation* is not considered standard terminology. Herniation may then be subclassified as *broad-based* protrusion if it involves 25% to 50% of the disc margin or *focal* protrusion if it involves less than 25% of the disc margin. The term *extrusion* applies when the broadest diameter of the herniation lies away from the underlying disc rather than at the base of herniation (Fig. 7-14D). The terms *sequestration* and *free fragment* apply when a herniated portion of the disc no longer has contact with the parent disc. Not all disc margin abnormalities are reliably classified into one of the categories by means of this system.

Disc herniations may also be classified by their location vis à vis the central and lateral spinal canals. Use of the terms *midline* or *paramidline* indicates that the disc extends into the spinal canal in or near the midline. Use of the term *lateral* indicates that the disc extends into the neural foramen. The term *far lateral* indicates extension of the disc herniation lateral to the neural foramen. When the disc fragment has a location above or below the parent disc level it is said to have *migrated*. Disc herniations may also be described by their relation to nerve roots. A herniation may displace, compress, stretch, or obscure a spinal nerve in the neural foramen or the central spinal canal, potentially indicating that the affected spinal nerve root is the cause of the patient's pain. When the herniation does not affect an adjoining spinal nerve or spinal cord (and even when it does), other mechanisms of pain production should be considered.

MRI has a nearly perfect accuracy for detecting disc herniations.[31] In the lumbar region, MRI shows the disc fragment, because it is outlined by the fat of the epidural space. In the cervical spine, which contains less fat, MRI shows the displaced disc margin and spondylosis, because they are outlined by the CSF of the subarachnoid space. MRI helps differentiate herniated discs from epidural tumors such as lymphoma and schwannoma, epidural hematoma, cavernous hemangioma, and synovial cyst. In uncertain cases, use of intravenous contrast medium helps to distinguish (usually) enhancing neoplastic processes from (usually) nonenhancing disc herniations. Differentiation of an epidural hematoma from disc herniation requires a high index of suspicion for the epidural hematoma, because neither enhance.[55] In the anterior lumbar spinal canal, an epidural hematoma is usually midline, homogeneous in signal intensity, and (usually) closer in signal intensity to fluid than to disc material (Fig. 7-15).

Osseous Changes Related to Disc Degeneration

The vertebral end plates adjoining a degenerating disc also undergo degeneration and show three types of change[56]: bone marrow edema (type I), fatty conversion of bone marrow (type II), and bony sclerosis (type III) (Fig. 7-16). Type I end plate changes represent water, and perhaps granulation tissue, so the end plates exhibit low signal on T1W imaging and high signal on T2W imaging. Type II end plate changes represent fat, so the end plates exhibit high signal on T1W imaging and slightly less high signal on T2W imaging. Type III end plate changes represent bone, so the end plates exhibit low signal intensity on both T1W and T2W imaging.[56] The clinical significance of these changes is uncertain. Some correlation of type II changes with spinal instability has been suggested,[57] but additional confirmation is needed.

Additional MRI Features in Disc Degeneration

Degeneration may result in foci of increased T2 signal intensity within a disc, reflecting fluid that collects within a fissure or cavity. These foci may be difficult to distinguish from pus accompanying discitis-osteomyelitis, espe-

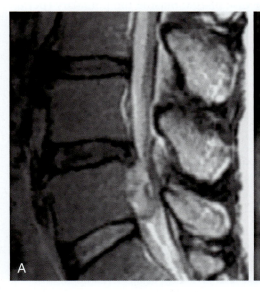
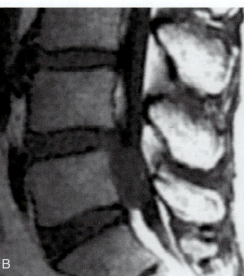

■ **FIGURE 7-15** Sagittal T1W (**A**) and T2W (**B**) MR images demonstrate an epidural hematoma anterior to the dural sac at L5-S1. The collection of blood has longer T1 and T2 relaxation times than most disc fragments, occupies a position slightly below the disc, and has rounded borders.

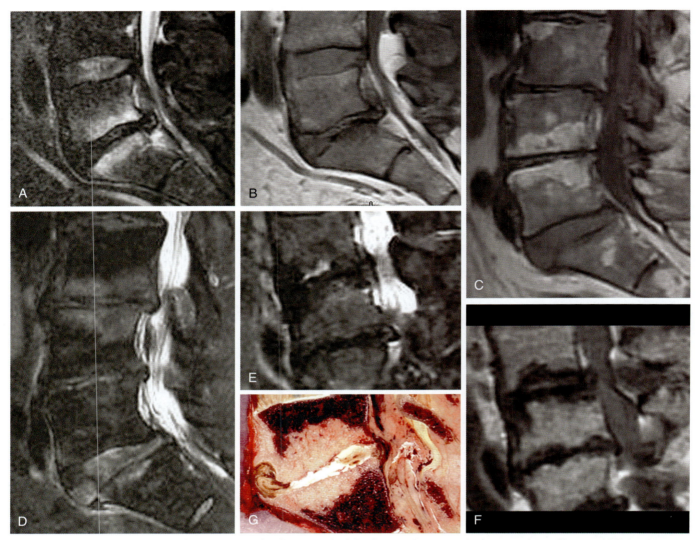

■ FIGURE 7-16 Vertebral end plate changes associated with intervertebral disc degenerations. **A,** Sagittal T2W MR image illustrates high signal intensity adjacent to the degenerating disc characteristic of type I vertebral end plate changes. **B,** Sagittal T1W MR image demonstrates isointensity or hypointensity in the type I changes. The signal intensity changes reflect edema or hyperemia in the marrow. Type II changes, characterized by conversion of red marrow to fatty marrow, result in high signal intensity in T1W images (**C**) and hypointensity in T2W spin-echo images or fast spin-echo images with fat suppression (**D**). Type III changes display low signal intensity in T2W (**E**) and T1W images (**F**). The low signal intensity results from the sclerotic changes in the end plate and often in the adjacent vertebral cortex, shown in a sagittal anatomic section through the lumbar spine (**G**).

cially if the adjoining vertebral margins show type I end plate changes. Contrast enhancement, extensive end plate destruction, and edema within the adjacent soft tissue usually signify infection rather than degenerative disc disease. Disc degeneration may also result in foci of increased T1 signal intensity from calcium salts deposited within the disc.[58] MRI may show a region of absent signal when gas is present within the degenerating disc ("vacuum phenomenon").

Imaging Intervertebral Disc Degeneration with Newer MRI Strategies

Dynamic imaging, in which rotational torque is applied to the spine during an imaging study, may be used to measure the mobility of the spinal motion segment. Dynamic imaging shows that aging discs normally allow the motion segment to rotate less than 1 degree, whereas degenerating discs allow it to rotate up to 6 degrees.[24,36] Diffusion-weighted imaging shows significant changes in the magnitude and anisotropy of water diffusion in discs that contain a radial tear versus those that do not.[16] T2 relaxation times are significantly shorter in discs with a radial tear than in discs with an intact annulus.[6,16] Quantitative MR techniques such as the measurement of T2 relaxation times in the disc may facilitate the distinction between aging and degenerating intervertebral discs.

CERVICAL INTERVERTEBRAL DISC DEGENERATION

The anatomic, biochemical, and biomechanical features of cervical disc degeneration are less well documented than those of lumbar disc degeneration. Degenerating cervical

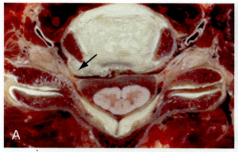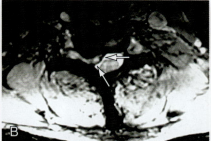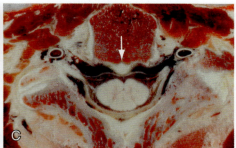

■ **FIGURE 7-17** Herniated intervertebral discs in the cervical spine. **A,** Axial anatomic cadaver section shows a disc herniation in the proximal part of the neural foramen (*arrow*). **B,** Axial T2W MR image shows a disc herniation in a similar location in a patient. Note that the borders of the herniation have a low signal intensity indicative of calcium or bone (*arrows*). **C,** Axial anatomic section in another cadaver illustrates central disc herniation (*arrow*) that does not affect the spinal nerve roots or spinal cord.

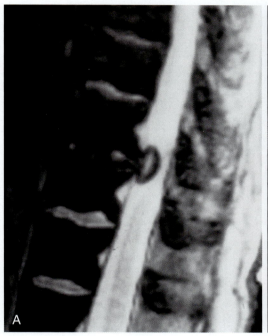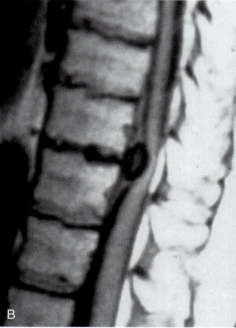

■ **FIGURE 7-18** Sagittal T2W (**A**) and T1W (**B**) MR images show a large, partially calcified disc herniation that displaces and compresses the thoracic spinal cord. The herniation was confirmed at laminectomy.

intervertebral discs are characterized on MRI by decreased signal intensity and reduced height. MRI may show sclerosis in vertebral end plates adjacent to the degenerating disc and in the region of the degenerating uncovertebral joints. Unlike herniations in the lumbar region, cervical herniations usually have concurrent osseous changes, creating an abnormal disc-osteophyte complex (synonyms: ventral ridge, osteochondrosis). Radial tears are common in the degenerating cervical disc, but high intensity zones are seen less frequently in cervical than lumbar discs. Extruded and migrated fragments of disc commonly seen with lumbar disc herniations are infrequent with cervical disc herniations.

In patients with cervical degenerative disc disease, MRI is used to determine the degree of nerve root and cord compression, to determine the size and proportions of disc and bone in the disc-osteophyte complex, and to detect secondary edema or myelomalacia in the compressed spinal cord (Fig. 7-17). High-resolution MR images help to determine whether the degree of canal/foramen narrowing is sufficient to affect a spinal nerve or spinal cord or is simply incidental to adjacent degenerative changes.

THORACIC INTERVERTEBRAL DISC DEGENERATION

Thoracic intervertebral discs degenerate less commonly than cervical or lumbar discs, perhaps because of the stabilizing effect of the ribs on forces affecting the disc. In the thoracic region, reduced height and signal intensity characterize degenerating intervertebral discs. With disc degeneration the posterior annulus fibrosus may extend posteriorly as a small symmetric or asymmetric bulge. These bulges do not commonly cause radicular pain and only questionably cause back pain. Free fragments do not occur commonly in the thoracic region. Some large herniated thoracic discs may contain calcification, mimicking a meningioma (Fig. 7-18). Thoracic disc degeneration may cause central spinal stenosis but rarely lateral spinal stenosis.

DEGENERATIVE CHANGES IN THE VERTEBRAE, INTERVERTEBRAL ARTICULATIONS, AND LIGAMENTS

Vertebral Bodies

Degenerative disease does not typically affect vertebral bodies. The nearly universal spondylosis deformans is better considered a sign of aging than a mark of degeneration. However, when focal spondylosis accompanies intervertebral disc degeneration it may be categorized as a manifestation of intervertebral disc degeneration. Uncovertebral joint degeneration and zygapophyseal (facet) joint degeneration will be considered in this section, recognizing the fact that the uncovertebral joint lacks the characteristics of a true joint and results primarily from degeneration in the intervertebral disc. Vertebral end plate changes that accompany intervertebral disc degeneration were described earlier in this chapter.

Uncovertebral Joint Degeneration

The cervical spine has a pair of uncovertebral joints at C3 through C7. Uncovertebral joints are characterized by the presence of fibrocartilage between the uncinate process below and a focal depression in the inferior end plate of the vertebra above, named the "echancrure," from the French word for notch or indentation. With age, small clefts or bursae develop in the fibrocartilage between the uncinate process and the adjacent vertebra. As the intervertebral discs narrow with age, the uncinate processes on the superior aspects of the lower vertebrae move closer to the upper vertebrae, narrowing the uncovertebral joints. This closer anatomic relationship stimulates bone resorption and subsequent bony overgrowth (Fig. 7-19). These osseous reactions constitute uncovertebral joint degeneration. Hypertrophic bone may contribute to neural foraminal narrowing. In the cervical spine, the spinal nerve roots course through the inferior portion of the neural foramina while the uncovertebral joints border the upper margin of the neural foramina. Therefore, early in the disease, the hypertrophic bone associated with uncovertebral degeneration usually does not affect the spinal nerves in the neural foramina. Vacuum phenomenon often occurs in the degenerating uncovertebral joint. The low signal gas is not easily distinguished from sclerotic bone by MRI but can be easily differentiated by CT.

Ligamentum Flavum (Yellow Ligament) Degeneration

In the process of degeneration, the ligamentum flavum develops calcification, small cysts, and fissures.[50] When cysts and fissures develop near the facet joint, they weaken the ligamentum flavum sufficiently to permit the synovium of the facet joint to herniate into the spinal canal, where if forms a synovial cyst (Fig. 7-20). Synovium may also invade the space between the ligamentum flavum and the neural arch, occasionally producing erosions that simulate a destructive process (Fig. 7-21). The most commonly identified pathologic change in the ligament is thickening, sometime designated hypertrophy. Thickening represents

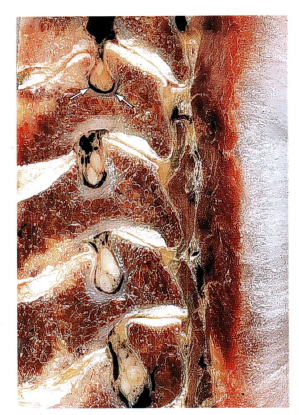

■ FIGURE 7-19 Oblique sagittal anatomic section perpendicular to the cervical neural foramina from a cadaver, showing normal and degenerated uncovertebral joints. Anterior is to the reader's left. The C4-C5 uncovertebral joint at the anterior margin of the neural foramen appears normal. At C5-C6 and C6-C7 mild hypertrophic changes at the uncovertebral joints narrow the neural foramina without affecting the emerging spinal nerves. At C3-C4 in association with the narrowing of the intervertebral disc, moderate sclerosis and hypertrophic changes in the uncovertebral joint and hypertrophy of the facet joint posterior to the neural foramen appear to affect the spinal nerve in the neural foramen (*arrows*).

an increase in width due to a decrease in the length of the ligament as the disc diminishes in height.

Thickening of the ligamentum flavum contributes to central and lateral spinal stenosis. Because the ligamentum flavum lines the posterior aspect of the central spinal canal, thickening of the ligament reduces the volume of the central spinal canal. A thickened ligamentum flavum may then compress the dural sac in the cervical or lumbar region (Fig. 7-22). Because the ligamentum flavum also lines the posterior aspect of the neural foramen, thickening of the ligamentum may also produce lateral spinal stenosis. Compression of a spinal nerve in the neural foramen more commonly results from thickening of the ligamentum flavum than from a bulging intervertebral disc (Fig. 7-23).

Zygapophyseal (Facet) Joint Degeneration

Degenerative changes in the zygapophyseal joints resemble degenerative changes in other synovial joints. The term *zygapophyseal joint degeneration* signifies greater thin-

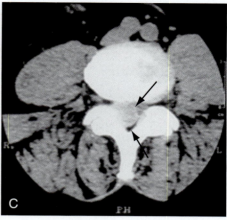

■ **FIGURE 7-20** MR images in three patients showing lumbar synovial cysts. **A,** Sagittal T2W MR image shows a synovial cyst (*arrow*) exhibiting central high signal from synovial fluid and peripheral low signal from a calcified cyst wall. **B,** Sagittal T1W MR image shows a high signal intensity from blood within the synovial cyst (*arrow*). **C,** Axial CT. The large synovial cyst (*arrows*) shows high density due to contrast material injected directly into the adjacent facet joint.

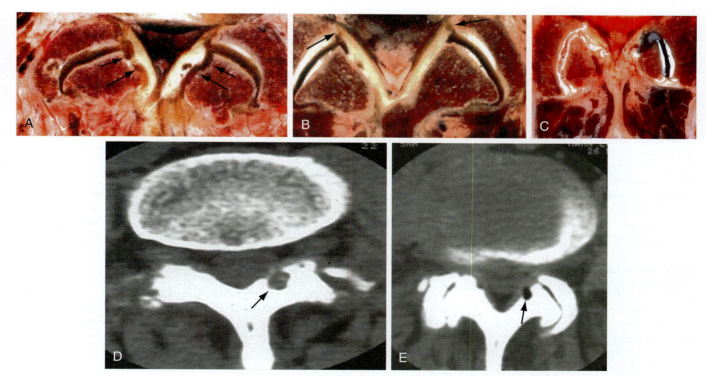

■ **FIGURE 7-21** Axial anatomic sections (**A-C**) and axial CT images (**D, E**) show various appearances of synovial cysts. **A,** Fluid-filled synovial cysts (*arrows*) lie between the ligamentum flavum and the vertebral lamina. **B,** The ligamentum flavum shows defects (*arrows*), through which synovium may herniate to produce an intraspinal synovial cyst. **C,** Dye injected into the left facet joint leaked into a synovial outpouching intruding into the ligamentum flavum. The opposite facet joint shows marked degeneration of the articular cartilage and degeneration of the ligamentum flavum with calcium deposits. **D,** Axial CT image demonstrates erosion of the lamina (*arrow*) secondary to an outpouching of the synovium. **E,** In another patient, an axial CT image shows a collection of gas adjacent to the lamina (*arrow*) owing to vacuum phenomenon in the adjacent joint with escape of gas into extra-articular synovium.

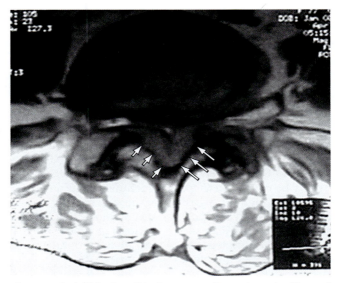

■ **FIGURE 7-22** Axial T1W MR image shows marked thickening of the ligamentum flavum (*arrowheads*) contributing to severe narrowing of the central spinal canal.

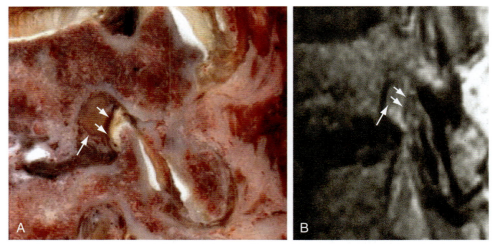

■ **FIGURE 7-23** **A,** Sagittal anatomic section through the neural foramen illustrates shortening and thickening of the ligamentum flavum (*arrowheads*), which contribute to the compression of the spinal nerve emerging at this level (*arrow*). The bulging intervertebral disc does not directly affect the spinal nerve. **B,** Similar sagittal T2W MR image in a different subject shows the thickened ligamentum flavum (*arrowheads*) and its relation to the emerging spinal nerve (*arrow*).

ning of cartilage and greater change in the articular processes than expected for normal aging (see Chapter 6).[59] In the lumbar spine, facet joint degeneration begins with superficial crevasses in the articular cartilage, described as "crab meat degeneration." With additional destruction of cartilage, the articular bone is exposed, leading to superficial erosions or deep cysts in the subarticular bone.[60] This process may stimulate an osteoblastic reaction, resulting in sclerosis and hypertrophy of the articular processes. In the thoracic and lumbar spines, the nerve roots that emerge through the neural foramina course through the superior portion of the neural foramina, immediately inferior to the upper pedicle. Significant bony hypertrophy of the facet joint narrows the neural foramen and may compress these emerging nerve roots within the foramen. High-resolution MRI and CT demonstrate the osseous and cartilaginous changes in the joint.[61]

In the lumbar spine, zygapophyseal joint degeneration causes back pain in a variety of ways. By one mechanism, hypertrophic changes in the joint may narrow the neural foramen to compress a spinal nerve, resulting in radicular pain. By another mechanism, subarticular inflammation stimulating nerve endings in the articular processes may cause pain that is referred in the distribution of the two adjacent spinal nerves that innervate the joint. This referred pain has a similar distribution and character to pain resulting from nerve root compression. Zygapophyseal joint degeneration may contribute to central spinal stenosis, producing symptoms of "pseudoclaudication." Zygapophyseal joint erosions also destabilize the motion segment, contributing to degenerative spinal instability.

Zygapophyseal joint arthropathy particularly affects the lower lumbar segments.[62-64] The arthropathy proceeds more rapidly at L4-5 than at other levels, probably because the stresses on the facet joints are greatest at this level. Degenerative spondylolisthesis, which results predominantly from facet joint degeneration, occurs almost exclusively at the L4-5 level.

Intraspinal synovial cysts result from degeneration of *both* the zygapophyseal joint and the ligamentum flavum. With excessive fluid in the joint, the synovium may herniate through a degenerated ligamentum flavum. The synovial cyst appears in images as an epidural soft tissue process adjacent to a degenerating facet joint, usually at L4-5 and less commonly at other lumbar, thoracic, or cervical levels (see Fig. 7-21). The capsule of the cyst may be calcified. The contents of the cyst may be clear fluid (high T2 signal intensity), proteinaceous fluid (high T1 signal intensity), gas (absence of signal), or blood (high T1 signal intensity and/or low T2 signal intensity). The capsule enhances markedly after administration of intravenous contrast medium. The enhancing capsule may mimic a meningioma or schwannoma.

IMAGING

MRI is frequently used to help diagnose the cause of back pain in patients with degenerative disease. Unfortunately, MRI accurately detects the anatomic and pathologic changes present but often fails to identify the cause of pain or to indicate a specific therapy. MRI may identify highly similar degenerative changes in patients with—and without—back pain. To increase the specificity of imaging, MRI and CT are often supplemented with other techniques such as discography and functional spinal imaging.

In cases imaged for possible disc herniation, sagittal and axial T1W and T2W MR images are inspected for evidence of an abnormal disc margin and evidence of nerve root compression. Patients with evidence of nerve root compression may be candidates for surgical decompression of the nerve and possible spinal stabilization. Demonstrating where the nerve is affected provides useful information for planning surgery. Inaccurate diagnosis of nerve root compression or displacement may contribute to the high incidence of "failed back surgery" in patients presenting with back pain. Identification of the cause of back pain in patients without nerve root compression or radicular signs is less clear. Disc fragments or bulging annuli that do not compress a spinal nerve may still be associated with pain, even pain that simulates very closely a herniated disc.[41] Pain in these cases likely results from the radial tear in the annulus fibrosus.

Therapies to preserve disc function without discectomy or fusion are under evaluation. Some experimental therapies target abnormal biochemistry in the degenerating disc and employ growth factors, genetic material, and genetic regulators injected into the disc to slow or reverse disc degeneration. Implantable devices to maintain the flexibility of the motion segment have completed initial clinical trials. Devices to repair radial tears in the annulus fibrosus have been described and tested. Which of these investigational devices or procedures may best serve the patient with back pain is not presently known. Ongoing research clearly demonstrates the need for better imaging criteria to identify discs that require intervention and to develop imaging strategies to monitor treatment.

In cases imaged for suspected spinal stenosis, the anatomic relationships in the central and lateral spinal canals are inspected. In patients with lower extremity weakness or cervical radiculopathy, the relationships of the spinal cord and nerves in the central and lateral cervical canal are assessed. In patients with low back pain, radicular pain, or pain exacerbated by walking and relieved by rest (pseudo-claudication), the relationship of lumbar nerve roots in the central and lateral spinal canals is assessed. In both regions, the spinal stenosis may be central, lateral, or both. MRI or CT findings that support a diagnosis of *central* spinal stenosis are obliteration of CSF in the subarachnoid space and (in severe cases) high signal intensity in the spinal cord due to myelomalacia (Fig. 7-24). CT and MRI findings that support a diagnosis of *lateral* spinal stenosis include foraminal narrowing sufficient to obliterate all fat around the exiting spinal nerve (Fig. 7-25).

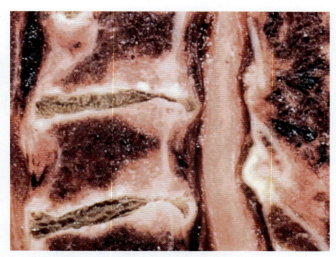

■ **FIGURE 7-24** Sagittal anatomic section through the cervical spine shows a congenitally narrow central spinal canal that is narrowed further anteriorly by disc/osteophyte complexes and posteriorly by buckling of the ligamentum flavum. The spinal cord is compressed.

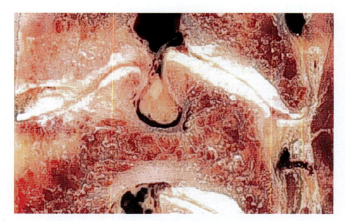

■ **FIGURE 7-25** Anatomic section perpendicular to a cervical neural foramen. Hypertrophic changes in the uncovertebral joint encroach on the anterior aspect of the neural foramen, and hypertrophic changes in the zygoapophyseal joint encroach on the posterior aspect of the spinal canal. Fat in the neural foramen is displaced, and the spinal nerve appears compressed.

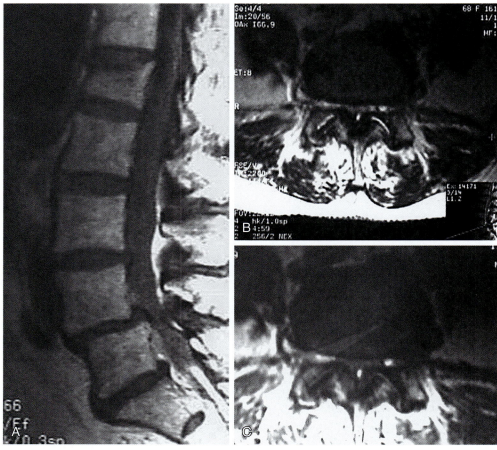

■ **FIGURE 7-26**   Degenerative spondylolisthesis. **A,** The sagittal T1W MR image shows grade 1 spondylolisthesis at L4-5. The axial T2W (**B**) and axial T1W (**C**) MR images at the L4-5 level demonstrate severe spinal stenosis due to the spondylolisthesis and thickening of the ligamentum flavum.

Acquisition of images in three planes facilitates the diagnosis of lateral spinal stenosis. Such images may be acquired sequentially as three separate single plane series in the axial, sagittal, and oblique planes or may be obtained simultaneously as a 3D dataset. Other signs of lumbar spinal stenosis include reduced lumbar epidural fat (Fig. 7-26) (except where excess epidural fat actually compresses the cauda equina, a condition designated epidural lipomatosis). In some cases, "redundant" or "serpentine" roots of the cauda equina cephalic and caudal to a severe stenosis may be seen. Increased T2 signal in the intrathecal CSF caudal to a stenotic level indicates that high-grade stenosis has reduced the CSF pulsations distal to that level. Narrowing of the central spinal canal sufficient to eliminate the high T2 signal intensity within the dural sac indicates critical central lumbar spinal stenosis. In the neural foramen, the fat and vascular tissue surrounding the nerve are obliterated in lateral spinal stenosis.

Spinal stenosis is often graded as mild, moderate, and severe on the basis of subjective criteria, with poor inter-rater and intra-rater agreement.[65] In patients with symptoms suggesting spinal stenosis, the most important role of MRI is to determine whether the narrowing of the canal/foramen is sufficient to compress spinal nerves (crit-ical stenosis) or not (noncritical stenosis). The accuracy of MRI for differentiating critical from noncritical stenosis has not been reported. The clinical diagnosis of spinal stenosis in any patient requires the correlation of imaging findings with clinical evaluation.

The diagnosis of degenerative spondylolisthesis with MRI is very important because surgical management may be especially effective in treating this condition. Spondylolisthesis is most frequent in the seventh and eighth decades of life and is more frequent in women than in men. It occurs almost exclusively at the L4-5 level. Additional study is needed to determine whether MRI can display worsening of the spondylolisthesis in the upright versus the supine scanning position. MRI typically shows severe destruction of the zygapophyseal joints at L4-5. MRI may also show a relatively sagittal orientation of the facets, which further predisposes the spine to spondylolisthesis. Together, the degenerative changes in the zygapophyseal joints and the spondylolisthesis combine to narrow the central spinal canal.

ANALYSIS

A sample report on the CT diagnosis of degenerative disease of the spine is provided in Box 7-1.

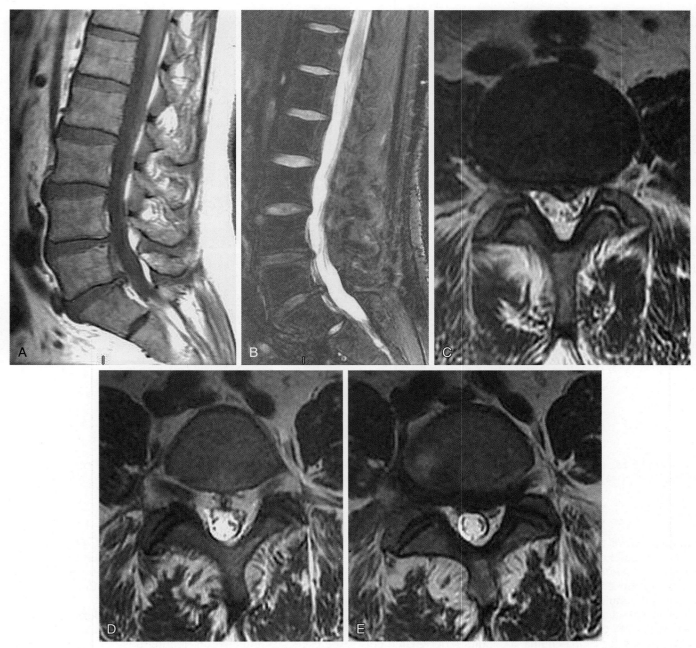

■ **FIGURE 7-27** Sagittal T1W (**A**) and T2W (**B**) MR images through the lumbar spine show loss of signal intensity in the L4-L5 and L5-S1 discs with loss of disc height. A radial tear is evident in the posterior annulus of the L5-S1 disc. The loss of signal intensity in the L4-L5 disc indicates the presence of a radial tear. A vestigial S1-S2 disc is present. The L1-L2, L2-L3, and L3-L4 intervertebral discs have normal signal intensity and height. **C,** Axial image shows a central protrusion of the disc at L4-L5 that indents the dural sac but does not appear to compress spinal nerve roots. At L5-S1, two axial slices (**D, E**) show mild intrusion of the disc into the central spinal canal but no compression of spinal nerves in the neural foramina or in the central spinal canal. This patient had disc degeneration at the two lower lumbar intervertebral disc levels without evidence of nerve root compression.

BOX 7-1   Imaging of Degenerative Disease of the Spine

PATIENT HISTORY

A 69-year-old woman presented with aching axial low back pain that had worsened over the previous 3 weeks.

TECHNIQUE

Serial axial CT sections were obtained through the distal thoracic, lumbar, and upper sacral spines at 0.75-mm collimation and reformatted into 3-mm thick axial, sagittal, and coronal sections using both soft tissue and bone algorithms. No contrast agent was administered.

FINDINGS

The aorta and iliac artery have mild atherosclerosis with no evidence of aneurysm. No hydronephrosis, mass, or lymphadenopathy is noted. The lumbar vertebrae show osteopenia with thickening of the vertical weight-bearing trabeculae, mild dextroscoliosis, slightly increased lordosis with minimal posterior offset of L5 behind S1, and mild osteophytic spurring at L4-L5. The paraspinal muscles show the asymmetric prominence typically seen along the convexity of a scoliosis.

The intervertebral discs at L3-4 and L4-5 are narrowed with calcification of the posterior margin of the L4-L5 disc and gas within a radial tear at L5-S1. The spinal canal shows small overall dimension with focal narrowing at L3-4, L4-5, and L5-S1 that is most severe at L4-5. The facet joints show mild degenerative change with thickening of the ligamentum flavum bilaterally. The prominent disc bulge, facet hypertrophy, and thick ligamentum flavum narrow the neural foramina bilaterally at L3-4, L4-5, and L5-S1. The spinous processes are normal.

IMPRESSION

1. Osteopenia
2. Mild dextroscoliosis
3. Mild degenerative spondylosis and spinal stenosis with narrowing of the neural foramina in the distal lumbar spine, most severe at L4-5
4. Radial tear of the annulus fibrosus at L5-S1

KEY POINTS

- Evaluate the spine for the presence of developmental, traumatic, or other gross changes.
- Evaluate the signal intensity and appearance of the high and low signal intensity tissues in the disc and its height.
- Inspect for fissures in the disc.
- Evaluate the margins of the disc for evidence of herniation, bulging, and nerve root compression.
- Evaluate the signal intensity of the vertebral bone marrow and end plates at each disc level.
- Inspect for thickening of the ligamentum flavum in the central spinal canal and neural foramina.
- Evaluate the size of the central spinal canal and neural foramina in multiple planes.
- Evaluate for evidence of erosions and bony hypertrophy and synovial cysts related to the zygapophyseal joints.
- Evaluate for bony hypertrophy of the uncovertebral joints and their effects on the neural foramen.
- Inspect the spinal cord and cauda equina for effects of degenerative changes.
- Inspect other tissues included in the spine images: prevertebral, vascular, organ, or nodal tissues.

SUGGESTED READINGS

Krueger EC, Perry JO, Wu Y, Haughton V. Changes in T2 relaxation times associated with maturation of the human intervertebral disk. AJNR Am J Neuroradiol 2007; 28:1237-1241.

Modic MT, Steinberg PM, Ross JS, et al. Degenerative disk disease: assessment of changes in vertebral body marrow with MR imaging. Radiology 1988; 166:193-199.

Monson NL, Haughton VM, Modl JM, et al. Normal and degenerating articular cartilage: in vitro correlation of MR imaging and histologic findings. J Magn Reson Imaging 1992; 2:41-45.

Ross JS, Modic MT, Masaryk TJ. Tears of the anulus fibrosus: assessment with Gd-DTPA-enhanced MR imaging. AJR Am J Roentgenol 1990; 154:159-162.

Yu SW, Haughton VM, Sether LA, et al. Comparison of MR and diskography in detecting radial tears of the anulus: a postmortem study. AJNR Am J Neuroradiol 1989; 10:1077-1081.

Yu SW, Sether LA, Ho PS, et al. Tears of the anulus fibrosus: correlation between MR and pathologic findings in cadavers. AJNR Am J Neuroradiol 1988; 9:367-370.

REFERENCES

1. Powell MC, Wilson M, Szyprt P, et al. Prevalence of lumbar disk degeneration observed by magnetic resonance imaging in symptomless women. Lancet 1986; 2:1366-1367.
2. Salminen J, Erkintal-Tertti MO, Paajanen HEK. Magnetic resonance imaging findings of lumbar spine in the young: correlation with leisure time physical activity, spinal mobility and trunk muscle strength in 15 year old pupils without back pain. J Spinal Disord 1993; 6:386-638.
3. Stroman P. Magnetic resonance imaging of neuronal function in the spinal cord: spinal FMRI. Clin Med Res 2005; 3:146-156.
4. Quigley MF, Iskandar B, Quigley ME, et al. Cerebrospinal fluid flow in foramen magnum: temporal and spatial patterns at MR imaging in volunteers and in patients with Chiari I malformation. Radiology 2004; 232:229-236.
5. Boos N, Wallin A, Schmucker T, et al. Quantitative MR imaging of lumbar intervertebral disk and vertebral bodies: methodology,

reproducibility, and preliminary results. Magn Reson Imaging 1994; 1:577-587.

6. Perry J, Haughton V, Anderson PA, et al. The value of T2 relaxation times to characterize lumbar intervertebral disks: preliminary results. AJNR Am J Neuroradiol 2006; 27:337-342.

7. Krueger EC, Perry JO, Wu Y, Haughton V. Changes in T2 relaxation times associated with maturation of the human intervertebral disk. AJNR Am J Neuroradiol 2007; 28:1237-1241.

8. Majumdar S. Magnetic resonance imaging and spectroscopy of the intervertebral disc. NMR Biomed 2006; 19:894-903.

9. Diamant B, Karlsson J, Nachemson A. Correlation between lactate levels and pH in discs of patients with lumbar rhizopathies. Experientia 1968; 24:1195-1196.

10. Haughton VM, Nguyen CM, Ho KC. The etiology of focal spinal arachnoiditis: an experimental study. Spine 1993; 18:1193-1198.

11. Scherer A, Wittsack HJ, Engelbrecht V, et al. Proton MR spectroscopy of the lumbar spine in patients with glycogen storage disease type Ib. J Magn Reson Imaging 2001; 14:757-762.

12. Kealey SM, Aho T, Delong D, et al. Assessment of apparent diffusion coefficient in normal and degenerated intervertebral lumbar disks: initial experience. Radiology 2005; 235:569-574.

13. Nguyen-Minh C, Riley L 3rd, Ho KC, et al. Effect of degeneration of the intervertebral disk on the process of diffusion. AJNR Am J Neuroradiol 1997; 18:435-442.

14. Hsu EW, Setton LA. Diffusion tensor microscopy of the intervertebral disk anulus fibrosus. Magn Reson Med 1999; 41:992-999.

15. Tertti M, Paajanen H, Laato M, et al. Disk degeneration in magnetic resonance imaging: a comparative biochemical, histologic, and radiologic study in cadaver spines. Spine 1991; 16:629-634.

16. Boos N, Wallin A, Schmucker T, et al. Quantitative MR imaging of lumbar intervertebral disk and vertebral bodies: methodology, reproducibility, and preliminary results. Magn Reson Imaging 1994; 12:577-587

17. Robson MD, Bydder GM. Clinical ultrashort echo time imaging of bone and other connective tissues. NMR Biomed 2006; 19:765-780.

18. Mistretta CA, Wieben O, Velikina J, et al. Highly constrained backprojection for time-resolved MRI. Magn Reson Med 2006; 55: 30-40.

19. Bowen BC, Fraser K, Kochan JP, et al. Spinal dural arteriovenous fistulas: evaluation with MR angiography. AJNR Am J Neuroradiol 1995; 16:2029-2043.

20. Willen J, Danielson B. The diagnostic effect from axial loading of the lumbar spine during computed tomography and magnetic resonance imaging in patients with degenerative disorders. Spine 2001; 26:2607-2614.

21. Schonstrom NR, Lindahl S, Willen J, Hansson T. Dynamic changes in the dimensions of the spinal canal: an experimental study in vitro. J Orthop Res 1989; 7:115-121.

22. Vitzthum HE, Konig A, Seifert V. Dynamic examination of the lumbar spine by using vertical, open magnetic resonance imaging. J Neurosurg 2000; 93(1 Suppl):58-64.

23. Haughton VM, Rogers B, Meyerand ME, Resnick DK. Measuring the axial rotation of lumbar vertebrae in vivo with MR imaging. AJNR Am J Neuroradiol 2002; 23:1110-1116.

24. Blankenbaker DG, Haughton VM, Rogers BP, et al. Axial rotation of the lumbar spinal motion segments correlated with concordant pain on discography: a preliminary study. AJR Am J Roentgenol 2006; 186:795-799.

25. Weishaupt D, Schmid MR, Zanetti M, et al. Positional MR imaging of the lumbar spine: does it demonstrate nerve root compromise not visible at conventional MR imaging? Radiology 2000; 215:247-253.

26. Pope MH, Panjabi M. Biomechanical definitions of spinal instability. Spine 1985; 10:255-256.

27. Panjabi MM, Thibodeau LL, Crisco JJ 3d, White AA 3d. What constitutes spinal instability? Clin Neurosurg 1988; 34:313-339.

28. Shaffer WO, Spratt KF, Weinstein J, et al. The consistency and accuracy of roentgenograms for measuring sagittal translation in the lumbar vertebral motion segment: an experimental model. Spine 1990; 15:741-750.

29. Nowicki BH, Haughton VM, Schmidt TA, et al. Occult lumbar lateral spinal stenosis in neural foramina subjected to physiologic loading. AJNR Am J Neuroradiol 1996; 17:1605-1614.

30. Axelsson P, Karlsson BS. Intervertebral mobility in the progressive degenerative process: a radiostereometric analysis. Eur Spine J 2004; 13:567-572.

31. Jarvik JG, Deyo RA. Diagnostic evaluation of low back pain with emphasis on imaging. Ann Intern Med 2002; 137:586-597.

32. Jensen MC, Brant-Zawadzki MN, Obuchowski N, et al. Magnetic resonance imaging of the lumbar spine in people without back pain. N Engl J Med 1994; 331:69-73.

33. Modic MT, Obuchowski NA, Ross JS, et al. Acute low back pain and radiculopathy: MR imaging findings and their prognostic role and effect on outcome. Radiology 2005; 237:597-604.

34. Puschel J. Der Wassergehalt normaler und degenerierter Zwischenwirbelscheiben. Beitr Path Anat 1930; 84:123-130.

35. Antoniou J, Steffen T, Nelson F, et al. The human lumbar intervertebral disc: evidence for changes in the biosynthesis and denaturation of the extracellular matrix with growth, maturation, ageing, and degeneration. J Clin Invest 1996; 98:996-1003.

36. Schmidt TA, An HS, Lim TH, et al. The stiffness of lumbar spinal motion segments with a high-intensity zone in the anulus fibrosus. Spine 1998; 23:2167-2173.

37. Rogers BP, Haughton VM, Arfanakis K, Meyerand ME. Application of image registration to measurement of intervertebral rotation in the lumbar spine. Magn Reson Med 2002; 48:1072-1075.

38. Fardon DF, Milette PC. Nomenclature and classification of lumbar disk pathology: recommendations of the Combined Task Forces of the North American Spine Society, American Society of Spine Radiology, and American Society of Neuroradiology. Spine 2001; 26: E93-E113.

39. Yu S, Sether L, Wagner M, Haughton V. Tears of the anulus fibrosus: correlation between MR and pathologic findings in cadavers. AJR Am J Roentgenol 1988; 9:367-370.

40. Schmidt H, Kettler A, Heuer F, et al. Intradiscal pressure, shear strain, and fiber strain in the intervertebral disk under combined loading. Spine 2007; 32:748-755.

41. Fernstrom U. Discographical study of ruptured lumbar intervertebral discs. Acta Chir Scand Suppl 1960; Suppl 258:1-60.

42. Goldie I. Granulation tissue in the ruptured intervertebral disc. Acta Pathol Microbiol Scand 1958; 42:302-304.

43. Crock HV. Internal disk disruption: a challenge to disk prolapse fifty years on. Spine 1986; 11:650-653.

44. Fujiwara A, An HS, Lim TH, Haughton VM. Morphologic changes in the lumbar intervertebral foramen due to flexion-extension, lateral bending, and axial rotation: an in vitro anatomic and biomechanical study. Spine 2000; 25:3036-3044.

45. Nowicki BH, Haughton VM, Schmidt TA, et al. Occult lumbar lateral spinal stenosis in neural foramina subjected to physiologic loading. AJNR Am J Neuroradiol 1996; 17:1605-1614.

46. Smyth MJ, Wright V. Sciatica and the intervertebral disc. J Bone Joint Surg 1958; 40:1401-1418.

47. Devor M. Neuropathic pain and injured nerve: peripheral mechanisms. Br Med Bull 1991; 47:619-630.

48. Buirski G. Magnetic resonance signal patterns of lumbar discs in patients with low back pain: a prospective study with discographic correlation. Spine 1992; 17:1199-1204.

49. Vanharanta H, Sachs BL, Spivey MA, et al. The relationship of pain provocation to lumbar disk deterioration as seen by CT/discography. Spine 1987; 12:295-298.

50. Kang CH, Kim YH, Lee SH, et al. Can magnetic resonance imaging accurately predict concordant pain provocation during provocative disc infection? Skeletal Radiol 2009; 38:877-885.

51. Yu SW, Haughton VM, Sether LA, Wagner M. Comparison of MR and diskography in detecting radial tears of the anulus: a postmortem study. AJNR Am J Neuroradiol 1989; 10:1077-1081.

52. Ross JS, Modic MT, Masaryk TJ. Tears of the anulus fibrosus: assessment with Gd-DTPA-enhanced MR imaging. AJR Am J Roentgenol 1990; 154:159-162.

53. Schneiderman G, Flannigan B, Kingston S, et al. Magnetic resonance imaging in the diagnosis of disk degeneration: correlation with discography. Spine 1987; 12:276-281.

54. Pfirrmann CW, Metzdorf A, Zanetti M, et al. Magnetic resonance classification of lumbar intervertebral disk degeneration. Spine 2001; 26:1873-1878.

55. Gundry CR, Heithoff KB. Epidural hematoma of the lumbar spine: 18 surgically confirmed cases. Radiology 1993; 187:427-431.

56. Modic MT, Steinberg PM, Ross JS, et al. Degenerative disk disease: assessment of changes in vertebral body marrow with MR imaging. Radiology 1988; 166:193-199.

57. Toyone T, Takahashi K, Kitahara H, et al. Vertebral bone marrow changes in degenerative lumbar disk disease. J Bone Joint Surg 1995; 765:757-764.

58. Major NM, Helms CA, Genant HK. Calcification demonstrated as high signal intensity on T1-weighted MR images of the disks of the lumbar spine. Radiology 1993; 189:494-496.

59. Fletcher G, Haughton VM, Ho KC, Yu SW. Age-related changes in the cervical facet joints: studies with cryomicrotomy, MR, and CT. AJR Am J Roentgenol 1990; 154:817-820.

60. Yu SW, Sether L, Haughton VM. Facet joint menisci of the cervical spine: correlative MR imaging and cryomicrotomy study. Radiology 1987; 164:79-82.

61. Monson NL, Haughton VM, Modl JM, et al. Normal and degenerating articular cartilage: in vitro correlation of MR imaging and histologic findings. J Magn Reson Imaging 1992; 2:41-45.

62. Grogan J, Nowicki BH, Schmidt TA, Haughton VM. Lumbar facet joint tropism does not accelerate degeneration of the facet joints. AJNR Am J Neuroradiol 1997; 18:1325-1329.

63. Carrera GF, Haughton VM, Syvertsen A, Williams AL. Computed tomography of the lumbar facet joints. Radiology 1980; 134:145-148.

64. Yong-Hing K, Kirkaldy-Willis WH: The pathophysiology of degenerative disease of the lumbar spine. Orthop Clin North Am 1983; 14:491-504.

65. Stafira JS, Sonnad JR, Yuh WT, et al. Qualitative assessment of cervical spinal stenosis: observer variability on CT and MR images. AJNR Am J Neuroradiol 2003; 24:766-769.

PART FIVE

Normal Vascularization and Ischemia

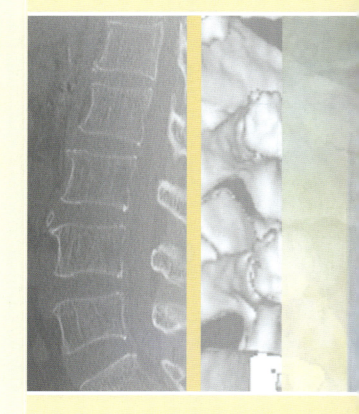

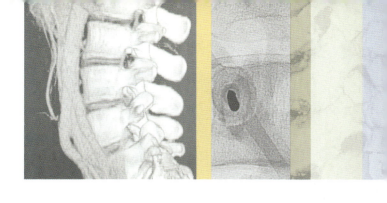

CHAPTER 8

Spinal Vascular Anatomy

Timo Krings, Sosikhan Geibprasert, and Armin K. Thron

The normal vascular anatomy of the spine and spinal cord is described in this chapter as it follows the blood flow from large arteries to smaller arterial trunks and through the capillaries to venous drainage channels of progressively larger size. The application of this anatomy to the imaging of spinal cord pathology is reviewed elsewhere.

ARTERIES

Segmental Arteries and Their Anastomoses

In the segmented spine, the metamere consists of the vertebral body, the paraspinal muscles, the dura, the spinal cord, and the nerve roots for that segment. The blood supply to each metamere derives from the corresponding segmental artery. In the fetus, segmental arteries are present for each of the 31 spinal segments. After intrauterine vascular rearrangement, however, the typical segmental supply is preserved only in the thoracic and lumbar regions: in most of the thoracic region these segmental arteries are the intercostal arteries. In the uppermost thoracic region, several thoracic segments evolve into a common feeder, designated the supreme intercostal artery. In the lumbar region, the four or five lumbar arteries represent the segmental arteries on each side.

The segmental arteries typically supply all the tissues on one side of a given metamere, except for the spinal cord. Because of its embryologic origin, each metamere is centered at the level of the vertebral disc and includes two half vertebrae: the half vertebra above the disc and the half vertebra below the disc. Therefore, each vertebra is supplied by two sequential segmental arteries on each side. These segmental arteries anastomose extensively across the midline; they also anastomose above and below the segmental boundaries via an extraspinal longitudinal

system that interconnects neighboring segmental arteries longitudinally (Figs. 8-1 and 8-2).

This system is highly developed in the cervical region, where the vertebral artery, the deep cervical, and ascending cervical arteries form the most effective chain of longitudinal anastomoses. On each side, the vertebral artery, the deep cervical artery, and the ascending cervical artery provide three potential sources of blood supply to the cervical spine. The vertebral arteries constitute a chain of intersegmental anastomoses, each able to supply a cervical segment. The most prominent cervical arterial anastomosis is the arcade of the dens. In the upper cervical region, potential sources of metameric blood supply include the anastomoses with the external carotid artery via (1) the occipital artery (the C1 and C2 anastomoses) and (2) the ascending pharyngeal artery (the hypoglossal artery that anastomoses with the C3 collateral of the vertebral artery via the odontoid arterial arch). In the sacral and lower lumbar region, the most important supply to the caudal spine arises from the sacral arteries and the iliolumbar artery derived from the internal iliac arteries. These often supply the L5 level.

The segmental spinal vessels course on the lateral aspect of the vertebra or transverse process. They first pass posteriorly along the curve of the vertebral body to supply the periphery of the vertebral body via perforating arteries. At the neural foramen, the spinal branch of the segmental artery passes medially and enters the vertebral canal through the neural foramen. There it regularly divides into three branches: an anterior and a posterior artery of the vertebral canal that supply the bony spinal column and a radicular artery that supplies the dura and nerve root at every segmental level. The muscular branch of the segmental artery continues on, posterior to the neural foramen, to supply the paraspinal musculature.

Within the spinal canal, an intraspinal extradural system establishes transverse anastomoses between sides and

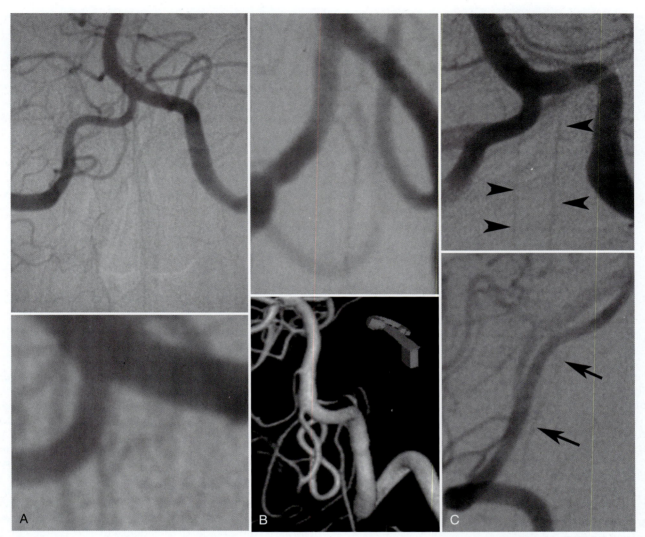

■ **FIGURE 8-1**   The origin of the anterior spinal artery from the vertebral artery varies. It may arise from one or both vertebral arteries. Its junction in the midline is variable, ranging from early fusion in the anterior sulcus to a long unfused segment along the anterior surface of the cord. **A,** "Classic" textbook appearance of a bilateral supply to the anterior spinal artery with a proximal fusion along the midline. **B,** Unilateral supply to the anterior spinal artery. **C,** Bilateral unfused supply to the anterior spinal artery in AP (*arrowheads*) and lateral (*black arrows*) views.

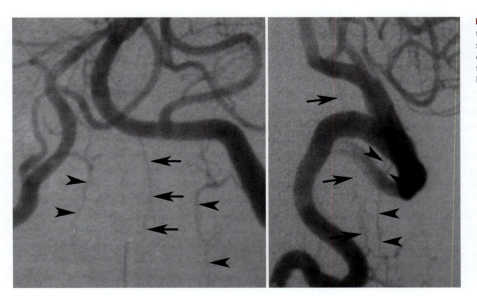

■ **FIGURE 8-2**   In addition to its supply from the anterior spinal artery (*arrows*), the cervical spinal cord may be supplied from the posterolateral spinal arteries (*arrowheads*) that may arise from the posteroinferior posterior inferior cerebellar artery or the vertebral artery directly.

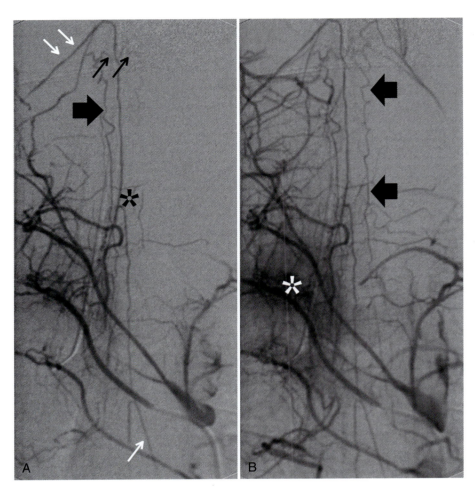

■ **FIGURE 8-3** At various, unpredictable levels, flow within the anterior spinal artery is reinforced by additional metameric arterial supply. In this young patient with suspected arteriovenous malformation, injection of the right segmental artery at the T4 level (A: early arterial, B: late arterial phase) displays the anterior spinal artery, its division into superior and inferior branches (A, *black asterisk*), and retrograde filling of additional feeders both superior and inferior to the T4 level (A, *white arrows*). In addition, radiculopial arteries (*thick black arrows*) fill via an extensive collateral supply with longitudinal and transverse paravertebral anastomoses and via the anastomotic network of the vasocorona (A, *small black arrows*). The level of the injected segmental artery can be deduced from the extensive vertebral blush (B, *white asterisk*).

longitudinal anastomoses among segments. The retrocorporeal and prelaminar arteries supply the bone and dura and interconnect with neighboring and contralateral segmental arteries. These anastomoses provide an excellent collateral circulation. The multiple bilateral, intersegmental, intraspinal and extraspinal anastomoses explain why many segmental arteries can be visualized after injection of just one segmental artery. The extensive network of anastomoses protects the spinal cord against ischemia due to segmental arterial occlusion (Figs. 8-3 and 8-4).

Arteries of the Spinal Cord

Perimedullary Contributing Arteries

In the embryo each radicular artery gives rise to a radiculomedullary artery to supply the segmental spinal cord. Ontogenic transformation and fusion then reduces the number of radicular arteries supplying the spinal cord, so, in postnatal life, only limited—and unpredictable—numbers of segmental radicular arteries continue to reach the spinal cord. Some course along the ventral nerve root to supply the anterior surface of the cord. Others continue along the dorsal nerve root to supply the posterolateral surface of the spinal cord. The medullary vascular tree is pruned more extensively anteriorly than posteriorly. Only 2 to 14 (average, 6) anterior radiculomedullary arteries persist to supply the anterior cord, whereas 11 to 16

posterior radiculomedullary arteries persist to supply the posterolateral cord on each side (Box 8-1).

Different nomenclatures and classifications have been used to describe the arteries of the spinal cord, potentially leading to confusion. The original classification was based on the location and course of the arteries to the spinal cord. It identifies and distinguishes the anterior spinal artery from the posterior or posterolateral spinal arteries. A second classification proposed by Lasjaunias and Berenstein differentiates three types of spinal radicular arteries on the basis of the region they supply. This system identifies and distinguishes radicular, radiculopial, and radiculomedullary vessels. The spinal radicular artery is a small branch, present at every segmental level, which supplies only the segmental nerve root. The radiculopial artery supplies both the nerve root and the dorsolateral superficial pial system (e.g., posterior radicular artery). The radiculomedullary artery supplies the nerve root, the superficial pial system, and the medulla (e.g., anterior radicular artery). This classification offers advantages for the interventional neuroradiologist when compared with the classic nomenclature because it stresses the importance of the anterior spinal arteries for supply to the gray matter of the spinal cord parenchyma. However, because the anterior spinal artery has radicular, radiculopial, and medullary supply and the "radiculopial" posterolateral arteries may provide limited medullary supply (e.g., to part of the posterior horns), this classification may result in misunder-

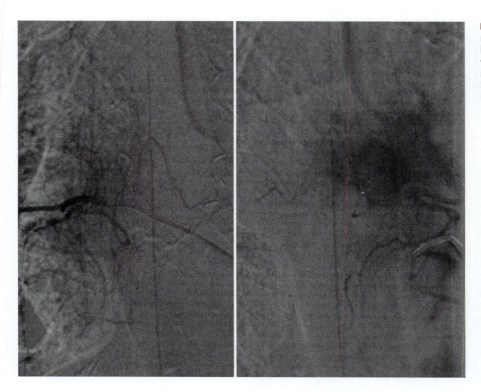

■ **FIGURE 8-4** The blood supply to the anterior spinal artery is highly variable. In this case, bilateral symmetric blood supply to this artery was found after injection in the left and right segmental arteries at the T8 level. Both injections led to retrograde filling of the same but contralateral anterior spinal artery supply.

BOX 8-1   Key Points of Spinal Arterial Anatomy

■ Anterior radiculomedullary arteries: 2-14, average 6
   Always follow nerve roots
   Supply a number of feeders to the
      Cervical cord: 2-3 on average
      Thoracic cord: 1-3 on average
      Lumbar enlargement/conus: 1-2 on average
   These supply the anterior spinal artery and vasocorona.
■ Single anterior spinal artery (ASpA): diameter 0.2-1.0 mm
■ Sulcal branches of ASpA: diameter 0.1-0.25 mm
■ The number of sulcal arteries varies with the spinal level:
   Cervical enlargement: ~5 per longitudinal cm
   Thoracic spinal cord: ~2-3 per longitudinal cm
   Thoracolumbar enlargement: ~6-8 per longitudinal cm
■ Posterior radiculomedullary arteries: 11-16, average 14
   These supply the paired posterior and posterolateral spinal arteries and vasocorona.
■ Paired posterolateral spinal arteries: Diameter 0.1-0.4 mm
■ Penetrating branches of the vasocorona:
   These are numerous: diameter 0.05 mm

---

standings. To prevent potential error, we recently proposed a slight modification to the classification system to overcome the anatomic overlap (Figs. 8-5 and 8-6):

● The term *radicular artery* signifies an artery that supplies the nerve root and the dura mater but not the spinal cord. Radicular arteries are present at every segmental level.
● The term *anterior radiculomedullary artery* signifies a radicular artery in which the persistent medullary branch courses with the anterior nerve root to join the longitudinal arterial trunk running on the anterior

surface of the spinal cord (i.e., the anterior spinal artery). The anterior radiculomedullary artery may also give a minor lateral contribution to the superficial pial network. The anterior radiculomedullary artery is not present at all levels.
● The term *posterior radiculomedullary artery* signifies a radicular artery in which the persistent medullary branch courses with the posterior nerve root to join the longitudinal systems of (1) the posterolateral spinal arteries (situated lateral to the entry zone of the dorsal nerve root) and/or (2) the posterior spinal arteries (situated medial to the entry zone of the dorsal nerve root). These arteries mainly supply the superficial pial network of vessels but may give small branches to the gray matter of the posterior horns (hence their designation radiculo*medullary* arteries). The posterior radiculomedullary artery is not present at all levels.

In using this classification, one must bear in mind that the posterior radiculomedullary arteries predominantly supply the surface of the spinal cord (i.e., the white matter) whereas the anterior radiculomedullary arteries predominantly supply the gray matter of the spinal cord (Figs. 8-7 and 8-8).

Superficial Spinal Cord Arteries

Both the anterior and posterior radiculomedullary arteries supply a system of superficial longitudinal anastomoses that are called the anterior and posterior (or posterolateral) spinal arteries. The anterior spinal artery typically originates from the two vertebral arteries and travels along the anterior median sulcus of the spinal cord (see Fig. 8-1). It has a diameter of 0.2 to 1.0 mm. The paired posterolateral spinal arteries typically originate from the

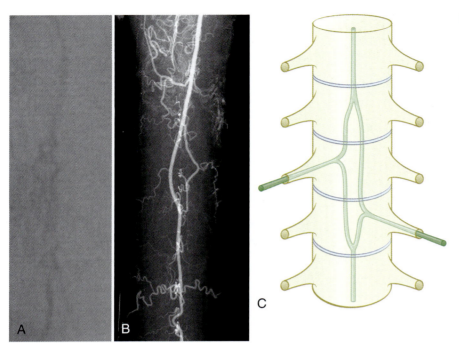

■ **FIGURE 8-5** Angiography. Microradiography (**A**, **B**) and schematic drawing (**C**) of segmental nonfusion of the anterior spinal artery due to segmental rearrangement and fusion of the initially paired anterior longitudinal axes. In the cervical region, the anterior spinal artery frequently shows segmental nonfusion over substantial distances.

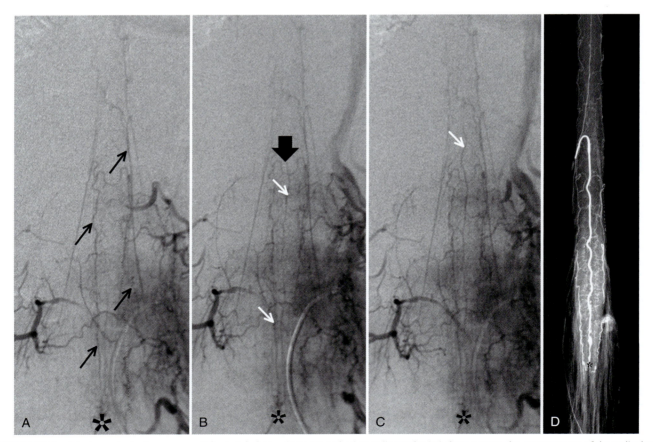

■ **FIGURE 8-6** Arteriography in three sequential arterial phases (**A** to **C**) and microradiography (**D**) demonstrate the anastomoses of the radiculopial network with the anterior spinal artery at the level of the conus medullaris. The posterior radiculomedullary arteries (*black arrows*) are connected to the anterior spinal artery (*white arrows*) through two anastomotic semicircles at the level of the conus (*asterisk*). These are known as the conal "arcade." Note the ladder-like anastomoses between paired lateral radiculopial dorsolateral arteries (*thick black arrow*).

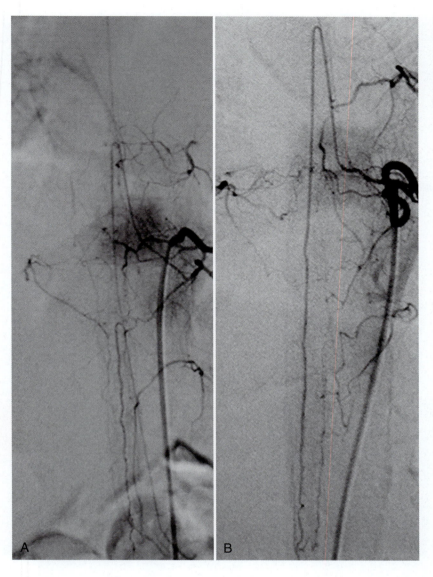

A

B

■ **FIGURE 8-7** Demonstration of the conal arcade by injection into the segmental artery that gives rise to the anterior spinal artery axis. **A** and **B**, Two examples are shown. In both patients the anterior spinal artery can be identified by its characteristic hairpin curve at the midline and its dominant descending branch. At the level of the conus, the anterior spinal artery curves lateral and posterior to anastomose with the posterolateral radiculopial network, which ascends bilaterally.

pre-atlantal portion of the vertebral artery or from the posterior inferior cerebellar artery of each side (see Fig. 8-2). They typically have a diameter of 0.1 to 0.4 mm. These three arteries run continuously from the cervical spine to the conus medullaris but, by themselves, cannot supply the entire spinal cord. Instead, they are reinforced at inconstant levels and intervals by flow from the anterior and posterior radiculomedullary arteries (see Fig. 8-3). For that reason the direction of blood flow in the anterior and posterior/posterolateral spinal arteries may be both caudocranial and craniocaudal at different levels.

The cervical spinal cord has anterior feeders derived from many vessels. The anterior feeders to the upper cervical cord originating from the intracranial segment of the vertebral artery may be very small. They can be unilateral or bilateral and may or may not fuse with each other. Nonfusion of the anterior spinal artery over some distance is frequent in this region. The number of anterior radiculomedullary feeders to the cervical cord averages two to three. One anterior radiculomedullary feeder between C5 and C8 is often distinctly larger (0.4-0.6 mm) than the others. This larger artery is designated the artery of the

cervical enlargement. It arises from the deep and ascending cervical arteries more often than from the vertebral artery (Figs. 8-9 and 8-10).

In the thoracic and lumbar levels, the anterior radiculomedullary arteries branch to reach the spinal cord in a very typical, asymmetric fashion (see Figs. 8-4 and 8-5). The anterior radiculomedullary arteries always reach the cord at the midline. There, a smaller ascending branch continues along the direction of the radicular artery in the midline of the anterior surface. A larger dominant descending branch forms a hairpin curve as soon as it reaches the midline at the entrance of the anterior fissure (see Fig. 8-8). The posterior radiculomedullary arteries reach the dorsal surface of the spinal cord slightly short of the midline (see Figs. 8-9 and 8-11). The major anterior radiculomedullary artery is the artery radiculomedullaris magna (of Adamkiewicz) (see Fig. 8-10). This artery arises close to the thoracolumbar enlargement (between T9 and L1 [exceptionally at L2 or L3], more often on the left side). It is unusual to have additional significant anterior radiculomedullary feeders inferior to the artery of Adamkiewicz.

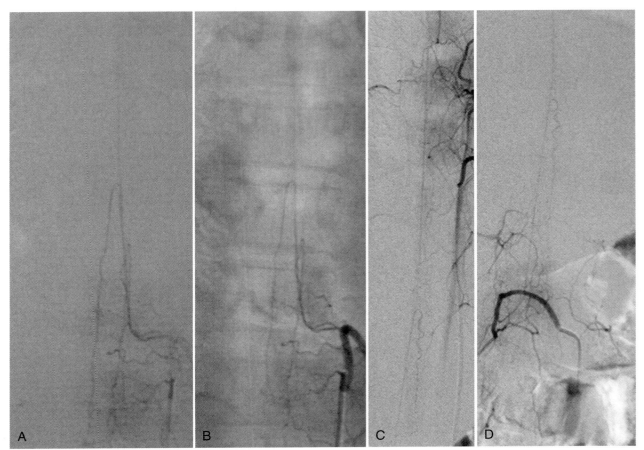

■ **FIGURE 8-8** Typical course of the anterior spinal artery. **A** and **B,** In the first patient the hairpin curve with the dominant descending branch is well seen. The half-translucent bone overlay demonstrates that the hairpin curve occurs close to the midline and that the anterior spinal artery descends exactly in the midline. **C** and **D,** In the second patient, injection into a segmental artery that supplies the anterior spinal artery demonstrates retrograde filling of a second more caudal contributor that was injected subsequently (**D**).

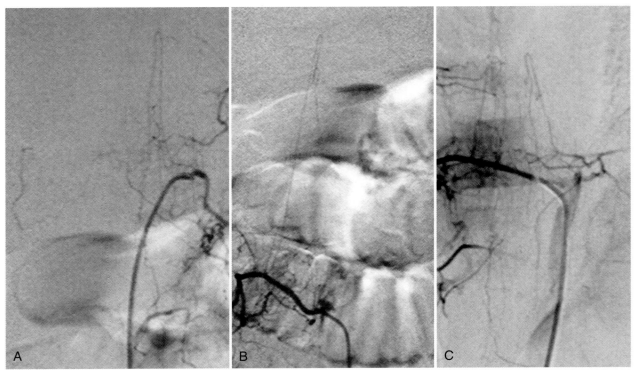

■ **FIGURE 8-9** Four radiculopial arteries in three different patients. **A** and **B,** The hairpin curve of a radiculopial artery is typically steeper and lies off the midline. An ascending branch is not always visualized. In **C,** the contralateral segmental artery that gives rise to a radiculopial artery is visualized via a retrocorporeal anastomosis of the segmental artery.

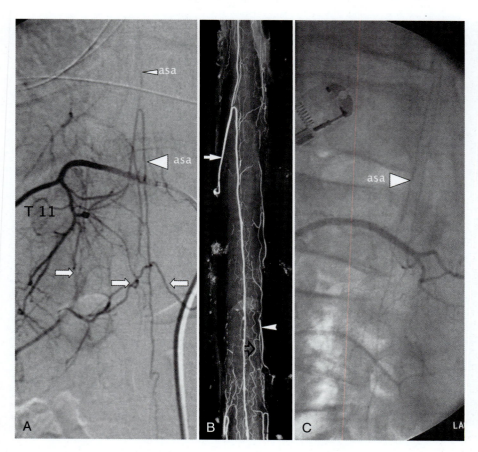

■ **FIGURE 8-10** **A,** At the thoracolumbar level, the great radiculomedullary artery (of Adamkiewicz) gives rise to the anterior spinal artery with its small ascending branch (*small arrowhead*) and dominant descending branch (*large arrowhead*). Other segmental arteries fill via longitudinal and transverse retrocorporeal anastomoses (*small white arrows*). **B,** The microradiograph demonstrates the great radiculomedullary artery (*white arrow*) and the posterior (*white arrowhead*) and posterolateral (*open arrow*) arteries. **C,** The lateral view demonstrates the anterior course of the anterior spinal artery (*white arrowhead*).

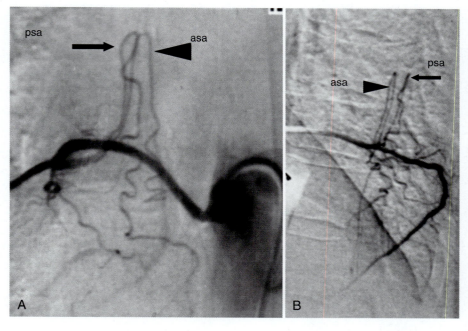

■ **FIGURE 8-11** **A,** In this patient, both the anterior (*arrowhead*) and the posterior (*arrow*) spinal artery arise from the same segmental artery. Anterior radiculomedullary arteries always reach the cord at the midline, whereas posterior arteries reach the cord slightly off midline. **B,** The lateral view clearly demonstrates the position of both spinal cord feeders (*arrowhead* and *arrow*).

The posterior radiculomedullary arteries connect to the anterior spinal artery through two semicircular anastomoses at the level of the conus, known as the "arcade" of the conus (see Figs. 8-6 and 8-7). The anterior and posterior arterial systems also anastomose via an extensive pial network to which they both contribute. This superficial pial network encircles the spinal cord and has been called the vasocorona. The major contribution to this superficial *pial* system derives from the posterior radiculomedullary arteries (Fig. 8-13). The anterior radiculomedullary arteries contribute to the pial system just before they enter the subpial space in the central sulcus (Fig. 8-14). The branches to the pial system on the anterior and lateral surfaces supply the ventral two thirds of the vasocorona (see Figs. 8-11 and 8-12).

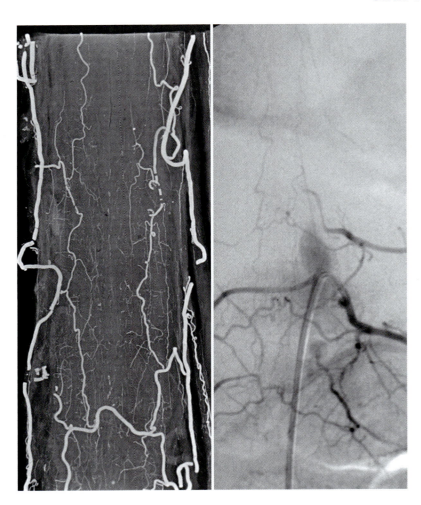

■ **FIGURE 8-12** A radiculopial dorsolateral feeder often demonstrates characteristic ladder-like anastomoses along the posterior surface of the spinal cord.

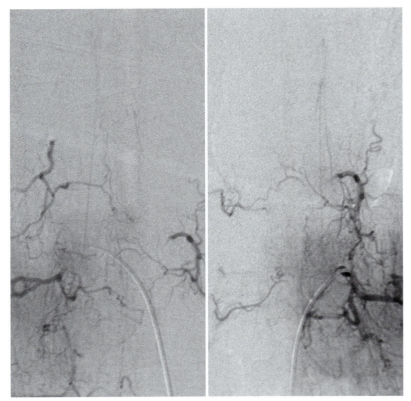

■ **FIGURE 8-13** Two radiculopial dorsolateral feeders anastomose via dorsal ladder-like connections. The arteries supplying the cord always follow the nerve root. At the lumbar and lower thoracic levels, therefore, they always follow a steeply ascending course before they reach the surface of the cord.

Intrinsic Arteries

The anterior spinal artery (ventral axis) provides the main arterial supply to the spinal cord (Fig. 8-15). This artery has a multisegmental distribution of blood and a distinct territory of supply. The arteries directly supplying the spinal cord are the (1) central (sulcal and sulcocommissural) arteries that originate from the anterior spinal artery and (2) the perforating branches that arise from the superficial pial network covering the spinal cord. Sulcal arteries are centrifugal, have a diameter of 0.1 to 0.25 mm, and supply the largest part of the gray matter. They penetrate the parenchyma to the depth of the anterior fissure, course to one side of the cord, and branch mainly within the gray matter (Fig. 8-16). The number of central arteries varies in the different levels: at the cervical enlargement about five central arteries are present per (longitudinal) centimeter. They take a horizontal course. The number of central arteries is two to three per centimeter for the thoracic region with a relatively high prevalence of steeply ascending and descending central artery branches. The densest concentration of central arteries is found in the thoracolumbar enlargement, where six to eight vessels can be found per centimeter (see Figs. 8-13 and 8-14).

The central arteries can anastomose via transmedullary arteries with deep perforating arteries entering from the vasocorona or the posterolateral arteries. The perforating

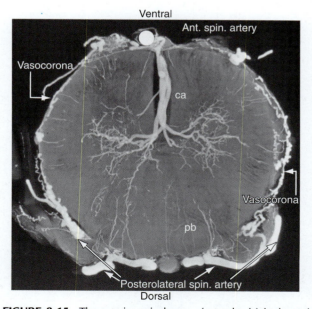

■ **FIGURE 8-15**   The anterior spinal artery (ventral axis) is the major arterial supply to the spinal cord. It irrigates a distinct multisegmental territory. The anterior spinal artery gives rise to central branches (ca, central artery), designated sulcal and subcommissural arteries, which branch outward into the spinal cord centrifugally. The anterior and posterior spinal arteries contribute to the superficial pial network that surrounds the spinal cord. This network gives rise to perforating branches (pd), which enter the cord from the surface and irrigate the cord centripetally.

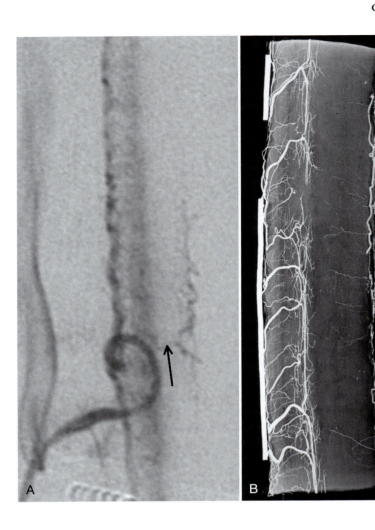

■ FIGURE 8-16 Selective spinal angiogram in lateral view (**A**) and sagittal microradiograph (**B**) of an anterior spinal artery injection demonstrate the sulcocommissural arteries that enter the spinal cord via the anterior sulcus. Note the anastomosis with the posterior spinal network via the vasocorona (**A**, *black arrow*).

arteries that arise from the superficial pial covering of the cord (vasocorona) penetrate into the white matter tracts from the periphery and therefore constitute a centripetal system. These vessels are numerous with a diameter of up to 0.05 mm. The posterior and posterolateral spinal arteries distribute blood to the dorsal one third of the vasocorona. They share with the central artery branches in the supply of the posterior horn and marginal portions of the central gray matter. The posterior/posterolateral arteries do not have as distinct a territory of supply as the anterior spinal artery. Instead, they appear to predominantly reinforce the ladder-like network of posterior pial arteries (see Figs. 8-15 and 8-16).

VEINS

The pattern of venous drainage deviates substantially from that of the arteries. The most important difference is that the spinal arteries always follow the nerves whereas the veins do not necessarily do so (Fig. 8-17; Box 8-2). The arrangement of the veins will be described in the direction of venous drainage from the spinal cord parenchyma toward the epidural venous plexus (see Fig. 8-17).

BOX 8-2   Key Points of Spinal Venous Anatomy

- The veins do not always follow the nerve roots.
- They drain the spinal cord segmentally with horizontal, radial course.
- They drain into two (sometimes discontinuous) longitudinal feeders:
  1. Anterior median vein, which lies deep to the anterior spinal artery in the subpial space
  2. Posterior median vein, which lies in the subarachnoid space and courses independent of the posterior and posterolateral spinal arteries
- At the thoracolumbar enlargement, the veins lie in the perimedullary subarachnoid space. These veins are the largest perimedullary vessels (up to 1.5 mm), larger than the adjacent spinal arteries.
- Transmedullary venous anastomoses (0.3-0.7 mm) interconnect the anterior and posterior median veins.
- Venous outlets are numerous on the surface of the spinal cord:
  Anterior surface: 6-11 veins ≥0.25 mm in diameter
  Posterior surface: 5-10 veins ≥0.25 mm in diameter

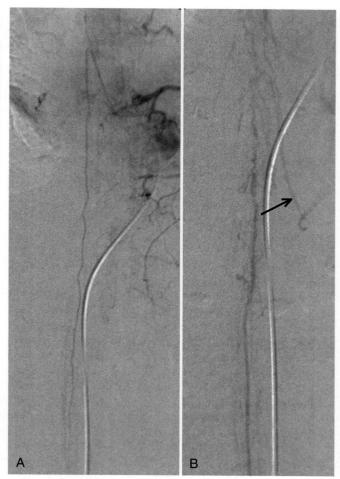

■ **FIGURE 8-17** A and B, Arterial and venous phases of a superselective injection in the segmental artery supplying the anterior spinal artery. Note the artery is smaller than the vein. The spinal radicular vein (**B**, *arrow*) can form a hairpin curve when it leaves the spinal cord to follow the nerve. This is superficially similar to the hairpin curve of the artery.

The blood of the spinal cord parenchyma is drained centripetally, from the depth of the cord to the surface of the cord, by intrinsic veins arrayed in a radial pattern. In axial sections, these intrinsic veins exhibit a horizontal, radial, and symmetric course in most parts of the spinal cord. Only in the lower thoracic cord, from the lower lumbar enlargement to the conus, are the sulcal veins (0.1-0.25 mm) larger than the numerous radial veins.

At the level of the spinal pia mater, blood accumulates into two longitudinal collectors: the anterior and posterior median spinal veins. The anterior median vein is located deep to the anterior spinal artery in the subpial space. Its diameter is largest in the lumbosacral region. In about 80% of cases it runs together with the filum terminale as a sometimes very large terminal vein to reach the end of the dural sac. The longitudinal venous system on the anterior and posterior surfaces of the cord is more variable in course, size, and location than the arterial system (Fig. 8-18). The longitudinal midline veins are not always continuous and may be replaced by secondary systems of smaller caliber. The posterior median spinal vein follows a course that is independent of the posterolateral arteries. It is especially large cranial to the thoracolumbar enlarge-

ment. Varicose convolutions are frequent. The posterior veins of the thoracolumbar enlargement are located in the perimedullary subarachnoid space. They have the largest diameter of all perimedullary vessels (including the arteries) (up to 1.5 mm), so they are the vessels most likely to be seen on normal MRI evaluation (Figs. 8-19 and 8-20). The vessels are part of a pial vascular network that has been called the venous or coronal plexus of the pia mater (see Fig. 8-18).

Intraparenchymal transmedullary venous anastomoses are often present, especially in the thoracic region. They lie in the midline, interconnect the anterior and posterior median veins, but receive no tributaries from the intrinsic spinal cord veins. These midline anastomoses easily direct blood from one side of the cord to the other. They measure 0.3 to 0.7 mm in diameter, so they may be seen on contrast-enhanced MRI. At the cervical level, the anterior and posterior median veins connect to the brain stem veins and basal sinuses around the foramen magnum.

The superficial venous blood collectors drain into the epidural venous plexus through radicular veins. The midline vein transitions to the radicular vein through a venous hairpin curve similar to the arterial hairpin curve described earlier. On angiographic images, therefore, the vein may be mistaken for an artery, particularly when an arteriovenous malformation causes venous enlargement and early venous filling. For the same reason it may be impossible to distinguish the anterior spinal artery from a radicular spinal vein on non–time-resolved MR angiography or CT angiography. The number of venous outlets is high. In some studies an average number of 25 radicular veins was counted on the anterior and posterior surfaces of the cord. If smaller veins (<0.25 mm diameter) are excluded, the number of radiculomedullary veins draining the spinal cord is 6 to 11 for the anterior system and 5 to 10 for the posterior systems. It is likely that the number of radicular veins decreases with age as the veins become fibrotic (see Figs. 8-19 and 8-20).

Drainage of blood from the spine and spinal cord is directed from the multiple radicular veins toward the epidural plexus. Retrograde flow from the epidural venous plexus to veins of the spinal cord (as during spinal epidural phlebography, for example) is very unusual and has only rarely been described in the literature. In anatomic cadaver studies it is nearly impossible to fill veins of the spinal cord by injecting into peripheral veins (e.g., intercostal veins). Anatomic studies show that there are no classic valves in these veins. Instead, microangiography and histology demonstrate substantial narrowing and zigzagging of the veins as they cross the dura (Fig. 8-21). These structural features seem to establish a functional anti-backflow system. The bends of the veins were seen to result either from close vicinity of a vein to a nerve root or from the presence of a bulge of dural collagenous fibers with a glomus-like appearance. Therefore, a distinction can be drawn between slit-type and bulge-type transdural venous "valves." Because epidural shunts without reflux to the perimedullary veins may occasionally be found during spinal angiography, this mechanism normally works even if the epidural plexus is arterialized.

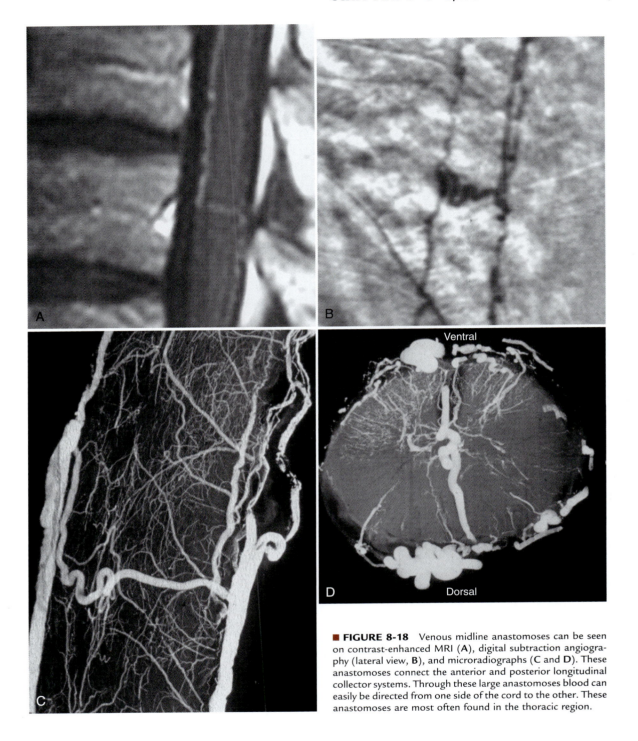

■ FIGURE 8-18 Venous midline anastomoses can be seen on contrast-enhanced MRI (**A**), digital subtraction angiography (lateral view, **B**), and microradiographs (**C** and **D**). These anastomoses connect the anterior and posterior longitudinal collector systems. Through these large anastomoses blood can easily be directed from one side of the cord to the other. These anastomoses are most often found in the thoracic region.

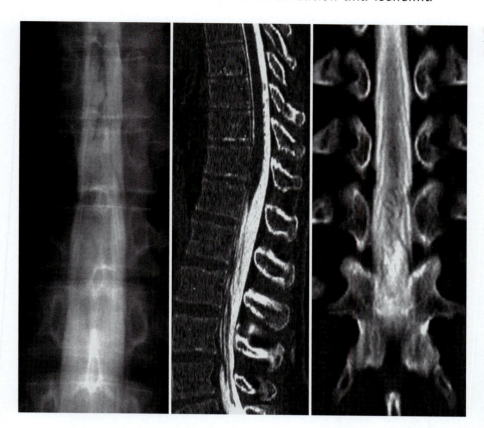

■ **FIGURE 8-19**   Perimedullary veins may be visualized on myelography and CT myelography because they have a diameter of up to 1.5 mm.

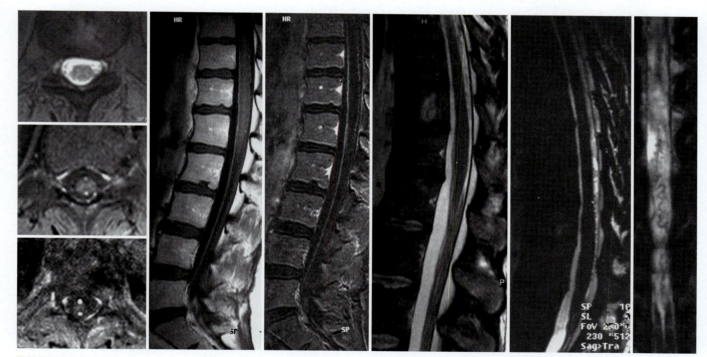

■ **FIGURE 8-20**   MRI displays the posterior veins of the thoracolumbar enlargement in axial, sagittal, and coronal sections. The anterior median vein lies deep to the anterior spinal artery in the subpial space. It has its largest diameter in the lumbosacral region. In about 80% of cases, the vein of the anterior median vein descends with the filum terminale as a (sometimes very large) terminal vein to reach the end of the dural sac. Varicose convolutions of the posterior veins are frequent and should be differentiated from dilated veins due to spinal arteriovenous shunts.

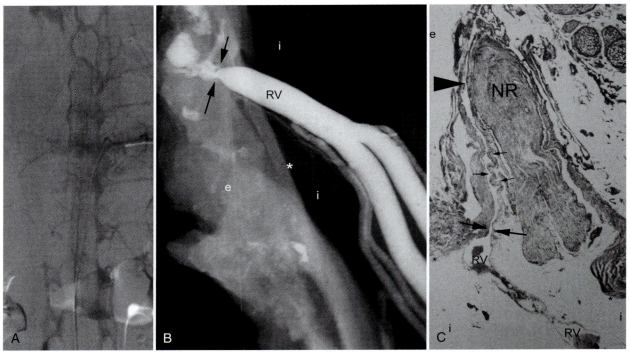

■ FIGURE 8-21 Before the blood enters the epidural venous plexus (**A**), it must traverse a valve-like intradural segment, formed by distinct narrowing (*large black arrows* in B and C) and zigzagging (*small black arrows*) of the radicular vein (RV) as it crosses the dura, as demonstrated on the microradiograph (**B**) and microscopic histology (**C**). Further narrowing of the radicular vein is seen (*arrowhead*) in the proximity of the nerve root (NR).

The epidural venous plexus is a valveless system composed of thin-walled elastic vessels that extend as a continuous system from the sacrum to the base of the skull within the fatty and fibrous tissue of the epidural space. In the lumbar region, the epidural venous plexus connects with the ascending lumbar vein via segmental veins and ultimately joins the azygos (right side) and hemiazygos veins (left side). In the thoracic region, the epidural venous plexus is connected with the azygos and hemiazygos venous systems by the intercostal veins. In the cervical region, the epidural venous plexus is connected with the vertebral and deep cervical veins (see Fig. 8-21).

KEY POINTS

- For each hemi-segment of the spine and spinal cord a metameric artery supplies the bone, the adjacent soft tissue, and the dural sleeve of the nerve root.
- The metameric arteries are densely interconnected via various longitudinal and transverse anastomoses.
- Blood supply to the spinal cord may arise from a variable number of metameric arteries. The specific segments at which the individual metameric arteries arise are unpredictable.
- Arteries supplying the spinal cord connect with either the posterolateral surface or the anterior surface to join the posterolateral or anterior spinal arteries, both systems being a series of longitudinal anastomoses that are reinforced from various levels and that interconnect with each other.
- The anterior spinal artery mainly supplies the gray matter deep in the cord via perforating sulcocommissural arteries, whereas the posterolateral arteries supply the white matter of the cord periphery via pial coronal arteries.
- Veins collect the blood of the spinal cord in a centrifugal pattern and join longitudinal collectors at the cord surface that further drain via radicular veins to the epidural venous plexus.

SUGGESTED READINGS

Lasjaunias P, Berenstein A, Ter Brugge KG. Surgical Neuroangiography, 2nd ed, Vol 1, Clinical Vascular Anatomy and Variations. Berlin, Springer, 2001.

Thron A. Vascular Anatomy of the Spinal Cord: Neuroradiological Investigations and Clinical Syndromes. Berlin, Springer, 1988.

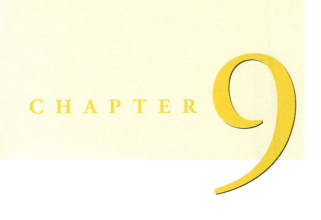

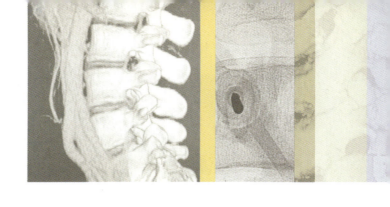

CHAPTER 9

Spinal Cord Arterial Ischemia

Timo Krings, Sasikhan Geibprasert, and Armin K. Thron

Spinal cord ischemia is caused by deficient spinal arterial blood flow secondary to occlusion of intercostal/lumbar arteries or to involvement of the intrinsic arteries of the cord. It is also referred to as ischemic myelomalacia of the spinal cord.

Epidemiology

The precise epidemiology of spinal cord arterial ischemia is unknown. In our experience, men and women are affected equally and age range is highly variable: 0.5 to 82 years, mean age 48 years. Based on the approximately 40 cases we have seen over the past years, we estimate the incidence to be close to 1 in 100,000 people per year. Approximately two thirds of spinal cord arterial infarctions involve the thoracolumbar enlargement and the conus medullaris (Fig. 9-1). The cervical region is less commonly affected.

Pathophysiology

Conditions that commonly cause *cerebral* infarction cause *spinal cord* infarction far less often.

Atherosclerosis rarely affects the spinal arteries. Simple occlusion of a spinal artery rarely causes spinal infarction because of the multiple anastomoses present among the spinal arteries. Watershed ischemia is similarly less common.

The traditional hypothesis of a watershed zone ischemic vulnerability near T4 is not supported by the relatively low incidence of spinal cord infarctions at that level in clinical and imaging analyses (Fig. 9-2). Thus, the concept of a vulnerable watershed zone at T4 seems no longer to be valid in acute spinal cord ischemia.

Instead, a wide variety of less usual diseases cause arterial infarction of the cord, including aortic dissection, surgery for aortoiliac occlusive disease, thromboembolism to the spinal arteries, coagulopathy, vasculitis, radiation-induced vasculopathy, toxic effects of contrast media, epidural anesthesia, periradicular nerve root therapy with corticosteroids, decompression illness (caisson disease, "the bends"), shock or cardiac arrest, lumbar artery compression, spinal tumors, and vascular malformations. Embolism of intervertebral disc cartilage may be a specific cause of arterial infarction of the spinal cord, because postmortem studies have shown cartilaginous material within the lumina of spinal arteries when spinal ischemia is associated with spinal trauma and increased axial loading. It is postulated that acute vertical herniations of disc material into the vertebral bodies increase intraosseous pressure and cause retrograde embolism of cartilaginous tissue into the arteries supplying the spinal cord.

Compression of a lumbar artery by the crus of the diaphragm is another, exceptionally rare, cause of spinal cord ischemia. The first right and left lumbar arteries and the second right lumbar artery course through an osteotendinous canal between the vertebral body and the crus of the diaphragm. If the artery of Adamkiewicz (great radiculomedullary artery of the lumbar enlargement) arises at these levels, the arterial supply of the spinal cord could be compromised by prolonged hyperlordosis, which kinks and compresses the lumbar arteries as they cross through the diaphragmatic crus (Fig. 9-3).

Clinical Presentation

Acute arterial ischemia of the spinal cord commonly presents as pain and acute onset of transverse cord symptoms. The specific neurologic deficits depend on the level and extent of cord damage. Symptoms may include nerve root deficits and sphincter disturbances. Because the arterial supply to the spinal cord is highly variable and because the anastomotic network is so extensive, true clinical spinal cord syndromes, such as the anterior spinal artery syndrome, are not often seen (Fig. 9-4).

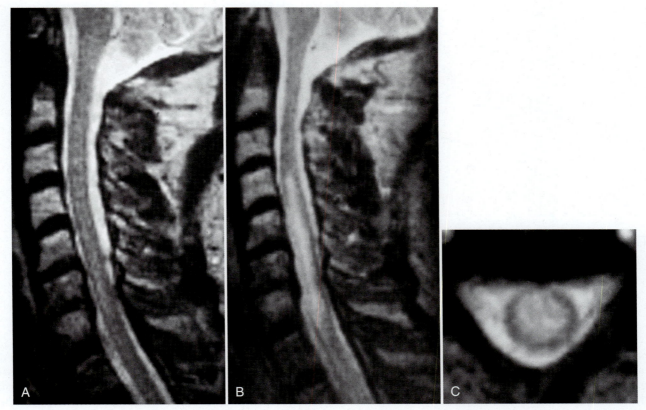

■ **FIGURE 9-1**   A 53-year-old man presented with acute tetraparesis. **A,** T2W MR image 5 hours after symptom onset demonstrates no cord abnormality. Follow-up 3 days later in sagittal (**B**) and axial (**C**) planes demonstrates an extensive infarction in the territory of the anterior spinal artery.

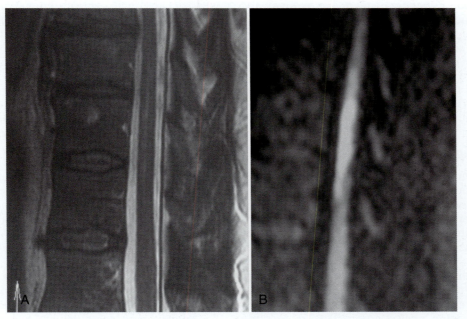

■ **FIGURE 9-2**   This 55-year-old man experienced acute onset of severe stabbing back pain followed by subacute onset of paraplegia. **A,** Eight hours after onset of the symptoms sagittal T2W MR image shows a subtle pencil-shaped hyperintensity of the spinal cord. **B,** Diffusion-weighted sagittal MR image shows a large area of diffusion restriction indicating spinal cord ischemia.

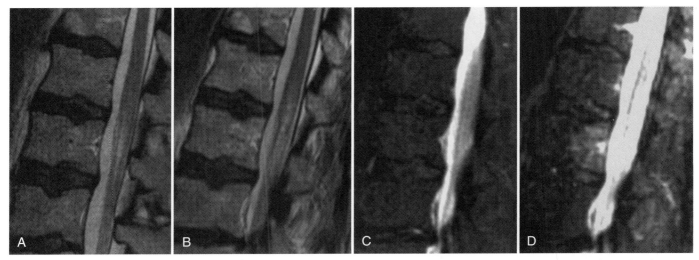

■ **FIGURE 9-3** Evolution of signal changes after spinal cord ischemia with an associated vertebral body infarction. **A to C,** At 1 hour after the onset of acute stabbing back pain and paraplegia, T2W and STIR images are essentially normal. **D,** Follow-up 3 days later with STIR MRI shows increased signal within the ischemic conus medullaris and the associated vertebral body infarction, indicating that the infarctions arose by occlusion of a segmental artery.

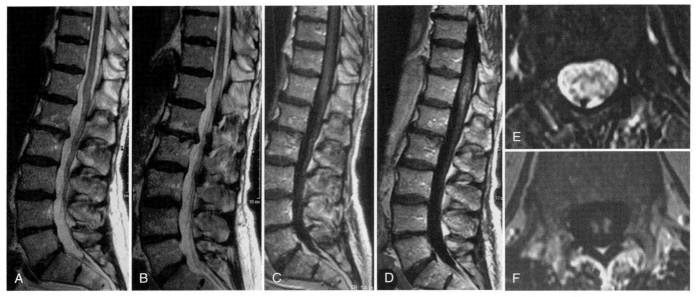

■ **FIGURE 9-4** This 62-year-old patient experienced acute onset of a conus medullaris syndrome. MRI was performed 4 hours (**A, C**) and then 7 days (**B, D, E, F**) after symptom onset. **A, B,** and **E** are T2W sequences. **C, D,** and **F** are contrast-enhanced T1W sequences. The initial MR images are normal. Appearance of hyperintensity and contrast enhancement at 7 days confirms that the patient suffered acute ischemia of the conus medullaris.

Imaging

Acute arterial ischemia of the spinal cord is best evaluated by MRI not CT. The field of view should include the aorta to rule out acute dissections that may occlude the segmental arteries. Only 50% of patients show demarcation of spinal ischemia within the first 24 hours. Thus, imaging studies are used mainly to rule out other potential causes of acute transverse cord symptoms, such as hyperacute hemorrhage. Areas of spinal cord ischemia usually appear as pencil-shaped zones of increased signal on T2-weighted (T2W) imaging within the anterior two thirds of the spinal cord. Circumscribed infarctions affect the posterior one

third of the spinal cord in the distribution of the radiculopial dorsolateral spinal arteries only rarely. Acute infarctions show moderate cord swelling that evolves into atrophy over the subsequent years. Acute cord infarctions show no enhancement, but subacute infarctions typically do enhance (usually beginning after 5 days and persisting for up to 3 weeks after the onset of ischemia). Therefore, contrast-enhanced T1-weighted (T1W) images help to date the injury. The enhancement seen along the periphery of the central gray matter is due to resorption of the damaged tissue by the infiltrating macrophages (as in the brain). The enhancement seen in the cauda equina results from disruption of the blood-cord barrier and reactive

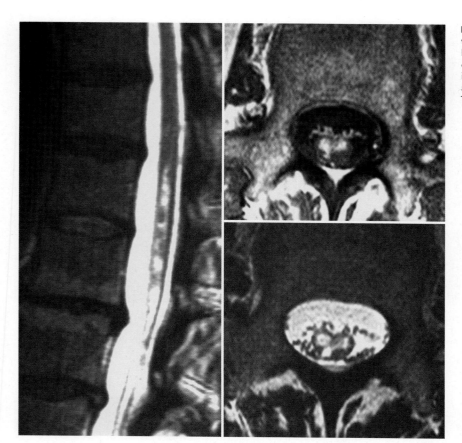

■ **FIGURE 9-5** A 55-year-old woman presented with acute onset of paraplegia and sphincter disturbances, indicating a transverse lesion of the spinal cord. On day 3, MRI demonstrates a patchy area of increased signal intensity in the conus medullaris and associated contrast enhancement on T2W imaging. The affected nerve roots also enhance.

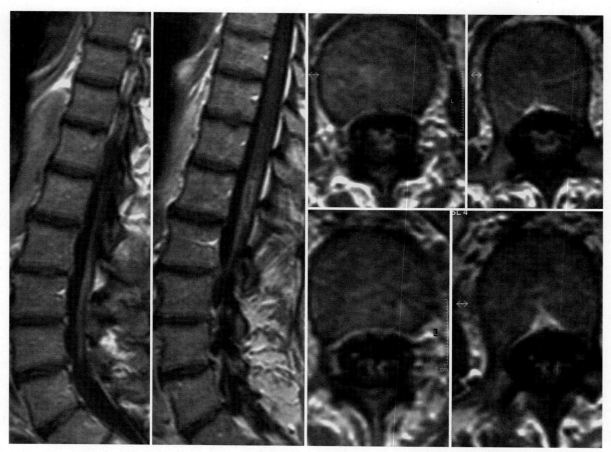

■ **FIGURE 9-6** MRI performed 19 days after spinal ischemic injury demonstrates contrast enhancement of the conus medullaris and the filum terminale. Contrast enhancement can persist for up to 3 weeks after the ischemic insult. The enhancement at the periphery of the central gray matter is due to resorption of damaged tissue by infiltrating macrophages (as in the brain). The enhancement of the cauda equina indicates disruption of the blood-cord barrier and reactive hyperemia.

hyperemia. Fat-suppressed MR sequences are essential for evaluating acute spinal cord ischemia. Demonstration of concurrent or evolving signal abnormality in the adjacent vertebral bodies is highly suggestive of acute cord infarction with concurrent infarction of the vertebral body from occlusion of the segmental artery. Vertebral body infarctions are present in approximately one third of all patients with spinal ischemia. The vertebral end plates and the deep medullary portion of the vertebrae are most vulnerable to ischemia (Figs. 9-5 to 9-8).

Other MRI techniques may help to establish the correct diagnosis of arterial infarction of the spinal cord: fluid-attenuated inversion recovery (FLAIR) sequences can help to detect subarachnoid hemorrhage as a rare differential diagnosis for acute onset of painful spinal symptoms. During the first week only, diffusion-weighted MRI (DWI) may show the restricted diffusion early in the course of the infarction; however, DWI is difficult to perform in the spine because of susceptibility artifacts.

ANALYSIS

Clinical findings of acute radicular pain with, or shortly followed by, spinal neurologic symptoms suggest possible spinal cord infarction. In the acute phase, the major role of imaging is to rule out other causes of nontraumatic acute transverse cord symptoms, especially hemorrhage. If imaging findings are normal in the acute stage and symptoms persist, follow-up imaging is recommended to establish spinal cord ischemia (see Box 9-1).

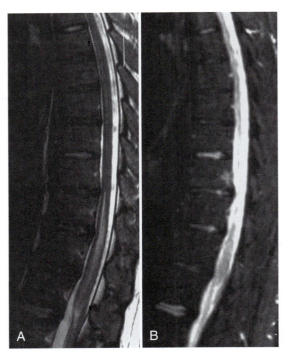

■ **FIGURE 9-7** While lifting a heavy weight from the ground, this 23-year-old student experienced severe stabbing back pain. Four hours later, he reported paresthesias of both legs, ascending paraparesis, and numbness below T10. Thirty minutes thereafter pain subsided, but the patient became paraplegic with bladder dysfunction. Cerebrospinal fluid studies and initial MRI were normal. **A, B,** Follow-up MRI on day 2 shows spinal cord ischemia and vertebral body infarction.

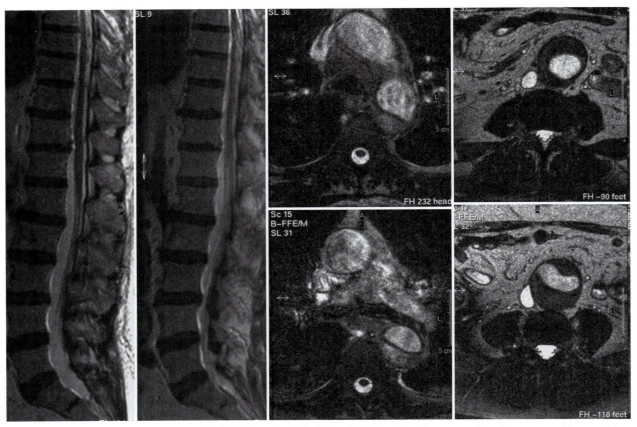

■ **FIGURE 9-8** Spinal cord ischemia due to aortic dissection. The field of view should be always large enough to demonstrate this potential cause of spinal cord ischemia.

BOX 9-1   MRI for Spinal Cord Ischemia

PATIENT HISTORY

While lifting weights, this patient, a 28-year-old man, developed severe stabbing back pain, followed by subacute paraparesis with loss of bladder and bowel control.

COMPARISON STUDY

Initial acute MRI (STIR and T2WI; Fig. 9-9A,B) was normal.

TECHNIQUE

Follow-up MRI (T2WI and STIR) was done 2 days later (Fig. 9-9C,D).

FINDINGS

There is extensive cord edema and a new hyperintensity in the dorsal portion of the 12th thoracic vertebra, consistent with a vertebral body infarction.

IMPRESSION

The clinical history, delayed appearance of positive MRI findings, and associated infarction of the vertebral body are classic manifestations of acute spinal cord ischemia.

KEY POINTS: DIFFERENTIAL DIAGNOSIS

- Spinal ischemia is a rare cause of acute nontraumatic transverse cord symptoms.
- Clinical differential diagnoses include infection; inflammatory or postinfectious acute transverse myelitis; hematomyelia; multiple sclerosis; spinal cord compression due to a neoplasm, a disc herniation, or a subdural/epidural hematoma; abscesses; delayed radiation myelopathy; or acute thrombosis of a spinal arteriovenous malformation. Most of these processes can be excluded by MRI.
- Imaging differential diagnoses of a pencil-shaped area of hyperintensity are spinal glioma and acute transverse myelitis. Spinal gliomas can usually be excluded by clinical criteria. Cerebrospinal fluid examinations may be needed to differentiate transverse myelitis from acute arterial infarction of the spinal cord.
- In patients with potential spinal cord ischemia, serial follow-up MRI should be performed *at short time intervals* because the serial changes in the pattern of contrast enhancement and the changes in the vertebral bodies help to document the correct diagnosis (Fig. 9-10).

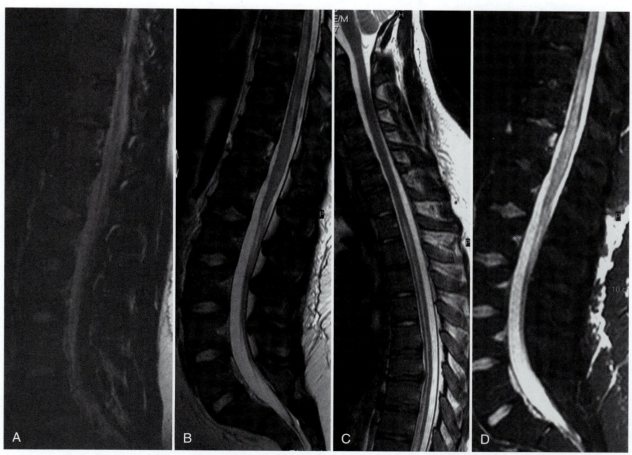

■ **FIGURE 9-9** A 48-year-old patient presented with severe stabbing back pain, followed by subacute paraparesis with loss of bladder and bowel control, after an exercise of weight lifting. Initial acute MRI was normal (**A, B**). Follow-up on day 2 demonstrates extensive cord edema and a new hyperintensity in the dorsal portion of 12th thoracic vertebra, consistent with a vertebral body infarction (**C, D**).

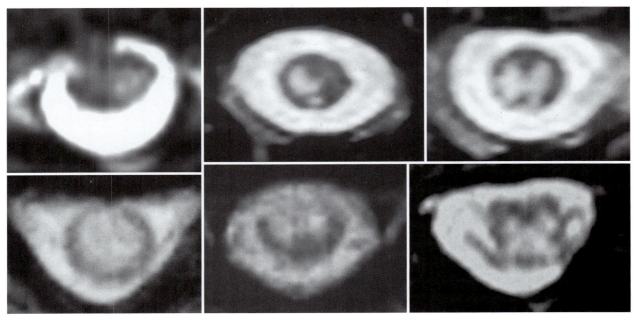

■ **FIGURE 9-10** Variable patterns of spinal cord infarction: six different patients. The marked variability stems from the unpredictable anastomoses in the intrinsic spinal arterial system.

SUGGESTED READINGS

Gravereaux EC, Faries PL, Burks JA, et al. Risk of spinal cord ischemia after endograft repair of thoracic aortic aneurysms. J Vasc Surg 2001; 34:997-1003.

Mikulis DJ, Ogilvy CS, McKee A, et al. Spinal cord infarction and fibrocartilaginous emboli. AJNR Am J Neuroradiol 1992; 13:155-160.

Mull M, Thron A. Spinal infarcts. In Von Kummer R, Back T: Magnetic Resonance Imaging in Ischemic Stroke. Berlin, Springer, 2006, pp 251-269.

Rogopoulos A, Benchimol D, Paquis P, et al. Lumbar artery compression by the diaphragmatic crus: a new etiology for spinal cord ischemia. Ann Neurol 2000; 48:261-264.

Weidauer S, Nichtweiss M, Lanfermann H, Zanella F. Spinal cord infarction: MR imaging and clinical features in 16 cases. Neuroradiology 2002; 44:851-857.

PART SIX

Spinal Trauma

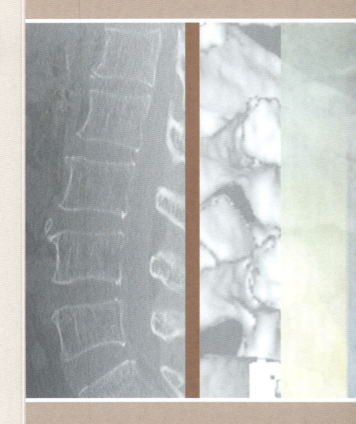

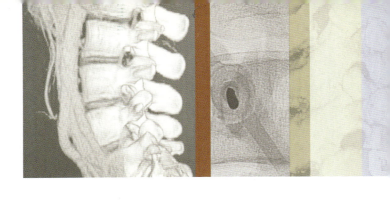

CHAPTER 10

Extra-axial Hemorrhages

Francis Michael Castellano

Spinal epidural hematoma and spinal subdural hematoma are accumulations of blood within the epidural or subdural spaces of the spinal canal or both. They may appear "spontaneously," result from trauma, or arise secondary to coagulopathy, vascular malformation, neoplasm, or another cause. The clinical symptoms are similar in both spinal epidural and spinal subdural hematomas and include local pain, extremity weakness, sensory loss, and bladder or bowel dysfunction. In the setting of trauma, CT is often the first imaging modality utilized for evaluation of the spinal axis. When spinal epidural or subdural hemorrhage is suspected, MRI becomes the modality of choice for prompt diagnosis, assessment of mass effect, and determination of treatment. Severe and/or progressive neurologic signs and increasing size of the hemorrhage usually lead to surgical evacuation of the clot. Mild, stable symptoms and stable clot size permit conservative management.[1]

SPINAL EPIDURAL HEMATOMA

Accumulation of blood within the spinal epidural space is referred to as spinal epidural hematoma (SEH).

Epidemiology

The majority of spinal epidural hemorrhages are "spontaneous."[1] Post-traumatic SEH is reported in as few as 1.7% of all spine injuries and is less common than spontaneous SEH.[1] However, recent reports suggest that traumatic SEH is more frequent than previously thought, especially in conjunction with spinal fractures or spinal soft tissue injuries.[1,3,4]

Clinical Presentation

SEH is an emergent condition that can result in progressive spinal cord or cauda equina compression and potentially devastating neurologic impairment. There are many causes. Most of these lesions appear to be "spontaneous." Nonspontaneous, secondary causes of SEH include trauma, coagulopathy, pregnancy, disc herniation, tumor, and arteriovenous fistula or malformation.[2] Clinical signs and symptoms of SEH include back pain, extremity weakness, sensory loss, and bladder or bowel dysfunction. The location and the degree of spinal cord/nerve root compression determine the severity of neurologic symptoms. SEHs resulting in acute or severe neurologic compromise are typically treated by prompt surgical evacuation. If symptoms are not severe or progressive, conservative management may be employed. Close follow-up with frequent clinical examinations and repeat MRIs of the spine ensure that the hematoma is not increasing in size.[1] Follow-up imaging may show reduced size or resolution of the hematoma within 2 weeks.[5] Patients may recover completely without neurologic deficit after conservative management. Patients older than 65 years have an increased incidence of residual symptoms, but there is no correlation between initial size of hematoma and the presence or severity of residual symptoms.[6]

Pathophysiology

SEHs are thought to result from venous hemorrhage. The epidural venous plexus gives rise to the basivertebral veins and communicates freely with both the intracranial venous sinuses and the azygous venous system.[7] The epidural plexus is valveless, rendering it susceptible to rupture from sudden increase in intra-abdominal or intrathoracic pressure.[2,8-10] The epidural venous plexus is most prominent in the thoracic spine.[8,10] Perhaps for that reason spontaneous SEHs are more common in the thoracic and cervicothoracic regions than the lumbar spine. The ventral aspect of the dural sac is strongly adherent to the posterior longitudinal ligament.[11] Therefore, spontaneous SEHs most commonly collect in the dorsal epidural space.[1,2,8]

Imaging

CT

In the setting of trauma, CT is often performed before MRI as either the initial screening examination of the spinal column or for further evaluation of an abnormality detected on plain radiographs. On CT, SEHs typically appear as extradural soft tissue masses with attenuation

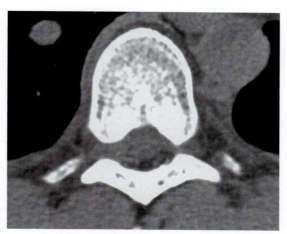

■ **FIGURE 10-1**   Axial CT image through the midthoracic spine demonstrates a hyperdense extramedullary mass ventral to the thoracic cord with severe mass effect on the cord.

similar to the intervertebral discs (60-70 HU).[12] When the abnormality is ventral, it may be impossible to differentiate a hematoma from an extruded disc fragment (Fig. 10-1). MRI is the most appropriate next step for further evaluation.

MRI

MRI is the primary diagnostic study for evaluating the soft tissues of the spine and spinal cord. It provides rapid, non-invasive evaluation of the entire spinal column and demonstrates any compression of the spinal cord or nerve roots that may necessitate emergent surgical decompression.[5,6,12] The craniocaudal extent of an epidural hematoma is variable. Most SEHs extend over two to four vertebral segments.[13] Some are limited to a single vertebral level, whereas others extend the length of the vertebral column. On axial sections, SEHs are most often biconvex with tapered cranial and caudal ends (Fig. 10-2).[11] Replacement of the normal epidural fat signal confirms that the hematoma lies in the epidural space (Fig. 10-3).[14]

The MRI appearance of SEH varies with the age of the lesion. In the hyperacute state (<6 hours), intracellular oxyhemoglobin predominates, so the signal is isointense on T1-weighted (T1W) images and mildly hyperintense on T2-weighted (T2W) images, relative to the spinal cord. From 6 to 72 hours, intracellular oxyhemoglobin within the hematoma deoxygenates to intracellular deoxyhemoglobin. This change causes the characteristic "acute"

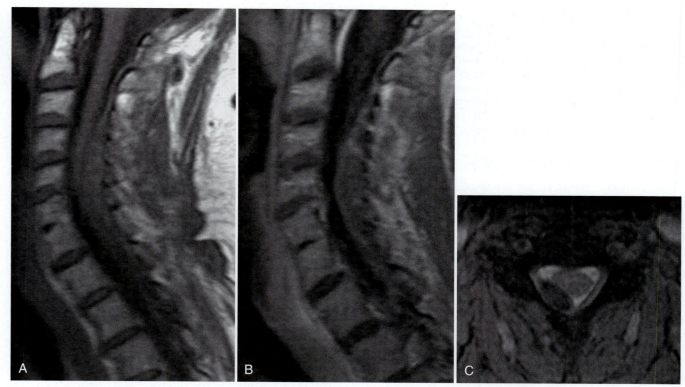

■ **FIGURE 10-2**   **A,** Sagittal T1W MR image of the cervical spine demonstrates a collection of blood in the dorsal epidural space. This hematoma is isointense to mildly hyperintense relative to the adjacent spinal cord. **B,** Sagittal T1W postgadolinium MR image of the cervical spine demonstrates peripheral enhancement of a dorsal epidural hematoma. This should not be confused with an extramedullary neoplasm. **C,** Axial T2W MR image through C5 in the same patient as in **A** and **B** shows a biconvex epidural hematoma of low signal intensity displacing the cervical cord.

■ **FIGURE 10-3 A,** Sagittal T1W MR image through the lower thoracic and lumbar spine demonstrates a ventral epidural hematoma with mildly increased signal relative to the spinal cord. Note how the hematoma replaces the normal epidural fat, confirming its location in the epidural space. The hematoma is secondary to an acute traumatic Chance type fracture of T12. **B,** Sagittal T2W MR image through the same level demonstrates that the hematoma has heterogeneous signal with predominantly increased signal intensity. Concomitant Chance fracture is present at L1, further compressing the spinal cord. **C,** Axial T1W MR image through L2 in the same patient as in **A** and **B** clearly demonstrates the ventral hyperintense epidural hematoma (*arrow*) and mass effect on the adjacent cauda equina. **D,** Axial T2W MR image at the same level demonstrates high signal intensity within the hematoma (*arrow*).

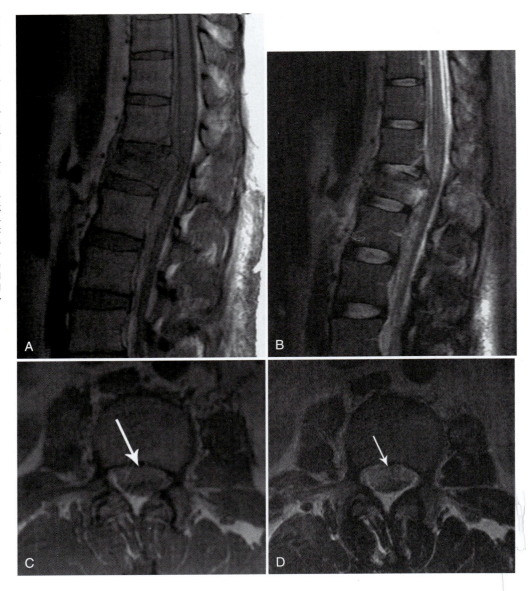

appearance: isointense to spinal cord on T1W images and markedly hypointense to spinal cord on T2W images.[5,6,12] The isointensity on T1W images has been reported to last up to 5 days after the initial trauma.[5] From 3 to 5 days onward, progressive formation of methemoglobin causes high signal intensity on T1W imaging relative to the spinal cord, with variable signal intensity on T2W imaging (depending on the proportions of intracellular and extracellular methemoglobin). In patients followed conservatively, increase in the signal intensity with time is virtually pathognomonic of an epidural hematoma on T1W imaging.[6] Chronic blood products are typically low in signal intensity on both T1W and T2W imaging.

Special Procedures

Angiography

Catheter angiography may be helpful in cases of unexplained or spontaneous epidural hematoma to exclude a spinal arteriovenous malformation, fistula, or hypervascular tumor.

Myelography

In some patients with unexplained back pain, myelography may be the initial test performed. An effaced thecal sac or constricted subarachnoid space could indicate a SEH. If there are medical contraindications to performing MRI, the spine can be evaluated by CT myelography.

SPINAL SUBDURAL HEMATOMA

Accumulation of blood in the spinal subdural space is referred to as spinal subdural hematoma (SSH).

Epidemiology

SSH is a rare lesion. Most spinal subdural hemorrhages are nontraumatic. Specific causes include spinal or intracranial surgery, lumbar puncture, anticoagulant therapy, hematologic disorders, vascular malformations, and tumors. Far fewer cases are post-traumatic.[15] Patients may be affected at any age, pediatric to elderly. There is a slight male predominance.[16]

Clinical Presentation

The clinical presentation of SSH resembles that of SEH. Patients typically present with acute neurologic symptoms from compression of the spinal cord or cauda equina.[17] Depending on the size and location of the SSH, there may be back pain, progressive extremity motor or sensory loss, and autonomic dysfunction with bowel or bladder incontinence. In the setting of trauma, it is important to maintain a high suspicion of possible SEH or SSH, even when other injuries such as fractures or ligamentous disruption are more immediately apparent.

Chosen appropriately, both surgical and conservative management may be used to treat SSH. Conservative management requires close clinical monitoring, often with serial follow-up MRIs.[17] The prognosis is worse for patients with cervical or thoracic SSHs and better for lumbar SSH.[15] The larger size of the lumbar canal and the termination of the spinal cord at L1-L2 probably protect the central nervous system from compression in the lumbar spinal canal, accounting for the better prognosis of lumbar SSH. Duration of symptoms for longer than 3 months is associated with a poorer prognosis.[15] In the absence of progressive or significant neurologic symptoms, spontaneous resolution has been reported.

Pathophysiology

Unlike the spinal epidural space, the spinal subdural space has no major blood vessels or bridging veins.[18] The avascular nature of the spinal subdural space and possible protection of the space by the vertebral column and paraspinal muscles may explain the low incidence of SSH.[16]

Several pathogeneses have been proposed for SSHs:

1. Abnormal increased intracranial pressure may tear the inner dura and cause bleeding by shearing forces.[15] This theory would also account for the relative frequency of concomitant intracranial hemorrhage in patients with SSHs.
2. At least some SSHs represent intraspinal decompression of intracranial subdural hemorrhage to a dependent location in the spinal subdural space. Since 2004, there have been 10 reported cases of post-traumatic SSHs.[19] Six of these 10 cases had associated intracranial hemorrhage. One case report described a temporal relationship between the rapid resolution of an intracranial subdural hematoma and subsequent development of an SSH.[19] Ultrastructural findings demonstrating the continuity of the intracranial and spinal subdural space[20] lend support to this theory.
3. Dissection of subarachnoid blood into the subdural space is another possible cause of SSH.[21] Failure to show concurrent subarachnoid blood in patients with SSHs may result from the dispersion of the subarach-

noid blood throughout the spinal subarachnoid space.[16]

Regardless of the cause, SSHs are far less common than SEHs.

Pathology

SSH is more often located in the thoracic or thoracolumbar region than the lumbar region alone.[22] The craniocaudal extent of SSH varies from 1 to 18 vertebral segments. The SSH is often located in the dorsal subdural space, but ventral and circumferential encasement of the thecal sac also occurs.[14]

Imaging

CT

An acute SSH appears as a hyperdense mass.[23] A chronic SSH often appears as an isodense mass relative to the spinal cord.[23] On CT, it can be difficult to determine whether a hematoma is located solely within the intradural space or the extradural space.[22] Demonstration that low-density epidural fat delimits the posterolateral borders of a hyperdense hematoma confirms that the hemorrhage is subdural. SSHs are often crescent shaped but can be biconvex.[13] Although CT may be the initial imaging study performed in the setting of trauma, clinical or imaging findings that suggest possible SSH warrant further investigation with MRI.

MRI

MRI is superior to other modalities for detecting an SSH. Multiplanar, multisequence MRI delimits the craniocaudal extent of the hematoma and the degree of any spinal cord/nerve root compression.[24] The MRI appearance of SSH depends on the age of the blood products. Hyperacute blood is typically isointense on T1W images and hyperintense on T2W images. In the first 72 hours after hemorrhage, SSH are isointense on T1W images and most often hypointense on T2W images owing to the presence of intracellular deoxyhemoglobin within intact red blood cells (Fig. 10-4).[25,26] After the first 3 days, methemoglobin causes hyperintensity on T1W images. The appearance on T2W images depends on the intracellular versus extracellular location of methemoglobin. Intracellular methemoglobin manifests as hypointensity on T2W imaging. As red blood cells lyse, extracellular methemoglobin accumulates and results in increased signal intensity on T2W imaging (Fig. 10-5).[25] Therefore, in the late subacute state, SSHs are hyperintense on both T1W and T2W images. As is true elsewhere in the body, chronic blood products are low in signal intensity on both T1W and T2W images.

Special Procedures

Angiography

Catheter-directed angiography may be helpful in cases of unexplained or spontaneous subdural hematoma to exclude a spinal arteriovenous malformation.

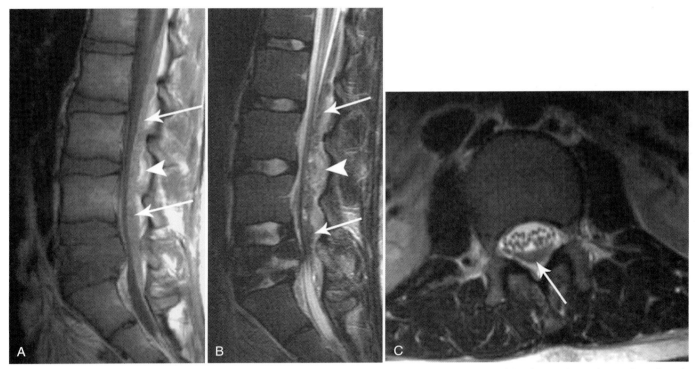

■ **FIGURE 10-4** **A,** Sagittal T1W MR image of the lumbar spine shows a hyperintense mass in the dorsal subdural space (*arrows*). Note how the epidural fat posterior to the hematoma is maintained (*arrowhead*), hence the location of the hematoma in the subdural space. **B,** Sagittal T2W MR image through the same level shows fairly uniform low signal intensity of the subdural hematoma (*arrows*) adjacent to high signal epidural fat (*arrowhead*). An acute traumatic compression fracture of L5 is present. **C,** Axial T2W MR image through L3 demonstrates the crescentic appearance of the subdural hematoma (*arrow*).

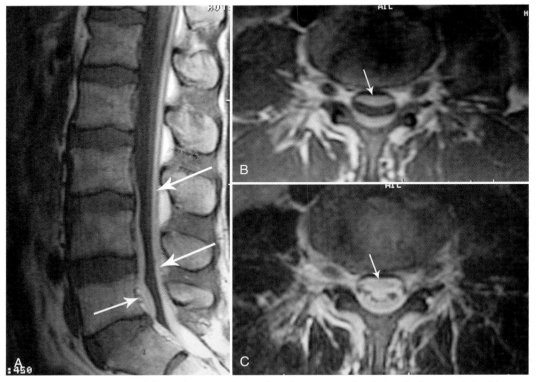

■ **FIGURE 10-5** **A,** Sagittal T1W MR image of the lumbar spine shows a hyperintense ventral and dorsal subacute subdural hematoma (*arrows*) in an anticoagulated patient. **B,** Axial T1W MR image through L5 shows striking increased T1 signal intensity consistent with the presence of methemoglobin in the ventral subdural hematoma (*arrow*). **C,** Axial T2W image through L5 shows increased signal intensity due to extracellular methemoglobin within the subacute subdural hematoma (*arrow*).

Myelography

In some patients with unexplained back pain, myelography may be the initial test performed. An effaced thecal sac or constricted subarachnoid space could indicate a SSH. If MRI is contraindicated, further evaluation with CT and/or CT myelography should be performed to characterize the nature, size, and position of the extramedullary mass and its effect on the underlying neural structures.

ANALYSIS

Differential diagnostic considerations for SEHs and SSHs include other extramedullary lesions, such as epidural abscess, disc herniation, or tumor, especially lymphoma. In the setting of trauma, the most common diagnostic problem is correct differentiation of acute disc herniation from SEH or SSH. Both may present as acute neurologic symptoms. An epidural mass will either have chronic progressive symptoms or be asymptomatic, depending on the extent of central canal and neural foraminal narrowing.

SEH vs. Disc

Several imaging features of epidural hematomas help to differentiate lumbar SEH from extruded lumbar disc fragments.[27] On T1W imaging EDHs typically show increased signal different from, and higher than, the adjacent disc. The length of epidural hemorrhages is greater than one half of the height of the adjacent vertebral body. SEHs have an egg-drop (teardrop) shape, and the height of the adjacent disc is preserved with SEH.[27] However, acute traumatic disc herniations and SEH may develop concurrently, owing to tearing of epidural veins adjacent to the displaced disc fragment.[12] In these cases, the diagnostic problem is to recognize the presence of both, not to choose between them.

SEH vs. Epidural Abscess

Although there is overlap in the imaging appearance of epidural hematoma and abscess, epidural abscesses are usually associated with concomitant discitis/osteomyelitis, which can be readily identified on MRI. Clinically, there is usually no history of trauma in patients with abscess. A diagnosis of SEH can be suspected when imaging identifies an epidural mass different from disc in a patient with no history of trauma and no clinical signs of infection.[6]

SEH vs. Tumor

Even in the setting of trauma, it is important to consider the possibility of an incidentally discovered mass, such as isolated epidural lymphoma, metastasis, or epidural angiolipoma. The presence and pattern of enhancement on gadolinium-enhanced MRI may help to document the presence of tumor.[6] Spinal epidural angiolipomas, for example, most often demonstrate intense homogeneous enhancement on fat-saturated T1W images.[28] However, some acute SEHs show a peripheral pattern of enhancement due to hyperemic dura mater and adjacent meninges

(see Fig. 10-2C).[29] Epidural hematomas older than 48 hours may show mixed or central enhancement.[5] Therefore, the presence of heterogeneous or peripheral contrast enhancement does not exclude an epidural hematoma.

BOX 10-1 MRI of Cervical Spine for Evaluation of a Spinal Epidural Hematoma

PATIENT HISTORY

A 28-year-old man presented after a motor vehicle accident.

COMPARISON STUDY

CT of the cervical spine was performed $3^1/_2$ hours earlier.

TECHNIQUE

Multiplanar multisequence MRI of the cervical spine without administration of a contrast agent was performed, including sagittal T1W, T2W, STIR, and axial T1W and T2W sequences.

FINDINGS

There is an abnormal extra-axial collection in the dorsal spinal epidural space extending from C4 to C7. The collection is biconvex on axial imaging. It replaces the normal fat signal within the dorsal epidural space. It displaces the cervical spinal cord ventrally, resulting in moderate to severe central canal stenosis. There is no abnormal intramedullary signal present within the spinal cord. The collection demonstrates isointense signal on T1W imaging and low signal on T2W imaging relative to the spinal cord.

The craniocervical, cervical, and cervicothoracic portions of the spine show normal alignment. Vertebral body height and disc spaces are preserved. No fracture or ligamentous injury is identified.

IMPRESSION

There is an acute cervical spinal epidural hematoma extending along the dorsal epidural space from C4 to C7, resulting in moderate to severe central canal stenosis and compression of the cervical spinal cord.

Emergent neurosurgical consultation is recommended.

These findings were discussed with Dr. (x) by me personally at (hour) on (date) with read-back confirmation.

KEY POINTS: DIFFERENTIAL DIAGNOSIS

■ Traumatic spinal epidural and subdural hematomas can cause potentially devastating neurologic compromise if not diagnosed and treated promptly.

■ On MRI, spinal epidural hematomas replace the normal epidural fat signal.[14] Because spinal subdural hematomas are located within the thecal sac, the adjacent epidural fat is maintained and delimits the posterolateral border of the hematoma.[25]

■ On axial imaging, spinal epidural hematomas are often biconvex whereas spinal subdural hematomas are most often crescent shaped.[13]

■ The craniocaudal extent of spinal epidural and subdural hematomas varies. On average, spinal subdural hematomas extend two to four vertebral segments whereas spinal subdural hematomas average seven segments in length.[14]

SUGGESTED READINGS

Buchowski JM, Riley LH. Epidural hematoma after immobilization of a "hangman's" fracture: case report and review of the literature. Spine J 2005; 5:332-335.
Kuker W, Thiex R, Friese S, et al. Spinal subdural and epidural haematomas: diagnostic and therapeutic aspects in acute and subacute cases. Acta Neurochir (Wien) 2000; 142:777-785.
Miller DR, Ray A, Hourihan MD. Spinal subdural haematoma: how relevant is the INR? Spinal Cord 2004; 42:477-480.

REFERENCES

1. Lefranc F, David P, Brotchi J, De Witte O. Traumatic epidural hematoma of the cervical spine: magnetic resonance imaging diagnosis and spontaneous resolution: case report. Neurosurgery 1999; 44:408-410; discussion 410-411.
2. Sklar EM, Post JM, Falcone S. MRI of acute spinal epidural hematomas. J Comput Assist Tomogr 1999; 23:238-243.
3. Soundappan SV, Darwish B, Chaseling R. Traumatic spinal epidural hematoma—unusual cause of torticollis in a child. Pediatr Emerg Care 2005; 21:847-849.
4. Cuenca PJ, Tulley EB, Devita D, Stone A. Delayed traumatic spinal epidural hematoma with spontaneous resolution of symptoms. J Emerg Med 2004; 27:37-41.
5. Fukui MB, Swarnkar AS, Williams RL. Acute spontaneous spinal epidural hematomas. AJNR Am J Neuroradiol 1999; 20:1365-1372.
6. Holtas S, Heiling M, Lonntoft M. Spontaneous spinal epidural hematoma: findings at MR imaging and clinical correlation. Radiology 1996; 199:409-413.
7. Hogan Q. Lumbar epidural anatomy: a new look by cytomicrotome section. Anesthesiology 1991; 75:767-775.
8. Szkup P, Stoneham G. Case report: spontaneous spinal epidural haematoma during pregnancy: case report and review of the literature. Br J Radiol 2004; 77:881-884.
9. Cheng-Ta Hsieh, Yung-Hsiao Chiang, Chi-Tun Tang, et al. Delayed traumatic thoracic spinal epidural hematoma: a case report and literature review. Am J Emerg Med 2007; 25:69-71
10. Groen RJ, Ponssen H. The spontaneous spinal epidural hematoma: a study of the etiology. J Neurol Sci 1990; 98:121-138.
11. Chang F-C, Lirng J-F, Luo C-B. Evaluation of clinical and MR findings for the prognosis of spinal epidural haematomas. Clin Radiol 2005; 60:762-770.
12. Gundry CR, Heithoff KB. Epidural hematoma of the lumbar spine: 18 surgically confirmed cases. Radiology 1993; 187:427-431.
13. Boukobza M, Guichard JP, Boissonet M, et al: Spinal epidural haematoma: report of 11 cases and review of the literature. Neuroradiology 1994; 36:456-459.
14. Boukobza M, Haddar D, Boissonet M, Merland JJ. Spinal subdural haematoma: a study of three cases. Clin Radiol 2001; 56:475-480.
15. Hung KS, Lui CC, Wang CH, et al: Traumatic spinal subdural hematoma with spontaneous resolution. Spine 2002; 27:E534-E538.
16. Jimbo H, Asamoto S, Mitsuyama T, et al: Spinal chronic subdural hematoma in association with anticoagulant therapy: a case report and literature review. Spine 2006; 31:E184-E187.
17. Sari A, Sert B, Dinc H, Kuzeyli K. Subacute spinal subdural hematoma associated with intracranial subdural hematoma. J Neuroradiol 2006; 33:67-69.
18. Nicholas DS, Weller RO. The fine anatomy of the spinal meninges. J Neurosurgery 1988; 69:276-282
19. Bortolotti C, Wang H, Fraser K, Lanzino G. Subacute spinal subdural hematoma after spontaneous resolution of cranial subdural hematoma: causal relationship or coincidence? J Neurosurgery (Spine 4) 2004; 100:372-374
20. Reina MA, De Leon Casasola O, Lopez A, et al: The origin of the spinal subdural space: ultrastructure findings. Anesth Analg 2002; 94:991-995.
21. Vinters HV, Barnett HJ, Kaufmann JC. Subdural hematoma of the spinal cord and widespread subarachnoid hemorrhage complicating anticoagulant therapy. Stroke 1980; 11:459-464.
22. Shimada Y, Sato K, Abe E, et al. Spinal subdural hematoma. Skeletal Radiol 1996; 25:477-480.
23. Tillich M, Kammerhuber F, Reittner P, et al. Chronic spinal subdural haematoma associated with intracranial subdural haematoma: CT and MRI. Neuroradiology 1999; 41:137-139.
24. Morandi X, Riffaud L, Chabert E, Brassier G. Acute nontraumatic spinal subdural hematomas in three patients. Spine 2001; 26: E547-E551.
25. Kulkarni AV, Willinsky RA, Gray T, Cusimano MD. Serial magnetic resonance imaging findings for a spontaneously resolving spinal subdural hematoma: case report. Neurosurgery 1998; 42:398-400; discussion 400-401.
26. Post MJ, Becerra JL, Madsen PW, et al. Acute spinal subdural hematoma: MR and CT findings with pathologic correlates. AJNR Am J Neuroradiol 1994; 15:1895-1905.
27. Dorsay TA, Helms CA. MR imaging of epidural hematoma in the lumbar spine. Skeletal Radiol 2002; 31:677-685. Epub 2002; Nov 12.
28. Leu NH, Chen CY, Shy CG, et al: MR imaging of an infiltrating spinal epidural angiolipoma. Am J Neuroradiol 2003; 24:1008-1011.
29. Caldemeyer KS, Mocharla R, Moran CC, Smith RR. Gadolinium enhancement in the center of a spinal epidural hematoma in a hemophiliac. J Comput Assist Tomogr 1993; 17:321-323.

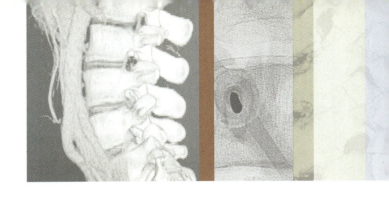

CHAPTER 11

Trauma to the Spinal Column

Michael Christian Hollingshead and Mauricio Castillo

Traumatic injuries of the spinal column reflect the mechanisms that produced them. The patterns of these injuries on imaging studies, therefore, help to predict the underlying mechanisms of trauma and lead, in turn, to more complete description of the pathologic process, more thorough search for associated abnormalities, and better patient prognostication. Differences in the anatomy and mobility of each spinal segment influence the pathologic process suffered.

Cervical spine injuries are typically classified as craniocervical or as subaxial. The craniocervical injuries are usually distractions at the atlanto-occipital and atlantoaxial junctions. These distractions are rare but are identified with increased frequency.[1] The subaxial cervical spine injuries are predominantly flexion and extension injuries. Because the ribs stabilize the upper thoracic spine, few injuries are seen there.[2] Spinal mobility increases further inferiorly, however, so fractures and fracture-dislocations occur more often in the lower thoracic and lumbar spine, especially at the thoracolumbar junction.[2,3]

Spinal *stability* indicates that the bony and ligamentous elements of the spinal column will remain in the same relative positions without shifting or separating from each other over time. Spinal *instability* indicates that, without stabilization, the spinal elements may shift and, by shifting, induce additional neurologic, soft tissue, or osseous injury.[4,5] A number of radiographic and CT signs suggest the presence of concurrent ligamentous injuries and high likelihood of instability.[4] MRI visualizes many ligaments directly, leading to better diagnosis of ligamentous injuries. MRI shows injuries of spinal ligaments as thinning of the ligaments, separations of the ligaments from the underlying bone, areas of discontinuity within the ligaments, and perifocal edema. MRI also shows concurrent injuries of the spinal cord. Therefore, MRI is particularly useful in patients with suspected unstable injuries, in patients with neurologic deficits, and in patients who are obtunded.

The *three-column model* is often used to assess and characterize stability of the spinal column.[5,6] In this model, the spinal column is considered to have three stability elements or "columns." The anterior column consists of the anterior longitudinal ligament plus the anterior two thirds of the vertebral bodies, discs, and annuli. The middle column consists of the posterior third of the vertebral bodies and discs, the posterior longitudinal ligament, and the posterior portion of the annuli. The posterior column includes all of the osseous and ligamentous structures posterior to the posterior longitudinal ligament. Denis described unstable injuries as either an injury involving all three columns or an injury that involves two contiguous columns, that is, the anterior and middle columns or the middle and posterior columns.[5]

Associated injuries include disc injuries or herniations, vertebral artery injuries, spinal cord injuries, intramedullary and extramedullary hematomas, meningeal tears, and nerve root trauma.[7,8] Identification of these injuries affects patient management and outcome.

ATLANTO-OCCIPITAL DISSOCIATION INJURIES

Atlanto-occipital dissociations are dislocations or subluxations of the occiput from C1 (the atlas). The direction of dissociation varies with the specific conjunction of vertical distraction with anterior, posterior, or lateral shear force.[9,10] Atlanto-occipital dissociations can be combined ligamentous and osseous injuries of the craniocervical junction or may be purely ligamentous. These dissociations may also be referred to as dislocations or subluxations.

Epidemiology

Atlanto-occipital dislocation is seen in 8% to 35% of deaths related to motor vehicle accidents.[9] The 30-day mortality of those patients who survive the injury is 35%.[11] The majority of patients present after a motor vehicle accident, but atlanto-occipital dislocation may also result from pedestrian injury.[9] Gregg and associates reviewed 135 survivors of atlanto-occipital dislocations. Of these, 80 were children and 55 were adults.[11] There were 53 females, 79 males, and 3 cases with no gender specified.[11] Bucholtz and colleagues reviewed 112 trauma victims post mortem and identified 9 patients (8%) with atlanto-occipital injuries. All were male.[12] Three victims were children younger than 18 years of age; 4 were between 18 and 24 years of age, and 2 were older.[12]

Clinical Presentation

Atlanto-occipital dislocations are usually fatal. Improved imaging and better initial emergency management, however, have led to increased numbers of survivors.[1] These patients typically present to the emergency department with spinal cord and other neurologic injuries, especially brain stem dysfunction and palsies of the lower cranial nerves V through XII.[9,11] They may also have significant vascular injuries.[13] Because the radiographic and CT presentation of purely ligamentous injuries can sometimes be subtle, clinical identification of signs and symptoms of brain stem injury can help to suggest this diagnosis.[1]

Pathophysiology

Atlanto-occipital dislocations most commonly result from distraction with either hyperflexion or hyperextension.[6] The major ligaments likely to be injured include the anterior atlanto-occipital membrane, the tectorial membrane, the transverse ligament, and the alar ligaments.[13,14] The tectorial membrane is believed to counter hyperextension, whereas the dens and foramen magnum counter hyperflexion.[12] These structures must be injured, therefore, by hyperextension and hyperflexion injuries.

Pathology

Atlanto-occipital injuries can be associated with skull fractures, most often involving the occipital condyles and including avulsion fractures of the alar ligaments.[13]

Because this injury involves the craniocervical junction, injury can damage the cranial nerves, especially lower cranial nerves V through XII.[9,11] The injury may involve the nucleus of the cranial nerve or its peripheral portion, such as with injury of the hypoglossal canal (cranial nerve XII) or the jugular foramen (cranial nerves IX-XI).[9]

Imaging

CT

The craniocervical region is often difficult to display on plain radiographs because the anatomy is complex and many significant structures overlap.[14] Patient condition may preclude optimal positioning for the radiographs. Obtunded patients cannot cooperate with the examination.[14] Spasm of the cervical musculature often elevates the shoulders to overlap the neck. When seen, prevertebral soft tissue swelling suggests adjacent spinal injury.[11]

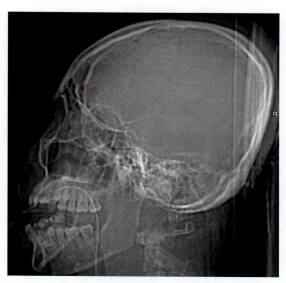

■ **FIGURE 11-1** Atlanto-occipital dislocation. Lateral scout radiograph from head CT demonstrates abnormal separation between the skull base and C1.

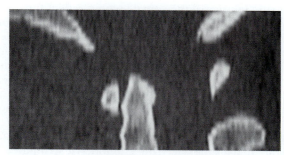

■ **FIGURE 11-2** Atlanto-occipital dislocation. Sagittal CT image demonstrates an abnormally increased basion-dental interval.

CT is easier to perform, displays the bony anatomy and fractures better, and, with multiplanar reformatting, can be used to image any portion of the spine at the precise angle needed. There may be prevertebral soft tissue swelling and separation of the occipital condyles from the lateral masses of C1.[11] Possible ligamentous injuries may be inferred by identifying increased lengths of two intervals: the basion-dental interval and the basion-axial interval (Figs. 11-1 to 11-3).[15] The basion-dental interval is the measurement from the basion to the superior tip of the dens.[15] The basion-axial interval is the perpendicular measurement from the basion to a line parallel to the posterior cortex of the axis.[15] Normally, these intervals should both be less than 12 mm. The Power ratio (the distance from basion to the posterior arch of C1 divided by the distance from the opisthion to the anterior arch of C1) has also been employed but can be more difficult to determine on plain films.[15]

MRI

MRI depicts the tectorial membrane, alar ligaments, and anterior atlanto-occipital membrane as well as other ligamentous and soft tissue structures of the craniocervi-

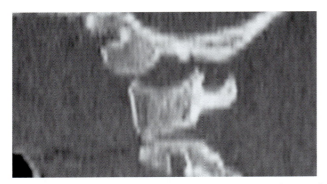

■ **FIGURE 11-3** *Atlanto-occipital dislocation (same patient as in Fig. 11-2). Off-midline sagittal CT image demonstrates posterior dislocation of the C1 lateral mass with respect to the occipital condyle.*

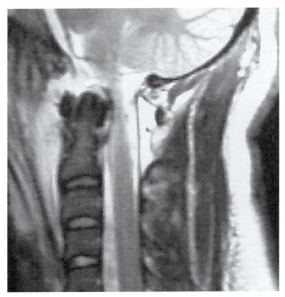

■ **FIGURE 11-4** *Atlanto-occipital dislocation. Sagittal T2W MR image demonstrates abnormal basion-dental interval. There are disruptions of the tectorial membrane, apical ligament, and anterior atlanto-occipital ligament. Prevertebral soft tissue edema is also noted.*

cal region (Fig. 11-4).[13] Abnormal separation between the occiput and C1 and increased signal within the joint capsules on T2-weighted (T2W) and short tau inversion recovery (STIR) MR sequences also suggest atlanto-occipital injuries.[13] MRI may also show hemorrhage and edema in the soft tissues, subarachnoid and epidural hemorrhages at the craniocervical junction, and contusion, edema, and hemorrhage of the spinal cord.[11,13]

Special Procedures

The walls of the vertebral arteries can be injured by stretching due to atlanto-occipital distraction, with subsequent dissection, thrombosis/obstruction, and pseudoaneurysm formation.[16] CT angiography (CTA), MR angiography (MRA), or conventional angiography may be employed to detect and characterize these vascular injuries.

ATLANTOAXIAL DISSOCIATION INJURIES

Atlantoaxial dissociation injuries are dislocations or subluxations of C1 on C2 due to injuries of the ligaments and osseous structures of the atlantoaxial (C1-C2) articulations. Because these injuries involve the craniocervical junction, consequences of injury and instability can be severe. These injuries are also referred to as distractions or subluxations.

Epidemiology

Post-traumatic atlantoaxial distraction injuries most frequently result from motor vehicle accidents, falls, and sports.[17] Overall, post-traumatic atlantoaxial distractions and subluxations are not common.[10,17]

Clinical Presentation

These patients typically present with neck pain in the setting of trauma.[17] With advanced degrees of subluxation, patients may also suffer neurologic injuries due to spinal cord damage or vertebral artery injury.[17] Concurrent head trauma may cause additional intracranial injury.[10,17]

Pathophysiology

The mechanism of injury typically involves distraction with extension or flexion.[13] The transverse ligament normally prevents anterior displacement of the atlas, so the transverse ligament is often seen to be injured in these cases.[10] The alar ligaments help maintain stability but may not be able to support the C1-C2 articulation when the transverse ligament is injured.[10] The anterior longitudinal ligament, posterior longitudinal ligament, tectorial membrane, and other cruciate ligaments also provide support for the C1-C2 articulation. Disruption of these ligaments can lead to subluxation or dislocation. Type II fractures of the odontoid process may also lead to subluxation or dislocation of C1 on C2.[10] Underlying inflammatory arthritides, infections, or neoplasms weaken these ligaments, so they may become disrupted by relatively mild injuries.[10]

White and associates describe five major types of atlantoaxial injury: bilateral anterior displacement, bilateral posterior displacement, unilateral anterior displacement, unilateral posterior displacement, and unilateral combined anterior and posterior C1-C2 subluxations and dislocations.[10]

Pathology

If the mechanism of trauma includes an anteroposterior force or lateral force, fractures of the odontoid may be seen in association with atlantoaxial subluxation or dislocation.[10]

Imaging

CT

Prevertebral soft tissue swelling usually signifies prevertebral edema and/or hemorrhage, suggesting possible subtle

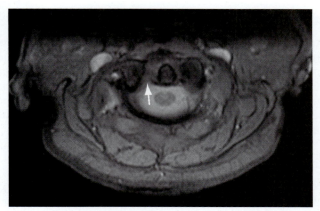

■ **FIGURE 11-5** Atlantoaxial instability. Axial T2*W MR image demonstrates a tear involving the right lateral portion of the transverse ligament (*arrow*).

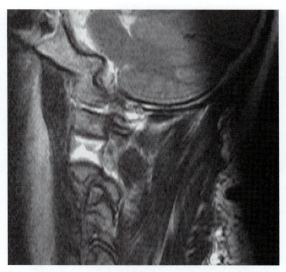

■ **FIGURE 11-6** Atlantoaxial dislocation. Off-midline sagittal T2W MR image demonstrates abnormal signal within the C1-C2 facet joint, which is also widened.

atlantoaxial subluxation.[6,13] Other signs of atlantoaxial subluxation on axial and reformatted CT images include displacement of the C1 lateral masses with respect to the C2 lateral masses, widening between the facets of C1 and C2, and widening of the anterior atlantodental interval.[15] The normal anterior atlantodental interval measures up to 3 mm in adults and 5 mm in children, so measurements greater than these indicate possible subluxation.

MRI

MRI displays the C1-C2 supporting ligaments directly, including the transverse ligament, tectorial membrane, anterior atlantodental ligament, and the alar ligaments (Fig. 11-5). In injured patients, MRI shows disruption, avulsion, or thinning of these ligaments plus any concurrent injuries of the anterior or posterior longitudinal ligament. Prevertebral soft tissue hemorrhage and edema may be identified directly. Injury of the facet joints manifests as abnormal separation of the facets and as increased signal on STIR and T2W images within the facet joints from fluid within the joints (Figs. 11-6 and 11-7). MRI also identifies signal abnormalities of the spinal cord and meninges such as cord contusion and intramedullary and extramedullary hemorrhages.[13]

Special Procedures

The walls of the vertebral arteries can be stretched and injured by abnormal motion at the C1-C2 articulation, leading to thrombosis, dissection, or pseudoaneurysm formation.[16] CTA, MRA, or conventional angiography may be employed.

FRACTURES OF THE ATLAS

Osseous injuries of the atlas include fractures of the anterior arch, the posterior arch, and the lateral masses. These C1 fractures may be accompanied by injury to the transverse ligament.[10,18] Alternate names include Jefferson burst fracture, anterior or posterior arch fractures, and lateral mass fractures.

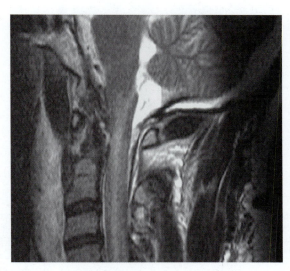

■ **FIGURE 11-7** Atlantoaxial dislocation (same patient as in Fig. 11-6). Parasagittal T2W MR image demonstrates disruption of the anterior longitudinal ligament, anterior atlanto-occipital ligament, and tectorial membrane. There is inferior dislocation of the axis with abnormal atlantodental interval. Prevertebral soft tissue edema is also noted. There is abnormal signal intensity in the cord, which proved to be infarct.

Epidemiology

Two to 13 percent of cervical spine fractures involve C1.[19]

Clinical Presentation

Modes of injury include motor vehicle accidents, falls, and diving.[18] Neurologic deficits are uncommon with these injuries, because the fragments typically disperse.[18,19] Neck pain and posterior headaches are the more common symptoms.[10]

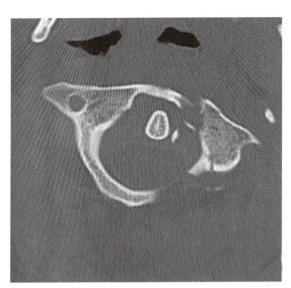

■ **FIGURE 11-8** Comminuted lateral mass atlas fracture with transverse ligament avulsion. Axial CT image demonstrates comminuted fractures of the anterior and posterior arches with abnormal lateral atlantodental interval.

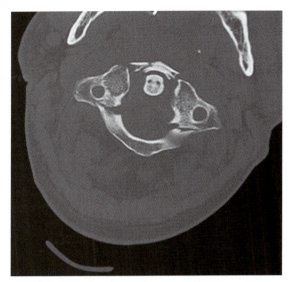

■ **FIGURE 11-10** Jefferson burst fracture. Axial CT image demonstrates dispersed fracture fragments from multiple fractures of the anterior and posterior arches.

Imaging

CT

Differentiation of the Jefferson fracture from an isolated fracture may be difficult with plain radiographs. CT demonstrates the fracture pattern more clearly (Fig. 11-10).[14] If the fracture involves the anterior arch, there is usually prevertebral soft tissue swelling due to prevertebral hematoma.

In Jefferson fractures, one should evaluate the integrity of the transverse ligament. One useful indicator involves measurement of the lateral displacement of the C1 lateral masses with respect to the C2 lateral masses. Cadaver studies have shown that a total lateral displacement of both lateral masses greater than 6.9 mm indicates possible disruption of the transverse ligament.[15,19] Heller and associates report that the proper value in living patients should be taken as more than 8.1 mm to allow for the magnification inherent in obtaining open mouth odontoid radiographs in patients.[15,20] CT can be used to measure this displacement accurately without concern for magnification.[15] Abnormal widening of the anterior atlantodental interval may also be used to suggest ligamentous injury.[19]

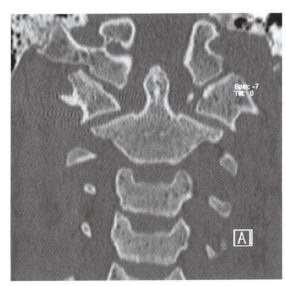

■ **FIGURE 11-9** Comminuted lateral mass atlas fracture with transverse ligament avulsion (same patient as in Figure 11-8). Coronal CT image demonstrates abnormally increased lateral atlantodental interval. There is a small osseous fragment medial to the left C1 lateral mass.

Pathophysiology

Because C1 is a ring there will typically be two or more fracture lines through it. Usually, the mechanism of injury involves vertical compression. The pattern of the fractures depends on the position of the head at impact and the degree of rotational force applied (Figs. 11-8 and 11-9).[10] The Jefferson burst fracture typically involves marked axial loading, which is of greater force and in a more vertical direction than seen with other types of C1 fractures. Four fragments usually result.[10,18] The transverse ligament may be injured.

MRI

MRI displays the transverse ligament and any associated injury directly. Type I injury involves disruption of the ligament, whereas type II injury involves an avulsion.[21] The distinction is clinically significant because type I injuries are typically treated with surgery.[21]

DENS FRACTURES

Fractures of C2 may involve the dens or pass inferior to the dens. Nonetheless, three of these injuries are designated dens fractures types I to III. Type I fractures involve only the superior portion of the dens. Type II fractures involve the base of the dens where the dens joins with the vertebral body. Type IIa fractures are comminuted type II fractures.[22] Type III fractures involve the body of C2 inferior to the insertion of the dens itself (Figs. 11-11 to 11-13).[22]

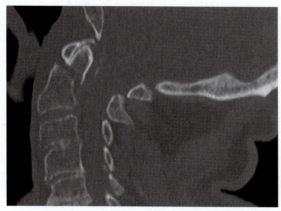

■ **FIGURE 11-11** Type II dens fracture. Sagittal CT image demonstrates an oblique fracture of the dens with posterior displacement of the superior portion of the dens.

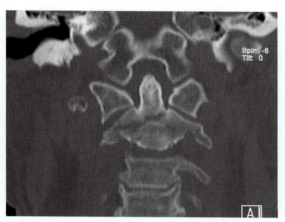

■ **FIGURE 11-12** Type III dens fracture. Coronal CT image demonstrates an oblique fracture through the dens and body of C2.

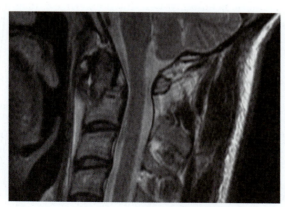

■ **FIGURE 11-13** Type III dens fracture with cruciate ligament injury. Sagittal T2W MR image demonstrates a fracture involving the dens with anterior displacement of the dens. This patient also had a cruciate ligament injury. Prevertebral soft tissue edema is noted.

Epidemiology

C2 fractures constitute about 20% of cervical spine fractures.[23] Greene and associates found that dens fractures occurred in 59% of 340 patients with C2 (axis) fractures.[23] Of these, type II fractures were the most common (120 of the 199 dens fractures, 60%). Only 2 patients had type I fractures.[23] Patients older than 50 years of age tended to have type II injuries, whereas younger patients more often had type III injuries.[23] Typical modes of injuries involved motor vehicle accidents, falls, and diving injuries.[22,23]

Clinical Presentation

Patients present with neck pain after trauma. There may be associated facial injuries. Spinal cord injury may complicate the fracture when there is sufficient displacement.[22]

Pathophysiology

Mechanisms suggested to cause dens fractures include anterior to posterior or posterior to anterior shear/translational injuries as well as hyperextension.[10] An important factor to consider is the stability of the transverse ligament, which can be injured in a similar fashion.[23] Type II fractures have a higher rate of nonunion than other dens fractures.[23]

Imaging

CT

Plain radiographs may show prevertebral soft tissue swelling, separation of the dens from the anterior arch of C1, angulation of the dens on the base of C2, and the actual fracture line(s).[14] These must all be identified and described.[15] Comminuted dens fractures usually require surgical fixation.[23] Displacement of the dens fragment grater than 6 mm usually indicates injury to the transverse ligament and also requires surgical fixation.[23] As with atlantoaxial dissociations, evaluation of the anterior atlantodental interval can help to identify ligamentous injury (see Fig. 11-13).[15] One should distinguish an acute fracture from an os odontoideum. The os odontoideum typically demonstrates sclerotic, corticated margins, whereas the dens fracture demonstrates an acute fracture line with cortical disruption.[6]

MRI

MRI is usually successful for demonstrating injury or disruption of the transverse ligament. This can alter management. Most dens fractures are managed with external fixation. Concurrent transverse ligament injury, however, usually requires surgical fixation.[23]

TRAUMATIC SPONDYLOLISTHESIS OF C2

Traumatic spondylolisthesis of C2 is a fracture of the pars interarticularis of C2. Other names for this entity include hangman's fracture and hangee's fracture. This injury is

Type I

Type IIa

Type II

Type III

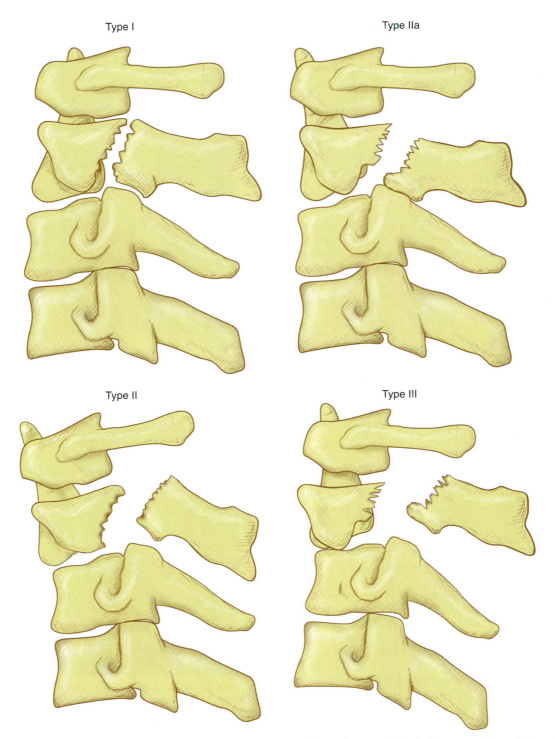

■ **FIGURE 11-14** Levine and Edwards' modification of the system of Effendi and coworkers. *Angulation* indicates angulation of C2 on C3. *Translation* indicates horizontal displacement of C2 on C3. Type I—less than 3-mm translation and no angulation. Type II—angulation and translation. Type IIa—angulation with mild translation. Type III—angulation and translation with facet dislocation. *(Redrawn from Levine AM, Edwards CC. The management of traumatic spondylolisthesis of the axis. J Bone Joint Surg Am 1985; 67:217-226.)*

commonly classified by the Levine and Edwards system or the Francis system.[23] The Levine and Edwards system is a modification of an earlier classification by Effendi and classifies traumatic spondylolisthesis based on four patterns/mechanisms of injury (Fig. 11-14).[24]

The system of Francis and coworkers describes the degree of injury and involves measurement of the displacement of C2 with respect to C3 in an anteroposterior direction as well as the angulation between C2 and C3.[23,25] Class I Francis injuries involve less than 3.5 mm of displacement and less than 11 degrees of angulation. Class II Francis injuries involve similar displacement but greater than 11 degrees of angulation. Class III injuries involve greater than 3.5 mm of displacement (but not more than 50% of the anteroposterior width of C3) with less than 11 degrees of angulation. Class IV injuries involve a similar degree of displacement with greater than 11 degrees of angulation. Class V injuries involve disruption of the disc.[25] However, not all injuries can be easily categorized in any of the available classification schemes.[22]

Epidemiology

Hangman's fractures constituted 22% of C2 fractures in the 340 patients reviewed by Greene and associates.[23] The most common type using the Francis classification was Francis grade I (65% of the 74 patients with traumatic spondylolisthesis of the axis).[23] Modes of injury include motor vehicle accidents, diving, and falls.[22,23]

Clinical Presentation

These patients typically present with neck pain. The incidence of neurologic compromise varies from 6% to 57%. The severity of the injury varies from mild urinary retention to nerve root injury to paralysis.[22] Neurologic injuries are seen more often with unstable fractures and those with fractures of C1.[22]

Pathophysiology

Different mechanisms of injury have been postulated to contribute to these C2 fractures, leading investigators to propose different classification systems for the injuries.[22] In Levine and Edwards' modification of the Effendi classification, type I injuries involve hyperextension and axial loading, type II injuries involve initial hyperextension and axial loading then anterior flexion and compression, type IIa injuries involve flexion and distraction, and type III injuries involve flexion and compression (see Fig. 11-14).[24] The appearance of the fracture and associated displacement/angulation of the fragments can indicate the mechanism involved.[24]

The origin of the eponym "hangman's fracture" or "hangee's fracture" is from judicial hangings in which the knot of the noose was placed beneath the jaw (submental knot) to increase the hyperextension.[10] The predominant mechanism in hanging with a submental knot is hyperextension with distraction, as opposed to the mechanisms given earlier for traumatic spondylolisthesis.[10]

Pathology

Concurrent fractures most often involve C1 but may affect C3 and the spinous processes of adjacent vertebrae.[22,23] The hyperextension force may be transmitted through the face, leading to soft tissue injuries and maxillofacial fractures.

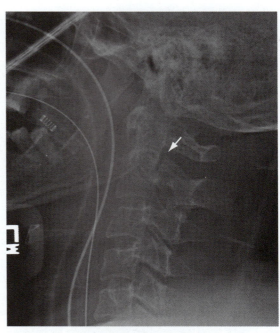

■ **FIGURE 11-15**   Traumatic spondylolisthesis of C2. Lateral radiograph demonstrates bilateral pars interarticularis fractures with minimal displacement (*arrow*).

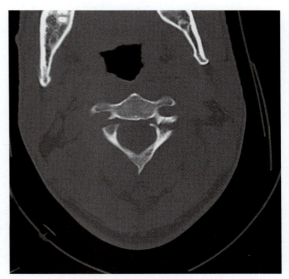

■ **FIGURE 11-16**   Traumatic spondylolisthesis of C2. Axial CT image demonstrates the bilateral pars interarticularis fractures with mild displacement. The fracture on the right involves a portion of the foramen transversarium.

Imaging

CT

Prevertebral soft tissue swelling is a helpful secondary sign of injury (Figs. 11-15 to 11-17). Hangman's fractures are coronally oriented, involve the pars interarticularis of C2, and may extend into the C2 body. There is variable angulation and displacement of C2 on C3, with possible interfacetal dislocation.[15,26] The C2-3 disc space may be widened.[26] Greene and associates found that higher-grade

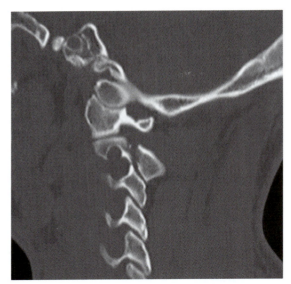

■ **FIGURE 11-17** Traumatic spondylolisthesis of C2 on CT (same patient as in Fig. 11-16). Off-midline sagittal CT image demonstrates one of the pars interarticularis fractures that extends into the facet joint.

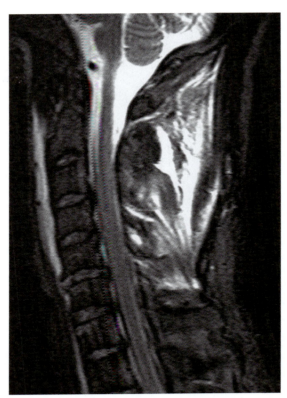

■ **FIGURE 11-18** Hyperextension injury with anterior longitudinal ligament disruption. Sagittal STIR image demonstrates diffuse prevertebral soft tissue edema. At the level of C5-6 there is disruption of the anterior longitudinal ligament with increased signal involving the disc, consistent with injury. There is high signal within the posterior ligamentous complex indicative of injury as well.

injuries typically required surgical fusion, regardless of whether the injuries were classified by the Effendi or the Francis system.[23]

MRI

MRI demonstrates the soft tissue injuries directly. Injury to the C2-C3 disc manifests as increased signal intensity within the disc on T2W or STIR images. Intradiscal hemorrhage shows increased signal on T1W imaging. With interfacetal dislocation there may be injuries of the facet joints, the posterior ligamentous complex, or the anterior or posterior longitudinal ligaments. Uncommonly, there is spinal cord contusion/edema or hemorrhage or nerve root injury.[22]

HYPEREXTENSION INJURIES OF THE SUBAXIAL CERVICAL SPINE AND HYPEREXTENSION TEARDROP INJURIES

These injuries involve hyperextension of the cervical spine. With low levels of force there may only be a ligamentous sprain. As the force increases, more damage occurs, leading to disruption of the anterior longitudinal ligament and eventual dislocation (Figs. 11-18 and 11-19).[26,27] These injuries are also known as hyperextension dislocations, laminar fractures, or pedicolaminar separation fractures.

Epidemiology

Hyperextension injuries of the cervical spine typically result from frontal head trauma or a rear-impact motor vehicle accident.[27] Older patients have increased risk of hyperextension because degenerative disease limits the extent of free spinal motion and because they have increased risk of these forms of trauma.[26]

Clinical Presentation

The clinical presentation depends on the degree of hyperextension force endured. In older patients, the teardrop hyperextension injury requires less force, usually occurs at C2, and usually does not result in spinal cord or nerve root injury.[6,26] Hyperextension teardrop injuries of vertebrae below C2 and hyperextension dislocations are commonly associated with neurologic injuries, especially the "central cord syndrome."[10,26] This "syndrome" causes (1) motor deficits that are greater in the upper extremities than the lower extremities, (2) sensory deficits involving loss of pain and temperature sensation without loss of sensitivity to touch, and (3) with progressive injury, loss of bladder function and lower extremity deficits.[10]

Other types of subaxial hyperextension injuries such as laminar or pedicle fractures are not typically associated with neurologic injury unless osseous fragments enter the canal or a pedicolaminar fracture-separation occurs.[26]

Pathophysiology

With the exception of the hyperextension teardrop injury in older patients, these hyperextension forces typically lead to injuries in the lower cervical spine, usually at C5-6.[10,27] As the hyperextension force increases, the number of injured structures also increases. Initially, there is

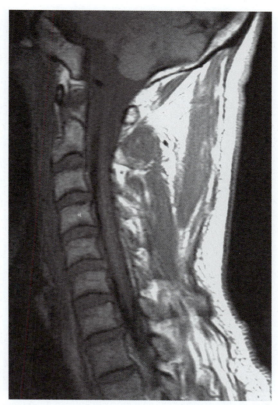

■ **FIGURE 11-19**   Hyperextension injury with anterior longitudinal ligament disruption (same patient as in Fig. 11-18). Sagittal T1W MR image demonstrates prevertebral soft tissue edema. The injury to the anterior longitudinal ligament is identified, but the disc injury is not well seen.

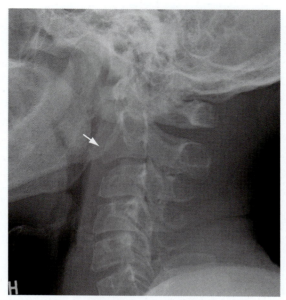

■ **FIGURE 11-20**   Hyperextension teardrop injury. Lateral radiograph demonstrates a small triangular fragment from the anteroinferior corner of C2 (*arrow*).

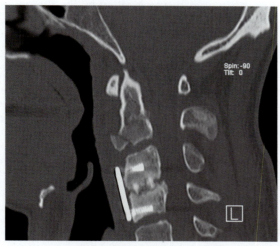

■ **FIGURE 11-21**   Hyperextension teardrop injury (different patient from Fig. 11-20). Sagittal CT image demonstrates a small, mildly displaced triangular fragment from the anteroinferior corner of the dens. There has been prior anterior fixation of C3 and C4.

prevertebral soft tissue injury, then injury to the anterior longitudinal ligament and discs. There may be disc herniation(s), or the discs may be avulsed from their endplates.[27] Still greater force injures all three columns of the spine, causing hyperextension dislocation with concurrent fractures and possible cord injury. Although laminar fractures may occur with flexion and compression injuries, they may also be seen in isolation or with other hyperextension injuries.[26] Pedicolaminar fracture-separations extend through the pedicles and laminae, separating the articular pillar from the rest of the vertebra.[26] The pedicolaminar fractures are unstable injuries that can also involve damage to the anterior and posterior longitudinal ligaments and the posterior ligamentous complex.[26]

Pathology

When these injuries involve a frontal blow, there can be associated injuries to the face.

Imaging

CT

The hyperextension teardrop injury usually involves C2 in older patients but the lower cervical spine in younger patients.[6] The fracture fragment typically breaks away from the anteroinferior corner of the vertebral body due to avulsion by the anterior longitudinal ligament (Figs. 11-20 and 11-21).[26] Frequently, the fragment appears "vertical" with a longer craniocaudal dimension than an anteroposterior dimension.[26] Subaxial teardrop injuries usually show prevertebral soft tissue swelling or hemorrhage.[6,26]

After severe hyperextension dislocations, the spinal column may "realign" spontaneously, masking the severity of injuries. Subtle signs of hyperextension injury include prevertebral soft tissue swelling and anterior widening ("anterior gaping") of the disc space at the level of injury.[26,27] The fracture fragment associated with this type of hyperextension injury usually appears horizontal, with a longer anteroposterior dimension than craniocaudal

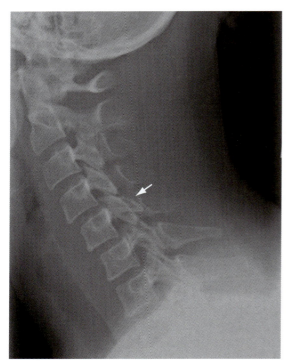

■ **FIGURE 11-22** Pedicolaminar fracture separation. Lateral radiograph demonstrates abnormal rotation of one of the C5 articular pillars (*arrow*).

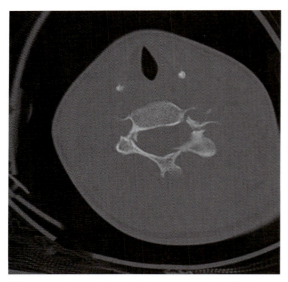

■ **FIGURE 11-23** Pedicolaminar fracture separation (different patient from Fig. 11-22). Axial CT demonstrates comminuted fractures of the left lamina and pedicle resulting in pedicolaminar fracture separation. The fractures involve the left foramen transversarium. There is also a fracture of the right pedicle.

dimension. This is the reverse of the appearance seen with hyperextension teardrop injuries.[26]

Laminar fractures and pedicolaminar separation-fractures are easily diagnosed with CT.[26] With these fractures, one must accurately identify the fracture fragments and determine whether they have narrowed the neuroforamen or the spinal canal (Figs. 11-22 and 11-23).[26]

MRI

MRI is very helpful for identifying soft tissue injuries involving the intervertebral discs, ligaments, and spinal cord.[27] Injured discs exhibit abnormally increased signal on STIR or T2W images. Intradiscal hemorrhage may appear bright on T1-weighted (T1W) images. MRI allows visualization of disc herniations and resultant canal narrowing.

In pedicolaminar separation-fractures, MRI is useful to identify concurrent injuries of the anterior and posterior longitudinal ligaments, posterior ligamentous complex, and facets.[26]

HYPERFLEXION INJURIES OF THE SUBAXIAL CERVICAL SPINE

Hyperflexion injuries encompass the spectrum of damage caused by progressive flexion force on the cervical spine below C2. Initially, the force may only damage the posterior ligamentous complex or cause simple compression fracture. Progressive force eventually leads to the unstable ligamentous and osseous injuries, including dislocations and flexion teardrop injury. Alternate names used include posterior ligamentous complex strain, compression fracture, unilateral interfacetal dislocation, bilateral interfacetal dislocation, and flexion teardrop injury.

Epidemiology

Modes of injury include motor vehicle accidents, diving, and falling.[28]

Clinical Presentation

The clinical presentation varies with the severity of injury. Isolated injuries such as sprains of the posterior ligamentous complex and simple compression fractures are stable and may present as only neck pain. Unilateral interfacetal dislocation usually does not cause a neurologic deficit but occasionally is associated with nerve root injuries and disc injuries.[6,29]

The flexion teardrop injury and bilateral interfacetal dislocation typically are associated with severe neurologic deficits.[6,28] One presentation of the flexion teardrop injury is the "anterior cord syndrome."[10,28] This involves quadriplegia and sensory deficits, such as loss of touch, pain, and temperature sensation with preservation of position and vibration sensation (which are carried in the dorsal columns of the spinal cord).[10,28] In a review of 45 patients with flexion teardrop injuries, Kim and coworkers reported that only 13% (6/45) were neurologically intact.[28] The remainder had either complete (56%) or incomplete (31%) quadriplegia.[28]

Pathophysiology

Flexion injuries tend to occur in the lower cervical spine. The simple compression fracture involves flexion with injury to the anterior portion of the vertebral body.[10] Further flexion and distraction eventually lead to bilateral

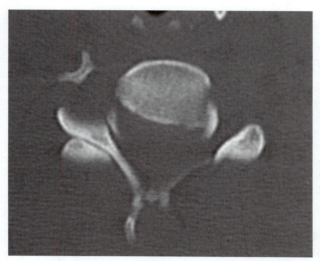

■ FIGURE 11-24 Unilateral interfacetal dislocation. Axial CT image demonstrates unilateral facet dislocation on the right with "uncovered" facets.

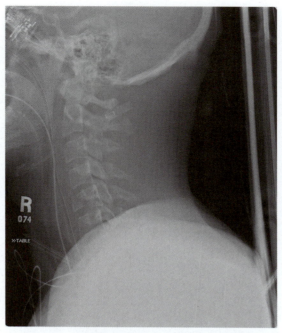

■ FIGURE 11-25 Flexion teardrop fracture. Lateral radiograph demonstrates a triangular fragment involving the anteroinferior corner of C5 with posterior displacement of the posterior portion of the vertebral body. Note prevertebral soft tissue swelling.

interfacetal dislocation and the flexion teardrop injury. Bilateral interfacetal dislocation is a severe injury that involves most of the soft tissue structures and ligaments, including the posterior ligamentous complex, facet joints, posterior longitudinal ligament, disc, and anterior longitudinal ligament.[6,29] The flexion teardrop injury involves injury of the ligaments and soft tissues of all three columns.[6] The mechanism for unilateral interfacetal dislocation is believed to be hyperflexion and distraction combined with rotation.[29] Unilateral interfacetal dislocation typically involves injury of the posterior ligaments, disc, and joint capsules and may involve the anterior longitudinal ligament.[6]

Imaging

CT

Posterior ligamentous complex sprain usually shows widening of the interspinous distance.

Simple compression fracture is seen on CT as compaction of the vertebra with greatest loss of height anteriorly (anterior wedging).

Unilateral and bilateral interfacetal dislocations manifest as uncovered facets on one or both sides (Fig. 11-24).[6] Unilateral dislocation typically shows less than 50% anterior subluxation of the vertebral body at the level of injury, whereas bilateral dislocation typically shows more than 50% anterior subluxation.[6] Both types may have associated facet fractures.[6]

Flexion teardrop injuries usually show a triangular fracture fragment that arises from the anteroinferior portion of the vertebral body, posterior displacement of the posterior portion of the injured vertebral body, narrowing of the posterior portion of the disc space below the level of injury, widening of the facet joint between the inferior facets at the level of injury and the superior facets of the next level below, kyphotic deformity at the level of injury, and posterior displacement of the upper cervical spine above the level of the injury (Fig. 11-25).[28]

MRI

MRI demonstrates the soft tissue and ligamentous injuries directly. In sprains of the posterior ligamentous complex there will be increased signal on T2W and STIR images within the substance of the complex, indicating edema. Unilateral and bilateral interfacetal dislocations and flexion teardrop injuries may demonstrate injuries to the disc, anterior and posterior longitudinal ligaments, posterior ligamentous complex, and facets (Figs. 11-26 to 11-29). However, the individual ligamentous injuries are not always easily identifiable by MRI.[29]

Special Procedures

Vertebral artery injuries including thrombosis/occlusion and dissection are seen in association with fracture-dislocations and interfacetal dislocations.[16] Therefore, MRA, CTA, or conventional angiography may be indicated in such patients.

VERTEBRAL ARTERY INJURY

The types of vertebral artery injuries after blunt trauma include thrombosis/occlusion, dissection, transection, and pseudoaneurysm formation. Other names used include vertebral artery thrombosis/occlusion, vertebral artery dissection, and vertebral artery pseudoaneurysm.

Epidemiology

Cervical spine injuries are associated with vertebral artery injuries. As the severity of trauma increases, the risk of vertebral artery injury also increases.[7] The incidence of

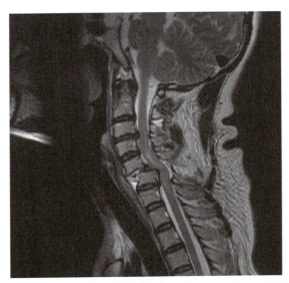

■ **FIGURE 11-26** Bilateral interfacetal dislocation. Sagittal T2 MRI demonstrates anterior dislocation of C5 on C6. The posterior and anterior longitudinal ligaments are disrupted. There is abnormal increased signal in the prevertebral soft tissues and involving the posterior ligamentous complex. Also note cord edema/contusion.

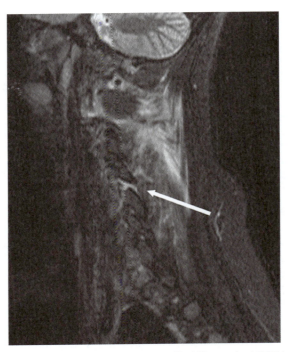

■ **FIGURE 11-28** Hyperflexion injury. Off-midline sagittal STIR image demonstrates edema involving the posterior ligamentous complex and cervical facet joint with subluxation of the facet (*arrow*).

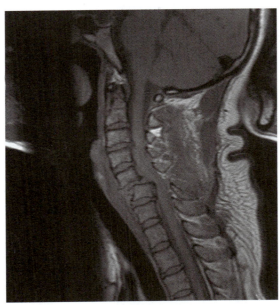

■ **FIGURE 11-27** Bilateral interfacetal dislocation (same patient as in Fig. 11-26). Sagittal T1W MR image demonstrates anterior dislocation of C5 on C6 with ligamentous disruption.

vertebral artery injury after cervical spine trauma ranges from 19% to 75%, depending on the specific types of cervical spine injuries included in the studies.[30] Dislocation injuries, for example, clearly increase the risk of arterial injury.[16] MRA is estimated to detect vertebral artery thrombosis in 13% to 16% of blunt trauma.[7,30] However, the true accuracy of MRA in this setting is not known.[7,30] Vertebral artery injuries arise in the same settings as cervical fractures, including motor vehicle accidents, hanging, diving, and falling, but vertebral artery injuries are also reported with minor trauma such as chiropractic adjustment and seizures.[16,30]

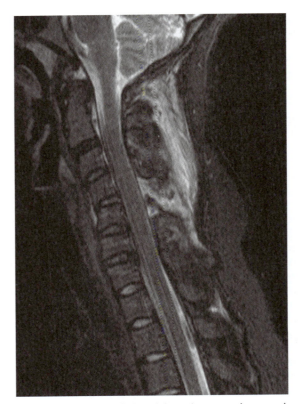

■ **FIGURE 11-29** Hyperflexion injury (same patient as in Fig. 11-28). Sagittal STIR image demonstrates similar injury involving the posterior ligamentous complex with prevertebral edema and focal kyphosis in the midcervical spine.

Clinical Presentation

Unilateral vertebral artery injury usually does not lead to neurologic deficit. Bilateral injury can lead to stroke and death.[30] Ren and associates argue for close monitoring of patients with unilateral vertebral artery injury, because after thrombosis the thrombus may embolize from the vertebral artery into the posterior circulation.[30] The neurologic sequelae will typically include posterior circulation symptoms such as ataxia or dizziness.[7,30] This diagnosis can be subtle and may be missed if suspicion or actual symptoms do not prompt specific search for it.[30]

Pathophysiology

The mechanism of injury in nonpenetrating trauma is believed to most likely be stretching/tearing of the vessel.[30] Points of specific vulnerability for vascular injury include the entry and exit points into the foramina transversaria at C6 and C1 and anywhere along the course between C1 and the foramen magnum.[16] Fracture-dislocations, distraction injuries, and fractures that extend into the foramina transversaria specifically increase the risk for arterial injury.[16] The relative absence of neurologic deficit after unilateral injury is believed to be due to preservation of flow through the contralateral vertebral artery.[16]

Pathology

Trauma to the vessel may injure the intima and media, leading to intraluminal thrombus and occlusion.[30]

Imaging

Ultrasonography

Doppler ultrasonography can identify lack of flow, indicating thrombosis. Ultrasonography may identify the thrombus within the lumen, irregularity of the wall, or the dissection flap itself.

CT

Noncontrast CT can identify the injuries that place patients at risk for vertebral artery injury. However, noncontrast CT has limited utility for this diagnosis. CTA can be used in the diagnosis and can be performed at the same time as other contrast-enhanced studies. Typical findings include occlusion, dissection, and pseudoaneurysm formation.

MRI

Noninvasive MRA is thought to be a useful screening study for vertebral artery injury. However, its accuracy is uncertain in subtle cases, and it may not differentiate spasm from mechanical injury successfully.[7,30] The MRA techniques include 2D and 3D time-of-flight MRA and contrast-enhanced MRA (Figs. 11-30 and 11-31).

It is useful to employ additional MRI sequences when there is suspicion of thrombosis or dissection of the vertebral artery. These include axial T2W images with fat

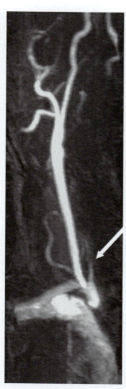

■ **FIGURE 11-30** Right vertebral artery occlusion. MIP image from MRA demonstrates an occluded right vertebral artery just after its origin (*arrow*). This patient had a facet dislocation injury.

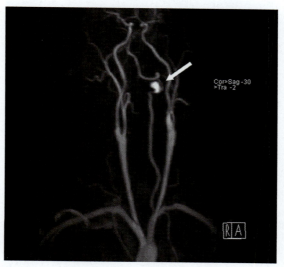

■ **FIGURE 11-31** Left vertebral artery pseudoaneurysm. MIP image from MRA demonstrates a saccular pseudoaneurysm arising from the distal left vertebral artery (*arrow*).

saturation and axial T1W images with and without fat saturation. In cases of dissection, maximum intensity projection (MIP) images may show nothing more than luminal narrowing. The T1W images (especially T1W fat saturation images) display adjacent crescent-shaped high signal consistent with acute thrombus in the false lumen. Together, fat saturation axial T1W and T2W sequences may visualize the dissection flap. Studies of arterial dissection should include MRI of the brain to identify infarcts in the areas supplied by the posterior circulation.[7]

Special Procedures

In traumatized patients at risk for arterial injury, conventional angiography can display gross injuries such as luminal narrowing, occlusion/thrombosis, and pseudoaneurysm. Conventional catheter angiography can also document subtle but significant irregularities that MRA could miss.[30] Use of conventional angiography for diagnosis also provides the opportunity for immediate interventional therapy of any vascular lesions detected.

CHANCE-TYPE INJURIES

Chance fractures or "lap belt fractures" classically were described as transverse fractures of the vertebral body and posterior elements.[3] Used more generally, the term *Chance fracture* describes a spectrum of flexion-distraction injuries that are purely osseous, purely soft tissue (rarely), or a combination of both. Recognition of Chance-type fractures raises suspicion of associated abdominal visceral injuries.[31]

Epidemiology

Chance fractures constitute 5% to 15% of thoracolumbar fractures.[3] These thoracolumbar fractures typically result from motor vehicle accidents, falls, and sports injuries.[3]

Clinical Presentation

These patients may present with a broad spectrum of abdominal injuries.[31] Neurologic deficits may also be present, because this injury involves the entire spinal column, including the spinal canal and cord.[31]

Pathophysiology

The mechanism of injury is flexion with distraction. Typically, these injuries occur at the thoracolumbar junction.[2] Chance fractures occur in a transverse or oblique plane, involve all three columns of the spine, and are consequently unstable.[2] The complex forces create an injury that may involve the spinous process and pedicles and extend anteriorly through the vertebral body. The antero-superior portion of the vertebral body may be compressed.[31] This injury should be distinguished from the burst fracture, which results from axial loading. Features that suggest a Chance-type injury include disruption of the posterior osseous and ligamentous structures with preservation of posterior vertebral body height.[3,31] However, Bernstein and colleagues describe a "burst" *component* to some Chance-type injuries with retropulsion of fragments.[3] Groves and coworkers found a high incidence of adjacent vertebral body injuries.[31]

Pathology

There can be widespread injury to the paraspinal musculature and subcutaneous tissues.[31]

Imaging

CT

CT with multiplanar reformatted images demonstrates the fractures and displays signs of concurrent soft tissue injury, such as widened interspinous distance and widened facet joints.[3] Usually, there is a transverse fracture through the posterior elements extending forward into the vertebral body. An important factor distinguishing Chance fractures from burst injuries is the preservation or even increased height of the posterior vertebral body seen with Chance fractures.[31] However, some Chance-type fractures have a "burst" component with retropulsion of fragments.[3]

MRI

MRI displays the extent of injury more fully. The fracture can be identified by the "sandwich sign": high T2 signal of edema above and below the low signal of hemorrhage within the fracture line (Fig. 11-32).[3,31] Typical findings include injury to the posterior ligamentous and/or osseous structures, associated vertebral body injuries, and soft tissue injuries.[31] MRI can identify disc herniation or injury, muscular and subcutaneous tissue injury, extramedullary hemorrhage, as well as spinal cord contusion or hemorrhage.[31]

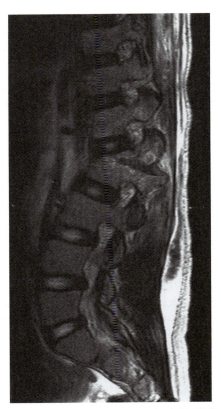

■ **FIGURE 11-32** Chance-type fracture. Sagittal T2W MR image demonstrates the "sandwich sign" with edema surrounding the transversely oriented fracture that involves the posterior elements, pedicle, and vertebral body. Note that the posterior vertebral body height is increased by the distraction component of the injury.

MISCELLANEOUS FRACTURES OF THE THORACOLUMBAR SPINE

Compression fractures involve loss of anterior vertebral body height.[2] Burst fractures are due to axial loading and involve loss of anterior vertebral body height as well as fracture of the posterior cortex and retropulsion of the posterior vertebral body fragments with possible loss of posterior vertebral body height.[32] Fracture-dislocations involve more severe trauma.

Epidemiology

Compression fractures are a common type of thoracolumbar injury. Burst fractures make up 64% to 81% of traumatic thoracolumbar injuries.[32] Fracture-dislocations are the least common of these three.

Clinical Presentation

Compression fractures may present as back pain. Because of the severity of injury, burst fractures and fracture-dislocations have a significant incidence of neurologic injury.[32]

Pathophysiology

The typical mechanisms of these injuries include various degrees of flexion and axial compression.[2] Lateral forces lead to different patterns of compression injuries, including lateral dislocation.

Compression fractures usually involve the anterior column alone and so are stable injuries. When they cause marked kyphosis (>40 degrees), they may become unstable.[2]

Burst fractures involve compression of the vertebral body with retropulsion of bone fragments.[32] Classification of burst fractures is a point of some contention.[2,32] Progressive force can lead to fracture-dislocations.

Because of stabilization by the ribs, fractures of the thoracic spine typically require more force to produce and are correspondingly less common than fractures of the thoracolumbar junction and lumbar spine.[2] The overall increased incidence of fractures at the thoracolumbar junction may be due to increased mobility at this level.[2]

Imaging

CT

Compression fractures can be easily diagnosed on radiographs. However, one must scrutinize the posterior portion of the vertebral bodies and the posterior elements to exclude a more severe injury. CT accurately depicts retropulsed fragments and the subsequent canal compromise, which result from burst injuries and fracture-dislocations (Fig. 11-33).[32] Fracture-dislocations are often obvious but may be subtle if the dislocation has spontaneously reduced.

MRI

MRI is not typically used for evaluating compression fractures but can be helpful in attempts to distinguish benign

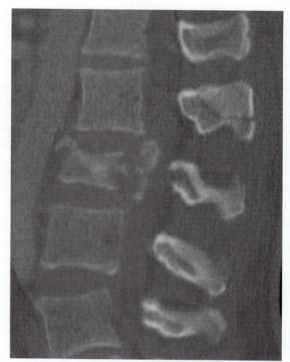

■ **FIGURE 11-33** Burst fracture. Sagittal CT image demonstrates a burst fracture involving L3 with retropulsion of fragments into the canal. There is a spinal process fracture at the level above.

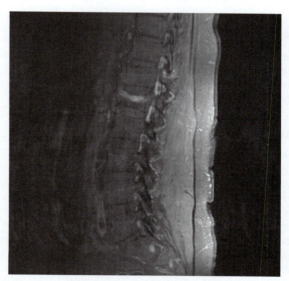

■ **FIGURE 11-34** Benign compression fracture. Sagittal T2W MR image demonstrates increased signal consistent with edema involving the superior portion of the L1 vertebral body.

from pathologic fracture (Fig. 11-34).[2] In burst fractures, MRI can identify posterior longitudinal ligament injury, cord injury, extramedullary hemorrhage, as well as other soft tissue injuries, including disc herniation (Fig. 11-35).[32] In fracture-dislocations, MRI allows identification of specific ligamentous injury as well as the extent of spinal cord injuries (Fig. 11-36).

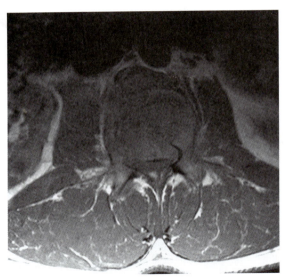

■ **FIGURE 11-35** Burst fracture (same patient as in Fig. 11-33). Axial T1W MR image demonstrates the burst fracture with marked central canal narrowing due to retropulsed fragments.

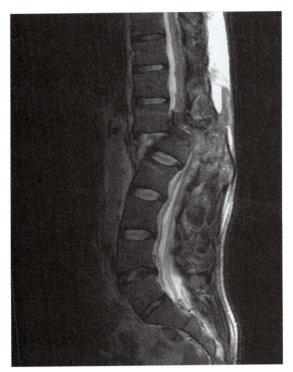

■ **FIGURE 11-36** Fracture-dislocation. Sagittal T2W MR image demonstrates posterior dislocation of L1 with respect to T12. There is transection of the cord at this level with extensive ligamentous injury and soft tissue injury involving all three columns.

ANALYSIS

In the cervical spine, one can consider the craniocervical junction and subaxial spine separately. Distraction type injuries include atlantoaxial and atlanto-occipital subluxation and dislocation (see Figs. 11-4 and 11-7). Osseous injuries include atlas injuries such as the Jefferson burst fracture as well as axis injuries, including dens fractures and traumatic spondylolisthesis of C2 (see Figs. 11-10,

11-11, and 11-16). In the subaxial cervical spine, differentiation between hyperflexion and hyperextension injuries is important and can be made based on the pattern of injury to the osseous and soft tissue structures (see Figs. 11-18 and 11-29).

Compression and burst fractures can occur throughout the spinal column (see Figs. 11-33 and 11-34). In the thoracolumbar spine, fracture-dislocations and Chance type injuries can be identified. Because of the association with abdominal visceral injury, Chance fractures need to be differentiated from other types of trauma, such as the burst fracture (see Fig. 11-32).[31] A sample report of a C5 fracture and ligamental tears is presented in Box 11-1.

BOX 11-1   MRI of Ligamental Tears and C5 Fracture

PATIENT HISTORY

A 22-year-old man presented after a motorcycle accident.

TECHNIQUE

Sagittal T1W, T2W, and STIR images as well as axial T1W, T2W, and T2*W images were obtained without administration of a contrast agent.

FINDINGS

There is normal alignment at the craniocervical junction. There is focal kyphosis and 5-mm anterolisthesis of C5 on C6, where there is focal disruption of the posterior longitudinal ligament. The anterior longitudinal ligament is buckled at this level but appears intact. Posterior to the C5 vertebral body, blood and disc material are noted deep to the posterior longitudinal ligament within the ventral epidural space and cause no cord compression. Interspinous edema is present at C5-6. There is widening of the facet joints at this level with associated abnormal STIR signal. Prevertebral edema is present from C4 through C7. The fractures involving C5 vertebral body and pedicles are more easily identified and described on the recent CT. Extensive edema is present in the paravertebral musculature posteriorly above and below the level of injury. There is moderate central canal stenosis from the focal kyphosis at C5-6 and a focus of increased signal within the spinal cord on T2W and STIR images at the same level suggestive of edema. Flow voids are present in both vertebral arteries.

IMPRESSION

- Focal disruption of the posterior longitudinal ligament occurs at C5-6, where there is focal kyphosis and anterolisthesis. Interspinous ligament tears are present at this level and the anterior longitudinal ligament is buckled.
- Known C5 fractures are better evaluated by the recent CT.
- There is a small focus of spinal cord edema at C5-6.

SURGICAL REPORT

Surgery involved C4-C6 anterior cervical decompression and arthrodesis. Findings included C5-C6 traumatic anterior spondylolisthesis with bilateral C5-C6 facet dislocations. There were bilateral C5 comminuted pedicle and lateral mass separation fractures and a spinal cord injury.

KEY POINTS: DIFFERENTIAL DIAGNOSIS

- Utilization of radiography, CT, and MRI will allow for accurate diagnosis and description of the various injuries.
- Recognition of the mechanism of injury can aid in accurate description of the injury and identification of associated injuries.

- Unstable injuries must be identified to help guide therapy.
- MRI can identify soft tissue trauma such as disc, ligamentous, and vascular injuries.

SUGGESTED READINGS

Bagley LJ. Imaging of spinal trauma. Radiol Clin North Am 2006; 44:1-12.

Cohen WA, Giaque AP, Hallam DK, et al. Evidence-based approach to use of MR imaging in acute spinal trauma. Eur J Radiol 2003; 48:49-60.

Daffner RH. Controversies in cervical spine imaging in trauma patients. Semin Musculoskelet Radiol 2005; 9:105-115.

Provenzale J. MR imaging of spinal trauma. Emerg Radiol 2007; 13:289-297.

Sliker CW, Mirvis SE, Shanmuganathan K. Assessing cervical spine stability in obtunded blunt trauma patients: review of medical literature. Radiology 2005; 234:733-739.

REFERENCES

1. Hosalkar JS, Cain EL, Horn D, et al. Traumatic atlanto-occipital dislocation in children. J Bone Joint Surg Am 2005; 87:2480-2488.
2. Gray L, Vandemark R, Hays M. Thoracic and lumbar spine trauma. Semin Ultrasound CT MR 2001; 22:125-134.
3. Bernstein MP, Mirvis SE, Shanmuganathan K. Chance-type fractures of the thoracolumbar spine: imaging analysis in 53 patients. AJR Am J Roentgenol 2006; 187:859-868.
4. Daffner RH, Deeb ZL, Goldberg AL, et al. The radiologic assessment of post-traumatic vertebral stability. Skel Radiol 1990; 19:103-108.
5. Denis F. Spinal instability as defined by the three-column spine concept in acute spinal trauma. Clin Orthop Relat Res 1984; (189):65-76.
6. Harris JH, Harris WH. The Radiology of Emergency Medicine. Baltimore, Lippincott Williams & Wilkins, 2000.
7. Torina PJ, Flanders AE, Carrino JA, et al. Incidence of vertebral artery thrombosis in cervical spine trauma: correlation with severity of spinal cord injury. AJNR Am J Neuroradiol 2005; 26:2645-2651.
8. Demaerel P. Magnetic resonance imaging of spinal cord trauma: a pictorial essay. Neuroradiology 2006; 48:223-232.
9. Fisher CG, Sun JCL, Dvorak M. Recognition and management of atlanto-occipital dislocation: improving survival from an often fatal condition. Can J Surg 2001; 44:412-420.
10. White AA, Panjabi MM. Clinical Biomechanics of the Spine. Philadelphia, JB Lippincott, 1978.
11. Gregg S, Kortbeek JB, du Plessis S. Atlanto-occipital dislocation: a case study of survival with partial recovery and review of the literature. J Trauma 2005; 58:168-171.
12. Bucholz RW, Burkhead WZ. The pathological anatomy of fatal atlanto-occipital dislocations. J Bone Joint Surg Am 1979; 61:248-250.
13. Deliganis AV, Baxter AB, Hanson JA, et al. Radiologic spectrum of craniocervical distraction injuries. RadioGraphics 2000; 20: S237-S250.
14. Harris JH. The cervicocranium: its radiographic assessment. Radiology 2001; 218:337-351.
15. Bono CM, Vaccaro AR, Fehlings M, et al. Measurement techniques for upper cervical spine injuries—consensus statement of the Spine Trauma Study Group. Spine 2007; 32:593-600.
16. Weller S, Rossitch E, Malek AM. Detection of vertebral artery injury after cervical spine trauma using magnetic resonance angiography. J Trauma 1999; 46:660-666.
17. De Beer JDV, Thomas M, Walters J, Anderson P. Traumatic atlanto-axial subluxation. J Bone Joint Surg Br 1988; 70:652-655.
18. Levine AM, Edwards CC. Fractures of the atlas. J Bone Joint Surg Am 1991; 73:680-691.
19. Isolated fractures of the atlas in adults. Neurosurgery 2002; 50(Suppl):S120-S124.
20. Heller JG, Viroslav S, Hudson T. Jefferson fractures: the role of magnification artifact in assessing transverse ligament integrity. J Spinal Disord 1993; 6:392-396.
21. Dickman CA, Greene K, Sonntag V. Injuries involving the transverse atlantal ligament: classification and treatment guidelines based upon experience with 39 injuries. Neurosurgery 1996; 38:44-50.
22. Isolated fractures of the axis. Neurosurgery 2002; 50(Suppl): S125-S139.
23. Greene KA, Dickman CA, Marciano FF, et al. Acute axis fractures: analysis of management and outcome in 340 consecutive cases. Spine 1997; 22:1843-1852.
24. Levine AM, Edwards CC. The management of traumatic spondylolisthesis of the axis. J Bone Joint Surg Am 1985; 67:217-226.
25. Francis WR, Fielding JW, Hawkins RJ, et al. Traumatic spondylolisthesis of the axis. J Bone Joint Surg Br 1981; 63:313-318.
26. Rao SK, Wasyliw C, Nunez DB Jr. Spectrum of imaging findings in hyperextension injuries of the neck. RadioGraphics 2005; 25:1239-1254.
27. Davis SJ, Teresi LM, Bradley WG, et al. Cervical spine hyperextension injuries: MR findings. Radiology 1991; 180:245-251.
28. Kim KS, Chen JJ, Russell EJ, Rogers LF. Flexion teardrop fracture of the cervical spine: radiographic characteristics. AJR Am J Roentgenol 1989; 152:319-326.
29. Vaccaro AR, Madigan L, Schweitzer M, et al. Magnetic resonance imaging analysis of soft tissue disruption after flexion-distraction injuries of the subaxial cervical spine. Spine 2001; 26:1866-1872.
30. Ren X, Wang W, Zhang X, et al. The comparative study of magnetic resonance angiography diagnosis and pathology of blunt vertebral artery injury. Spine 2006; 31:2124-2129.
31. Groves CJ, Cassar-Pullicino VN, Tins BJ, et al. Chance-type flexion-distraction injuries in the thoracolumbar spine: MR imaging characteristics. Radiology 2005; 236:601-608.
32. Petersilge CA, Emery SE. Thoracolumbar burst fracture: evaluating stability. Semin Ultrasound CT MR 1996; 17:105-111.

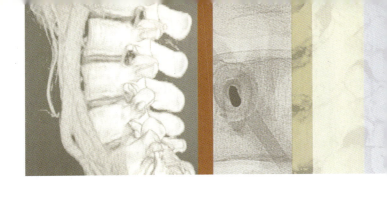

CHAPTER 12

Trauma to the Spinal Cord

Matthew F. Omojola

Spinal cord trauma is the application of excess force to the spinal cord and the consequences of that force for the cord. Traumatic spinal cord injury (SCI) may result from an acute blow to the spine, resulting in fracture or dislocation of the vertebrae, rupture of intervertebral discs and ligaments, occlusion or rupture of blood vessels of the spine or the spinal cord, and/or formation of extra-axial collections or hematoma. These processes can compress, bruise, expand, or tear the spinal cord. Nontraumatic SCI injury can result from many different preexisting diseases, including neoplasm, vascular stenoses and malformations, inflammatory disease, degenerative change, and radiation injury. The emphasis in this chapter is on trauma to the spinal cord, which invariably leads to SCI.

SCI can lead to cord concussion, contusion, hematoma, swelling, edema, transection, or a combination of these entities. Injury to the vascular supply of the spinal cord may lead to ischemia or infarction of the spinal cord, whereas extramedullary vascular injury may cause extra-axial hematomas, which compress the spinal cord. In some cases of SCI there is no evidence of bone injury on plain radiography or CT. These cases are referred to as *spinal cord injury without radiographic abnormality* (SCIWORA). Cases of SCIWORA do show evidence of injury to the spinal cord on MRI. SCIWORA occurs almost exclusively in young children and adolescents owing to the flexibility and elasticity of the immature spine, but it can also be seen in adults.[1,2]

Epidemiology

There are 10,000 to 11,000 new cases of traumatic SCI in the United States each year.[3,4] That number has increased slightly over the past two decades.[3,4] The average age at injury has increased during that period from 28.7 years in 1973-1979 to 37.6 years in 2000-2003.[5,6] There is substantial geographic variation in the incidence of SCI particularly in children, with the South and Midwest recording the highest frequency of these injuries.[7] C5 is the most common level of SCI, whereas the most common level to produce paraplegia is T12.[1]

For the general population, the causes of traumatic SCI have been motor vehicle accidents in about 50%, falls in 24%, violence including gunshot injuries in 11%, sports-related activities in 9%, and diverse other causes in 5%.[4,5] Men are affected disproportionately more than women (80:20). Factors contributing to SCI during motor vehicle accidents include not wearing seat belts and alcohol/drug use.

In children, the overall incidence of SCI in the United States is estimated at 1.99 cases per 100,000 children. Boys are twice as likely as girls to suffer SCI: 2.79 cases/100,000 boys versus 1.15 cases per 100,000 girls.[7] African-American children suffer the highest rate of injury (1.53 cases/100,000 children), whereas Asian-American children experience a significantly lower incidence than all other ethnic groups (0.36 cases/100,000 children).[7] In children, the mechanisms of injury include motor vehicle accident, 56%; accidental fall, 14%; firearm injury, 9%; sports-related injury, 8%; and others, 13%.[7]

Clinical Presentation

Patients presenting with possible SCI may be conscious or show impaired consciousness. The conscious patient typically complains of pain and loss of neurologic function or responds to inquiry about them. In these patients, neurologic evaluation discloses the level and density of the SCI. Inebriated, obtunded, or semiconscious patients may be unable to complain or respond appropriately to neurologic testing.[8] This second group of patients should be examined with suspicion of SCI until proven otherwise. Impaired patients impose special requirements. They should be imaged thoroughly to ensure that all significant injuries are defined and must be handled especially carefully to ensure that they are protected against excess manipulation during the period of impairment.[8] It is essential to determine the existence and extent of SCI at the earliest possible time because this will determine the appropriate management and outcome of this injury.

Local pain and tenderness may identify the level of anatomic injury. The level of anatomic injury, however, does not always correspond to the level of neurologic dysfunction. Severe injury to the T10-12 region may cause local spinal cord contusion, compression, and/or hematoma, whereas concurrent injury to the artery of Adamkiewicz causes infarction of an extensive segment of the spinal cord remote from the level of bone injury. Expanding compressive epidural hematoma may also produce a neurologic level far removed from the local injury.

Two major classifications have begun to standardize the evaluation and reporting of SCI to ensure adequate documentation of the extent of SCI: the Frankel classification[9] and the more recent, more comprehensive impairment scale by the American Spinal Injury Association (ASIA).[10] Radiologists should be familiar with the broad outlines of these classifications to communicate effectively with their colleagues (Tables 12-1 and 12-2).

Acute SCI usually presents as an acute neurologic deficit. The deficit is designated complete when there is absence of sensory and motor function below the level of injury resulting in paraplegia or tetraplegia. The deficit is classified as incomplete when there is (partial) sparing or asymmetric involvement below the level of injury. Incomplete clinical presentations include specific syndromes such as central cord syndrome, mixed cord syndrome, anterior cord syndrome, and Brown-Séquard syndrome.[4,10]

Months or years after the acute phase of the injury, SCI patients may show improvement, remain neurologically stable, or suffer new symptoms. New pain syndromes or spasms may suggest post-traumatic myelopathy from adhesions tethering or compressing the cord at the original site of injury or from cyst formation within (syringomyelia) or outside the spinal cord (arachnoid cyst). Scarring

usually affects the cord at the site of the initial injury. Cysts and syringes may enlarge and extend away from the original injury for long distances, leading to signs and symptoms remote from the site of first injury.[11]

Pathophysiology

Spinal cord trauma can be direct, indirect, or a combination of both depending on the causative mechanism.[12] Direct trauma is caused by violence, principally penetrating knife wounds or missiles that pass into the spinal cord. Knives tend to injure the dorsolateral portion of the spinal cord, where the cord is least protected by bone.[12] Knife injuries generally cause local edema and minimal hemorrhage confined to the level of injury. They usually are clinically incomplete. Occasionally, the penetrating implement may sever the spinal cord and cause complete SCI. Penetrating missiles may find their way into the spinal cord via the dorsolateral route or by exploding through the bony spine, causing shrapnel and/or bone fragments that lacerate the spinal cord. The explosion/laceration often creates a more severe and ragged SCI that extends far beyond the entry site. In this situation, the entry hole in the dura may be small, with minimal hemorrhage within the cord or within the subarachnoid, subdural, or epidural space around the cord.[12] Chronically, extensive adhesions and gliosis in the medullary and perimedullary spaces may lead to cyst formation within the spinal cord, encystment of the subarachnoid space, and tethering of the spinal cord to the dural-bony canal at the level of injury. Concurrent vascular injury may cause ischemia and infarction of the spinal cord. Spinal subluxation and dislocation may produce additional compressive injuries to the spinal cord.

Indirect injury to the spinal cord is the more common injury and is due to compression and/or stretching of the spinal cord by fracture-dislocation, subluxation, ruptured discs and ligaments, and epidural hematomas.[1,3,12] These injuries usually result from motor vehicle accidents, falls, sports injury, and so on. In some of these patients there may be no detectable bone abnormality (SCIWORA). Cervical fracture-dislocation is especially common at the C5-6 level, where it produces tetraplegia. Fracture-dislocation of the thoracic spine is more common in the lower thoracic spine (T11-12 level), where it causes paraplegia.

Pathology

Trauma to the spinal cord may cause contusion, hematoma, or a combination of both, resulting in cord swelling and/or interruption of fiber tracts.[12] The spinal cord may also be compressed and flattened by a large epidural hematoma, buckled or swollen ligaments, herniated disc material, and/or retropulsed bone fragments. The cord may be lacerated or transected by bone fragments, subluxation, or dislocation of vertebrae. Complete transection is said to be rare, however, because some viable neuronal tissue is almost always visible at autopsy even when there appears to be absence of tissue radiographically.[3] Depending on the extent of injury and the collateral circulation, areas of ischemia or infarction may extend far beyond the initial site of injury.

TABLE 12-1. Frankel Classification

Frankel A	Complete motor and sensory loss
Frankel B	Preserved sensation only
Frankel C	Sensation normal, no voluntary motor function
Frankel D	Motor function lower grade
Frankel E	Complete motor and sensory function

TABLE 12-2. ASIA Impairment Scale

A	Complete: No motor or sensory function is preserved in the sacral segments S4-S5.
B	Incomplete: Sensory but not motor function is preserved below the neurologic level and includes the sacral segments S4-S5.
C	Incomplete: Motor function is preserved below the neurologic level, and more than half of key muscles below the neurologic level have a muscle grade less than 3.
D	Incomplete: Motor function is preserved below the neurologic level, and at least half of key muscles below the neurologic level have a muscle grade of 3 or more.
E	Normal: Motor and sensory function are normal.

Chronic changes include atrophy, myelomalacia, cyst formation, cord tethering, and wallerian degeneration. These changes are related to resorption of hematoma, formation of perimedullary fibrous tissue, edema and swelling of the cord, accumulation of fluid within the spinal cord, and axonal death, in varying proportions. Acute spinal cord hematomas frequently lead to late spinal cord atrophy.[13]

Fractures, subluxation, and dislocation can cause indirect injury to the spinal cord. Comminuted or burst fractures tend to compromise the spinal canal and compress the spinal cord. Subluxed and dislocated vertebrae behave in similar fashion.

The initial damage to the meninges depends on the form of injury. Knife injuries tend to produce a small hole in the dura. Exploding missiles may tear a large hole in the dura, whereas bone fragments cause varying degrees of laceration. Bleeding occurs in and around the meninges and may accumulate into large hematomas, which not uncommonly compress the spinal cord. In the chronic stage, the meninges may become scarred, sclerotic, or calcified with obliteration of the perimedullary space and formation of adhesions. The adhesions loculate the subarachnoid space to form secondary arachnoid cysts and/or tether the spinal cord to the bony wall of the spinal canal. Tethering itself may impede cerebrospinal fluid (CSF) pulsations around the cord and lead to hydrosyringomyelia of the spinal cord at the level of injury and for long distances above and below the injury.[12]

Imaging

Ultrasonography

Ultrasound has no place in the initial evaluation of the acutely injured spinal cord. The bony spine serves as an impediment to ultrasound. However, intraoperative ultrasonography is highly useful for distinguishing between cord cyst and myelomalacia.

CT

CT has become the primary technique for evaluating injury to the spinal column, but it is inadequate for evaluating injury to the cord itself. CT is better than MRI for depicting underlying bone abnormalities and most indirect causes of SCI, particularly fractures and dislocations. CT shows the direct causes of SCI, including shrapnel or other metal fragments, bone fragments, and air bubbles. These help to document the trajectory of the impacting force.[14,15] Multidetector CT provides exquisite sagittal and coronal reformatted spine images, leading to better understanding of the injury of the spinal column. CT is not adequate for evaluating spinal and perispinal soft tissue injuries, particularly of the ligaments and spinal cord. Epidural hematomas are also poorly imaged by CT. The presence of a neurologic deficit is an indication for MRI.

MRI

The accuracy of MRI for assessing the acutely injured spinal cord has been documented by several authors.[3,13]

Goradia and coworkers correlated MRI findings with intraoperative findings in cervical spine trauma and discovered that MRI was highly sensitive for detecting the lesions that cause *indirect* SCI, such as disc injuries (93%), posterior longitudinal ligament injury (93%), and interspinous ligament injury (100%). MRI was less sensitive for detecting injuries of the anterior longitudinal ligament (71%) and ligamentum flavum (67%).[16]

Performing MRI safely in the acute spinal cord–injured patient can be technically challenging. It requires coordination among dedicated groups of care providers—from the transport team, to the nursing staff, to the technologists—to ensure the safe performance of high-quality diagnostic examinations. The many life support and immobilization devices pose significant problems for patient safety, for correct patient positioning within the narrow bore of the scanner, and for placement of suitable radiofrequency (imaging) coils. These life support devices include monitoring devices, ventilatory devices, external fixation devices, traction devices, cervical collars, spine boards, and body casts, among others. Because it is essential to minimize motion as much as possible to ensure examination quality and patient safety, sedation and pain medication may be required to keep the patient relatively quiet.

Consideration must also be given to the fact that unknown foreign bodies have the potential to create additional injury to the patient in the magnetic environment and/or to produce significant artifact, resulting in degradation of images. If there is any doubt about the safety of the patient or the equipment, alternative imaging techniques such as CT with or without myelography should be employed. However, such instances should be rare. Myelography may itself be difficult to perform in this group of patients and is notorious for inadequate characterization of spinal cord lesions. Suspicion for vascular injury may require some form of MR angiography, particularly when spinal arterial or vertebral artery injuries are suspected.

At 1.5 T, routine MR studies for SCI usually include sagittal T1-weighted (T1W), sagittal T2-weighted (T2W), sagittal short tau inversion recovery (STIR) images [or other forms of T2 fat suppression], axial T2W and/or axial gradient-recalled-echo (GRE) images in the cervical spine, and axial T2W images [or axial GRE images] in the thoracic spine. These are usually sufficient for the evaluation of the spinal cord (Table 12-3). When patient motion is a problem, fast imaging sequences such as fast spin-echo (FSE) T2W and half-Fourier single-shot turbo spin-echo (HASTE) images could be useful. These routine techniques provide sufficient detail about the spinal cord, ligaments, disc abnormalities, and soft tissue changes. Apart from bone contusion and fractures, bone injuries are not adequately addressed by MRI. Hence, CT will still be necessary to provide details that may be important for planning surgical intervention. CT has become the primary modality for evaluating the injured spine.[1]

Recent technologic advances have made it possible to apply advanced MRI techniques such as diffusion-weighted imaging (DWI), diffusion tensor imaging (DTI), diffusion tensor tractography, and perfusion imaging to the spine. These techniques have been less useful for the spinal cord

TABLE 12-3. Magnetic Resonance Sequences Used in Imaging Cervical Spine Injury

Type of MRI Sequence	Utility
Sagittal T1	Epidural hematoma, cord swelling
Sagittal T2 Turbo SE	Cord edema, spondylosis, cord compression, ligament injury
Sagittal Turbo STIR	Bone marrow edema, ligamentous and soft tissue injury
Sagittal T2* GRE	Cord hematoma, disc herniation, bone fragments
Axial T1	Epidural hematoma, posterior element fractures
Axial T2 Turbo SE	Cord edema, cord compression

Modified from Mhuircheartaigh NN, Kerr JM, Murray TG: MR imaging of traumatic spinal injuries. Semin Musculoskelet Radiol 2006;10:293-307.

than for the brain, however. The length of the spinal cord, its narrow cross section, the artifacts arising from CSF motion, and artifacts resulting from the multiple interfaces of bone, fat, and other soft tissue presently limit their success in the spine.[17,18] These techniques are, therefore, not routinely used in the evaluation of the injured spine.[17,18] Other technologic developments such as 3-T imaging and advanced coil design have achieved better signal-to-noise ratio and improved spatial resolution, whereas new imaging sequences such as parallel imaging have shortened scan times.[17,18] All these are expected to result in improved spinal evaluation in this special group of injured patients.

MRI changes of SCI will be addressed in two broad categories: acute SCI and chronic SCI.

Changes in Acute Spinal Cord Injury

Acute spinal injuries include intrinsic spinal cord injuries that cause direct neurologic deficit and indirect injuries to the surrounding structures such as ligaments, discs, hematoma, and bone fragments, which may compress the spinal cord secondarily. These indirect compressive lesions hamper adequate management and may cause permanent damage to the spinal cord if they are not recognized. Such extrinsic compressive lesions can be found in over 70% of spinal cord injuries on MRI.[13]

Kulkarni and colleagues[13] analyzed the MRI findings in 24 patients with acute SCI, classified the MR signal pattern on T1W and T2W imaging, and correlated these with their anatomic substrates. Four distinct patterns were found (including normal):

1. *Pattern 1:* 5 patients (21%). These patients showed a swollen spinal cord with inhomogeneous signal on T1W images. T2W imaging showed a large central area of hypointensity with surrounding hyperintense rim, interpreted as hemorrhage within a swollen spinal cord (Fig. 12-1). The signal changes resolve after a few weeks, revealing the underlying cord damage. Type 1 patients who were followed up tend not to improve or recover and more frequently exhibit complete SCI, Frankel A.

2. *Pattern 2:* 12 Patients (50%). These patients show normal cord signal on T1W imaging with diffuse high signal on T2W imaging extending slightly up and down

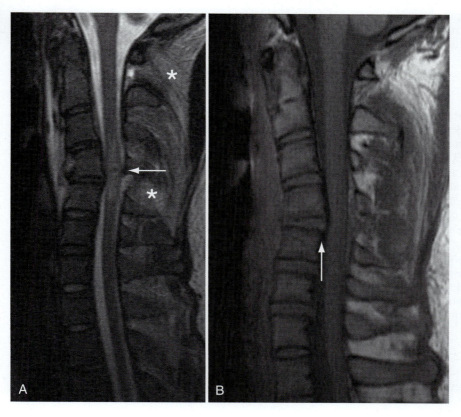

■ **FIGURE 12-1** Pattern 1 cord injury. **A,** Sagittal T2W MR image of the cervical spine showing a focal low intensity signal within the spinal cord at the C4-5 level (*arrow*). There is a surrounding rim of high intensity signal with another thin rim of hypointensity before the rather extensive smudgy high signal up and down the cord to C3 and C5. This is associated with a mild kyphosis and a ruptured ligamentum flavum at the C4-5 level. There is extensive paraspinal soft tissue edema (*asterisks*). **B,** Sagittal T1W MR image in this case shows a rather normal-appearing spinal cord, not heterogeneous signal as expected. C4-C5 disc herniation (*arrow*) is shown.

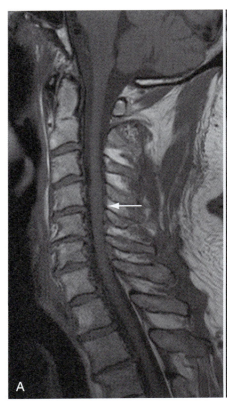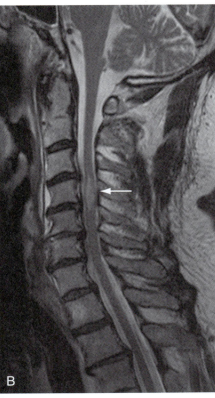

■ FIGURE 12-2 Pattern 2 cord injury. **A,** Midline sagittal T1W MR image of the cervical spine after a motor vehicle accident. The CT scan (not shown) revealed a C4 laminar fracture. The spinal cord shows mild fusiform swelling behind C4 with no signal abnormality (*arrow*). There is multi-level disc herniation with degenerative changes in the spine. **B,** Sagittal midline T2W MR image at the same time shows a focal fusiform swelling of the spinal cord behind C4 and upper C5 (*arrow*) with homogeneous high signal changes in the spinal cord. You could almost see speckled low intensity in these kind of lesions.

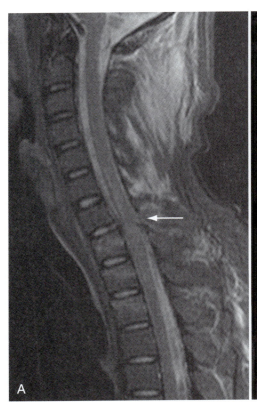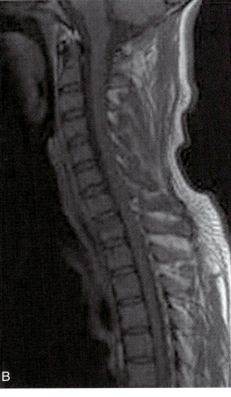

■ FIGURE 12-3 Pattern 3 spinal cord injury. **A,** A sagittal STIR MR image of the cervical spine in an unrestrained passenger after a motor vehicle accident shows heterogeneous signal changes in the spinal cord from about the C5-6 level to the T2-3 level. There is rupture of the posterior longitudinal ligament and the ligamentum flavum at C7-T1 (*arrow*), bone edema at T1-3, and extensive paraspinal muscle injury. **B,** Sagittal T1W MR image shows a normal-appearing spinal cord. Note that the ligament injuries are not visible.

the spinal cord from the level of injury, interpreted as spinal cord edema (Fig. 12-2). Follow-up usually reveals rapid resolution of the signal abnormality. These patients tend to have incomplete injury with subsequent improvement, Frankel B, C, or D. Two of these

patients had normal neurologic examination or Frankel E on follow-up.

3. *Pattern 3:* 2 patients (about 8%). These patients show normal signal on T1W imaging with heterogeneous signal on T2W imaging (Fig. 12-3). These lesions are

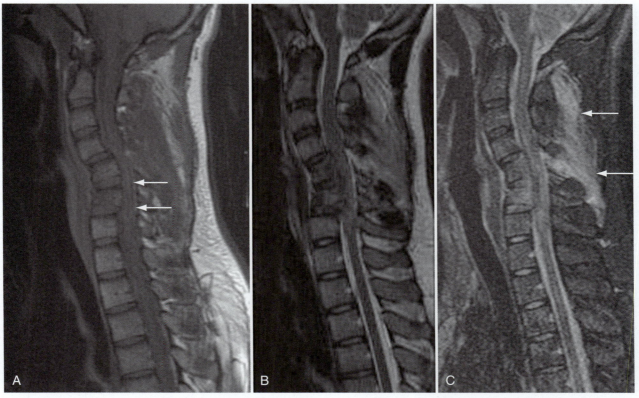

■ **FIGURE 12-4**   **A,** Sagittal T1W MR image of the cervical spine showing a C5-C6 traumatic kyphosis with high-signal changes in the spinal cord behind C5 and C6 (*arrows*) with a linear high signal extending cranially behind C4 to C1. **B,** Sagittal T2W MR image of the cervical spine in the same patient shows a heterogeneous signal abnormality in the spinal cord from C4 to C7. There is a thin high-signal epidural hemorrhage behind C2 and C3. Note the rupture of the C4-5 ligamentum flavum and the multilevel vertebra bone signal changes and the paraspinal soft tissue injury and spinous process fractures. **C,** Sagittal STIR image of the cervical spine exaggerates the high-signal changes within the injured area of the spinal cord and the paraspinal soft tissue changes (*arrows*).

thought to represent a combination of hemorrhage and edema. One patient in this group who was followed up showed clinical improvement.

4. *Pattern 4:* 5 patients (21%). These patients showed normal cord size and signal. Of the 3 patients in this group who were followed up, 2 had Frankel E whereas 1 had incomplete transection on follow-up neurologic examination.

Another pattern recently observed by me is high signal in the spinal cord on T1W imaging with a heterogeneous but predominantly low signal abnormality on T2W imaging (Fig. 12-4). This is thought to represent diffuse hemorrhage.

Overall, Kulkarni and colleagues found T1W imaging most useful for evaluating cord size and T2W imaging best for determining the characterizing signal abnormalities.[13] Flanders and associates correlated the MRI features of SCI with the extent of neurologic recovery[19] and confirmed Kulkarni and colleagues' findings. Patients with type 1 features on MRI have a poor chance for recovery after cervical SCI. Type 2 and type 4 patients tend to improve or recover completely. The number of type 3 patients was too small to be stratified reliably at this time.

Multiple series document that an apparently normal spinal cord on MRI may hide significant SCI. Five patients with neurologic deficit in Kulkarni and colleagues' series, for example, showed no demonstrable abnormality of cord signal or size on MRI. Kalfas and coworkers found an apparently normal MRI in 6 of 62 patients with SCI (9.7%) with varied spinal cord syndromes: 4 with incomplete mixed cord syndromes, 1 with central cord syndrome, and 1 with a complete cord syndrome.[3]

SCI may also cause transection or infarction of the spinal cord. Complete anatomic transection is rare. However, Kalfas and coworkers found a gap in cord continuity on sagittal T1W images in 7/62 patients (11.3 %); this was confirmed at surgery in 5 of the 7 and considered to represent complete cord transection.[3] Abnormally elevated T2 signal that extends far beyond the site of injury, both superiorly and inferiorly, and that appears to conform to a vascular territory suggests cord infarction (Fig. 12-5).

Extrinsic compression of the spinal cord may result from subluxed vertebrae, retropulsed bone fragments, ruptured disc materials, ruptured ligaments, spinal epidural hematoma, or a combination of all these. Subluxed vertebrae and retropulsed bone fragments are easy to identify on MRI (Fig. 12-6) and easily confirmed on CT. Epidural hematoma appears as a compressive epidural lesion with heterogeneous signal abnormality on all MRI sequences (Fig. 12-7). Small epidural hematomas,

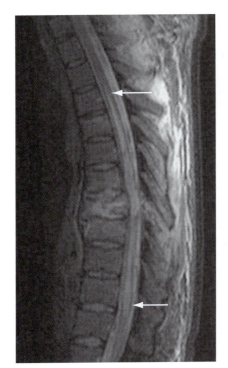

■ **FIGURE 12-5** Possible infarction. Midline sagittal STIR image of the thoracic spine showing a burst T9 fracture with mild fragment retropulsion and adjacent T8 and T10 vertebral body fractures and rupture of the T9-10 ligamentum flavum. There is extensive high signal within the spinal cord that extends cranially to T5 level and caudally to the conus medullaris (*arrows*). The distribution of abnormality beyond the site of original injury and the consideration that the artery of Adamkiewicz may have emanated from this region suggest that this pattern of signal change may represent ischemic infarction on top of the original spinal cord injury.

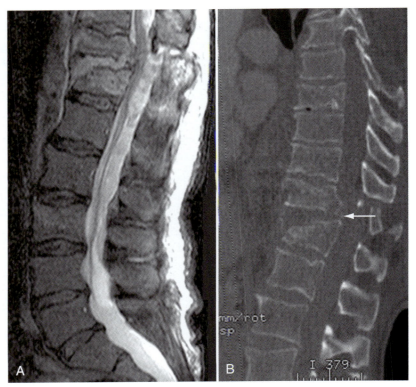

■ **FIGURE 12-6** Fracture subluxation. **A,** Sagittal T2W MR image of the thoracolumbar spine showing acute fracture subluxation of T11-12 with the spinal cord sandwiched between the retropulsed T12 vertebral body and posterior epidural hematoma and anteriorly displaced T11 laminae. Note the high signal intensity in the T11-12 disc extending behind the T11 inferior vertebral end plate where it contributes to the cord compression. **B,** A corresponding thoracic CT sagittal reformatted image shows the fracture subluxation in greater detail; it is clear that the signal change behind T11 is actually a bone fragment from the inferoposterior aspect of T11 (*arrow*).

■ **FIGURE 12-7** Epidural hematoma. **A,** Sagittal T1W MR image of the thoracic spine shows multilevel vertebral injuries with a transverse fracture dislocation through T11-12 vertebrae and posterior elements. T8 and T10 are also fractured (*arrows*). There is a large posterior epidural hematoma (*arrowheads*) of mild high signal intensity compared with the spinal cord and also compression of the spinal cord and thecal sac. **B,** Sagittal T2W MR image at the same time shows the epidural hematoma (*arrows*). Observe the high intensity signal lesion, with some heterogeneity, compressing the spinal cord.

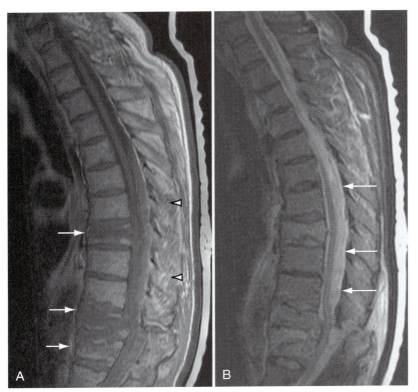

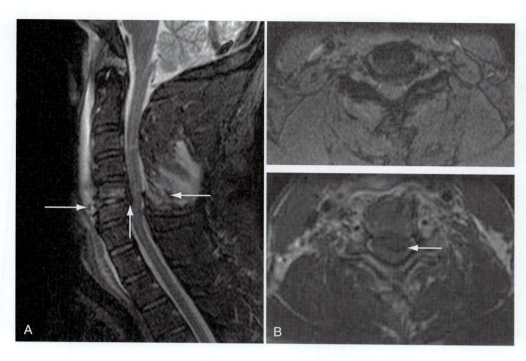

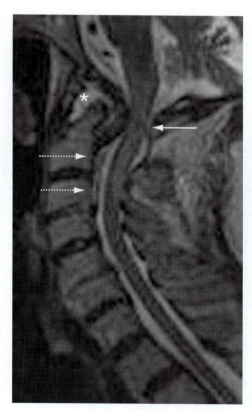

■ **FIGURE 12-9** SCIWORA. Midline sagittal cervical spine T2W MR image in a 91-year-old woman who was quadriplegic after a motor vehicle accident. There is heterogeneous mostly high signal within the spinal cord extending from the medulla down to C3 (*arrow*). There is thickening with abnormal high signal within the posterior longitudinal ligament at C1 consistent with injury to the ligament; note compression of the spinal cord. Note the fluid (high signal) around the odontoid process (*asterisk*) with a small epidural collection behind C2 and C3 (*stippled arrows*). CT did not reveal a fracture in this region.

particularly in the cervical region, may display homogeneous high signal abnormality on T2W images and slightly high signal intensity or isointensity with the spinal cord on T1W images (see Fig. 12-4). These could be the equivalent of hygroma in the head.

Disc injuries are equally well shown on T1W and T2W images, typically presenting as widening of the disc space, frank disc herniation, or abnormal signal within the disc space suggesting edema or hemorrhage (Fig. 12-8).[3,16] Ligament injuries such as rupture of the ligamentum flavum or of the anterior or posterior longitudinal ligament are often better shown on T2W sagittal images, where they may present as thickening, buckling, or frank discontinuity of structure. Invariably, there is high signal in the tissue surrounding the ruptured ligament. The low signal normally associated with the ligament itself may persist within the larger area of edema (Figs. 12-8 and 12-9).[16] On T1W imaging ligament injury tends to be underestimated. Although SCIWORA is common in adolescents, it does occur in adults and is invariably associated with ligament injury (see Fig. 12-9).

Chronic Trauma of the Spinal Cord

The technical challenges of imaging chronic SCI are less daunting than for imaging acute SCI. In most patients the condition has been stabilized. The fractures have healed or are healing. Spinal instrumentation may cause artifact and degrade the images, but most spinal instruments are now made from non-ferromagnetic material, so they do not endanger the patient in the MR environment. Patients on life support pose specific challenges for maintaining that support during MRI. These patients may be paralyzed and require help with mobility. Anesthesia may be required to ensure adequate ventilatory support and patient coop-

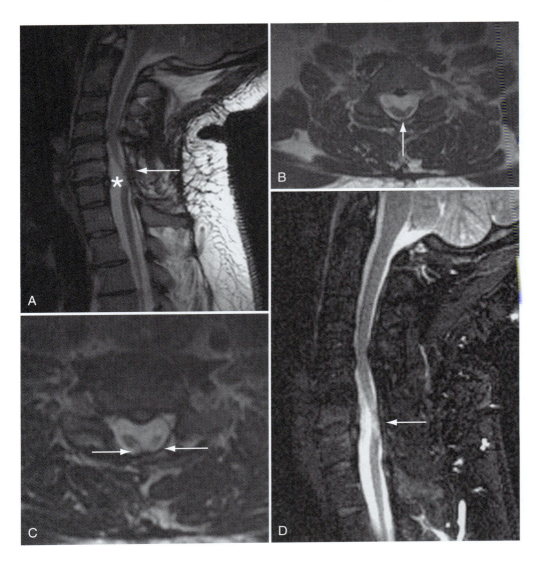

■ FIGURE 12-10 Postsurgical cord atrophy and tethering. **A,** Sagittal T2W MR image of the cervical spine some years after surgery for cord mass showing focal cord atrophy and tethering at C6-7 disc level (*arrow*). There is enlargement of the subarachnoid space anterior to the atrophied tethered cord (*asterisk*). Multilevel laminectomy was done from C5 to C7. **B,** Transverse T2W MR image through C6-7 level reveals a crescent-shaped atrophied spinal cord tethered posteriorly to the thecal sac (*arrow*). **C,** Transverse T2W MR image through the inferior C6-7 level showing apparent diplomyelia with each side tethered to the thecal sac (*arrows*). **D,** Sagittal fat-suppressed T2W MR image showing the tethered spinal cord at C6-7 with high signal at the site, suggesting gliosis or CSF between the diplomyelia (*arrow*).

eration. Surgical outcomes may have been suboptimal and require later imaging for proper evaluation and planning of new treatment options. The most common reason for imaging patients with chronic SCI is the onset of new symptoms, particularly post-traumatic myelopathy. MRI offers the best option for imaging these patients and is judged superior to CT or CT myelography.[20,21]

SCI may progress to spinal cord atrophy, myelomalacia, cyst or syrinx, spinal cord tethering, and/or wallerian degeneration. Spinal cord atrophy is diagnosed when MRI demonstrates focal reduction in the size of the spinal cord as compared with areas above or below the site of injury (Fig. 12-10). Quantitatively, a cervical or thoracic spinal cord that measures 5 to 6 mm or less in the sagittal dimension is considered atrophic.[22] Myelomalacia is diagnosed when MRI shows low signal on T1W imaging and high signal on T2W imaging, but the signal is different than CSF (Fig. 12-11). Cyst of the spinal cord is diagnosed when MRI shows a well-defined lesion with signal intensity that parallels CSF intensity on T1W and T2W imaging (Fig. 12-12). The distinction between myelomalacia and cord cyst is relatively easy when the lesions are large but difficult when the lesions are small and focal. Nonetheless, it is important to

try to distinguish the two, because their management differs significantly. Myelomalacia usually requires no surgical intervention, whereas spinal cord cyst may require surgical drainage.[11,20] In the very difficult case, intraoperative ultrasonography may establish the correct diagnosis before the cord is explored.

Tethering of the spinal cord is usually due to perimedullary adhesions. These frequently kink or tug at the spinal cord and deform the surrounding CSF space, leading to asymmetry of the subarachnoid space (see Fig. 12-10C). Such adhesions may themselves lead to syringomyelia.

ANALYSIS

SCI can be direct and/or indirect (see Box 12-1). How SCI is managed depends on those changes that are demonstrated at imaging and the clinical condition of the patient. The following are important in the interpretation of the images:

● Is there a focal spinal cord abnormality?

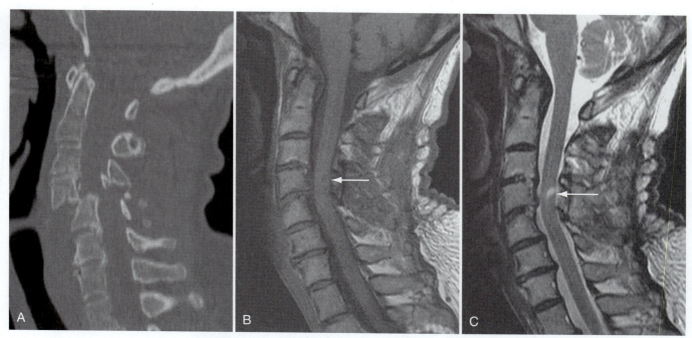

■ **FIGURE 12-11**   **A,** Sagittal reformatted multidetector CT scan of the cervical spine in this patient after a motor vehicle accident shows a grade 5 C4-C5 fracture-dislocation and locked facets with severe spinal canal stenosis. At the time of injury, the patient was unable to move all extremities but regained upper extremity movement on arrival at the hospital. Fracture-dislocation was reduced surgically without initial MRI. On day 3 after surgery the patient remained quadriplegic but recovered sensation at level C4-5. **B,** T1W cervical spine midline sagittal MR image on day 10 after surgical reduction with two-level laminectomy, and posterior spinal instrumentation shows a tiny, low-intensity signal posteriorly in the spinal cord at C4 (*arrow*). One would ordinarily expect a rather substantial cord injury from this sort of massive fracture-dislocation. Is this a cyst or myelomalacia? **C,** Sagittal T2W MR image on day 10 at same time as **B** shows a small, high-signal focus posteriorly in the spinal cord behind C4 (*arrow*). Margin is poorly defined. There is no obvious expansion or distention. It was interpreted as myelomalacia.

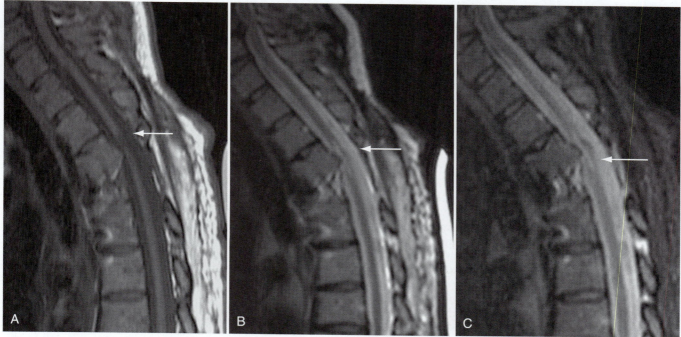

■ **FIGURE 12-12**   Cord cyst. **A,** Sagittal T1W MR image of the thoracic spine in a 40-year-old woman with a remote history of spinal cord injury causing paraplegia. She remains paraplegic and developed what was described as new symptoms of complex regional pain syndrome. There is susceptibility artifact at the site of T3/T4/T5 vertebral body fusion with posterior laminectomy. This image shows an ovoid low-intensity signal within the spinal cord as it passes over the short T3 kyphosis (*arrow*). It looks like there is loss of volume in the spinal cord at this level. **B,** Midline sagittal T2W MR image at same time as **A** shows the spinal cord "attached" to the T3 kyphosis. There is a small ovoid high signal within the spinal cord at T3-4 over the kyphosis separating a posterior irregular thin cord tissue from the kyphosis. The cord at this level does not show volume loss as suggested on the T1W image. The good definition of the margin of the signal change along with the slight posterior bowing at the site and the CSF signal intensity within the cord suggest a cyst or a syrinx. Spinal cord size proximal and distal to the signal change appears normal. **C,** Sagittal midline STIR confirms presence of central fluid within the spinal cord with a slight focal posterior bulge (*arrow*). It appears as if there is anterior tethering of the spinal cord to the T3 vertebral body.

BOX 12-1   CT and MRI of Spinal Cord Trauma

PATIENT HISTORY

A 37-year-old man fell out of bed backward and immediately experienced neck pain and dysesthetic pain in his hands and his triceps. There is no known history of underlying disease. Neurologic evaluation reveals a central cord syndrome with slight worsening of neurologic dysfunction throughout the day.

TECHNIQUE: CT

CT of the cervical spine without administration of a contrast agent was acquired in the transverse plane with sagittal and coronal reformatted imaging. Images are viewed in bone and soft tissue windows (Fig. 12-13).

FINDINGS

There is fusion of vertebral bodies with bony bridging. Diffuse fusion of facets bilaterally is noted throughout the cervical spine except at C1-2. Transverse fracture of the superior aspect of C7 extends posteriorly through the bilateral fused C6-7 facet joints. There is a 4-mm anterior displacement of C6 on C7. There is a small bone density posterior to the C6 spinous process consistent with a fracture fragment. The spinal cord is surrounded by an isodense soft tissue effacing the subarachnoid space.

IMPRESSION

1. The patient has a transverse fracture of the superior aspect of C7 extending through the posterior elements.
2. There is 4-mm anterior displacement of C6 on C7 and a fracture of the C6 spinous process.
3. Underlying diffuse bone fusion is consistent with ankylosing spondylitis.
4. An epidural hematoma is compressing the spinal cord.

TECHNIQUE: MRI

Multiplanar, multisequence MRI of the cervical spine was performed without administration of a contrast agent (Fig. 12-14).

FINDINGS

Transverse fracture is noted through C6-C7 facets bilaterally with rupture of anterior and posterior longitudinal ligaments and the ligamentum flavum at the C6-7 disc level. There is high signal within, and widening of, the C6-7 disc space on T2W images. There is a 4-mm anterior displacement of C6 on C7. The C7 vertebral body signal abnormality is consistent with edema. Extensive paraspinal soft tissue edema is evident posteriorly. A large epidural hematoma extends from C3 to the T4-5 disc level that is about 1 cm at its widest and completely obliterates the subarachnoid space around and compresses the spinal cord at the C6-7 level. No obvious focal signal abnormality is evident in the spinal cord. Focal signal abnormality behind the C6 vertebral body without significant indentation on the thecal sac could represent disc material or fluid.

IMPRESSION

1. A C6-C7 fracture subluxation is present with rupture of the anterior and posterior longitudinal ligaments and the ligamentum flavum and possibly the ligamentum nuchae, resulting in an unstable injury.
2. There is a C6-C7 disc injury with possible disc material or fluid behind the C6 disc.
3. A large epidural hematoma is compressing the spinal cord.
4. There is no focal spinal cord signal abnormality.
5. Paraspinal soft tissue edema.

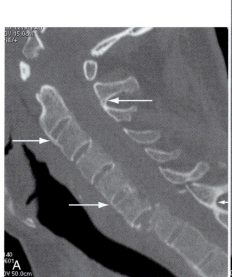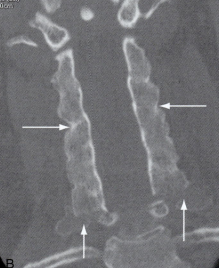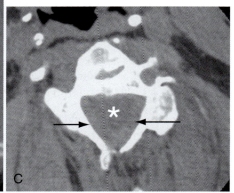

■ **FIGURE 12-13** Ankylosing spondylitis. **A,** Sagittal reformatted CT scan of the cervical spine showing C6-7 fracture subluxation with lamina line offset and tiny bone fragments at fracture sites. Observe the ligamental ossification at multiple levels (*arrows*) with relative preservation of disc spaces. **B,** CT coronal reformatted bone window of the cervical spine in the same patient as in A showing diffuse bony ankylosis of facet joints from C2 to C7 (*horizontal arrows*). Observe bilateral C6-7 facet joint transverse fractures (*vertical arrows*). **C,** CT transverse soft tissue window image through C5 showing a triangular high-density area (*arrows*) around the relatively low-density spinal cord/thecal sac (*asterisk*). The high-density structure correlates with the epidural hematoma seen on MRI.

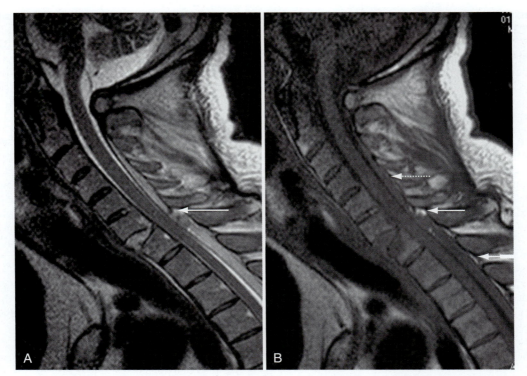

■ **FIGURE 12-14** Acute epidural hematoma in a 37-year-old man with ankylosing spondylitis. **A,** Sagittal T2W MR image of the cervical spine shows a fracture subluxation of C6-C7 vertebrae with rupture of anterior longitudinal and posterior longitudinal ligaments and the ligamentum flavum. There is C6-C7 lamina line offset. The C6-7 disc space is wide and bright with extension of the signal behind C6 (a disrupted disc was found in this location at surgery). There is a large, homogeneously high signal epidural hematoma posterior to the cord from C3 to T5. Note slight heterogeneity of signal within the epidural hematoma at the level of maximum spinal cord compression at C6-7 disc level (*arrow*). There is no obvious intrinsic spinal cord signal abnormality in this patient with incomplete spinal cord syndrome. The CT shows evidence of ankylosing spondylitis of which the patient was unaware. It is difficult to make that diagnosis on this MRI. **B,** Sagittal T1W MR image of the cervical spine in the same patient showing the C6-C7 subluxation and homogeneous isointense signal of the acute epidural hematoma (*banded arrow*). The focal high signal within the epidural hematoma at C6-7 is due to the bright signal intensity of fat herniated into the epidural hematoma (*arrow*).

A normal spinal cord on MRI is a good sign of a good prognosis. If the cord is abnormal, the pattern of signal abnormality may determine the prognosis. It is good to know this before treatment (see Figs. 12-1 to 12-4).

● What are the indirect causes of the injury?

A fracture subluxation may require reduction (see Fig. 12-6). The presence of disc injury or a traumatic disc herniation should be noted (see Figs. 12-2, 12-8, and 12-14). Fracture reduction without discectomy where disc herniation is present may result in poor outcome.

Ligament injury such as ligamentum flavum and anterior and posterior longitudinal ligament injuries should be described, if present (see Figs. 12-8, 12-9, and 12-14).

● Is there an epidural hematoma?

A large hematoma is readily visible. A small hematoma may be the sign of an unrecognized ligament injury (see Figs. 12-4 and 12-9).

● Is there evidence of underlying bone disease (see Figs. 12-13 and 12-14)?

Presence of underlying bone disease such as ankylosing spondylitis or local bone destruction due to other causes may determine the treatment option.

● In the chronically injured spinal cord, differentiation between myelomalacia and cord cyst or syrinx is important. This may not be difficult if the cyst is large, but a small cyst may not be readily distinguished from myelomalacia (see Figs. 12-11 and 12-12).

KEY POINTS

■ A normal spinal cord MRI does not exclude SCI. It only means recovery is likely to be complete.
■ Focal swelling of the spinal cord is the most common sign of acute SCI. The specific signal abnormality depends on whether there is edema, hemorrhage, or a combination of both.
■ It is important to look for subtle causes of indirect injury such as ruptured disc and ligaments and compressing extra-axial hematomas. These may affect how the patient is managed.
■ In patients with chronic SCI, it is important to distinguish between myelomalacia and cord cyst, because their management may differ significantly. On MRI, cord cyst is usually well defined with an intensity pattern that follows CSF.

SUGGESTED READINGS

Flanders AE, Croul SE. Spinal trauma. In Atlas SW (ed). Magnetic Resonance Imaging of the Brain and Spine. Philadelphia, Lippincott-Raven, 1996, pp 1161-1206.

Lammertse D, Dungan D, Dreisbach J, et al. National Institute on Disability and Rehabilitation. Neuroimaging in traumatic spinal cord injury: an evidence-based review for clinical practice and research. J Spinal Cord Med 2007; 30:205-214.

Slucky AV, Potter HG. Use of magnetic resonance imaging in spinal trauma: indications, techniques, and utility. J Am Acad Orthop Surg 1998; 6:134-145.

REFERENCES

1. Mhuircheartaigh NN, Kerr JM, Murray JG. MR imaging of traumatic spinal injuries. Semin Musculoskelet Radiol 2006; 10:293-307.
2. Hendey GW, Wolfson AB, Mower WR, Hoffman JR. Spinal cord injury without radiographic abnormality: result of the National Emergency X-Radiography Utilization Study in blunt cervical trauma. J Trauma 2002; 53:1-4.
3. Kalfas I, Wilberger J, Goldberg A, Prostko ER. Magnetic resonance imaging in acute spinal cord trauma. Neurosurgery 1988; 23:295-299.
4. Mayo Clinic. Spinal cord injury. Available at www.mayoclinic.com/health/spinal-cord-injury. Accessed 6/19/2007.
5. Ho CH, Wuermser L, Priebe MM, et al: Spinal cord injury medicine. 1. Epidemiology and classification. Arch Phys Med Rehabil 2007; 88(3 Suppl 1):S49-S54.
6. Jackson AB, Dijkers M, DeVivo MJ, Poczatek RB: A demographic profile of new traumatic spinal cord injuries: change and stability over 30 years. Arch Phys Med Rehabil 2004; 85:1740-1748.
7. Vitale MG, Goss JM, Matsumoto H, Roye DP Jr. Epidemiology of pediatric spinal cord injury in the United States. J Pediatr Orthop 2006; 26:745-749.
8. El Masry WS. Traumatic spinal cord injury: the relationship between pathology and clinical implications. Trauma 2006; 8:29-46.
9. Frankel HL, Hancock DO, Hyslop G, et al. The value of posterior reduction in initial management of closed injuries of the spine with paraplegia and tetraplegia. Paraplegia 1969; 7:179-192
10. American Spinal Injury Association. Standard neurological classification of spinal cord injury (revised 2000). Chicago, ASIA, 2002.
11. Stevens JM, Olney JS, Kendall BE. Post-traumatic cystic and non-cystic myelopathy. Neuroradiology 1985; 27:48-56.
12. Blackwood W, McMenemey WH, Meyer A, et al. Traumatic spinal lesions. In Greenfield's Neuropathology. London, Edward Arnold, 1963, pp 458-463.
13. Kulkarni MV, McArdie CB, Kopanicky D, et al. Acute spinal cord injury: MR imaging at 1.5 T. Radiology 1987; 164:837-843.
14. Hogan GJ, Mirvis SE, Shanmuganathan K, Scalea TM. Exclusion of unstable cervical spine injury in obtunded patients with blunt trauma: Is MR imaging needed when multi-detector row CT findings are normal? Radiology 2005; 237:106-113.
15. Schuster R, Waxman K, Sanchez B, et al. Magnetic resonance imaging is not needed to clear cervical spines in blunt trauma patients with normal computed tomographic results and no motor deficits. Arch Surg 2005; 140:762-766.
16. Goradia D, Linnau KF, Cohen WA, et al. Correlation of MR imaging findings with intraoperative findings after cervical spina trauma. Am J Neuroradiol 2007; 28:209-215.
17. Vertinski AT, Krasnokutsky MV, Augustin M, Bammer R. Cutting-edge imaging of the spine. Neuroimaging Clin North Am 2007; 17:117-136.
18. Ducreux D, Fillard P, Facon D, et al. Diffusion tensor magnetic resonance imaging and fiber tracking in spinal cord lesions: current and future indications. Neuroimaging Clin North Am 2007; 17:137-147.
19. Flanders AE, Spettell CM, Tartaglino LM, et al: Forecasting motor recovery after cervical spinal cord injury; value of MR imaging. Radiology 1996; 201:649-655.
20. Quencer RM, Sheldon JJ, Post JD, et al. MRI of the chronically injured cervical spinal cord. AJR Am J Roentgenol 1986; 147:125-132.
21. Yamashita Y, Takahashi M, Matsuno Y, et al. Chronic injuries of the spinal cord: Assessment with MR imaging. Radiology 1990; 175:849-854.
22. Lamount AC, Zachary J, Sheldon PWE. Cervical cord size in metrizamide myelography. Clin Radiol 1981; 32:409-412.

PART SEVEN

Spinal Vascular Malformations

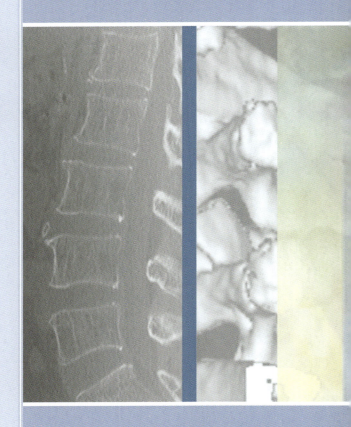

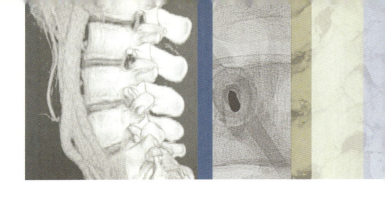

CHAPTER 13

Spinal Vascular Malformations

Timo Krings, Pierre L. Lasjaunias, and Armin K. Thron

Spinal vascular malformations are developmental derangements of the interconnections between arteries and veins, with secondary features of vascular enlargement, aneurysm and varix formation, mass effect from the enlarged vessels, excessively high flow with vascular steal and potential cardiac failure, and/or elevated venous pressure with low blood flow and backpressure ischemia due to venous congestion.

Multiple schemes have been proposed to classify spinal vascular malformations. Genetically, spinal cord arteriovenous malformations (AVMs) can be classified as:

- Hereditary lesions caused by a mutation in the vascular germinal cells, such as the spinal cord malformations associated with hereditary hemorrhagic telangiectasia
- Genetic nonhereditary lesions (i.e., somatic mutations) that share developmental metameric links, such as the spinal AV metameric syndromes (Cobb, Klippel-Trenaunay, and Parkes-Weber syndromes)
- Isolated sporadic spinal AV shunts not presently known to be associated with genetic defects and not due to trauma. Some of these may come to be reclassified as genetic or segmental over time.

Most spinal AVMs are sporadic. These are subclassified into congenital lesions such as AVMs and cavernous malformations (cavernomas) and acquired lesions such as dural AV fistulas (AVFs). Capillary telangiectases have not yet been found in the spine and will not be further discussed.

Congenital spinal cord AVMs are believed to represent populations of structurally unstable blood vessels with phenotypic evidence of upregulated angiogenesis. Specifically, excessive expression of endothelial growth factor in the setting of endoglin insufficiency may lead to the development of AV shunts. Although they are congenital lesions, they are rarely diagnosed antenatally. Patients are probably born with a propensity to form AV shunts, which becomes manifest only after a second or third event interferes with

vessel repair or angiogenesis. Animal models suggest that the Notch signaling pathway may malfunction, leading to errors in specifying arterial and venous identities. Deficiencies in the cytoskeleton of the vessels may also lead to disorganized, weak vessels. The segment of the affected vessel that first shows an abnormality is the postcapillary venule. Morphologically, spinal AV shunts appear to be centered in the proximal venous circulation.

The term *angioarchitecture* signifies the nature of the feeding arteries (radiculomeningeal versus radiculopial versus radiculomedullary), the morphology of the spinal AV shunt proper (nidus versus fistula, intranidal aneurysms, etc.), and the nature of the draining veins (medullary, perimedullary, radicular, epidural, or parachordal) at a given time. The term specifically incorporates the concept that the morphology of the AV shunt and the nature of the draining veins may change with time as the shunting causes increasing venous ectasias, rerouting of blood, changes in the intranidal architecture, or recruitment of additional arterial feeders.

The nature of the feeding artery is important to differentiate dural AV shunts from pial AV malformations. While the former are fed by *radiculomeningeal* arteries (i.e., arteries that normally feed the dura and nerve roots), the latter are fed by arteries that normally feed the spinal cord itself (i.e., *radiculomedullary* and *radiculopial* arteries). Concerning the morphology of the spinal AV shunt proper, two forms are found: (1) A *fistula* is a direct connection between the artery and vein with no interposed vessels. Fistulas are subclassified into low-flow microfistulas and high-flow macrofistulas that represent the extreme ends of a spectrum. (2) A *nidus* is a network of (pathologic) vessels interposed between the feeding artery and draining. Finally, the nature of the draining veins allows (at least in part) prediction of the clinical course, with a purely epidural or parachordal drainage only rarely leading to neurologic deficits (and, if so, in most instances due to mass effect of enlarged venous pouches on exiting nerve roots) while a medullary and perimedullary drainage may interfere with normal drainage of the cord leading to venous congestion.

The angioarchitecture is therefore defined to identify the specific nature of the shunt and its potential risks. These data are then integrated into a treatment plan on the basis of the known risks and (variable) success rates for each form of treatment for each type of malformation. Typically, consideration is given first to an endovascular approach to treatment, followed by consideration of direct surgical intervention.

SPINAL DURAL AV FISTULAS

A spinal dural AVF is an AV shunt between a radiculomeningeal artery and a radicular vein, which then drains retrograde to the perimedullary vessels, leading to venous congestion of the spinal cord.

Epidemiology

Spinal dural AVFs are the most frequent vascular malformation of the spine and account for 70% of all AV shunts of the spine. Presumably, they are acquired lesions, but the exact etiology is not known. The disease usually becomes symptomatic in older men (between ages 40 to 60 years). Most fistulas affect the thoracolumbar region.

Pathology

The AV shunt is located inside the dura mater, close to the spinal nerve root, where a radiculomeningeal artery lies near to a radicular vein. The radiculomeningeal artery supplies the nerve root and the meninges but not necessarily the spinal cord. The radicular vein drains into the spinal canal. Shunting of arterial blood into the venous system raises spinal venous pressure, diminishes the AV pressure gradient, impedes the drainage of normal spinal veins, and leads to venous congestion with intramedullary edema. There is stasis within the radiculomedullary arteries with delayed venous return. Together, these cause chronic hypoxia and progressive myelopathy.

Clinical Presentation

The clinical symptoms resulting from congestive myelopathy are not specific. They include hypesthesia, paresthesias, paraparesis, back pain that may radiate to the lower legs, impotence, and sphincter disturbances. The neurologic deficits are often slowly progressive, even insidious, so patients present with very long histories of vague but progressive symptoms. Less commonly, patients may have acute onset of symptoms or periodic remissions as the disease progresses. Without therapy, spinal dural AVF results in irreversible paraplegia or even tetraplegia.

Imaging

MRI

The characteristic MRI features of spinal dural AVF are cord edema and dilated perimedullary vessels (Figs. 13-1 to 13-9). T2-weighted (T2W) images typically show hyperintensity of the cord swelling. The centromedullary predominantly gray matter appears as a poorly marginated

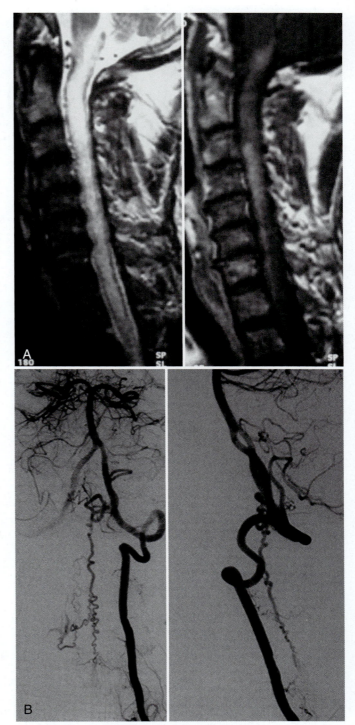

■ **FIGURE 13-1** A 62-year-old man presented with numbness of both legs for 3 months with progressive weakness for 1 month and hyperreflexia. Sensory function (pinprick sensation) was decreased below T9. **A,** MRI (T2 and T1 post contrast) demonstrated a contrast-enhancing, T2 hyperintense lesion extending from the craniocervical junction downward. Pathologic vessels are seen as flow voids ventral to the spinal cord on T2W imaging. **B,** Left vertebral arteriography revealed a dural AVF at the level of the foramen magnum.

"H-shaped" hyperintensity that extends over multiple segments. A hypointense rim surrounds the congested cord and most likely reflects deoxygenated blood within the congested capillaries. There may be contrast

Text continued on p. 259

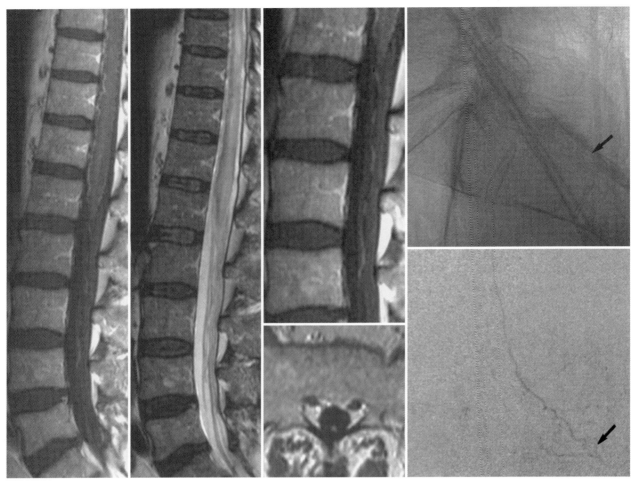

■ **FIGURE 13-2** Dural AVFs can be found from the level of the foramen magnum to the sacrum. In this patient, the dilated vein of the filum terminale suggested a deeply situated AV shunt, which was found at the S2-3 level in association with a thin, retrogradely ascending vein of the filum terminale (*arrows*).

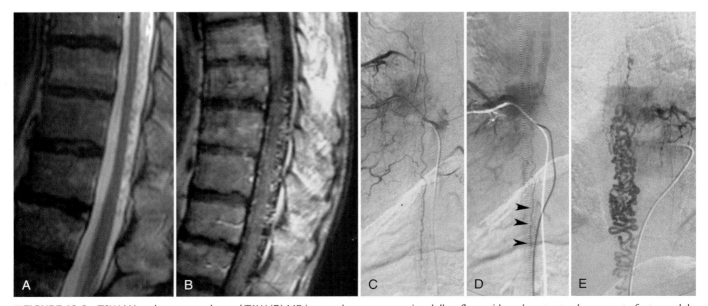

■ **FIGURE 13-3** T2W (**A**) and contrast-enhanced T1W (**B**) MR images demonstrate perimedullary flow voids and contrast enhancement of retromedullary vessels. Although no cord edema is yet present, these findings are highly suggestive of an AV shunt. Selective catheterization of the right T10 segmental artery demonstrates the anterior spinal artery at 8 seconds (**C**) and 23 seconds (**D**) after injection of contrast. Because the normal AV circulation time is 10 seconds, the arteriogram shows stasis in the anterior spinal artery (*arrowheads,* **D**), reflecting increased venous pressure, and confirms the diagnosis of a spinal AV shunt. The shunt is due to the dural AVF fed by the left T8 segmental artery (**E**).

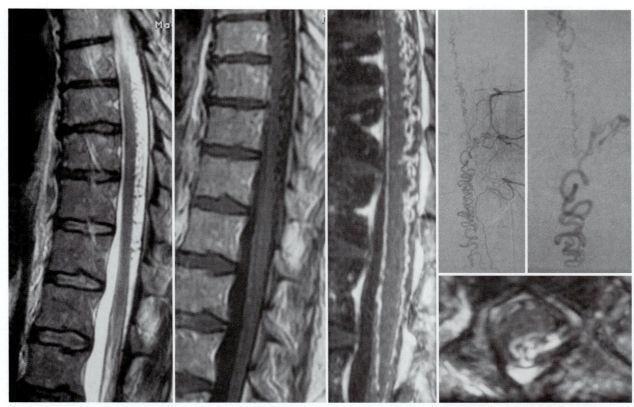

■ **FIGURE 13-4** MRI using T2W imaging and contrast-enhanced T1W imaging and contrast-enhanced MRA with sagittal and axial reconstructions demonstrate abnormally coiled vessels, especially on the dorsal aspect of the spinal cord. Slight cord edema and mild contrast enhancement of the conus indicate chronic cord ischemia from venous congestion. The global injection demonstrates the AV shunt, which is better appreciated on the superselective injection.

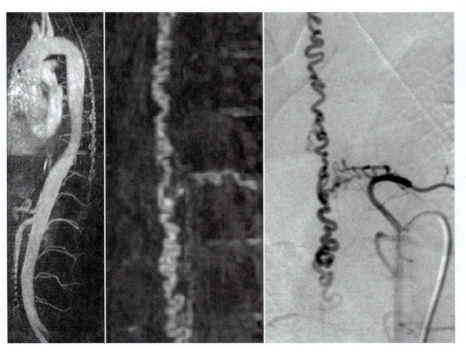

■ **FIGURE 13-5** Contrast-enhanced MR angiograms successfully show the presence of the AV shunt by detecting contrast agent within perimedullary veins in an early arterial phase. They document the precise level of the malformation, enabling the radiologist to target the late digital subtraction angiograms to the right level.

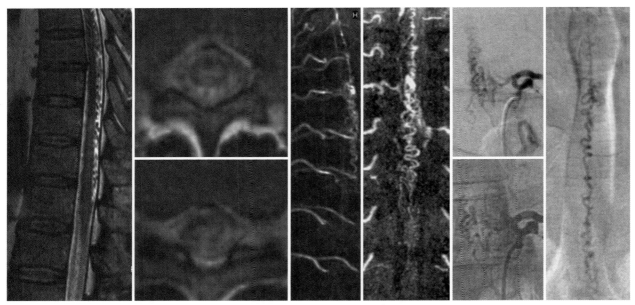

■ **FIGURE 13-6** Early arterial phase angiogram shows the typical appearance of a spinal dural AVF with cord edema, dilated perimedullary flow voids, and contrast material in perimedullary veins. The shunt typically lies just under the pedicle of the vertebral body. Venous drainage can be directed cranially, caudally, or both.

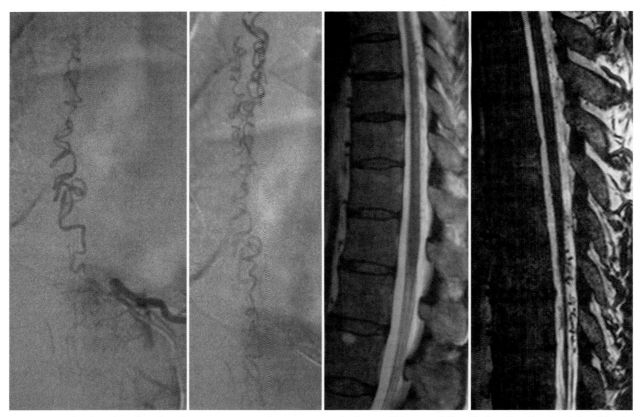

■ **FIGURE 13-7** Classic turbo spin-echo T2W MR sequences demonstrate cord edema well but may fail to display dilated perimedullary blood vessels. These are better demonstrated on heavily T2W sequences such as constructive interference steady-state (CISS) sequences.

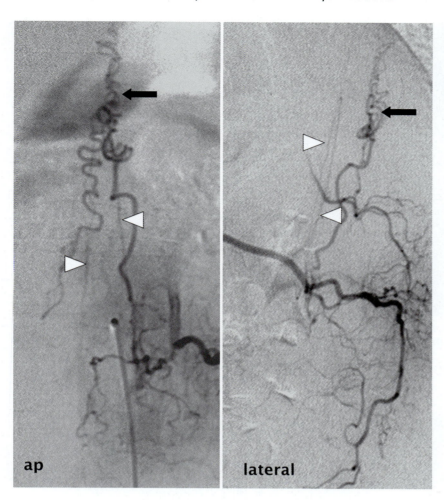

ap

lateral

■ **FIGURE 13-8** Because of the specific anatomic deposition of the spinal cord vascularization, the major supply to the anterior spinal artery (*white arrowheads*) may be derived from the same segmental artery that also feeds the dural AV shunt. The *black arrows* indicate dilated perimedullary vessels, which lie posterior to the spinal cord on the lateral view.

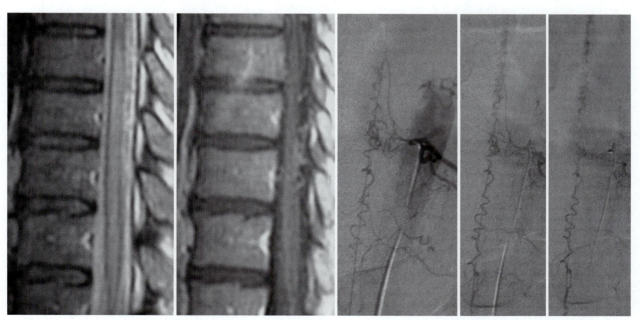

■ **FIGURE 13-9**   In this patient, the major supply to the anterior spinal artery arises from the same segmental artery as the dural AVF. The anterior spinal artery shows normal caliber and normal straight course. The arterialized spinal cord veins are dilated and coiled. This difference demonstrates that the anterior spinal artery does not contribute to the shunt. The shunt actually arises from the radiculomeningeal branch of the segmental artery.

enhancement from the chronic venous congestion. With disease progression, the cord will become atrophic. On T2W imaging the dilated and coiled perimedullary vessels usually appear as prominent flow voids. If the AV shunt volume is small, however, the perimedullary vessels may be seen only after enhancement with a contrast agent.

Angiography

Localization of the spinal dural AVF can be very difficult. Neither the location of the pathologic vessels nor the location of the intramedullary imaging abnormalities seems to be related to level of the fistula. Noninvasive diagnostic techniques such as contrast-enhanced MR angiography (MRA) with fast acquisition protocols have been developed, but lengthy, perhaps multiple catheterization procedures may still be required for diagnosis. Selective angiography shows stasis of contrast material in the radiculomedullary arteries, especially the anterior spinal artery. Injection into the segmental artery harboring the AVF depicts the early venous filling and retrograde flow of the opacified radiculomedullary veins into the spinal canal. An extensive network of dilated perimedullary veins is often visible.

Management

Spinal dural AVF may be treated in two ways (Figs. 13-10 to 13-12). The intradural vein that receives blood from the shunt may be occluded surgically. This is a relatively simple and safe intervention except for sacral fistulas. Alternatively, the fistula may be obliterated by superselective catheterization of the feeding radiculomeningeal artery and glue obliteration of the fistula (see Figs. 13-10 and 13-11). The embolic agent must pass the nidus and

reach and occlude the proximal segment of the draining vein to prevent subsequent intradural collateral filling of the fistula. The success rate of endovascular therapy varies from 25% to 75%. Complete occlusion of the fistula stops disease, but only two thirds of all patients have regression of motor symptoms and only one third show an improvement of their sensory disturbances. Impotence and sphincter disturbances are seldom reversible.

SPINAL CORD ARTERIOVENOUS MALFORMATIONS

Spinal cord AVMs are vascular malformations fed by radiculomedullary and/or radiculopial arteries intrinsic to the cord and drained by intrinsic veins of the spinal cord. The AV shunts may be intramedullary and/or perimedullary in location. Spinal cord AVMs include both glomerular (nidal) AVMs and AV fistulas of the cord.

Epidemiology

Arteriovenous malformations of the spinal cord constitute close to 20% of all vascular malformations of the spine. They typically present in the second decade of life. There is no gender difference in adults. Among children, however, boys are affected far more often than girls.

Clinical Presentation

Spinal AVMs may present as acute hemorrhage and sudden onset of neurologic symptoms and deficits. If there is no sudden hemorrhage, the symptomatology is nonspecific. Patients may complain of hypesthesia or paresthesia,

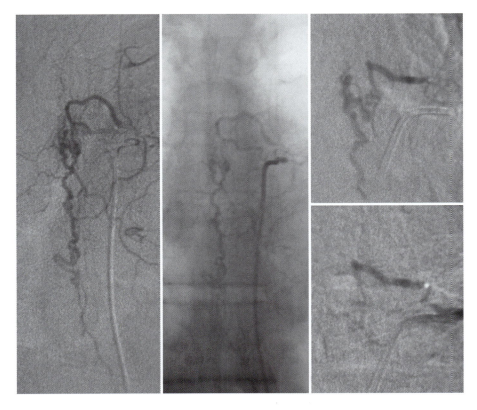

■ **FIGURE 13-10** One potential treatment option for spinal AV shunts is endovascular occlusion of the shunt with a liquid embolic agent (*N*-butyl cyanoacrylate, NBCA). To be successful, this glue has to pass from the artery through the shunt into the nidus. In this patient, the superselective injection demonstrates that the glue has not passed completely into the venous segment, so there will be delayed reopening of the fistula through the vast network of anastomoses in this region.

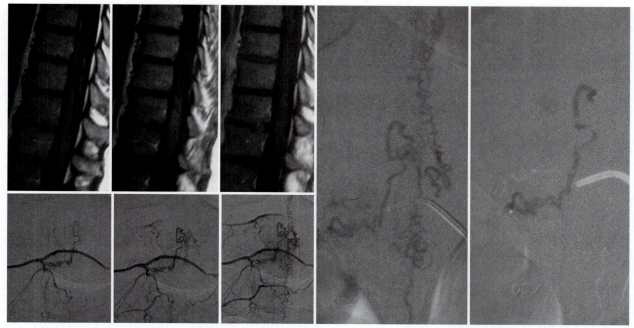

■ **FIGURE 13-11**   In this patient, the superselective injection of liquid embolic material has passed from the arterial to the venous site, securely closing the shunting zone.

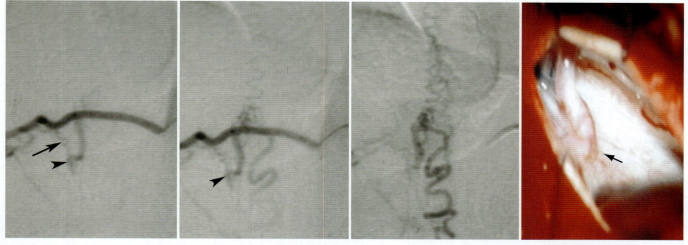

■ **FIGURE 13-12**   Selective injection into the segmental artery displays the radiculomeningeal branch (*arrow, first image*) that feeds the dural AVF. Later phase images show that this branch connects with a radicular vein (*arrowhead*) at the level of the nerve root sleeve just under the pedicle. The radicular vein (*arrowhead*) drains retrograde to fill the spinal epimedullary vessels, leading to venous congestion. Surgical exposure demonstrates the dilated and arterialized vein (*arrow, last image*).

weakness, and diffuse back and muscle pain. Progressive sensorimotor symptoms can slowly develop or acutely worsen followed by some improvements over time. Fistulous AVMs often present as symptoms of subarachnoid hemorrhage because of their intradural perimedullary location. Glomerular AVMs may become symptomatic by venous congestion alone, by intraparenchymal hemorrhage, and/or by subarachnoid hemorrhage.

Pathophysiology

Spinal cord AVMs may take glomerular or fistulous forms.

Glomerular AVMs (plexiform AVMs, nidal AVMs) are characterized by a vascular nidus similar to the nidus of cerebral AVMs. They are usually intramedullary, typically have multiple feeding arteries derived from both the posterior and anterior systems, and drain into dilated spinal cord vessels. Superficial compartments of the nidus can reach the subarachnoid space. The glomerular AVM is the most frequent spinal cord AVM.

Fistulous AVMs (intradural AVFs, AVMs of the perimedullary fistula type) are characterized by direct AV shunts located superficially on the spinal cord. There is no intervening nidus, and there is rarely any intramedullary compartment. Fistulous spinal AVMs fed by the *ventral* spinal arterial system are subpial. Fistulous spinal AVMs fed by the *dorsal* spinal arterial system are subarachnoid.

Fistulous spinal AVMS are subclassified into microfistulous and macrofistulous forms. These appear to be different types of lesion, because we have not observed any microfistulous AVMs to enlarge into a macrofistulous form nor any macrofistulous AVM to regress or spontaneously thrombose into a microfistulous form (unless it had been embolized). Furthermore, the two lesions behave differently in adults and children.

Microfistulous AVMs account for 90% of all adult spinal cord AVFs. They are distinguished from the dural AVFs, because they are fed by radiculo*medullary* arteries, not radiculo*meningeal* arteries. They are drained by superficial perimedullary veins, which may pass far superiorly within the spinal canal and even ascend through the foramen magnum into the posterior fossa. Microfistulous AVMs have low shunt volume, so they display only moderately enlarged feeding veins and arteries. They are distributed throughout the spinal cord: 10% cervical, 50% thoracic, and 40% lumbosacral (of which two thirds are located at the filum terminale). Cervical lesions typically present as progressive sensory deficits, whereas thoracic microfistulous AVFs most commonly present as hemorrhage (hematomyelia or subarachnoid hemorrhage) and often show progressive myelopathy. Lesions of the conus

and filum terminale fistulas manifest as progressive myelopathy or acute nonhemorrhagic paraplegia.

Macrofistulous spinal AVMs account for 10% of all adult spinal cord AVFs. They have a high shunt volume leading to massive remodeling of the blood vessels with markedly enlarged arteries and veins and variceal "pouches." Macrofistulous spinal cord AVMs are typically found in children with hereditary hemorrhagic telangiectasia (HHT).

Pathology

The AV shunting leads to vascular steal phenomena, elevated venous pressure with venous congestion and back-pressure ischemia, and mass effect from dilated arteries, flow-related aneurysms, dilated veins, and large varices.

Imaging

MRI

On MRI, spinal cord AVMs typically show conglomerate dilated, perimedullary and intramedullary vessels (Figs. 13-13 to 13-35). These appear as flow voids on T2W

Text continued on p. 274

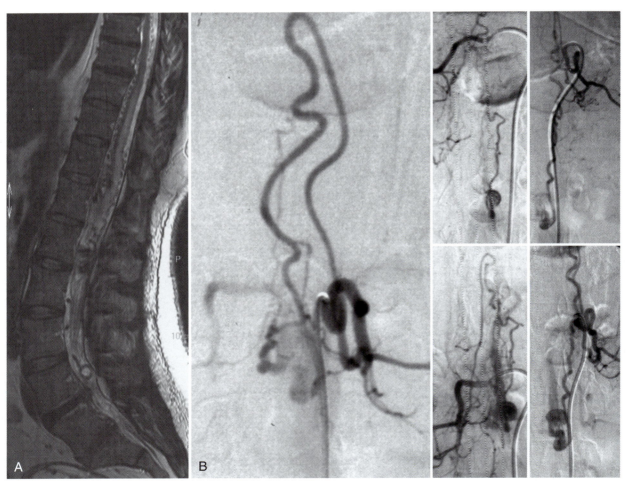

■ **FIGURE 13-13** **A,** T2W MR image demonstrates flow voids within dilated, coiled perimedullary vessels and cord edema from venous congestion. **B,** Angiography reveals a spinal perimedullary fistula or fistulous form of spinal AVM. Spinal AVMs are always fed by arteries that also supply the cord, that is, the anterior spinal or dorsolateral spinal arteries. The fistulous form has no nidus interposed between the artery and the vein. The degree of arterial dilatation depends on the rate of flow within the arteries. Multiple feeders may be present and most often converge to a single opening.

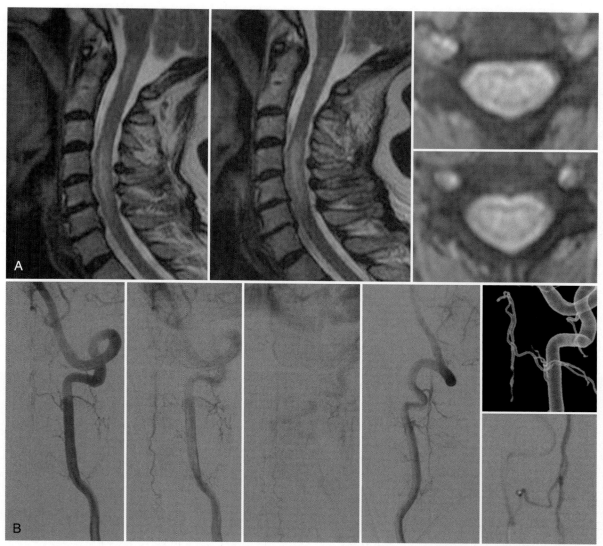

■ **FIGURE 13-14** Spinal perimedullary fistula with slow flow. **A,** In these patients, MRI may fail to demonstrate dilated or pathologic vessels, especially when the shunt is located anteriorly, because the vein anterior to the spinal cord runs in the subpial space. **B,** Angiography revealed the shunt, best seen after superselective injection.

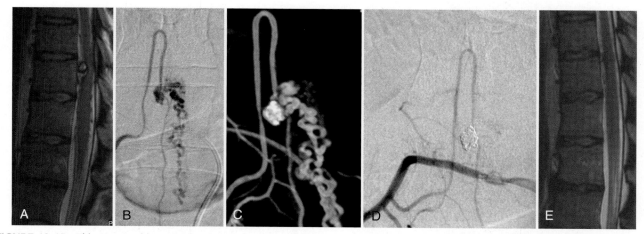

■ **FIGURE 13-15** This 23-year-old man suffered sudden onset of stabbing back pain, followed by acute paraplegia. **A,** Admission MRI demonstrated subarachnoid hemorrhage and a flow void anterior to the spinal cord. Angiography revealed a perimedullary fistula fed by the anterior spinal artery (**B**) with a venous aneurysm (varix) (**C**) at the transition between artery and vein. **D,** The varix was completely occluded using coils, leading to complete obliteration of the fistula with preservation of the flow in the anterior spinal artery. **E,** Follow-up MRI demonstrated complete regression of the varix, and the patient recovered completely from his deficit.

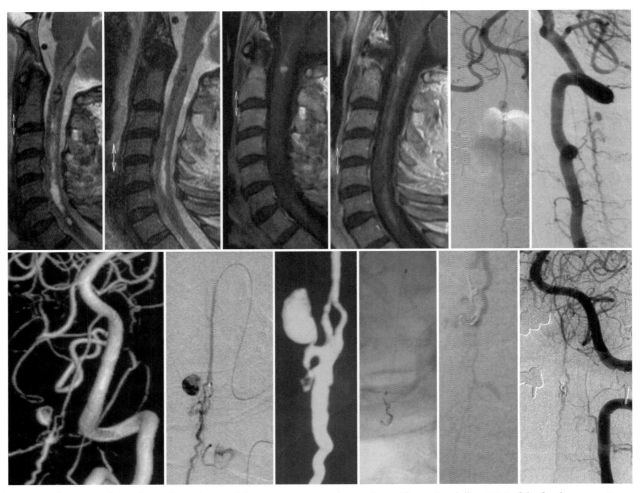

■ **FIGURE 13-16** Intramedullary hemorrhage due to a false venous aneurysm in a patient with a perimedullary AVM of the fistulous type. A segmental nonfusion of the anterior spinal artery can be seen just proximal to the transition from the artery to the vein. This angioarchitecure permitted occlusion of the feeding artery with two small soft coils.

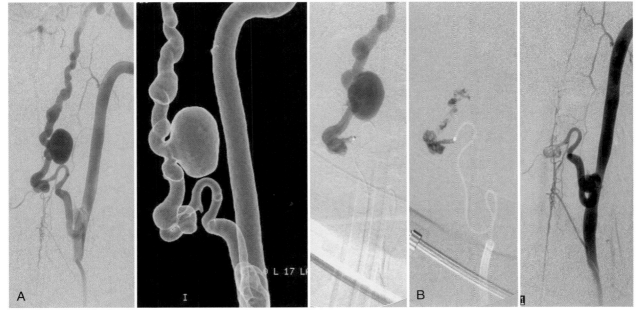

■ **FIGURE 13-17** Spinal perimedullary fistula. In most instances the venous aneurysm is located close to the transition from artery to vein. **A,** In this case, the varix lies more distal, farther from the AV transition, as shown by the sudden change in diameter of the vessels. **B,** Injection of a liquid embolic agent with passage of the glue from the arterial to the venous segment completely and permanently occluded the shunt.

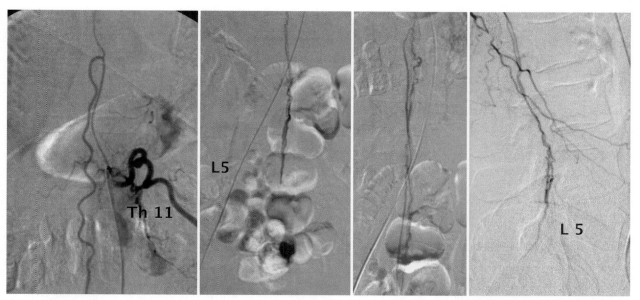

■ **FIGURE 13-18** Fistulas of the filum terminale are a special form of spinal perimedullary fistulas. These are invariably fed by the anterior spinal artery that descends and enters a vein at its distal portion. This vein then ascends to lead to progressive venous congestion of the conus and cord.

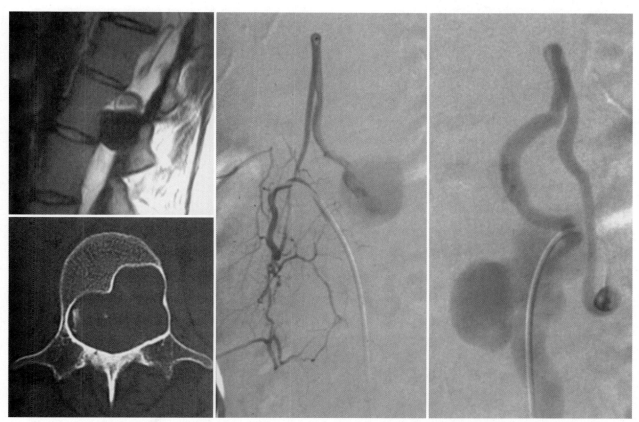

■ **FIGURE 13-19** Microfistulas and macrofistulas of the perimedullary type can be distinguished by the sizes of the feeding artery and draining veins. Macrofistulas associated with hereditary hemorrhagic telangiectasia are typically single-hole multifeeder malformations that may cause mass effect and posterior vertebral scalloping after pulsations.

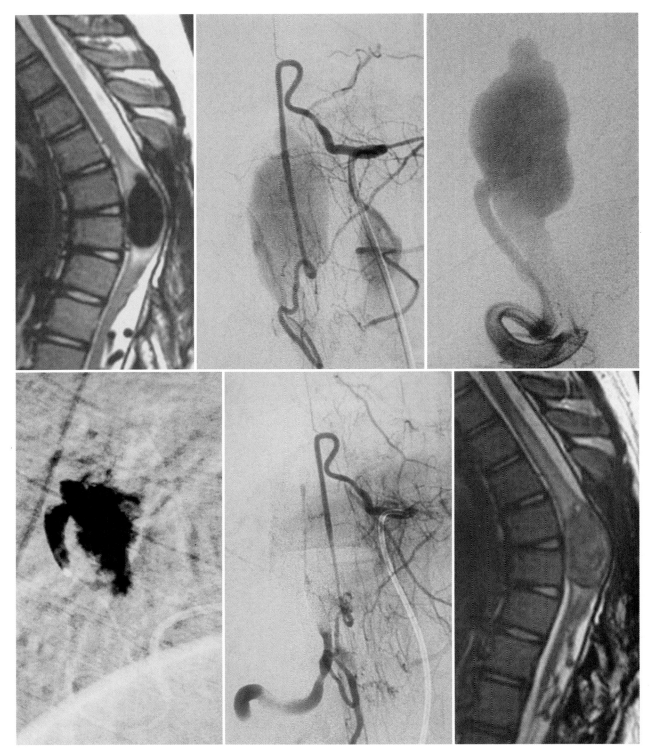

■ **FIGURE 13-20** Macrofistula in HTT. Both the anterior spinal artery and a posterolateral spinal artery converge to the same opening, leading into a massively dilated venous pouch that then drains into dilated perimedullary vessels. The safest endovascular approach is through the dorsolateral radiculopial arteries. Injection of a liquid embolic agent at that site occludes the inflow zone of the venous pouch, creating a "mushroom"-shaped glue mass. After occlusion, thrombosis of the venous pouch may cause mass effect with transient worsening of the symptoms.

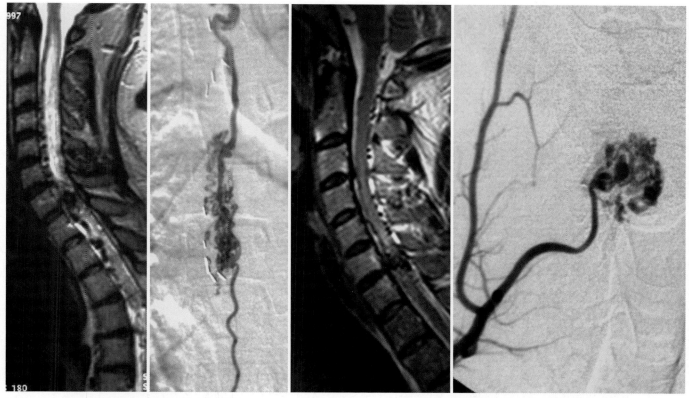

■ **FIGURE 13-21** T2W MR images in two different patients show glomerular AVMs with different degrees of cord edema. The location of the glomerular portion of the malformation within the cord is well displayed.

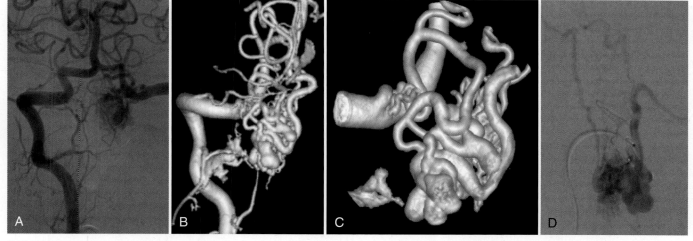

■ **FIGURE 13-22** Angiography (**A**), 3D rotational angiography (**B** and **C**), and superselective injection (**D**) of a glomerular AVM demonstrate the "nidal" aspect of the AVM. The 3D reconstructions show potential weak points of the AVM, such as intranidal aneurysms, better than conventional angiograms, permitting them to be targeted for subsequent treatment.

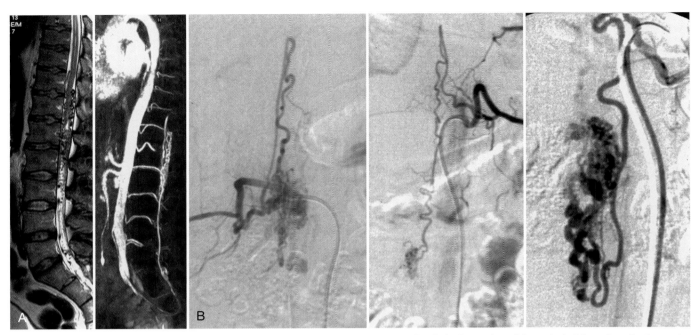

■ FIGURE 13-23 T2W MR images (**A**) and contrast-enhanced MRA (**B**) show the nidus of pathologic vessels and the early draining veins of a glomerular AVM. These malformations typically have multiple feeders, which may join to vascularize the same compartment or supply separate compartments of the AVM.

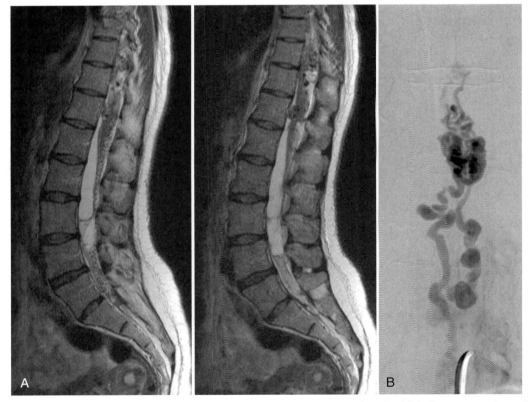

■ FIGURE 13-24 **A,** Sequelae of spinal subarachnoid hemorrhage with multiple septations and arachnoiditic change. **B,** Angiography reveals multiple outpouchings of vessels.

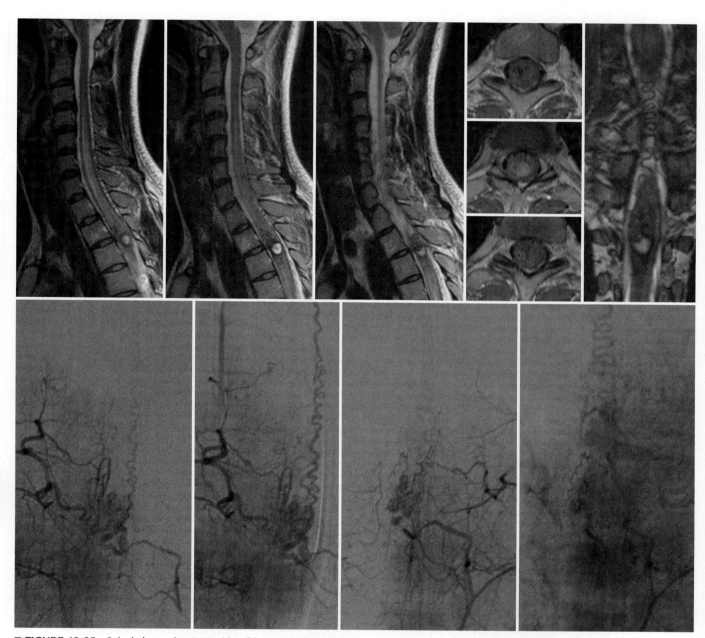

■ **FIGURE 13-25** Spinal glomerular AVM with a false, partly thrombosed aneurysm in the cord, leading to cord edema.

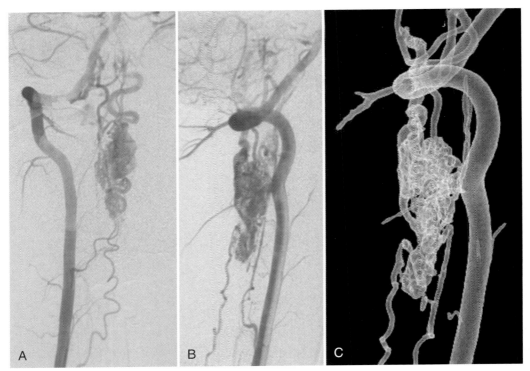

■ **FIGURE 13-26** Anteroposterior (**A**) and lateral (**B**) views and 3D rotational angiography (**C**) demonstrate the intranidal architecture of this cervical glomerular AVM.

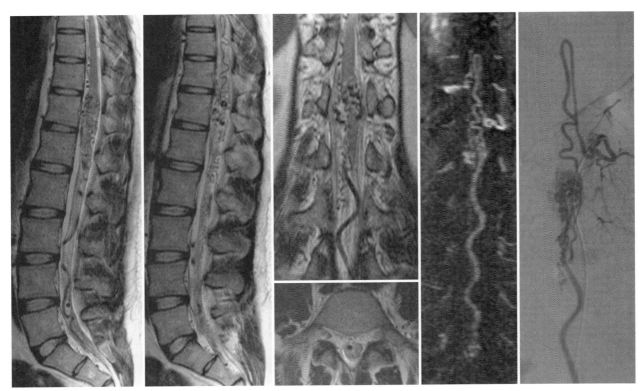

■ **FIGURE 13-27** T2W MR images and contrast-enhanced early arterial phase MRA demonstrate the dilated feeding vessels and draining veins of a glomerular AVM. Digital subtraction angiography confirms the architecture of the feeding arteries, the nidus, and the draining veins.

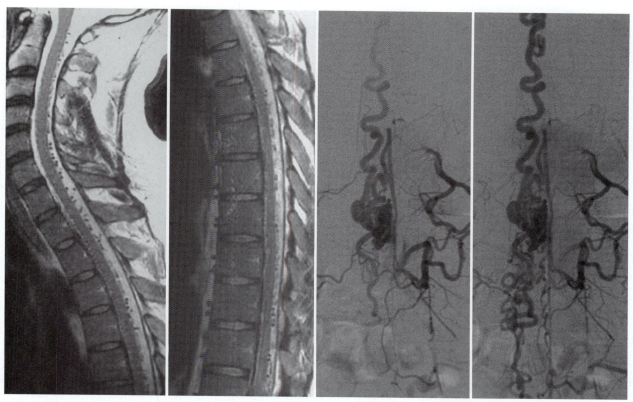

■ **FIGURE 13-28**   MRI does not always display the intramedullary nidus within a glomerular AVM. The flow voids of the dilated perimedullary veins may be visualized along the entire length of the spinal cord, depending on the individual drainage pattern of the malformation.

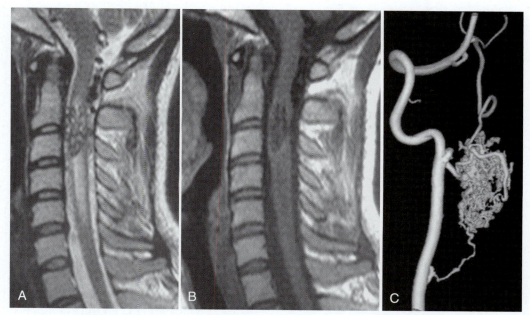

■ **FIGURE 13-29**   **A,** T2W MR image shows the intramedullary nidus, cord edema, and cranial venous drainage of the glomerular AVM. **B,** T1W image shows a variable signal depending on the flow velocity of the AVM. **C,** The 3D rotational angiography demonstrates the arterial feeder and the intranidal architecture.

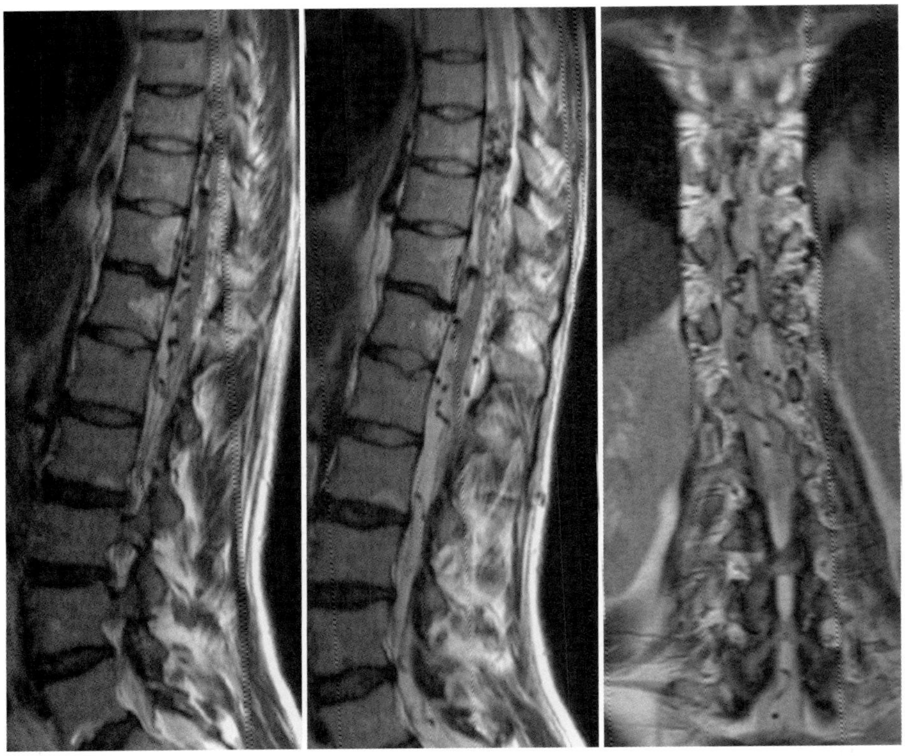

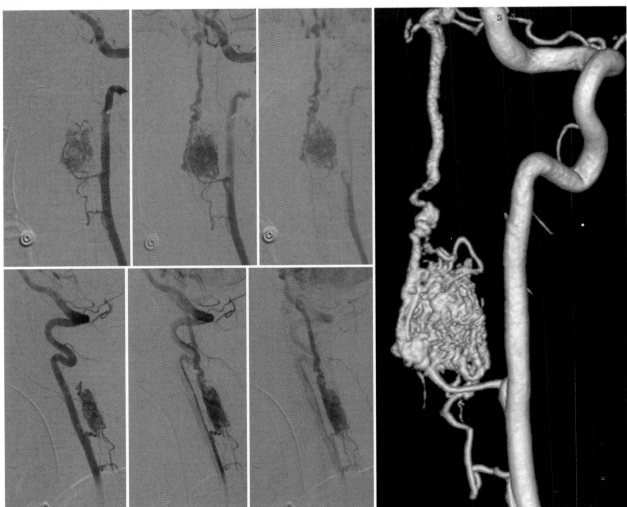

■ **FIGURE 13-30** Glomerular AVM of the lower thoracic spine demonstrating dilated vessels, venous outpouchings, and the nidus within the cord.

■ **FIGURE 13-31** Arterial and venous phases of a cervical glomerular AVM draining craniad. *Upper row,* Anteroposterior projection. *Lower row,* Lateral projection of a left vertebral angiogram.

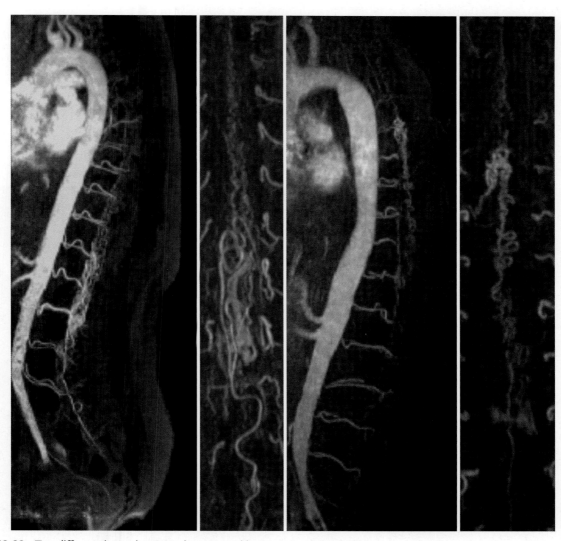

■ **FIGURE 13-32**　Two different glomerular AVMs demonstrated by contrast-enhanced MRA.

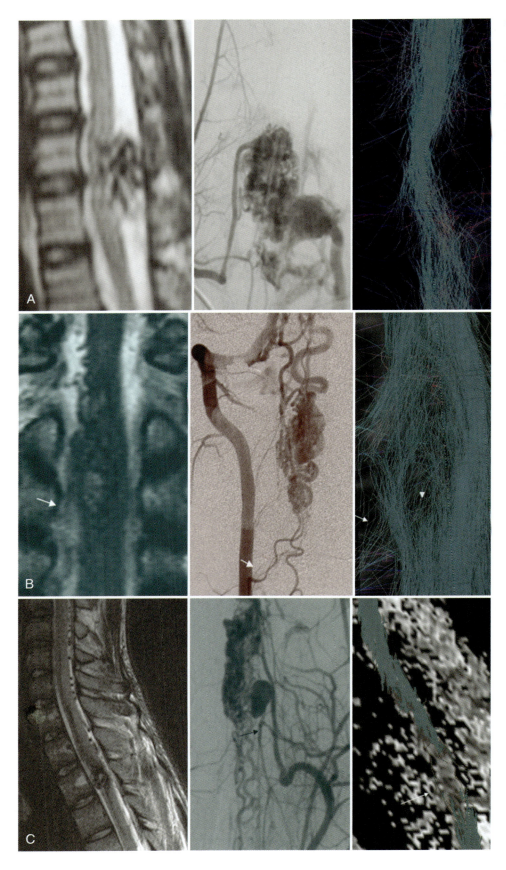

■ **FIGURE 13-33** Diffusion tensor imaging of three different glomerular AVMs. This new technique may shed light on the pathogenesis of each case. In **A** the fibers are displaced laterally. In **B** the fibers are dispersed, indicating cord edema (*white arrowhead*). The segmental artery supplying the AVM can be visualized (*white arrows*). In **C,** apparent disruption of the fibers (*white arrow*) is presumably related to susceptibility effects of hemoglobin degradation products close to the thrombosed pouch.

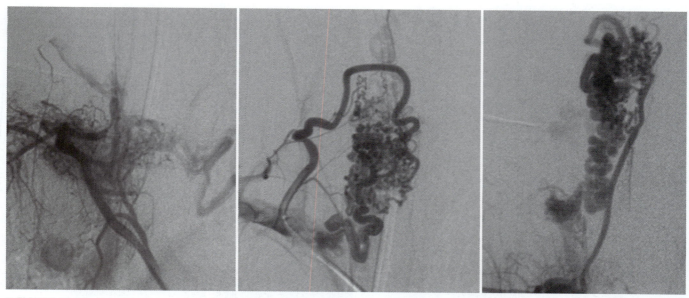

■ **FIGURE 13-34** Spinal AV metameric syndrome (SAMS) (Cobb's syndrome) with a glomerular AVM and a shunt along the nerve root.

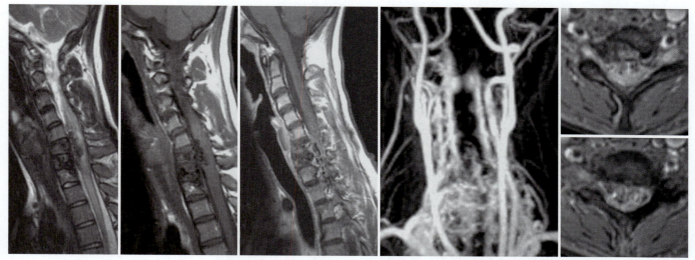

■ **FIGURE 13-35** Spinal AV metameric syndrome (SAMS) (Cobb's syndrome) with a glomerular AVM in the vertebral body, the spinal cord, and the adjacent paravertebral muscles, documenting the metameric distribution of this vascular malformation.

imaging and as mixed hyperintense to hypointense tubular structures on T1-weighted (T1W) imaging (depending on their flow velocity and direction). The venous congestion and edema manifest as cord swelling with intramedullary hyperintensity on T2W imaging. Contrast enhancement may vary. Concurrent intraparenchymal hemorrhages demonstrate signal intensity that varies with their age. There may be subarachnoid hemorrhage.

MRI usually cannot define the type of the spinal malformation, but it should define the location of the AVM in relation to the spinal cord and dura and distinguish between low-flow and high-flow forms of AVMs. Because small arterial feeders and draining veins may escape detection on noncontrast MRI, especially in low-flow perimedullary fistulous AVMs, contrast media must be given to detect subtle venous dilatations.

Angiography

Recently it has been shown that using fast MRA techniques can display the main arterial feeder of glomerular spinal AVMs and those of fistulous spinal AVMs that have a single large arterial feeder. Spinal cord AVMs with small or multiple feeders have not yet been investigated. Selective spinal angiography remains necessary to define the exact type of the AVM and to plan subsequent treatment.

Management

The proper management of asymptomatic spinal AVMs is uncertain, because the natural history of these lesions is poorly known. Symptomatic spinal AVMs should be treated to ameliorate symptoms and improve patient prognosis. The therapy of choice for all spinal cord AVMs is endovascular embolization. This should be performed only after selective spinal angiography, careful analysis of the specific angioarchitecture of the malformation, and selection of an embolic agent (coils, glue, particles) appropriate to that specific angioarchitecture.

In glomerular spinal AVMs, glue or particles can be employed to obliterate the nidus. Even partial embolization seems to improve the prognosis of these patients.

In low-flow perimedullary fistulas, glue (or sometimes coils) at the fistula zone can be used to obliterate the most proximal portion of the venous segment. Proximal arterial occlusion will not obliterate the fistula, because of collateral recanalization from the radiculopial network. If the proximal venous segment cannot be filled by the glue cast or the coils, endovascular therapy should be avoided and surgical resection considered instead.

Large high-flow fistulous spinal AVMs can easily be treated successfully in nearly all cases by superselective catheterization reaching close to the fistula and subsequent closure of the fistula with concentrated glue, coils, or other agent. Because the aim of embolization is to occlude the most proximal portion of the venous segment, glue embolization can be performed using a "mushroom-shaped" glue cast.

CAVERNOUS MALFORMATIONS (CAVERNOMAS)

Spinal cord cavernomas are intramedullary vascular malformations composed of dilated thin-walled capillaries and sinusoids with no intervening brain parenchyma, no identifiable feeding artery, and no specific draining vein. Alternate names include spinal cord cavernous malformation, cavernous hemangioma of the spinal cord, and intramedullary cavernous malformation.

Epidemiology

Cavernomas are estimated to constitute 5% of all spinal vascular malformations. They typically present first in middle-aged patients but may be found in all age groups. Females are affected more than males by 2:1. Familial occurrence, coexistent metameric vascular nevi, and concurrent intracranial cavernous malformations have been described. The thoracic spine is more often affected than the cervical spine.

Pathophysiology

Spinal cavernomas may cause symptoms by acute intramedullary hemorrhage or rarely by primary subarachnoid hemorrhage. Progressive myelopathy may result from lesion expansion by capillary dilatation or proliferation, repetitive small hemorrhages in or around the lesion, or (possibly) toxic effects of degradation products of the intramedullary blood.

Clinical Presentation

Spinal cavernomas may cause acute, recurrent, and/or progressive myelopathy. The typical clinical features of intramedullary cavernous malformations are sensorimotor deficits, usually appearing several hours after the onset of pain. Acute symptoms/deficits such as sudden quadriplegia are thought to indicate new hemorrhage within or around the lesion. Slowly progressive symptoms likely reflect repeated episodes of minor hemorrhage or local pressure effects on the surrounding spinal cord tissue due to capillary proliferation or dilatation. Once symptoms appear, the clinical course is typically one of progressive myelopathy.

Pathology

Grossly, spinal cavernomas are discrete, well-circumscribed, lobulated, red-purple raspberry-like lesions. Microscopically, cavernomas are composed of dilated, thin-walled capillaries that have a simple endothelial lining with variably thin fibrous adventitia. Residua of previous hemorrhage may be present, including scarring, collections of hemosiderin-laden macrophages, and calcification. The lesion is surrounded by variable degrees of gliosis and edema. The lining of the cavernoma is histologically indistinguishable from the lining of a capillary telangiectasia.

Imaging

CT

On CT, some cavernomas are detectable by virtue of recent hemorrhage or extensive calcification. Others remain indetectable by CT.

MRI

On MRI, cavernomas appear as well-defined, circumscribed lesions of varying size (Figs. 13-36 to 13-40). On T2W imaging they characteristically display a hypointense rim that circumscribes an inhomogeneous, often hyperintense "popcorn" center. The hypointense rim is due to magnetic susceptibility artifacts from hemosiderin deposits. The complex reticulated core with its typical mulberry-like appearance represents hemorrhage in different stages of evolution. T2W images tend to overestimate the size of the cavernoma, because the hemosiderin does not correspond to the lesion itself. The size of the cavernoma and its precise relation to the surface of the cord is best visualized on T1W images.

Angiography

Angiography may fail to display cavernomas, because they do not opacify in the time frame of typical angiographic runs. Very slow injection with a slow rate of filling occasionally rescues a negative study. Because cavernomas fill and drain slowly, they actually accumulate contrast agent during the whole angiographic procedure. Therefore, each new "scout" image for subtraction actually displays increasing concentrations of contrast that are then subtracted out from the new run. Using the very first scout image before injection of any contrast agent may disclose the opacity of a cavernoma not seen by standard

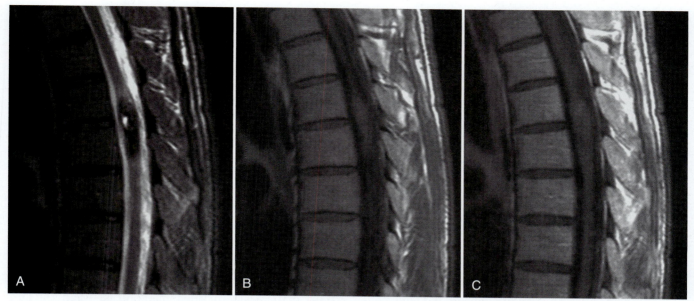

■ **FIGURE 13-36**   A, Classic T2W MR appearance of a spinal cord cavernous malformation with a hypointense rim and a reticulated hyperintense core reflecting blood degradation products at various stages of evolution. **B** and **C**, On T1W imaging, slight hyperintensity typically indicates methemoglobin. Edema surrounds the lesion. **C**, Post contrast study may show faint enhancement of the lesion.

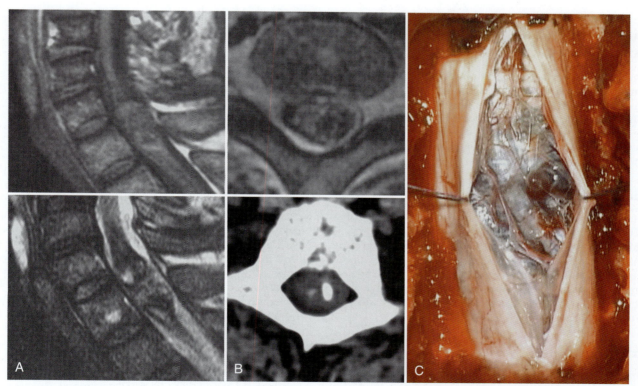

■ **FIGURE 13-37**   Giant, partially calcified cavernoma: MR images (**A**), CT scans (**B**), and surgical exposure (**C**). Blood products in different stages give this lesion a very heterogeneous appearance on imaging. As demonstrated here, cavernomas may rarely cause mass effect.

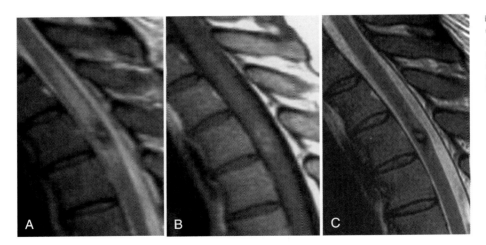

■ **FIGURE 13-38** Evolution of a cavernoma over time: The first two images (**A** and **B**) taken after the acute onset of spinal cord symptoms show fresh hemorrhage and edema. Repeat study after resolution of symptoms shows clearance of the edema and depicts the intramedullary cavernoma better (**C**).

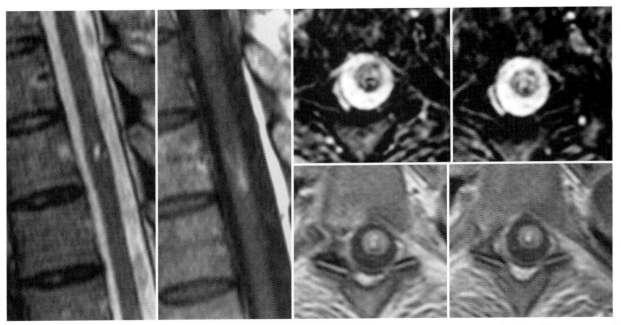

■ **FIGURE 13-39** Typical T2W and T1W MR appearance of a spinal cavernoma. T2W imaging tends to overestimate the size of the cavernoma, because the hemosiderin does not correspond to the lesion itself. The size of the cavernoma and its precise relation to the surface of the cord is best visualized on T1W images.

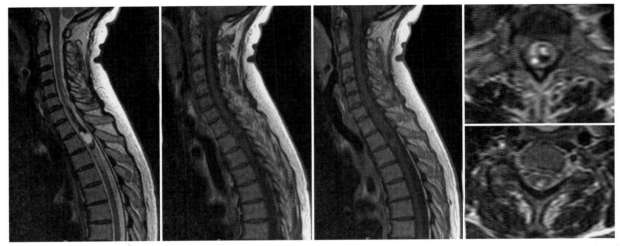

■ **FIGURE 13-40** T2W MR images of the spinal cord demonstrate a hypointense rim surrounding a nonenhancing intramedullary lesion histologically proven to be cavernoma. Differential diagnoses include micro AVMs and ependymomas.

BOX 13-1   MRI and Angiography of Suggested Dural AVF

PATIENT HISTORY

This 41-year-old female complained of slowly progressive weakness and paresthesias that were slowly ascending and gradually worsening. Associated nonradicular pain led to an initial diagnosis of degenerative disc disease.

FINDINGS

MRI with contrast enhancement showed edema of the spinal cord and enlarged enhancing pathologic intradural vessels in the perimedullary location and along the nerve roots (Fig. 13-41). No abnormal intramedullary vessels were detected. There were no signs of prior hemorrhage (e.g., arachnoiditis). Although the gender and the rather young age did not favor the diagnosis of a dural AVF, the imaging findings and clinical history were strongly suggestive. Digital subtraction spinal angiography showed rapid filling of the descending branch of a dilated anterior spinal artery. Because the anterior spinal artery stops at the conus and its descending branch (the artery of the filum terminale) is not normally visible, the early and dilated appearance of this vessel in addition to the pathologic vessels in the lumbar region seen on MRI indicated a fistula of the filum terminale. The hallmark of the filum terminale fistula is two vessels that run parallel to each other and that can be identified as artery and vein in time-resolved images. The point of fistulation is always located at the turn from the descending anterior spinal artery into the ascending vein of the filum terminale. Therapy must be aimed at occluding the fistulous point.

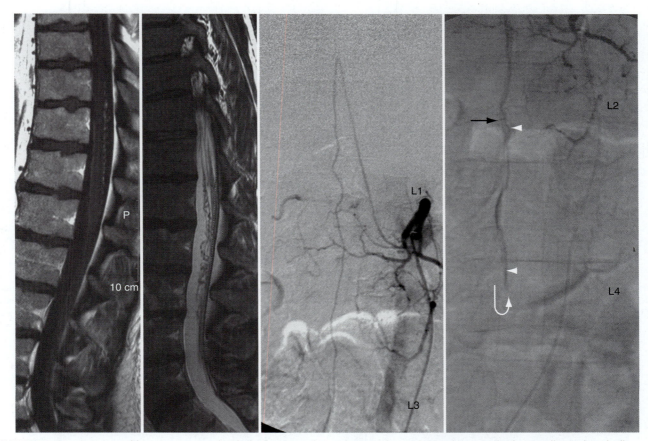

■ **FIGURE 13-41**   A 41-year-old woman presented with slowly progressive weakness and paresthesias that were slowly ascending and gradually worsening. MRI with contrast enhancement showed edema of the spinal cord and enlarged enhancing pathologic intradural vessels in the perimedullary location and along the nerve roots. No abnormal intramedullary vessels were detected. Spinal angiography showed rapid filling of the anterior spinal artery descending to the artery of the filum terminale (*black arrow*). A fistulous communication (*curved white arrow*) at L4 level before draining into the ascending vein of the filum terminale (*white arrowheads*) was noted.

subtraction technique. Despite the low yield, patients with acute spinal hemorrhage should still have spinal angiography to rule out a small glomerular AVM, which might not be detected by spinal MRI in the acute phase after a hemorrhage.

Differential Diagnosis

At present, imaging techniques cannot distinguish whether an acute spinal cord hemorrhage is due to a micro AVM or a single spinal cord cavernoma. If there are multiple lesions, however, the diagnosis of cavernoma is more likely. Serial follow-up imaging and selective spinal angiography may be necessary to determine the correct diagnosis. Spinal cord cavernomas may also mimic spinal cord tumors such as glioma, ependymoma, or anaplastic astrocytoma, especially if the cavernomas are large.

Management

Asymptomatic cavernomas are usually followed by serial imaging and not treated. Once cavernomas become symptomatic, however, they typically cause progressive myelopathy, so therapy becomes indicated. Endovascular techniques are not appropriate for cavernomas. Instead, surgical resection of cavernomas can be performed safely using meticulous microsurgical technique. First the lesion is localized carefully as to level and position within the spinal cord. If the lesion lies close to the surface of the cord, dissection is started directly over the lesion. If the lesion is located deep within the cord, it may be approached by myelotomy performed over an area of bluish discoloration or by standard approaches through the dorsal root entry zone or median sulcus. The lesion is then debulked gradually, using slight traction, coagulation, and gentle suction in the surrounding yellow plane of gliotic tissue to deliver the lesion without damage to the neighboring intact nervous tissue. The lesion bed should be carefully inspected after resection for small residual portions.

ANALYSIS

The key to diagnosing the type of spinal cord vascular malformations is careful characterization of their arterial supply. This differentiates the dural AVFs from the pial AVMs. This differentiation is important to determine the natural history of the patient and to plan subsequent treatment.

KEY POINTS: DIFFERENTIAL DIAGNOSIS

- The key diagnostic findings of spinal dural AVFs are dilated perimedullary vessels (seen as flow voids on T2W MRI) and cord. Caution must be taken not to misinterpret cerebrospinal fluid pulsation artifacts as flow voids. Contrast enhancement may help to distinguish between true vessels and artifacts.
- The major differential diagnoses of cord AVMs are spinal cord ischemia, glioma, and infection. In most cases, patient history and MRI demonstration of abnormal perimedullary vessels lead to the correct diagnosis. On MRI alone, slow flow perimedullary fistulas cannot be differentiated from spinal dural AVFs. On selective angiography, however, they can be easily differentiated by their feeding artery.
- Spinal cord vascular malformations are rare but treatable causes of progressive spinal cord symptoms.

- Initial diagnosis depends on MRI to demonstrate pathologic flow voids, cord edema, or spinal hemorrhage and to provide an initial assessment of which malformation to expect.
- The pathophysiology of many spinal vascular malformations is determined by their venous drainage. Elevated intravenous pressure impedes blood flow, leading to stasis, progressive venous congestion, congestive venous edema, and cord ischemia.
- Whereas dural AVFs never bleed and never demonstrate pathologic flow voids, cavernomas and spinal AVMs may bleed and do demonstrate pathologic flow voids.
- Spinal angiography still is necessary to determine the exact type of shunt and to plan subsequent treatment. Whereas spinal AVMs are supplied by arteries that normally also supply the cord, spinal dural AVFs are supplied by radiculomeningeal arteries that do not supply the cord.

SUGGESTED READINGS

Berenstein A, Lasjaunias P, Ter Brugge KG. Surgical Neuroangiography, 2nd ed. Vol 2, Clinical and Endovascular Treatment Aspects in Adults. Berlin, Springer, 2004.

Doppman JL, Di Chiro G, Dwyer AJ, et al. Magnetic resonance imaging of spinal arteriovenous malformations. J Neurosurg 1987; 66: 830-834.

Krings T, Mull M, Gilsbach JM, Thron A. Spinal vascular malformations. Eur Radiol 2005; 15:267-278.

Rodesch G, Hurth M, Alvarez H, et al. Embolization of spinal cord arteriovenous shunts: morphological and clinical follow-up and results—review of 69 consecutive cases. Neurosurgery 2003; 53:40-49.

Rosenblum B, Oldfield EH, Doppman JL, Di Chiro G. Spinal arteriovenous malformations: a comparison of dural arteriovenous fistulas and intradural AVMs in 81 patients. J Neurosurg 1987; 67:795-802.

Thron A, Caplan LR. Vascular malformations and interventional neuroradiology of the spinal cord. In Brandt T, Caplan LR, Dichgans J, et al. (eds). Neurological Disorders: Course and Treatment. Boston, Academic Press, 2003, pp 517-528.

Weinzierl M, Krings T, Korinth M, et al. MRI and intraoperative findings in cavernous haemangiomas of the spinal cord, Neuroradiology 2004; 46:65-71.

Zevgaridis D, Medele RJ, Hamburger C, et al. Cavernous haemangiomas of the spinal cord: a review of 117 cases. Acta Neurochir (Wien) 1999; 141:237-245.

PART EIGHT

Spinal Cysts and Tumors

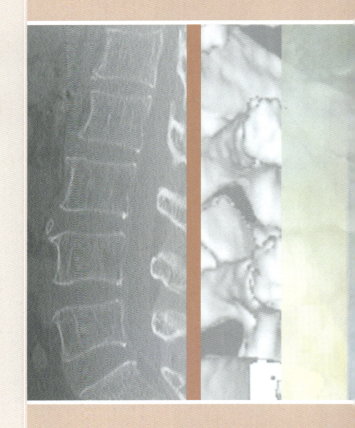

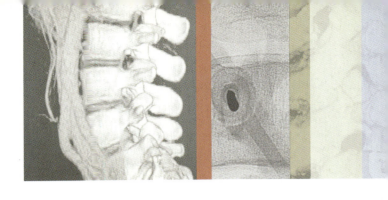

CHAPTER 14

Spinal Cysts

Krisztina Baráth, Michel Guy André Mittelbronn, Paola Carmina Valbuena Parra, and Spyros S. Kollias

Cystic lesions of the spine are a diverse group of infectious, post-traumatic, postinterventional, and degenerative abnormalities with the common feature of a fluid collection with a wall. The cellular linings of the walls may be squamous epithelium, columnar epithelium, arachnoid cap cells, ependymal cells, or collagenous fibrous tissue. The cyst may contain simple low protein fluid similar to cerebrospinal fluid (CSF), highly proteinaceous fluid, hemorrhagic fluid, or tumoral fluid and may even have solid components (e.g., dermal appendages, scolex, tumor-nodule) depending on the nature of the cyst. It may have enhancing inflammatory or tumoral walls or nonenhancing densely collagenous walls. MRI is not yet able to differentiate among the different cell linings, but it can identify the number and size of any cysts, the compartment in which they lie, any extension to adjacent compartments, any mass effect on the surrounding anatomic structures, and, to some extent, the nature of the intracystic contents. MRI and CT are both helpful in characterizing intracystic components (fat, blood, CSF, soft tissue, calcification) and perilesional contrast enhancement, which indicates an inflammatory/tumoral cyst wall. Together with the age, gender, and history of the patient, the neuroimaging features of the cyst help to establish the cause of the lesion and the opportunities available for treatment.

Spinal cysts may be grouped by their location into intramedullary, intradural extramedullary, and extradural lesions. Such classification helps in planning therapy, but it is less useful for differential diagnosis because almost all of the entities may occur in more than one anatomic compartment or may extend through several compartments. Therefore, we elect to discuss these lesions by their histologic type, as follows (the percentage relates to all primary spinal tumors):

- Dermoid cyst (dermoid + epidermoid: 0.8%-1.1%)
- Epidermoid cyst (dermoid + epidermoid: 0.8%-1.1%)
- Meningeal cyst (1%-3%)
  - Type I
  - Type II
  - Type III
- Ependymal cyst (0.2%-0.4%)
- Neurenteric cyst (0.7%-1.3%)
- Syringohydromyelia
- Degenerative cyst
  - Facet joint cyst
  - Ligamentum flavum cyst
  - Discal cyst

Parasitic cysts and cystic tumors must also be considered in the differential diagnosis.

DERMOID CYST

Dermoids are cystic lesions lined by squamous epithelium and containing dermal appendages. They are also sometimes called dermoid tumors.

Epidemiology

Spinal dermoids and epidermoids together account for 0.8% to 1.1% of primary spinal tumors. They are equally frequent in males and females. The majority of dermoid cysts (62%-84%) are intradural extramedullary lesions. Sixteen to 38% of dermoics are intramedullary. Extradural location is rare. About 5% of all dermoid and epidermoid cysts are multiple. The cranial to spinal ratio of dermoids is 6:1.

Clinical Presentation

Congenital dermoids may present in the newborn period or infancy. However, they may also grow very slowly and not cause symptoms until adulthood. Acquired lesions may cause symptoms years after lumbar puncture, surgery, or trauma. Patients commonly present with a several month history of backache or radicular pain and slowly progressive myelopathy. Because most spinal dermoid cysts arise in the lumbosacral area, they often present as a conus medullaris syndrome. Rupture of the lesion may be asymptomatic or cause acute aseptic (chemical) meningitis, with headache, seizure, hydrocephalus, and/or ischemic stroke (secondary to arterial vasospasm).

Pathophysiology

Dermoids are not true neoplasms. They arise from inclusion of dermis within adjacent tissue. The congenital form develops at the time of neural tube closure, between 3 and 5 weeks of fetal life. The acquired form develops after lumbar puncture, surgery, or trauma due to iatrogenic introduction of dermal elements into the spinal canal, most often into the subarachnoid space.[1] The incidence of dermoids after myelomeningocele or meningocele repair is about 2%.[2]

Congenital dermoids may be associated with a cutaneous "stigma," such as hypertrichosis in the overlying skin, with a dorsal dermal sinus, spina bifida, diastematomyelia, syringomyelia, and/or intradural extramedullary or intramedullary lipoma. The most frequent of these is the dermal sinus, which results from focal nondisjunction of neural ectoderm from cutaneous ectoderm. However, dermal sinuses are present in only a minority of cases (20%). Most dermoids have no associated dermal sinus.

Pathology

Dermoid cysts can be connected with the skin through a dermal sinus tract. When present, the tract shows an external ostium that may appear as a dimple in or adjacent to a midline cutaneous hemangioma. There may be a small patch of thin sparse wiry hairs within the ostium. Infrequently, the ostium lies to one side of the midline.

The surrounding bone of the spinal canal may evidence dysraphism and signs of pressure remodeling with canal enlargement due to chronic mass effect.

Dermoid cysts are filled with thick caseous material, which is an oily mixture of breakdown products of hair, secretions of sweat and sebaceous glands, teeth and nails, liquid lipid, and cholesterol. One can also observe skin appendages and, rarely, calcifications (Fig. 14-1). In contrast to epidermoid cysts, dermoid cysts are usually well demarcated from the surrounding tissue.

Dermoid cysts show stratified squamous epithelium plus adnexal appendages, especially hair follicles and sebaceous and sweat glands (Fig. 14-2). On immunohistochemistry, the epithelial lining usually stains for cytokeratins and epithelial membrane antigen (EMA).

Dermoids may occur anywhere along the craniospinal axis but are most often in the midline. In the spine, most dermoids are lumbosacral (60%), followed by sacrococcygeal, 25%; thoracic, 10%; and cervical, 5%.

Imaging

Ultrasonography

Dermoid cysts are usually hypoechoic fluid-containing structures with focal areas of hyperechogenicity representing fat.

CT

On CT, dermoids resemble fat and show a round, oval, or multilobular, well-delineated hypodensity with solid structures (hair, nail) and calcifications (see Fig. 14-1D). Larger cysts may be associated with focal bony erosion and widening of the spinal canal (see Fig. 14-1E, F).

MRI

The MRI appearance depends on the proportions of fat and dermal appendages contained within the cyst. The cyst signal is usually heterogeneous, with T1-weighted (T1W) and T2-weighted (T2W) imaging partly hyperintense from the fatty component and with T2W imaging partly iso/hypointense from the mixture of hair, glandular elements, cholesterol, and water content of the glandular secretions (see Fig. 14-1A-C). Dermoid cysts do not enhance, unless they are infected or have ruptured, causing sterile inflammation. Infection is more frequent in those dermoids linked to the skin surface by dermal sinuses. Infected dermoids may show ring enhancement that resembles an abscess or may convert into frank abscess. Ruptured dermoid cysts typically show multiple T1-hyperintense droplets of spilled lipid material within the perimedullary subarachnoidal space (see Fig. 14-1B), the central canal, and the intracranial CSF spaces.

EPIDERMOID CYST

Epidermoids are cystic lesions lined by squamous epithelium with no dermal appendages. By definition, the presence of dermal appendages makes the lesion a dermoid, not an epidermoid. They can also be called epidermoid tumors or pearly tumors.

Epidemiology

Together, spinal epidermoids and dermoids account for 0.8% to 1.1% of primary spinal tumors. They are more frequent in males. The distribution of epidermoids within the spinal canal is similar to that of spinal dermoids. About 60% of epidermoids are intradural extramedullary and 40% are intramedullary. Extradural epidermoids are very rare. Approximately 5% of all spinal dermoid and epidermoid lesions are multiple.

Clinical Presentation

Congenital epidermoids grow even more slowly than dermoids, so symptoms may not occur until age 30 to 50

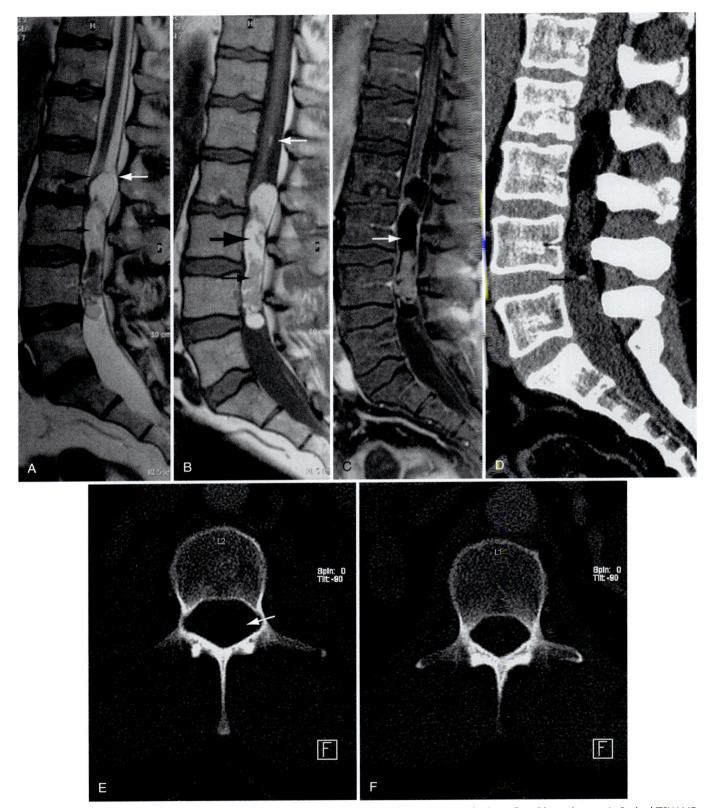

■ **FIGURE 14-1** Intradural extramedullary dermoid in a 52-year-old man with backache, leg paresthesia, and anal incontinence. **A**, Sagittal T2W MR image depicts a large cystic intradural mass (*thin black arrow*) in the region of the conus medullaris and cauda equina. Note displacement of the dura mater (*thin white arrow*) posteriorly and the conus medullaris (*thick black arrow*) anteriorly. **B**, Sagittal T1W MR image shows an isointense solid component (*thin black arrow*) and a hyperintense fatty component (*thick black arrow*). A small fatty droplet is also visible in the subarachnoidal space (*thin white arrow*). **C**, Sagittal T1W MR image with fat suppression and administration of gadolinium affirms the presence of fat (*arrow*) that is suppressed with this sequence. **D**, The sagittal CT image shows an additional small calcification (*arrow*). **E**, The axial CT with bone window depicts a spinal canal widening in the region of the hypodense fatty component (at the level of L2) (*arrow*). In **F**, the spinal canal above it (at the level of L1) looks normal. This is a sign of a slow-growing pathologic process with remodeling of the subjacent bony structures.

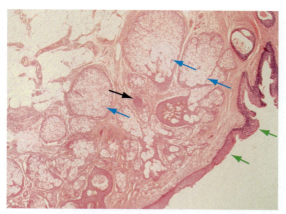

■ **FIGURE 14-2** Dermoid cyst. Note stratified squamous epithelium (*green arrows*) as well as hair follicles (*black arrow*) and sebaceous glands (*blue arrows*) (H&E).

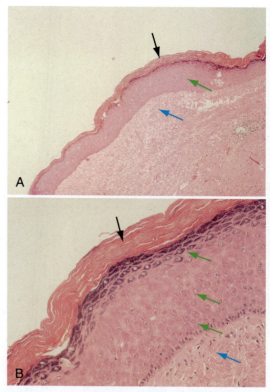

■ **FIGURE 14-3** Epidermoid cyst. A and **B,** Cyst wall consisting of stratified squamous epithelium (*green arrows*) mounted on connective tissue (*blue arrows*). The center of the cyst is filled by concentric lamellae of desquamated keratin (*black arrows*) (H&E).

years. Acquired epidermoids may not cause symptoms until 2 to 23 years after lumbar puncture, surgery, or trauma. Clinical symptoms are identical to those of dermoids, namely, back pain, radiculopathy, myelopathy (most often cauda equina syndrome), or symptoms of chemical meningitis from cyst rupture.

Pathophysiology

Epidermoids are not true neoplasms. Rather, they arise from inclusion of epidermis within the spinal canal. Enlargement of the cyst results from proliferation of the stratified squamous cells and from desquamation of keratinized debris into the center of the cyst. Congenital epidermoids develop at the time of neural tube closure, at between 3 and 5 weeks of fetal life. Acquired epidermoids develop after lumbar puncture, surgery, or trauma by introducing epidermis into the intradural space iatrogenically. In one study, 41% of all intraspinal epidermoids were caused by lumbar punctures.[3] Acquired epidermoid cysts may also develop after (myelo)meningocele repair (13%-27%), which is about six times more frequent than dermoid cysts.[2] Congenital epidermoids may be associated with hypertrichosis, posterior dermal sinus, spina bifida, diastematomyelia, syringomyelia, and intradural extramedullary or intramedullary lipoma. Dermal sinuses are less frequent with epidermoids than with dermoids.

Pathology

Epidermoids may cause remodeling of the spinal canal just as do dermoids. Epidermal cysts are encapsulated lesions. A smooth, glistening surface (capsule) encloses waxy material representing a mixture of keratin and cholesterin. There is a "mother-of-pearl" appearance that is almost pathognomonic and that leads to the synonym "pearly tumor." Often, no sharp border to the surrounding tissue is visible.

The cysts are lined by stratified squamous epithelium mounted on connective tissue. The center of the cyst is filled by concentric lamellae of desquamated keratin (Fig.

14-3). The epithelial lining shows positive immunohistochemical staining for cytokeratins and EMA.

Epidermoids can occur anywhere along the craniospinal axis. Unlike dermoids, which are most common in the midline, epidermoids tend to lie off midline. Spinal epidermoids most commonly affect the lumbosacral levels.

Imaging

Ultrasonography

Ultrasonography shows a hypoechoic cyst with internal echoes.

CT

On CT, epidermoids are well-circumscribed lesions that have low density very similar to CSF. They may be difficult or impossible to distinguish from arachnoid cysts by CT. Calcification is rare. Widening and remodeling of the spinal canal indicates a slowly growing lesion.

MRI

T1W and T2W MR images show a cystic lesion with signal intensity similar to CSF, that is, hypointense or isointense on T1W and hyperintense on T2W imaging (Fig. 14-4). As a result, epidermoids may be very difficult to detect and display on standard MRI, especially when the lesion is small. If the cyst is large, causing enlargement of the

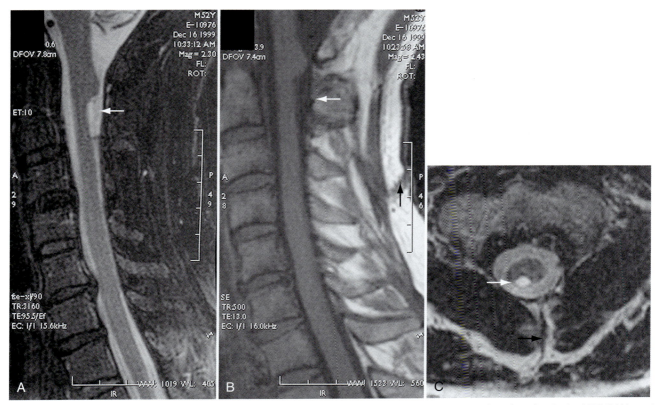

■ **FIGURE 14-4** Intradural extramedullary epidermoid in a 52-year-old man with slowly progressive cervical myelopathy. Sagittal T2W (**A**), sagittal T1W (**B**) and axial T2W (**C**) MR images show a liquor-intense cystic lesion (*white arrow*) with compression of the spinal cord from dorsal. The associated dermal sinus tract is well visible (*black arrow*): the subcutaneous segment is shown on **B**, and the paraspinal segment is evident on **C**.

subarachnoid space, eventually with deformation of the spinal cord, high suspicion has to be raised and additional sequences have to be performed. Diffusion-weighted imaging (DWI) provides a definitive diagnosis, because epidermoids cause diffusion restriction whereas free CSF and arachnoid cysts show no restriction of diffusion.[4] Fluid-attenuated inversion recovery (FLAIR) and constructive interference in steady-state sequence/fast imaging employing steady-state acquisition (CISS/FIESTA) sequences and magnetization transfer techniques are also useful for depicting the more viscous nature of the epidermoid cyst. Occasionally, epidermoids show high density on CT, hyperintense signal on T1W MRI, and hypointense signal on T2W MRI (compared with CSF). The precise signal depends on the chemical state of the cholesterol and/or on the proportion of cholesterol versus keratin (see Box 14-1). Methemoglobin from bleeding can also cause high signal on T1W MRI. Such atypical imaging features may make it difficult to differentiate epidermoid cysts from lipomas or dermoids, unless fat saturation sequences are incorporated into the study. Because epidermoids do not contain fat, they retain their high signal on fat-suppressed images, whereas lipomas and dermoids do not. Epidermoid cysts usually do not enhance, although a thin rim of enhancement may occasionally be observed at the periphery of the lesion, possibly representing compressed parenchyma or granulation tissue. Epidermoid cysts may become infected, especially if they are associated with a dermal sinus. When the lesion shows

a thick ring of enhancement, it may resemble an abscess, or have become one.

Special Procedures

In the past, myelography was useful for diagnosing the presence of an intradural extramedullary cystic lesion. Epidermoid cysts cause filling defect within the opacified CSF, often with concurrent mass effect on the spinal cord and nerve roots. Ruptured and infected epidermoids often obliterate the subarachnoid space focally or diffusely and cause extensive matting of the roots of the cauda equina. Myelography could not differentiate reliably between an epidermoid cyst and a noncommunicating arachnoid cyst. It has largely been replaced by MRI.

MENINGEAL CYST

Meningeal cysts may be completely loculated from the subarachnoid space or may form freely communicating pockets of CSF lined by arachnoid mater and/or a fibrocollagenous layer. They can be referred to as arachnoid cysts, diverticula, or pouches or as meningeal diverticula.

Epidemiology

Spinal meningeal cysts are uncommon lesions, accounting for 1% to 3% of all primary spinal tumors. There is no

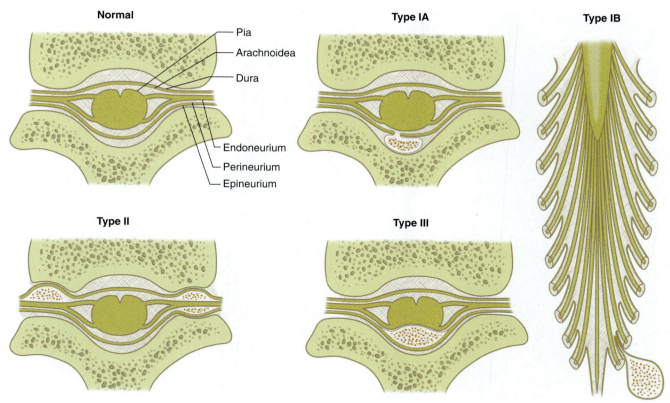

FIGURE 14-5 The Nabors classification of meningeal cysts.[6]

gender predilection. Thoracic meningeal cysts are more common in adolescents, whereas lumbosacral meningeal cysts are more common in adults, presenting usually at the age of 40 to 50 years. Meningeal cysts are more often extradural than intradural extramedullary.

Clinical Presentation

Most spinal meningeal cysts are asymptomatic and are discovered incidentally by MRI. The symptoms are dependent on the location as well as on the extension of the cyst. Cervical meningeal cysts present as spastic tetraparesis and sensory disturbances. Thoracic cysts cause progressive spastic paraparesis and sensory symptoms but usually not back pain. Lumbar or lumbosacral cysts typically present as low back pain, leg pain, leg weakness or numbness, gait disturbance, and urinary or stool incontinence.[5] Most meningeal cysts lie within the dorsal portion of the spinal canal, causing sensory symptoms. Rare anteriorly located cysts cause motor dysfunction instead. Symptoms can be exacerbated by changing posture and by Valsalva maneuver. Approximately 30% of patients show fluctuating levels of symptoms. On occasion, progressive symptoms lead the patient to fall, causing cyst rupture and "spontaneous" but transient cure.

Pathophysiology

The Nabors classification is based on intraoperative inspection combined with MRI findings and histologic characteristics and differentiates three types of meningeal cysts[6]:

Type I: Extradural meningeal cyst with no nerve root fibers
  Type IA: Extradural arachnoid cyst
  Type IB: Sacral meningocele
Type II: Extradural cysts with nerve root fibers running within the cyst cavity or within the cyst wall
Type III: Intradural cysts

Anatomically, a meningeal cyst is a diverticulum of the arachnoid mater/dura mater or the nerve root sheath. Figure 14-5 illustrates the normal anatomic relationships and the three types of meningeal cysts.[6]

Within the neural foramina, the meningeal layers of the thecal sac blend into the investments of the nerve roots. Normally, the dura mater blends into the epineurium, the arachnoid mater blends into the perineurium, and the pia mater blends into the endoneurium of the nerve roots.[7]

Type IA meningeal cysts (extradural arachnoid cysts) develop when a diverticulum of the arachnoid mater protrudes through a dural defect to herniate into the extradural space. These cysts occur most frequently in adolescents and are most commonly located in the thoracic spine.

Type IB meningeal cysts (sacral meningoceles) are anatomically meningoceles connected by a pedicle at the caudal tip of the dural sac, most often adjacent to the sacral or coccygeal nerve roots. They are found mostly in middle-aged or elderly adults and lie within the sacral canal.

Type II meningeal cysts are also extradural cysts. Anatomically, they are dilatations of the spinal nerve root sleeve. In this type, the nerve root fibers run either in the

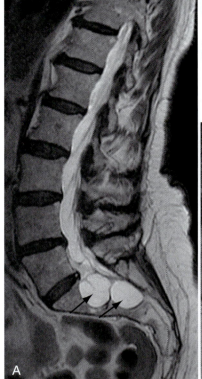
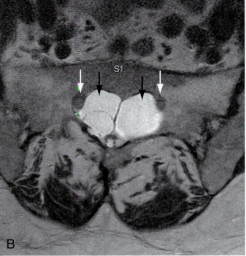
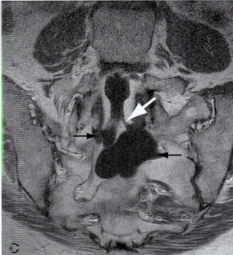
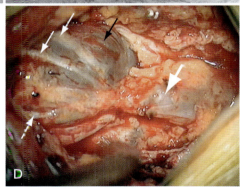

■ **FIGURE 14-6** Type II meningeal cyst in a 67-year-old woman with a 2-year history of backache and pain in the right leg. Sagittal T2W (**A**), axial T2W (**B**), and coronal T1W (**C**) MR images and intraoperative photograph (**D**) reveal two cysts along the S1 nerve roots on the right and on the left side (*thin black arrows*). The nerve roots run in the wall of the cysts (*thin white arrow,* **B, D**). On **A** and **B**, note the scalloping of the sacral vertebral bodies. The *thick white arrows* on **C** and **D** show the pedicle, which represents the continuity of the cyst with the subarachnoidal space. (**D**, *courtesy of Prof. Bertalanffy, Neurosurgery, University Hospital of Zürich.*)

cyst wall (Fig. 14-6) or centrally within the cyst (Fig. 14-7). They occur anywhere along the spinal canal, but they are most prominent and most commonly symptomatic in the sacral region. Multiple cysts are more frequent than single cysts. They occur most often in middle-aged adults and are usually diagnosed incidentally.

Type III meningeal cysts ("intradural cysts") (Fig. 14-8) lie within the subarachnoidal space (intradural extramedullary position). These cysts may or may not communicate with the subarachnoid space. They are most frequent in the thoracic spine dorsal to the spinal cord, rarely anterior, but may be found anywhere along the spinal subarachnoid space. These cysts are often multiple and asymptomatic. They may be congenital or may be acquired after trauma, postsurgical arachnoiditis, or other insults that cause inflammation and subarachnoid adhesions.[8]

All of the meningeal cysts (except the completely loculated cysts) communicate with the subarachnoid space

and contain CSF.[9] The pathophysiologic mechanism for these cysts may be proliferation of arachnoid granulations through a low-resistance dural area, with production of CSF that then becomes entrapped. Theories for the enlargement of these cysts include active fluid secretion from the cyst wall, osmotic pressure gradients between the subarachnoid space and the cyst, and a ball valve–like mechanism that allows inflow into the cyst but restricts outflow.[5] Intermittent elevations of pressure within the subarachnoid space (e.g., from coughing and changing posture) could also result in cyst expansion. This mechanism would also explain development of high intracystic pressures (see Fig. 14-7D). The fact that extradural cysts are most commonly found in the elderly or in patients with connective tissue disorders such as Marfan syndrome and neurofibromatosis points to the possibility of a congenital predisposition that allows the arachnoid to herniate through a weak point in the dura. Extradural arachnoidal cysts may also be associated with congenital neural tube

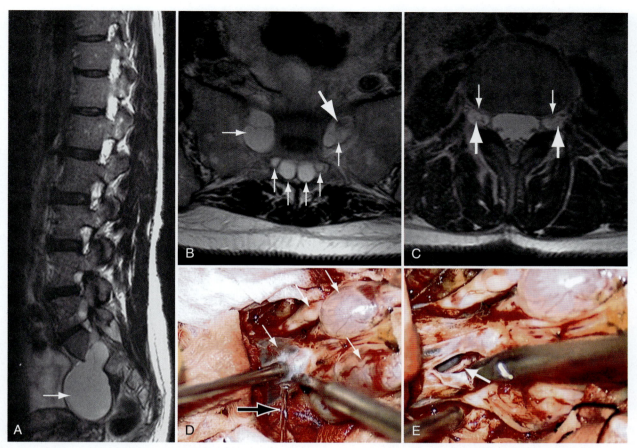

■ **FIGURE 14-7** Type II meningeal cyst in a 44-year-old woman with radicular symptoms of the left S1 and S2 nerve roots. Sagittal T2W (**A**), axial sacral T2W (**B**), and axial lumbar T2W (**C**) MR images and intraoperative photographs (**D, E**) show the multiple cysts (*thin white arrows*) with the nerve roots running centrally within the cysts (*thick white arrows*). Note the high pressure outflow of the CSF after incision of the cyst wall (*thick black arrow*, **D**). (**D and E**, *courtesy of Prof. Bertalanffy, Neurosurgery, University Hospital of Zürich.*)

■ **FIGURE 14-8** Type III meningeal cyst in a 52-year-old man, incidental finding. Sagittal T2W (**A**) and axial T2W (**B**) MR images show the deformation of the spinal cord from posterior at the level of T5-6, which suggests—although not well delineated—the presence of a cystic lesion (*black thin arrow*). Based on the signal intensities similar to CSF and the location of the cyst, the diagnosis of an arachnoid cyst was presumed. Note its location inside the dura mater (*thin white arrow*), clearly in the subarachnoid space.

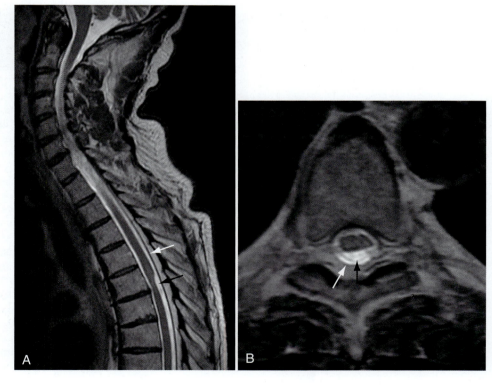

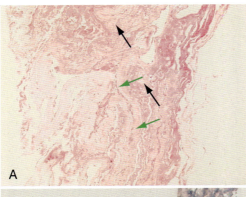
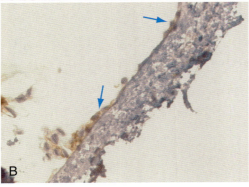

■ **FIGURE 14-9** Type III meningeal cyst. **A,** Arachnoid cap cells (*green arrows*) and the outer lining, which consist of collagenous connective tissue (*black arrows*) (H&E). **B,** Immunohistochemistry demonstrates positivity for EMA (*blue arrows*) but negativity for GFAP and S100.

defects. The syndrome of distichiasis, lymphedema, and extradural arachnoid cysts has been related to mutations of the gene for the transcription factor FoxC2 or a mutation at 16q24.

Pathology

Large meningeal cysts frequently scallop the surrounding bone, enlarging the spinal canal and/or neural foramina. In type IA meningeal cysts the arachnoid herniates through the disrupted dura mater. In type IB meningeal cysts, the lesion is essentially a dural diverticulum (sacral meningocele). Type II cysts represent a dilatation of the nerve root sleeve. Type III cysts are created by arachnoid duplications/dissections or adhesions. Depending on the cyst location, the subarachnoid space may be either widened or compressed. In type II meningeal cysts the nerve roots run either in the wall or in the center of the cyst.

Meningeal cysts present with a thin translucent membrane. The cysts contain clear fluid (CSF) or occasionally xanthochromic fluid. The CSF within the cyst may have slightly higher protein content than the rest of the subarachnoid space.

The inner lining of meningeal cysts consists of arachnoid cap cells. The outer lining consists of collagenous connective tissue (Fig. 14-9). The arachnoid layer is not always present.

Immunohistochemical staining is positive for EMA but negative for glial fibrillary acidic protein (GFAP) and S100 protein.

Spinal meningeal cysts occur most frequently in the thoracic spine (65%), followed by the lumbar and lumbosacral spine (13%), the thoracolumbar region (12%), the sacral spine (7%) and the cervical spine (3%).[5] Most are located dorsally within the spinal canal (80%). A ventral position is rare (20%). Most of the intradural cysts are located in the thoracic region and extend craniocaud over several vertebral body levels.

Imaging

CT

CT depicts scalloping of the bone with thinning of the pedicles and enlargement of the neural foramina, indicating a longstanding pathology.

MRI

MRI is useful to identify the cyst, to determine its precise anatomic location and extensions, and to define its relation to surrounding structures (nerves, spinal cord, and bone). On MRI meningeal cysts may be well circumscribed, oval, or elongated lesions. Sometimes the presence of a cyst is suggested only by slight mass effect on the spinal cord or splaying of nerve roots. In such cases, CISS/FIESTA pulse sequences may display the thin cyst wall that separates the cyst proper from the surrounding subarachnoid space. Combined intraforaminal and extraforaminal lesions may assume a dumbbell shape. The signal characteristics are consistent with CSF: hyperintense on T2W and hypointense on T1W images. No contrast enhancement is seen.

Special Procedures

CT myelography is essential to reveal any communication between the cyst and the subarachnoid space. However, CT may not show filling of the cyst immediately after the injection of iodinated contrast media in the subarachnoidal space. Instead, the cyst may fill only hours later (e.g., 3-24 hours).[9] CT myelography also demonstrates a partial or complete CSF block in the spinal canal.

EPENDYMAL CYST

Ependymal cyst is a developmental lesion lined with ependyma and derived from isolated ependymal tissue. It can also be called a neuroepithelial cyst, glioependymal cyst, or choroidal epithelial cyst.

Epidemiology

A spinal ependymal cyst is a very rare entity. Intradural extramedullary ependymal cysts comprise 0.2% to 0.4% of all primary spinal tumors. Fewer than 20 cases of intramedullary ependymal cysts have been reported.[10] Intradural extramedullary ependymal cysts show a 2:1 predilection for females and commonly present with symptoms after the fourth decade.[11] Intramedullary ependymal cysts show no gender or age predisposition.[10]

Clinical Presentation

Symptoms depend on cyst location and size and include slowly progressive myelopathy with or without radiculopathy (i.e., intermittent paraparesis or tetraparesis, paresthesia, and radicular pain).

Pathophysiology

Ependymal cyst is a developmental lesion. The pathogenesis is believed to be focal invagination of the floor plate during neural tube closure, with later formation of the cyst. The future intramedullary or extramedullary location of the cyst then depends on the site of the isolated ependymal tissue. Ependymal cysts are usually separated from the central canal of the spinal cord and are most frequently located in the anterior spinal cord. Extramedullary ependymal cysts may arise by glioependymal ectopia.

Pathology

Ependymal cysts have thin walls that are detached from the normal ependyma. The lining consists of columnar epithelium morphologically resembling normal ependymal cells (see Fig. 14-9). The epithelial cells can possess cilia, but goblet cells are absent. Immunohistochemistry is positive for GFAP and S100.

Among the intramedullary ependymal cysts, the thoracolumbar area is the most frequent location.[10] Intradural extramedullary cysts are most common in the region of the conus medullaris and cauda equina.[11] They are located most frequently in the anterolateral spinal cord or subarachnoid space.

Imaging

MRI

On MRI, ependymal cysts appear as well-defined lesions with low signal intensity on T1W and high signal intensity on T2W images, like CSF. They do not show contrast enhancement (Fig. 14-10).

NEURENTERIC CYST

Neurenteric cysts are congenital malformations lined by intestinal-like or respiratory-like, mucus-secreting epithelium. These lesions can also be called enterogenous cysts, endodermal cysts, or bronchogenic cysts.

Epidemiology

Neurenteric cysts are rare, comprising 0.7% to 1.3% of all primary spinal cord tumors. The age at presentation is usually 20 to 30 years. Most cases occur in men.[12]

Clinical Presentation

Common symptoms are backache associated with progressive myelopathy. Half the patients have urinary incon-

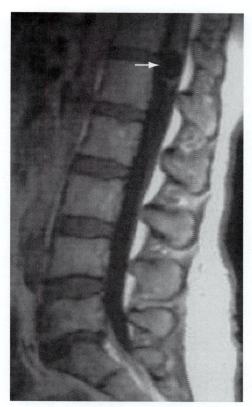

■ **FIGURE 14-10** Ependymal cyst in a 41-year-old woman. Sagittal T1W MR image shows a cystic lesion in the conus medullaris (*arrow*). *(Courtesy of Robert Veres, National Institute of Neurosurgery, Budapest.)*

tinence. The median duration of symptoms is 1 month. In intramedullary neurenteric cysts, the clinical course may fluctuate with changing rates of mucin production and absorption.[12]

Pathophysiology

The primary pathophysiologic event is a defect in the notochord and neural plate during the third week of fetal life. These defects allow an endodermal diverticulum to herniate through the defect and come into contact with the ectoderm. Vertebral column anomalies, such as spina bifida, Klippel-Feil syndrome, and hemivertebra occur in 30% of the cases. The vertebral anomalies are more common with cysts that are intradural extramedullary, cervicothoracic, and ventral. Neurenteric cysts may be associated also with midline cutaneous anomalies such as cutaneous groove, dermal sinus, pigmented skin, or hypertrichosis.

Pathology

There are associated midline cutaneous abnormalities, as discussed earlier. There may be midline dysraphism of the anterior and/or posterior elements of the spinal canal, perhaps reflecting persistence of the embryonic canal of Kovalevsky. Other vertebral column anomalies may occur (see earlier).

Neurenteric cysts are fluid-filled cysts with thin walls. The fluid can be clear (CSF-like) or proteinaceous (milky, creamy). The cyst wall consists of a single layer of pseudostratified columnar epithelium mounted on a basement membrane and covering collagenous fibrous tissue (Fig. 14-11). Often, cilia are found on epithelial cells. The epithelial lining shows gastrointestinal or respiratory differentiation. Mucous or serous glands, smooth muscle, lymphoid tissue, and nerve ganglia can also occur within the cyst walls. Rarely, ependymal or glial areas are observed. Immunohistochemistry is positive for cytokeratins and EMA but not for GFAP.

Neurenteric cysts are most commonly located in the cervicothoracic region (70%), in an intradural extramedullary (70%-95%) location, and in a ventral position to the spinal cord.[12] Intramedullary cysts are rare (5%-30%).

Imaging

Ultrasonography

A hypoechoic cyst can be imaged.

MRI

On MRI, neurenteric cysts are hyperintense to isointense on T2W imaging and hypointense to isointense on T1W imaging, depending on their protein content (Fig. 14-12). They are primarily nonenhancing lesions, but mild ring enhancement can be observed.

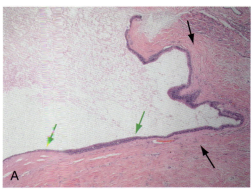

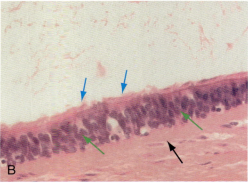

■ **FIGURE 14-11** Neurenteric cyst. **A**, Single layer pseudostratified columnar epithelium (*green arrows*) mounted on a basement membrane and covering collagenous fibrous tissue (*black arrows*). **B**, Presentation of the cilia (*blue arrows*) on epithelial cells (H&E).

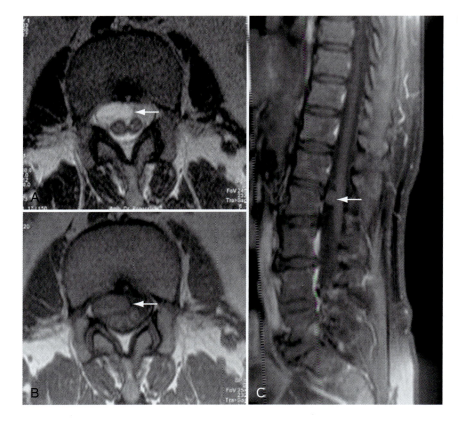

■ **FIGURE 14-12** Neurenteric cyst in a 42-year-old man with conus medullaris syndrome. Axial T2W (**A**), axial T1W (**B**), and sagittal T1W (**C**) MR images with gadolinium demonstrate an intradural extramedullary cyst that is anterolateral from the conus (*arrow*). The conus is light compressed. No contrast enhancement is seen.

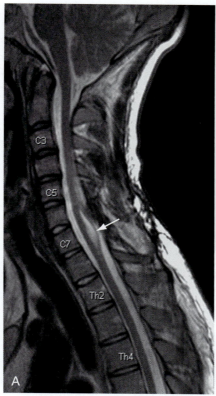
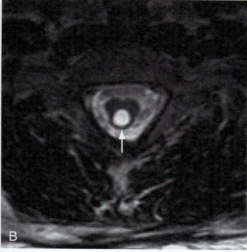

■ **FIGURE 14-13** Syringohydromyelia, Chiari II malformation, in a 25-year-old man. Sagittal (**A**) and axial (**B**) T2W MR images demonstrate the dilatation of the central canal (*arrow*). Observe the herniation of the cerebellar tonsilla.

SYRINGOHYDROMYELIA

Syringomyelia is a cystic cavity in the spinal cord that may or may not communicate with the central canal. Hydromyelia is a dilatation of the central canal. Because the differentiation with MRI is difficult, the term *syringohydromyelia* is often used to encompass both possibilities.

Epidemiology

Syringohydromyelia may arise in association with Chiari I malformation in 20% to 85% of cases and in association with Chiari II malformation in 48% to 88% of cases. Most cases present in late adolescence. No gender predilection is known. Post-traumatic syringohydromyelia is an uncommon complication after spinal trauma. Idiopathic syringohydromyelia has an estimated annual incidence of 8.4 new cases/100,000 people.

Clinical Presentation

Clinical symptoms vary with the longitudinal and axial location of the syrinx. Classically, the first manifestation is pain, followed by upper extremity weakness, lower extremity spasticity, paresthesias, and sphincter dysfunction. Sensory disturbances can appear as dissociated sensory loss with loss of pain and temperature sensation and preservation of proprioception.[13]

Because syringohydromyelia is a potential long-term complication of spinal trauma, late neurologic deterioration even years after spinal trauma needs careful evaluation to rule out syringohydromyelia (and secondary loculation of the subarachnoid space as well).[14]

Associated abnormalities include hydrocephalus, Chiari malformations, spinal dysraphism syndromes, tethered cord, scoliosis, and arachnoid cyst.

Pathophysiology

The most common cause of syringohydromyelia is caudal protrusion of posterior fossa contents into the upper cervical spinal canal, as in Chiari I and II malformations (Fig. 14-13), followed by tethered cord (Fig. 14-14). Most theories of the pathogenesis of syringohydromyelia in association with Chiari malformations emphasize impediment to the free passage of CSF (and CSF pulsations) through the foramen magnum, altering the balance of hydrostatic forces between the extramedullary CSF within the subarachnoid space and the intratissular force within the spinal cord. These may cause mechanical stress on the patent central canal or on the surface of the spinal cord.[15] The exact pathogenesis of post-traumatic syringohydromyelia is not known, but any adhesions or partial loculations of the subarachnoid space may impair CSF pulsations, leading to transient, repetitive pressure gradients from cord to subarachnoid space with each cardiac cycle.[14,16] In addition, coalescences of necrotic and/or hemorrhagic nests to form a syrinx have also been implicated as etiologic factors. The formation of the cavity may occur months or years after the trauma.

Syringohydromyelia is also observed in association with intramedullary spinal tumors (Fig. 14-15) and with spinal arachnoid cysts, suggesting a change in the CSF flow as pathogenesis.[17]

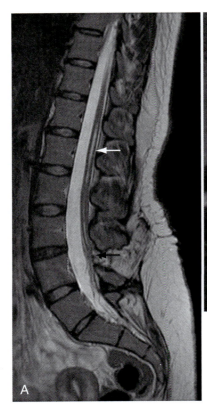

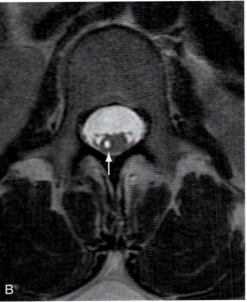

■ FIGURE 14-14 Syringohydromyelia, tethered cord, in a 21-year-old woman. Sagittal (**A**) and axial (**B**) T2W MR images show eccentric syringohydromyelia (*white arrow*) associated with tethered cord (*black arrow*).

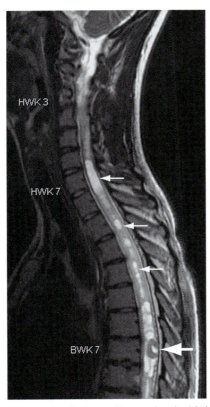

■ FIGURE 14-15 Syringohydromyelia associated with hemangioblastoma. T2W MR image shows the large sacculated syrinx extending in the thoracocervical spinal cord (*thin white arrows*), as well as thoracolumbar (not shown). Observe the nodule of the hemangioblastoma (*thick white arrow*).

Pathology

Syringohydromyelia is a tubular cavitation of the spinal cord, which is filled with clear or yellow fluid. In hydromyelia there is dilatation of the central canal, with retained (perhaps partially disrupted) ependymal lining. In syringomyelia there is a paracentral cavity lined by gliotic parenchyma. The walls show highly variable morphology ranging from gliotic CNS tissue to layers of collagen (Fig. 14-16). A communication with the central canal that can be detected by its ependymal lining is frequently seen.

Syringohydromyelia may occur anywhere along the spinal cord.

Imaging

Ultrasonography

A hypoechoic cavity can be seen.

CT

CT myelography can help in revealing arachnoid adhesions or cysts that may not be depicted on conventional MRI and can be the cause of syrinx formation.

MRI

MRI is the best imaging modality to identify the syrinx and the accompanying pathologic processes. Typically, a post-traumatic syrinx is central and round/oval below the injury site.[14] The syrinx shows high signal on T2W and low signal

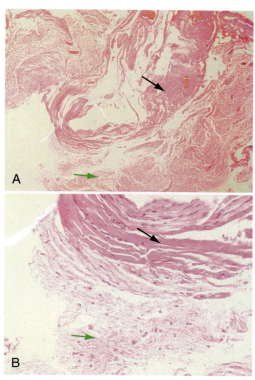

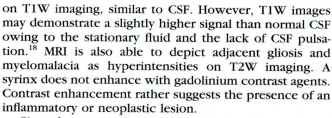

■ **FIGURE 14-16** Syringohydromyelia. **A** and **B**, Gliotic CNS tissue (*green arrow*) and layers of collagen (*black arrow*) (H&E).

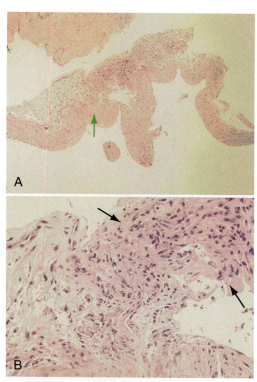

■ **FIGURE 14-17** Synovial cyst. Fibrous tissue (*green arrow*, **A**) and inflammation and chronic granulation tissue (*black arrows*, **B**) (H&E).

on T1W imaging, similar to CSF. However, T1W images may demonstrate a slightly higher signal than normal CSF owing to the stationary fluid and the lack of CSF pulsation.[18] MRI is also able to depict adjacent gliosis and myelomalacia as hyperintensities on T2W imaging. A syrinx does not enhance with gadolinium contrast agents. Contrast enhancement rather suggests the presence of an inflammatory or neoplastic lesion.

Cine phase-contrast MRI demonstrates obstruction of the craniocaudal CSF flow during cardiac systole. Demonstration of prominent CSF pulsations within a hydrosyringomyelia is proposed to indicate that the cavity will continue to grow unless decompressed surgically.[19] Postoperatively, cine MRI plays an important role in demonstrating the restoration of physiologic flow patterns, which has proven to be an important prognostic factor for symptom resolution.[20]

DEGENERATIVE CYSTS

This group of cystic lesions is formed as a result of degenerative changes of the lumbar spine. Degenerative cysts include facet joint cyst, ligamentum flavum cyst, and discal cyst (ganglion cyst).[21]

Epidemiology

Facet joint cysts and ligamentum flavum cysts present at ages 60 to 70 years with no gender predilection.[22] Discal cysts are rare, mostly reported in men between 20 and 40 years of age.[23]

Clinical Presentation

Some degenerative cysts are incidental findings; others cause acute or chronic symptoms identical to herniated disc or spinal canal stenosis.

Pathophysiology

The degenerative changes of the vertebrae, discs, and facet joints and the aging of the ligamentum flavum may cause cysts to form within the facet joint and ligamentum flavum. It is hypothesized that softening and fluid production within a degenerated disc causes fluid to spill into the paradiscal zone with later encapsulation to form a discal cyst.[24]

Pathology

Synovial cysts are sac-like protrusions within the synovium. Ligamentum flavum cysts represent a cyst formation within the ligamentum flavum.

Synovial "cysts" (Fig. 14-17) usually lack an epithelial wall, so they are not true cysts. Instead, they are pseudocysts enclosed by a wall of fibrous tissue with inflammation and chronic granulation tissue.

Ligamentum flavum "cysts" (Fig. 14-18) similarly lack an epithelial lining and are pseudocysts enclosed by a wall of degenerated/disrupted ligament, fibrous tissue, and chronic granulation reaction. These features are well shown by elastica–van Gieson stains that detect elastic and collagen fibers.

Synovial and ligamentum flavum cysts most often arise in the lumbar spine, with few cases reported in the thoracic and cervical regions.

Imaging

CT

Degenerative cysts are difficult to detect with CT unless there is secondary hemorrhage, calcification, or gas

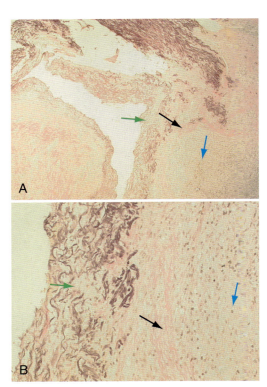

■ **FIGURE 14-18** Ligamentum flavum cyst. **A** and **B,** Elastica–van Gieson stain shows the degenerated or disrupted ligaments (*green arrow*) accompanied by a fibrous (*black arrow*) and chronic granulation reaction. This stain is useful to detect elastic (black staining) (*blue arrow*) and collagenous (blue staining) fibers.

evolved into the cyst from the facet joint. CT shows well the degenerative arthrosis of the facet joint (Fig. 14-19C) and may show mild ring enhancement of the inflamed tissue (Fig. 14-19B).

MRI

Facet joint cysts appear as well-defined, homogeneous lesions at the posterolateral aspects of the spinal canal (at the 5 or 7 o'clock position) adjacent to the facet joint (Fig. 14-19). They usually have CSF-like signal intensities (hypointense on T1W and hyperintense on T2W images) but may show reversed signal, with high signal on T1W and low signal on T2W images when there is hemorrhage or highly proteinaceous cyst fluid. Postcontrast studies usually show ring-like contrast enhancement. Ligamentum flavum cysts also lie within the posterolateral spinal canal, embedded within the ligament (Fig. 14-20). Discal cysts, however, present in the ventrolateral extradural space adjacent to a lumbar herniated disc (Fig. 14-21).

ANALYSIS

Dermoid cysts are easy to differentiate from other spinal cysts because of the fat content and dermal appendages. Dermoid cysts present heterogenous signal on MRI with solid, fluid, and fat components as opposed to other spinal cysts, which have signal intensities similar to CSF. If the patient is a young adult, the major differential diagnostic possibility is teratoma, which can look similar (Fig. 14-22). Dermoid cysts may usually be differentiated from lipomas, because dermoid cysts displace blood vessels and nerves whereas lipomas usually encompass the neurovascular structures (Fig. 14-23). After dermoid rupture or infection, however, the inflammatory mass may engulf all adjacent structures in continuity.

Epidermoid cysts show signal intensities similar to meningeal cyst, ependymal cysts, and parasitic and neurenteric cysts on conventional MRI (with T1 hypointensity and T2 hyperintensity). However, differentiation is possible with DWI, FLAIR, and CISS/FIESTA sequences:

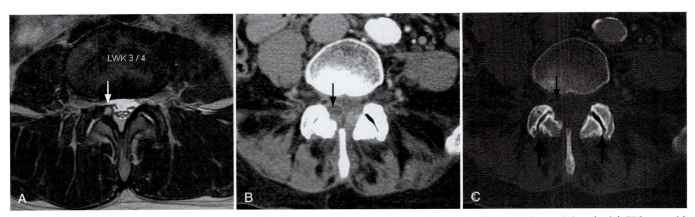

■ **FIGURE 14-19** Facet joint cyst (*thin arrows* in **A** to **C**) in a 73-year-old woman with a backache. Axial T2W MR image (**A**) and axial CT image with soft tissue window level (**B**) demonstrate the round cystic lesion with ring-like contrast enhancement on CT. The cyst is oriented to the facet joint and located posterolateral in the spinal canal, extradurally. **C,** CT with bone level window; note the facet joint arthrosis (*thick arrows*).

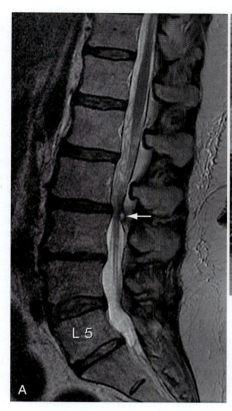

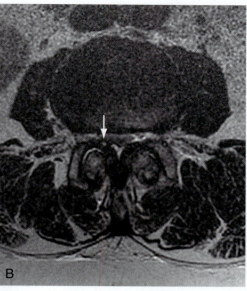

■ **FIGURE 14-20** Ligamentum flavum cyst in a 62-year-old woman with a backache. Sagittal (**A**) and axial (**B**) T2W MR images show a small cystic lesion embedded in the hypertrophic ligamentum flavum (*arrow*).

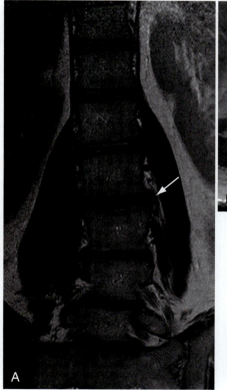

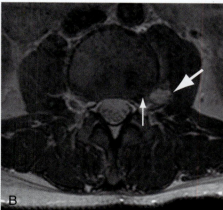

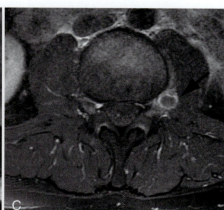

■ **FIGURE 14-21** Discal cyst in a 45-year-old man with a backache. **A,** Coronal T2W MR image shows the lateral discus hernia on the left (*thin white arrow*). **B,** After conservative therapy, 6 months later, axial T2W image shows new development of a cystic lesion (*thick white arrow*) next to the herniated disc (*thin white arrow*). **C,** Axial T1W MR image with gadolinium and fat suppression shows presentation of the ring-like contrast enhancement on the periphery of the cyst (*black arrow*).

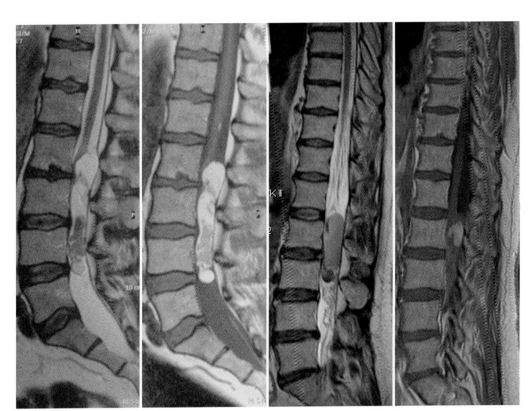

■ **FIGURE 14-22** Dermoid cyst. Note the similarity in appearance to teratoma.

Dermoid cyst

Teratoma

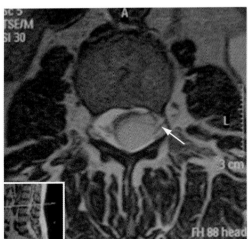

Dermoid cyst

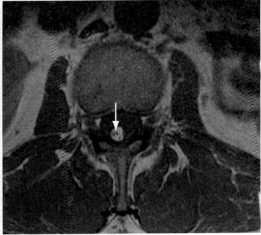

Lipoma

■ **FIGURE 14-23** Dermoid cyst. Note displacement of blood vessels and nerves (*arrow*). This distinguishes them from lipomas, which usually encompass the neurovascular structures (*arrow*).

epidermoids demonstrate restricted diffusion on DWI and show intracystic solid components with FLAIR and CISS/FIESTA, whereas meningeal cysts, ependymal cysts, and parasitic and neurenteric cysts all show nearly homogeneous clear fluid spaces. Demonstration of an associated sinus tract or thick pericystic ring enhancement suggests the diagnosis of epidermoid or infected epidermoid. Infected epidermoids with thick ring-like contrast enhancement may resemble or become abscesses.

Both epidermoid and abscess show restricted diffusion. Clinically, however, the abscess is usually associated with acute clinical onset and generalized symptoms of an infectious process, factors not seen with epidermoids.

Small meningeal cyst type II and traumatic pseudomeningocele caused by spinal nerve root avulsion are basically indistinguishable from each other (Fig. 14-24). The only clues are history or other imaging evidence of trauma or brachial plexus injury.

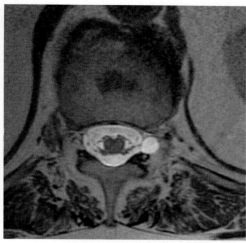
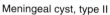

Meningeal cyst, type II

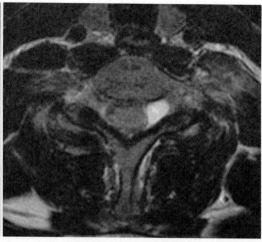

Traumatic pseudomeningocele

■ **FIGURE 14-24** Small meningeal cyst type II and traumatic pseudomeningocele caused by spinal nerve root avulsion are basically indistinguishable from each other.

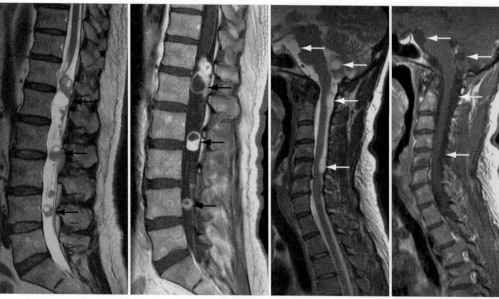

Multiple cystic tumor (presumed schwannoma)

Meningeal cyst, type III

■ **FIGURE 14-25** Cystic tumors usually show contrast enhancement (*black arrows*), whereas arachnoidal cysts (meningeal cyst type III) do not (*white arrows*).

Meningeal cyst type III may resemble epidermoid cyst. The differential diagnosis is based on DWI, because epidermoids show diffusion restriction whereas meningeal cysts do not. The location of a cyst relative to the spinal cord as well as the spinal level can help to differentiate among meningeal cyst type III (thoracic, dorsal), ependymal cyst (thoracolumbar, anterolateral), and neurenteric cyst (cervical, anterior).

Intramedullary ependymal cysts can be differentiated from cystic neoplastic lesions based on the lack of solid contrast enhancement and edema. Sometimes the differentiation from syringohydromyelia or ventriculus terminalis is difficult. In these cases, the off-center location, lack of spinal dysraphism, and late presentation of symptoms (in adulthood) favor the diagnosis of ependymal cyst.

Neurenteric cysts contain mucin as opposed to the CSF content of ependymal cysts, so they may present as higher signal intensity on T1W images. Differentiation from an anterior meningeal cyst may be impossible.

Syringohydromyelia must be evaluated carefully to exclude Chiari malformations, tethered cord, and neoplastic etiology. A contrast-enhancing nodule suggests tumor with associated syrinx.

Degenerative cysts are characteristically associated with degenerative changes of the spine and do not cause differential diagnostic problems.

Cystic tumors usually show contrast enhancement, whereas arachnoidal cysts (meningeal cyst type III) do not (Fig. 14-25).

A sample report is presented in Box 14-1.

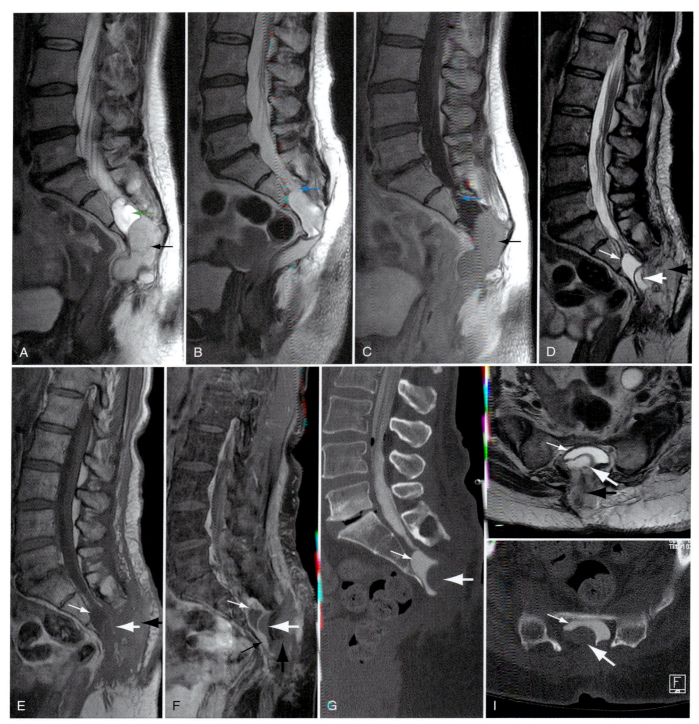

■ FIGURE 14-26 A 50-year-old woman presented with slowly progressive pain at the sacrum. The first MRI demonstrates a large sacral epidermoid with signal intensity slightly hypointense to CSF on T2W imaging (*black arrow*, **A**) and slightly hyperintense to CSF on T1W imaging (*black arrow*, **C**), representing xanthochromia or higher protein concentration. The CSF-like fluid-filled cystic lesion above the epidermoid (*green arrow*, **A**) communicates with the subarachnoidal space through a pedicle (*blue arrow*, **B**, **C**) and represents an associated meningocele. Contrast MRI 2 years after surgery: Two cystic lesions shown on sagittal T2W (**D**), sagittal T1W (**E**), and sagittal fat-suppressed T1W images after gadolinium injection (**F**); sagittal CT myelography (**G**); axial T2W image (**H**); and axial CT myelography (**I**). The anterior cyst (*thin white arrow on all images*) filled with iodinated contrast medium on the CT myelography (**G**, **I**) and proved to be a recurrent meningocele. The posteriorly located T1 isointense, T2 hyperintense cyst (*thick white arrow on all images*) did not fill with contrast media on the CT myelography and was histologically proved to be a recurrent epidermoid cyst. The thick contrast enhancement around the lesion (*thin black arrow*, **F**) is a sign of inflammation. Note the scar tissue in the region of the laminectomy (*thick black arrow*, **D**, **E**, **F**, **H**).

BOX 14-1 MRI of Epidermoid

PATIENT HISTORY

This 50-year-old woman presented with slowly progressive pain at the sacrum.

FINDINGS

The first MRI demonstrates a large sacral epidermoid with signal intensity slightly hypointense to CSF on T2W imaging (see Fig. 14-26A) and slightly hyperintense to CSF on T1W imaging (see Fig. 14-26C), representing xanthochromia or higher protein concentration. This feature helps to display the lesion better than typical epidermoids, which have signal intensities similar to CSF. No contrast enhancement is seen (gadoterate meglumine [Dotarem], 0.1 mmol/kg, was used). The CSF-like fluid-filled cystic lesion above the epidermoid communicates with the subarachnoidal space through a pedicle and represents an associated meningocele (see Fig. 14-26A to C).

OUTCOME

The sacral canal was widened, and the sacral and coccygeal vertebral bodies were eroded. The epidermoid cyst extended anteriorly into the anal region, without breaking through the wall of the rectum. The cyst was completely removed, and the meningocele was repaired.

COMMENT

Two years later the patient developed a sacral fistula that discharged fluid. The anterior cyst filled with iodinated contrast medium on CT myelography (see Fig. 14-26G, I) and proved to be a recurrent meningocele. The posteriorly located T1-isointense, T2-hyperintense cyst did not fill with contrast media on CT myelography and was histologically proved to be a recurrent epidermoid cyst. The thick contrast enhancement around the lesion (see Fig. 14-26F) is a sign of inflammation. Note the scar tissue in the region of the laminectomy (see Fig. 14-26D-F, H). The patient underwent a successful reoperation. The fistula and the epidermoid were removed, and the meningocele was repaired and covered with a muscle flap.

KEY POINTS: DIFFERENTIAL DIAGNOSIS

- Dermoid cyst: mainly intradural extramedullary dorsal, midline location in the lumbosacral region with mixed signal (fat, fluid, dermal appendages) on MRI.
- Epidermoid cyst: mainly intradural extramedullary dorsal, off-midline location in the lumbosacral region with MRI signal intensities similar to CSF but restricted diffusion on DWI.
- Meningeal cyst: Type IA cysts are mainly thoracic and posterior in location, type IB and II cysts are mainly sacral, and type III cysts are mainly thoracic and posterior. These cysts may have thin walls and contain CSF, so they may sometimes be detected only by the mass effect they exert. Dermoids can be differentiated by their fat content (T1 hyperintense, becoming hypointense on fat-suppression sequences), and epidermoids can be differentiated by their inhomogeneous higher signal on DWI, FLAIR, or CISS/FIESTA sequences.
- Ependymal cyst: mainly intradural extramedullary, thoracolumbar, and anterolateral in location, eccentric "off center" to the central canal, with signal intensity like CSF.
- Neurenteric cyst: mainly intradural extramedullary, cervico-thoracic (ventral position) or conal (dorsal position), with signal intensity like CSF. Diagnostic clues are evidence of midline dysraphic defects such as spina bifida and butterfly vertebrae.
- Syringohydromyelia: intramedullary, cervical, or thoracic in location. Except in cases of clear Chiari malformation, contrast-enhanced studies should be performed to exclude tumor.
- Degenerative cyst of the spine: lumbar position, ring-like contrast enhancement is common. Associated degenerative changes (facet joint arthrosis, ligamentum flavum hypertrophy, discal hernia) may be seen.
- Parasitic cysts: hydatid cyst (through several compartments; bony involvement is frequent) and cysticercosis (subarachnoid or intramedullary; leptomeningitis and pachymeningitis). In endemic areas, consider these cysts higher in the differential diagnosis.
- Cystic spinal tumor: nodular contrast enhancement and associated edema are the most important features.

SUGGESTED READINGS

ArunKumar MJ, Selvapandian S, Chandy MJ. Sacral nerve root cysts: a review on pathophysiology. Neurol India 1999; 47:61-64.

Brice G, Mansour S, Bell R, et al. Analysis of the phenotypic abnormalities in lymphoedema-distichiasis syndrome in 74 patients with *FOXC2* mutations or linkage to 16q24. J Med Genet 2002; 39:478-483.

Di Lorenzo N, Cacciola F. Adult syringomyelia: classification, pathogenesis and therapeutic approaches. J Neurosurg Sci 2005; 49:65-72.

Osenbach RK, Godersky JC, Traynelis VC, Schelper RD. Intradural extramedullary cysts of the spinal canal: clinical presentation, radiographic diagnosis, and surgical management. Neurosurgery 1992; 30:35-42.

Wang MY, Levi AD, Green BA. Intradural spinal arachnoid cysts in adults. Surg Neurol 2003; 60:49-55; discussion 55-56.

REFERENCES

1. Najjar MW, Kusske JA, Hasso AN. Dorsal intramedullary dermoids. Neurosurg Rev 2005; 28:320-325.
2. Yen CP, Kung SS, Kwan AL, et al. Epidermoid cysts associated with thoracic meningocele. Acta Neurochir (Wien) 2008; 150:305-308; discussion 308-309. Epub 2008; Jan 14.
3. Manno NJ, Uihlein A, Kernohan JW. Intraspinal epidermoids. J Neurosurg 1962; 19:754-765.
4. Gupta DK, Shilpa S, Amini AC, et al. Congenital adrenal hyperplasia: long-term evaluation of feminizing genitoplasty and psychosocial aspects. Pediatr Surg Int 2006; 22:905-909.
5. Gortvai P. Extradural cysts of the spinal canal. J Neurol Neurosurg Psychiatry 1963; 26:223-230.
6. Naborss MW, Pait TG, Byrd EB, et al. Updated assessment and current classification of spinal meningeal cysts. J Neurosurg 1988; 68:366-377.
7. Tarlov IM. Spinal perineurial and meningeal cysts. J Neurol Neurosurg Psychiatry 1970; 33:833-843.
8. Sklar E, Quencer RM, Green BA, et al. Acquired spinal subarachnoid cysts: evaluation with MR, CT myelography, and intraoperative sonography. AJNR Am J Neuroradiol 1989; 10:1097-1104.
9. DiSclafani A 2nd, Canale DJ. Communicating spinal arachnoid cysts: diagnosis by delayed metrizamide computed tomography. Surg Neurol 1985; 23:428-430.
10. Saito K, Morita A, Shibahara J, Kirino T. Spinal intramedullary ependymal cyst: a case report and review of the literature. Acta Neurochir (Wien) 2005; 147:443-446; discussion 446.
11. Fortuna A, Mercuri S. Intradural spinal cysts. Acta Neurochir (Wien) 1983; 68:289-314.
12. Garg N, Sampath S, Yasha TC, et al. Is total excision of spinal neurenteric cysts possible? Br J Neurosurg 2008; 22:241-251.
13. Rhoades CE, Neff JR, Rengachary SS, et al. Diagnosis of post-traumatic syringohydromyelia presenting as neuropathic joints: report of two cases and review of the literature. Clin Orthop Relat Res 1983; (180):182-187.
14. Hida K, Iwasaki Y, Imamura H, Abe H. Posttraumatic syringomyelia: its characteristic magnetic resonance imaging findings and surgical management. Neurosurgery 1994; 35:886-891; discussion 891.
15. du Boulay G, Shah SH, Currie JC, Logue V. The mechanism of hydromyelia in Chiari type 1 malformations. Br J Radiol 1974; 47:579-587.
16. Greitz D. Unraveling the riddle of syringomyelia. Neurosurg Rev 2006; 29:251-264.
17. Takeuchi A, Miyamoto K, Sugiyama S, et al. Spinal arachnoid cysts associated with syringomyelia: report of two cases and a review of the literature. J Spinal Disord Tech 2003; 16:207-211.
18. Reed CM, Campbell SE, Beall DP, et al. Atlanto-occipital dislocation with traumatic pseudomeningocele formation and post-traumatic syringomyelia. Spine 2005; 30:E128-E133.
19. Castillo M, Quencer RM, Green BA, Montalvo BM. Syringomyelia as a consequence of compressive extramedullary lesions: postoperative clinical and radiological manifestations. AJR Am J Roentgenol 1988; 150:391-396.
20. Tominaga T, Watabe N, Takahashi T, et al. Quantitative assessment of surgical decompression of the cervical spine with cine phase contrast magnetic resonance imaging. Neurosurgery 2002; 50:791-795; discussion 796.
21. Marshman LA, Benjamin JC, David KM, et al. "Disc cysts" and "posterior longitudinal ligament ganglion cysts": synonymous entities? Report of three cases and literature review. Neurosurgery 2005; 57: E818.
22. Epstein NE. Lumbar synovial cysts: a review of diagnosis, surgical management, and outcome assessment. J Spinal Disord Tech 2004; 17:321-325.
23. Tokunaga M, Aizawa T, Htodo H, et al. Lumbar discal cyst followed by intervertebral disc herniation: MRI findings of two cases. J Orthop Sci 2006; 11:81-84.
24. Kono K, Nakamura H, Inoue Y, et al. Intraspinal extradural cysts communicating with adjacent herniated disks: imaging characteristics and possible pathogenesis. AJNR Am J Neuroradiol 1999; 20:1373-1377.

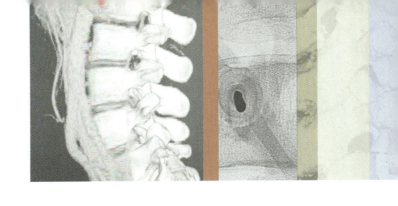

15

Spinal Tumors

Spyros S. Kollias, David Mark Capper, Nadja Saupe, and Krisztina Baráth

Spinal tumors comprise a large spectrum of distinct histologic entities that may arise primarily from the spinal cord (intra-axial or intramedullary space), the surrounding leptomeninges (intradural extramedullary space), or the extradural soft tissues and bony structures (extradural space). All three anatomic compartments may also be secondarily affected by metastatic disease from a known or unknown distant primary neoplasm. The same category also includes primary and metastatic bone tumors affecting the vertebrae and paraspinal soft tissue masses that extend into the spinal canal through the vertebral foramina or through direct infiltration of the vertebrae. Clinical signs and symptoms are variable and nonspecific, including back pain, weakness, radicular pain, and paresthesia, and all are often attributed to degenerative disease, which together with the relatively low incidence of spinal tumors frequently leads to a delayed diagnosis.

Spinal tumors account for 15% of all tumors of the central nervous system (CNS), with an incidence of 0.5 to 2.5 cases per 100,000 population. Both genders are usually equally affected, although meningiomas are more common in women and ependymomas are more common in men. Additionally, intramedullary tumors are more common in children, whereas extramedullary tumors are more frequent in adults. Almost 60% of the spinal tumors are located in the extradural space, whereas 40% are located within the thecal sac. Of the intradural tumors, the extramedullary ones represent the majority (80%) whereas intramedullary neoplasms are rare (10%). Approximately 10% of all spinal tumors, particularly schwannomas, may have concomitant intradural and extradural components at the time of diagnosis.

MRI is the diagnostic modality of choice for the neuroradiologic assessment of spinal neoplasia. Its superior soft tissue visualization and contrast differentiation between normal and pathologic tissues allow early diagnosis, assessment of associated edema, differentiation between solid and cystic components, and accurate anatomic localization of the neoplasm in one of the just-mentioned anatomic compartments (Fig. 15-1), thus facilitating characterization even of specific histologic subtypes. Ependymomas, astrocytomas, and gangliogliomas are the most common intramedullary tumors, followed by hemangioblastomas and metastases. The histologic spectrum of intradural extramedullary tumors is dominated by schwannomas and meningiomas. Leptomeningeal metastases are relatively less frequent but are increasingly recognized since the advent of MRI and paramagnetic contrast agents as well as the increasing life expectancy of patients with primary tumors in other locations. In the extradural space, metastatic disease involving the osseous spinal elements is the most common neoplastic cause of spinal myelopathy, with primary bone tumors such as osteoblastomas, giant cell tumors, or aneurysmal bone cysts being less common. Other neuroradiologic examinations such as CT, myelography, or CT myelography are useful if MRI is contraindicated. CT can provide additional information related to associated osseous changes (remodeling, erosion, sclerosis), potential intratumoral calcifications, and hemorrhage that may help the differential diagnosis and the planning of the surgical intervention. Selective angiography is performed only in hypervascular tumors, such as meningiomas or hemangioblastomas, in cases in which a preoperative embolization of the tumor is indicated. New research applications of MR technology such as diffusion tensor imaging (DTI) or magnetic resonance spectroscopy (MRS) are increasingly applied for aiding preoperative planning and for estimating prognosis.

A first step in the differential diagnosis of a spinal tumor is the correct localization of the lesion's origin to one of the anatomic compartments described earlier (see Fig. 15-1). This information together with the age of the patient greatly narrows the differential diagnosis to a group of histologic entities originating from a specific anatomic space. However, in large intradural tumors, differentiation between intramedullary or extramedullary origin is not always possible. Moreover, intradural extramedullary tumors may show an extradural, transforaminal extension and intramedullary tumors may be associated with an exophytic, perimedullary component. Visualization of the dural sac on high-resolution T2-weighted (T2W) images in the axial and sagittal planes is most valuable for an accurate anatomic localization.

A practical histologic/anatomic classification of spinal tumors is given in Table 15-1.

Spinal compartments

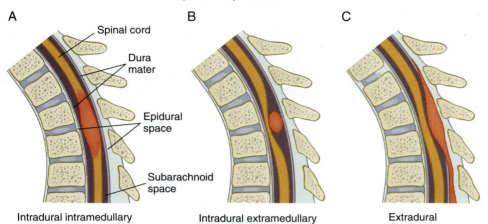

■ **FIGURE 15-1** Spinal compartments.

TABLE 15-1. Classification of Spinal Tumors

Intradural Intramedullary Neoplasms
Neuroepithelial Tumors (90%)
Ependymal cell tumors (60%)
   Ependymoma (WHO grade II)
   Anaplastic ependymoma (WHO grade III)
   Subependymoma (WHO grade I)
   Myxopapillary ependymoma of the filum terminale (WHO grade
     I) (often included in the intradural extramedullary category)
Astrocytic (glial) tumors (30%)
   Diffuse astrocytoma (WHO grade II)
   Pilocytic astrocytoma (WHO grade I)
   Anaplastic astrocytoma (WHO grade III)
   Glioblastoma multiforme (WHO grade IV)
   Pleomorphic xanthoastrocytoma (WHO grade II)
Oligodendroglial tumors
   Oligodendroglioma (WHO grade II)
   Anaplastic oligodendroglioma (WHO grade III)
Mixed glial tumor
   Oligoastrocytoma (WHO grade II)
   Anaplastic oligoastrocytoma (WHO grade III)
Mixed neuronal-glial tumors
   Ganglioglioma (WHO grade I)
   Gangliocytoma (WHO grade I)
   Ganglioneuroblastoma (WHO grade IV)
Neuroendocrine tumors
   Paraganglioma (WHO grade I)

Mesenchymal Tumors (7%)
Hemangioblastoma (2%-7%)
Lipoma
Sarcoma (mixed tumor-gliosarcoma)
Melanocytoma/malignant melanoma

Metastatic Tumors (2%)
Primary CNS tumor
Other primary tumors

Other Very Rare Tumors (1%)
Hematopoietic tumors
   Primary lymphoma
   Leukemia
Spinal nerve tumors
   Schwannoma
   Neurofibroma

Germ cell tumors
   Germinoma
   Teratoma
   Embryonal carcinoma
   Mixed germ cell tumors

Intradural Extramedullary Neoplasms
Meningeal tumors
   Meningioma* (WHO grade I)
   Atypical meningioma (WHO grade II)
   Anaplastic meningioma (WHO grade III)
Peripheral nerve tumors
   Nerve sheath schwannomas* (WHO grade I)
   Nerve sheath neurofibromas* (WHO grade I)
   Malignant peripheral nerve sheath tumor (WHO grade III/IV)
Mesenchymal and neuroendocrine tumors
   Lipomas
   Fibrosarcoma
   Hemangiopericytoma
   Paraganglioma
Hematopoietic tumors
   Primary or metastatic lymphoma*
Metastases

Extradural Neoplasms
Primary bone tumors
   Hemangioma
   Chordoma
   Aneurysmal bone cyst
   Chondrosarcoma
   Ewing's sarcoma
   Fibrosarcoma
   Giant cell tumor
   Lymphoma
   Plasmacytoma
   Myeloma
   Osteoid osteoma
   Osteoblastoma
   Osteosarcoma
Neuroblastic tumors
   Neuroblastoma*
Metastatic disease to the adjacent osseous elements

WHO, World Health Organization.
*May show more often a concomitant extension to both extradural and intradural spaces.

INTRADURAL INTRAMEDULLARY TUMORS OF THE SPINE

Spinal intramedullary tumors account for 5% to 10% of all spinal tumors in adults and approximately 35% in children. The intradural intramedullary compartment represents the spinal cord itself, which explains the predominance of glial tumors (90%) in this location. Nonglial neoplasms are much less common (10%).

MRI is the modality of choice for identifying internal structural abnormalities of the spinal cord, such as edema, hemorrhage, cyst, syringohydromyelia, and contrast enhancement. Most spinal cord tumors show some degree of enhancement after intravenous contrast agent administration; however, the absence of enhancement does not exclude an intramedullary neoplasm, especially in the presence of cord expansion, cyst formation, or edema.

Approximately 60% of intramedullary tumors are accompanied by either a reactive dilatation of the central canal (syringohydromyelia; also called polar cyst, satellite cyst, or reactive cyst) or intratumoral cysts. Reactive cysts develop above and below the solid tumor, and they do not enhance on MRI. Tumoral cysts, however, are associated with a variable surrounding solid component and, in most cases, show contrast enhancement of the cyst wall. Characterization of the nature of the cyst is important, because reactive cysts simply collapse after excision of the solid component whereas tumoral cysts have to be removed.

Focal spinal cord expansion with tapered narrowing of the adjacent subarachnoid (intradural) space but intact dura mater point to the location of a space-occupying mass within the spinal cord (Fig. 15-1A). Intramedullary signal alterations in the absence of spinal cord expansion favor a non-neoplastic etiology, such as motor neuron degenerative diseases (e.g., amyotrophic lateral sclerosis), inflammatory diseases (e.g., poliomyelitis, chronic demyelination associated with multiple sclerosis), vascular causes (e.g., nonhemorrhagic cord infarction, amyloid angiopathy), or gliosis (e.g., chronic compressive myelopathy) in the differential diagnosis. The differentiation between neoplastic and non-neoplastic diseases of the spine is crucial for therapeutic planning.

Ependymoma

An ependymoma is a neuroepithelial tumor derived from the ependymal cells of the central canal. Different histologic variants include myxopapillary ependymoma and subependymoma.

Epidemiology

Ependymomas are the most common intramedullary spinal tumors in adults, accounting for up to 60% of all intramedullary tumors.[1] The mean age at presentation is around 40 years, and there is a slight male predominance. Spinal ependymomas constitute 30% of all CNS ependymomas.

These tumors are usually solitary, but multiple ependymomas of the spinal cord, often in association with other spinal masses (i.e., meningiomas and schwannomas), may be present in patients with neurofibromatosis type 2 (NF2).[2] Multiple or isolated ependymomas in the intramedullary but most often in the extramedullary-intradural space may also appear as secondary metastases of a primary intracranial or spinal ependymoma (see Fig. 15-9C, D).

Myxopapillary ependymoma of the filum terminale is a histologic variant accounting for about 13% of all ependymomas but more than 80% of all ependymomas that are located in the conus medullaris and filum terminale. These tumors are located extramedullary and occur predominantly in males. The mean age at presentation is slightly younger than 35 years.

Subependymoma, another variant of ependymoma, appears rarely in the spinal cord, and only about 40 cases have been reported in the literature. It is estimated that because of their benign course 50% are asymptomatic during life and therefore mostly found incidentally at autopsies. When symptomatic, patients are usually male (2:1) and older than 40 years of age.

Primary low-grade ependymomas of the spine (World Health Organization [WHO] grade I and II, i.e., myxopapillary ependymoma and classic ependymoma, respectively) are far more common than high-grade lesions (WHO grade III, i.e., anaplastic ependymomas).

Clinical Presentation

Patients present with a history of mild and slowly progressive neurologic impairment. The tumor's slow growth rate and tendency to compress instead of infiltrate the adjacent neural tissue often lead to a delay in primary diagnosis. The mean duration of symptoms before diagnosis is 36 months. At diagnosis most patients complain of back pain and focal sensory and/or motor deficits, depending on the segmental location of the tumor. Sensory symptoms are the predominant complaints, probably due to compression or interruption of the crossing spinothalamic tracts around the central canal.[3] An unusual presentation reported in spinal ependymomas is cranial nerve palsy. Spinal ependymomas have a tendency for causing microhemorrhages, and a delay in diagnosis may lead to superficial hemosiderosis with involvement of the caudal cranial nerves around the brain stem, producing cranial nerve symptoms. An otherwise unexplained superficial hemosiderosis in a cranial MRI study should prompt a spinal investigation with MRI for the exclusion of a spinal ependymoma.

Myxopapillary ependymomas, owing to their most frequent caudal location, usually present as lower back and leg pain and sphincter dysfunction.

Approximately 50% of subependymomas are asymptomatic. If symptomatic, patients usually complain of a long history of progressive back pain. Motor or sensory deficit may also appear, according to the segmental localization.

Pathophysiology

Ependymomas are ependymal cell tumors and are classified according to the WHO grading system for spinal cord tumors as ependymoma (WHO grade II), myxopapillary ependymoma (WHO grade I), subependy-

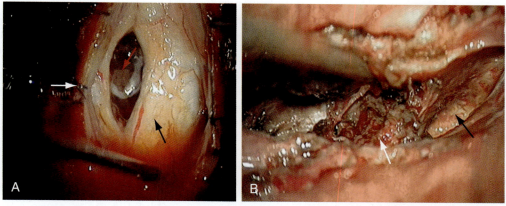

■ **FIGURE 15-2**   **A,** Macroscopic view of an intramedullary ependymoma. Retracted dura mater (*white arrow*), opened spinal cord (*black arrow*), and grayish, soft, well-demarcated intramedullary tumor (*red arrow*). **B,** Macroscopic view of a myxopapillary ependymoma. Sausage-like encapsulated tumor (*black arrow*) with compartments of less well-circumscribed, hemorrhagic, soft tumor (*white arrow*).   (*Intraoperative photographs:* **A** *courtesy of Dr. Réne-Ludwig Bernays, Neurosurgery, University Hospital, Zürich;* **B** *courtesy of Prof. Helmut Bertalanffy, Neurosurgery, University Hospital, Zürich.*)

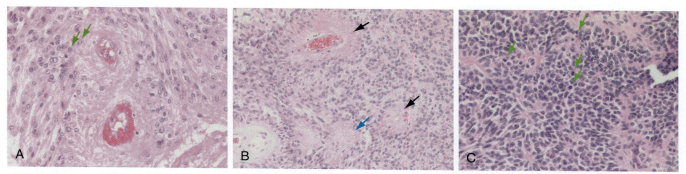

■ **FIGURE 15-3**   Ependymoma. Note uniform tumor cells with a round to oval nucleus and with speckled ("salt and pepper") chromatin (*green arrows,* **A**). The characteristic perivascular pseudorosettes (*black arrows*) or ependymal rosettes (*blue arrow*) are shown on **B**. Anaplastic ependymomas present with higher cell density and increased mitotic activity (*green arrows,* **C**). (H & E stain.)

moma (WHO grade I), and anaplastic ependymoma (WHO grade III).

Classic ependymomas originate from the ependymal cells of the central canal. Myxopapillary ependymomas arise from the ependymal glia of the filum terminale. The origin of subependymomas is uncertain. They may derive from cells of the subependymal plate or residual periventricular matrix or from tanycytes (bridging cells between the pial and ependymal layers).

Ependymomas have been documented to appear in up to 89% of patients with confirmed NF2, an autosomal dominant disorder caused by mutations of the *NF2* gene on chromosome 22q. On confirmation of NF2, clinical and radiologic evaluation, including MRI of the entire neuraxis, is crucial because presymptomatic diagnosis of spinal tumors improves the outcome of therapeutic management[4] and the prognosis.

Pathology

Ependymomas are usually well-demarcated, grayish, soft tumors (Fig. 15-2A). Myxopapillary ependymomas are often encapsulated, lobulated, sausage-shaped masses and show a soft, grayish appearance (see Fig. 15-2B). Subep-

endymomas usually present as well-demarcated, firm nodules of variable size.

Classic ependymomas are well delineated and moderately cellular. The tumor cells are uniform and mainly possess a round-to-oval nucleus with speckled ("salt and pepper") chromatin (Fig. 15-3A). A typical hallmark for ependymomas is the formation of perivascular pseudorosettes or ependymal rosettes (see Fig. 15-3B). Blood vessels are often hyalinized. If ependymomas undergo malignant transformation (anaplastic ependymoma), cell density, mitotic activity, and proliferative indices are higher (see Fig. 15-3C) and necroses and vascular proliferations are common features.

On immunohistochemistry ependymomas show positivity for glial fibrillary acidic protein (GFAP), S-100 protein, and vimentin in the majority of cases. They often show a typical dot-like staining pattern for epithelial membrane antigen (EMA).

In most myxopapillary ependymomas, areas with a papillary tumor pattern of columnar to cuboid tumor cells on a fibrovascular stroma (Fig. 15-4A) can be found. A myxoid matrix rich in microcysts is seen between tumor cells and blood vessels as well as in the tumor capsule (see Fig. 15-4B).

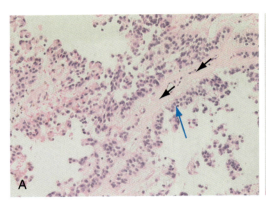

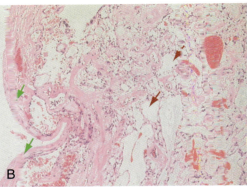

■ **FIGURE 15-4** Myxopapillary ependymoma. Note papillary tumor pattern of columnar to cuboid tumor cells (*blue arrow,* **A**) on a fibrovascular stroma (*black arrows,* **A**). A myxoid matrix with many microcysts (*red arrows,* **B**) is seen between tumor cells and blood vessels. The tumor is encapsulated (*green arrows,* **B**). (H & E stain.)

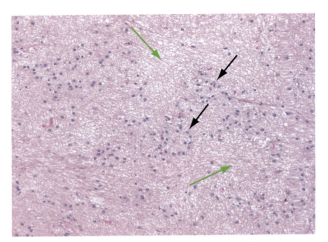

■ **FIGURE 15-5** Subependymomas have a typical appearance of clustered, relatively monomorphic tumor cells (*black arrows*) that are surrounded by a dense fibrillary matrix of glial processes (*green arrows*).

On immunohistochemical staining, myxopapillary ependymomas are typically positive for GFAP and S-100 and typically lack immunoreaction for cytokeratins.

Spinal subependymomas are characterized by clusters of cells surrounded by a dense fibrillary matrix (Fig. 15-5). The tumor cells exhibit ependymal and astrocytic differentiation markers. Microcystic changes are observed, although less commonly than in the other types of ependymomas. On immunohistochemistry they typically stain for GFAP and, to a lesser extent, for neuronal markers. Compared with the classic ependymoma, subependymomas have a very low rate of cellular proliferation, usually with an MIB-1 index below 1%.

Classic ependymomas are most commonly located in the cervical (67%) cord with or without extension into the upper thoracic region. Approximately 26% are located in the thoracic spine and 7% in the conus medullaris.[3]

Myxopapillary ependymomas are tumors of the filum terminale and the conus medullaris and, thus, they are the most common neoplasms of this region (83%).

The localization pattern of subependymomas is most often cervical and then thoracic and thoracolumbar.

Imaging

Ultrasonography

On ultrasound evaluation a sharply defined homogeneous echogenicity is seen.

CT

On CT, ependymomas show isodensity or slight hyperdensity relative to the spinal cord. Intense contrast enhancement is typical.

MRI

Ependymomas (except for the rare ectopically located ependymomas) arise from the ependymal cells of the central canal and, therefore, when small, have a central intramedullary location generating a focal, symmetric enlargement of the spinal cord. On MRI these tumors appear as circumscribed masses that are commonly hypointense/isointense to cord on T1-weighted (T1W) images and are typically hyperintense on T2W images. A variable degree of contrast enhancement is seen in more than 80% of cases (Fig. 15-6). About 80% of ependymomas are associated with cysts, which are most often reactive cysts (polar cysts) (see Box 15-1) as opposed to tumoral cysts, which occur more often with astrocytic tumors (see Fig. 15-11). Spinal cord edema surrounding the tumor to a variable extent is present in 60% of cases and more often evident in large lobular tumors (see Figs. 15-6C and 15-7C). In 20% to 30% of cases, ependymomas may be outlined by a linear T2 signal hypointensity showing hemosiderin deposition as a result of chronic microbleedings (see Fig. 15-7C), which helps in their differentiation from other contrast-enhancing glial tumors. Calcification is uncommon, as opposed to intracranial ependymomas. Owing to the central intramedullary location of the tumor, compression or disruption of medullary spinal tracts may be found on DTI (see Fig. 15-6D).

In contrast to other ependymomas, myxopapillary ependymomas show a predilection for the conus medullaris and filum terminale and are extramedullary. They appear as isointense/hypointense masses on T1W images and as isointense/hyperintense masses on T2W

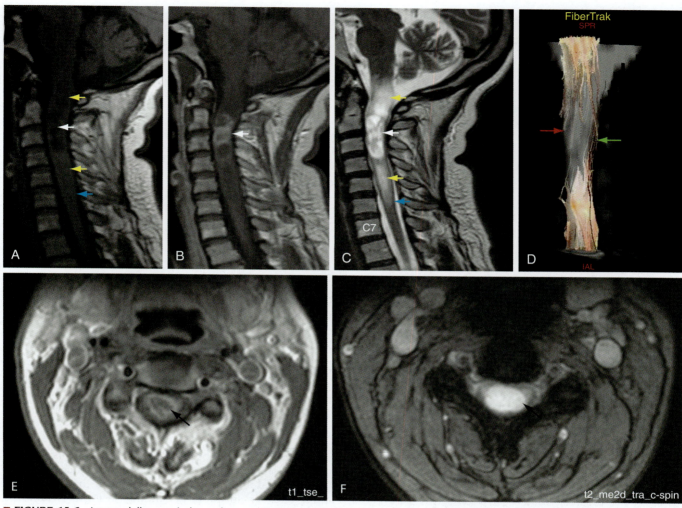

■ **FIGURE 15-6** Intramedullary cervical ependymoma. **A,** Sagittal T1W MR image demonstrates hypointense signal of the cervical cord at segment C2-C4 (*white arrow*) but also with abnormal low signal intensity in the adjacent cranial and caudal cord segments (*yellow arrows*) and associated diffuse enlargement of the cord down to segment C6 (*blue arrow*). **B,** Contrast-enhanced sagittal T1W image demonstrates inhomogeneous enhancing tumor (*white arrow*). **C,** Sagittal T2W image demonstrates relatively well-circumscribed inhomogeneous hyperintense mass that represents the tumor (*white arrow*) as well as diffuse hyperintense signal on the cranial and caudal cord by edema (*yellow arrows*) and cord enlargement down to segment C6 (*blue arrow*). **D,** Sagittal reconstruction of the longitudinal fibers shows the discontinuity of the fibers in the region of the anterior funiculus (*red arrow*) and the compression of the fibers in the region of the lateral and posterior funiculus (*green arrow*). Contrast-enhanced axial T1W image (**E**) and axial T2W STIR image (**F**) demonstrate intramedullary central location of the T2 hyperintense mass with inhomogeneous enhancement (*black arrows*).

images (Fig. 15-8). They are often associated with cystic components and invariably enhance after administration of gadolinium. Occasionally, hyperintensity on both T1W and T2W images is seen in the cystic components of the mass, reflecting mucin or hemorrhage.

Spinal subependymomas present on MRI as fusiform masses with well-defined borders. Enhancement is present in 50% of cases. This histologic subtype is often difficult to differentiate from other intramedullary tumors. A distinctive feature reported in subependymomas is their eccentric location in contrast to the central location of ependymomas.

Anaplastic ependymomas (WHO grade III) have a malignant behavior. At the time of diagnosis they tend to appear as multifocal lesions involving multiple segments of the spinal cord (Fig. 15-9). They are frequently associated

with prominent edema and hemorrhage and show a rapid progression on follow-up examinations.

Association with scoliosis, vertebral body scalloping, pedicle erosion, and laminar thinning has also been described in ependymal tumors, but these features are more often seen with extramedullary spinal neoplasms.

Spinal Cord Astrocytoma

Spinal cord astrocytoma is a neuroepithelial intramedullary tumor originating from astrocytic glial cells.

The histologic subtypes of low-grade (WHO grade I and II) astrocytomas in the spinal cord include pilocytic astrocytoma and diffuse astrocytoma, respectively, whereas the high-grade (WHO grade III and IV) subtypes include anaplastic astrocytoma and glioblastoma multiforme, respectively.

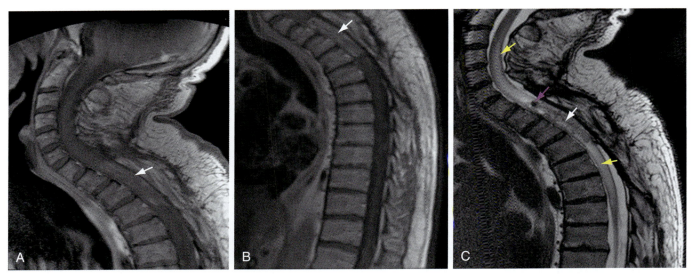

■ FIGURE 15-7 Hemorrhagic tumor recurrence of a thoracic intramedullary ependymoma. **A,** Sagittal T1W MR image demonstrates primary inhomogeneous mass with isointense/hypointense/hyperintense signal on segments T1 to T3 (*white arrow*). The hyperintense signal represents hemorrhage inside and on the margins of the mass. **B,** Contrast-enhanced sagittal T1W image demonstrates only minor inhomogeneous enhancement (*white arrow*). **C,** Sagittal T2W image demonstrates mixed isointense/hypointense and hyperintense signal of the mass (*white arrow*) and diffuse hyperintense signal cranial and caudal from the mass representing edema (*yellow arrows*). Observe the small hemosiderin cap on the cranial part of the tumor (*purple arrow*), representing chronic hemorrhage.

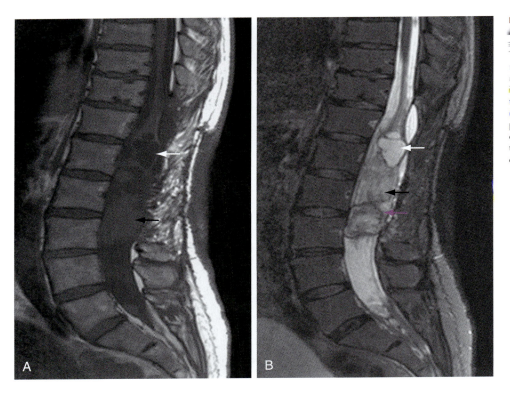

■ FIGURE 15-8 Recurrent myxopapillary ependymoma of the conus medullaris and filum terminale. Sagittal T1W (A) and sagittal T2W (B) MR images demonstrate heterogeneous mass with regions of T1 hypointense and T2 hyperintense signal (*white arrow*) corresponding to cysts and T1 and T2 isointense signal (*black arrows*) corresponding to solid parts of the tumor. Observe the hemosiderin ring on the surface of the tumor in the lower compartment representing chronic hemorrhage (*purple arrow*).

Epidemiology

Astrocytomas are the second most common intramedullary tumors after ependymomas in adults. In children, astrocytic gliomas seem to be the most commonly found intramedullary tumors, especially owing to the high frequency of pilocytic astrocytoma. The incidence of primary spinal cord astrocytoma is reported as 2.5 per 100,000 per year, being 10-fold less than primary astrocytomas of the brain.[5] Low-grade astrocytomas are more common than high-grade tumors. Primary glioblastoma multiforme of the spinal cord is very rare, accounting only for 0.2% to 1.5% of all spinal cord astrocytomas. Radiation-induced glioblastoma multiforme is extremely rare, with only a few reported cases in the literature.[6] Secondary spinal astrocytomas from metastatic dissemination of a primary

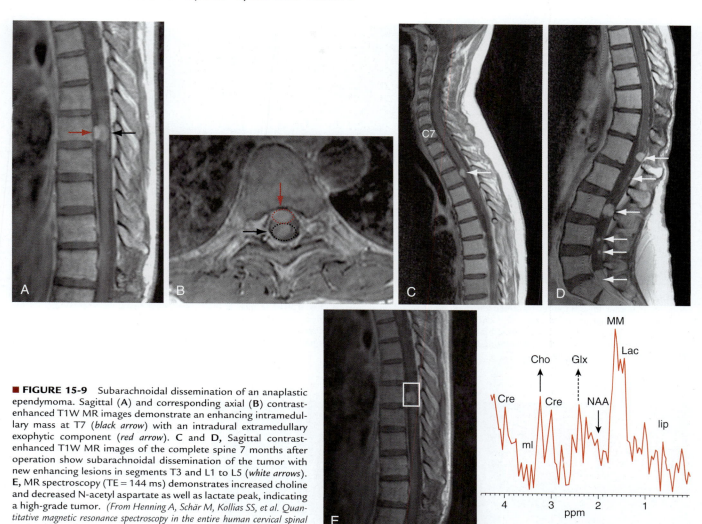

■ **FIGURE 15-9** Subarachnoidal dissemination of an anaplastic ependymoma. Sagittal (**A**) and corresponding axial (**B**) contrast-enhanced T1W MR images demonstrate an enhancing intramedullary mass at T7 (*black arrow*) with an intradural extramedullary exophytic component (*red arrow*). **C** and **D**, Sagittal contrast-enhanced T1W MR images of the complete spine 7 months after operation show subarachnoidal dissemination of the tumor with new enhancing lesions in segments T3 and L1 to L5 (*white arrows*). **E**, MR spectroscopy (TE = 144 ms) demonstrates increased choline and decreased N-acetyl aspartate as well as lactate peak, indicating a high-grade tumor. (*From Henning A, Schär M, Kollias SS, et al. Quantitative magnetic resonance spectroscopy in the entire human cervical spinal cord and beyond at 3T. Magn Reson Med 2008; 59:1250-1258.*)

intracranial malignant astrocytoma are more frequent than primary spinal cord astrocytic gliomas.

In adults, the average age at onset is 29 years, a presentation that is earlier than that for ependymomas. Men are more commonly affected.

Clinical Presentation

The course of disease is related to the histologic grade of the tumor. Patients with low-grade tumors have mild neurologic impairment and a slowly progressive course, whereas high-grade tumors are associated with rapidly progressing neurologic symptoms. The neurologic deficits depend on the segmental localization of the mass and are nonspecific. Chronic back pain and focal sensory and/or motor deficits are the most common complaints. Because conus medullaris involvement is rare, bowel and bladder dysfunctions are also uncommon.

Because of the infiltrative nature of astrocytomas, resection is not feasible and the prognosis is far worse than that for classic ependymomas.

Pathophysiology

Spinal cord astrocytomas are glial cell tumors and are classified according to the WHO grading system for spinal cord tumors as low grade, including pilocytic astrocytoma (WHO grade I) and diffuse astrocytoma (WHO grade II), and high grade, including anaplastic astrocytoma (WHO grade III) and glioblastoma multiforme (WHO grade IV).

Several genetic mutations have been reported in low- and high-grade tumors, including mutation of the well-known tumor suppressor *TP53*, growth factor receptors (platelet-derived growth factor/receptor [PDGF/R] over-expression and epidermal growth factor receptor [EGFR] amplification), *RB* mutation. cell cycle protein CDK4 amplification, PTEN loss, 19q loss, 11p loss, INK4a/ARF loss, gain of chromosome 7, and loss of chromosome 10 or 10q.[7]

Pathology

Pilocytic astrocytomas are usually sharply delineated and often show cystic formations.

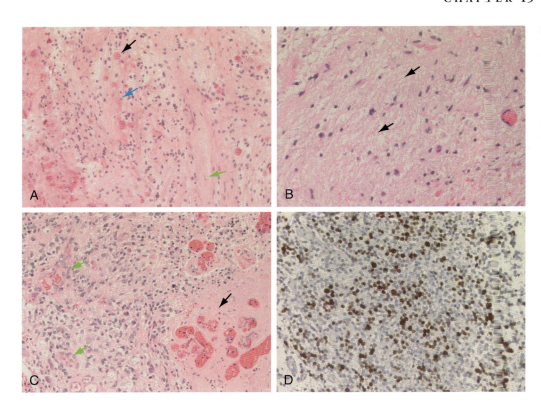

■ **FIGURE 15-10** A, Pilocytic astrocytoma showing low to moderate cell density with varying proportions of bipolar cells (*blue arrow*) with Rosenthal fibers (*green arrow*). Microcysts and eosinophilic granular bodies/hyaline droplets are frequently found (*black arrow*). B, Diffuse astrocytoma shows low cell density with tumor cells of uniform morphology within a dense fibrillary matrix (*black arrows*). C, Glioblastoma multiforme shows high cellularity. The hallmarks are necroses (*black arrow*), which are often accompanied by hypercellular pseudopalisading border zones, and vascular proliferations (*green arrows*). D, Proliferation index of glioblastoma multiforme is usually high; here, around 15% of the tumor cells stain for the proliferation marker MIB-1. (**A** to **C**, H & E stain.)

Diffuse astrocytomas show diffuse borders owing to their infiltrative growth pattern. The normal CNS tissue is usually infiltrated but not destroyed. Cyst formation is occasionally present.

Glioblastoma multiforme is usually poorly delineated. The internal composition of the lesion is very inhomogeneous, showing hemorrhages and necroses.

Pilocytic astrocytomas are of low to moderate cell density with varying proportions of bipolar cells with Rosenthal fibers. Microcysts and eosinophilic granular bodies/hyaline droplets are frequently found (Fig. 15-10A). On immunohistochemical stains the tumor cells are positive for GFAP and S-100. The MIB-1 proliferation index is usually low (up to 4%).

Low-grade diffuse astrocytomas show low cell density with tumor cells of uniform morphology within a dense fibrillary matrix (see Fig. 15-10B). On immunohistochemical staining the tumor cells are positive for GFAP and S-100. The MIB-1 proliferation index is usually low (less than 4%).

Glioblastomas are highly cellular pleomorphic astrocytic tumors. The hallmarks are necroses, which are often accompanied by hypercellular pseudopalisading border zones and vascular proliferations (see Fig. 15-10C). On immunohistochemistry a large fraction of tumor cells stain positive for GFAP and S-100. The MIB-1 proliferation index is usually high, often more than 15% (see Fig. 15-10D).

The thoracic cord is the most common site of involvement, followed by the cervical cord.

Imaging

CT

On CT, low-grade astrocytomas present as hypodense, homogeneous, ill-defined masses with minimal or absent contrast enhancement that cause an enlargement of the spinal cord. High-grade tumors may show areas of more intense contrast enhancement and internal heterogeneity. Mild bone scalloping with spinal canal widening can be seen, but less commonly than with ependymomas or with extramedullary intradural tumors.

MRI

On MRI, pilocytic astrocytomas may enhance homogeneously or heterogeneously or may show no enhancement at all (Figs. 15-11 and 15-12).

Diffuse astrocytomas also often present as hypointense to isointense masses on T1W images and appear hyperintense on T2W images. They have poorly defined margins, and differentiation of the tumor border from adjacent edema is difficult. Contrast enhancement is usually mild and may be focal or diffuse or may be completely absent (Fig. 15-13). Enhancement alone cannot be used to differentiate between low- and high-grade gliomas. The tumor may extend to several vertebral segments, and multifocal or even holocord variants have also been described (especially in association with pilocytic astrocytoma). Associated cysts are commonly observed (more frequently than in ependymomas), particularly with pilocytic type tumors, and they can be reactive or tumorous (see Fig. 15-1 C). Hemorrhage is uncommon, in contrast to ependymomas. As astrocytomas arise from the parenchyma of the cord, they are usually eccentrically located in the cord as opposed to ependymomas, which are typically centrally located (see Analysis and Fig. 15-97, later). The accurate cross-sectional localization of the tumor on axial T2W images is important for planning the operative approach and should always be

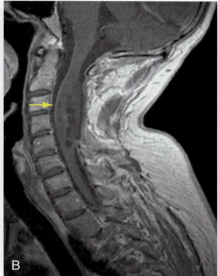
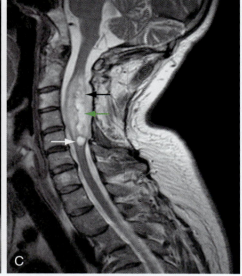

■ **FIGURE 15-11** Intramedullary cervical pilocytic astrocytoma. **A,** Sagittal T1W MR image demonstrates hypointense intramedullary mass at C2 to C5 (*black arrow*) leading to diffuse enlargement of the cord, with a garland-like hyperintense component representing blood (*purple arrow*). A tumorous cyst is also seen (*green arrow*). **B,** Contrast-enhanced sagittal T1W image demonstrates no enhancement of the tumor. Only the anterior spinal vein is seen on the anterior surface of the cord (*yellow arrow*). **C,** Sagittal T2W image demonstrates an inhomogeneous hyperintense mass (*black arrow*) with a polar cyst (*white arrow*) as well as a tumorous cyst (*green arrow*). This is an unusual case, regarding the hemorrhage and the nonenhancement of the tumor.

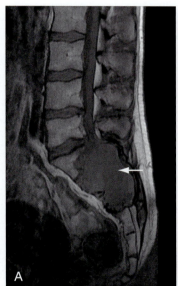
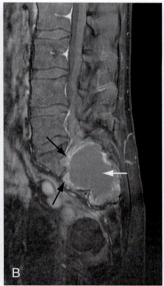
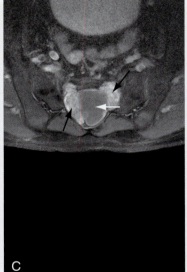
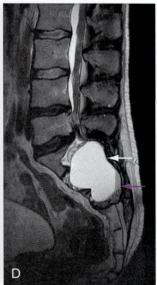

■ **FIGURE 15-12** Pilocytic astrocytoma of the lumbosacral junction. **A,** Sagittal T1W MR image demonstrates an intradural hypointense cyst at L5 to S3 (*white arrow*). **B,** Sagittal T1W contrast-enhanced, fat-saturated image demonstrates the cyst (*white arrow*) and some solid, contrast-enhancing parts (*black arrows*). **C,** Axial contrast-enhanced, fat-saturated T1W image demonstrates the cyst (*white arrow*) and the solid, enhancing tumor parts (*black arrows*). **D,** Sagittal T2W image demonstrates the hyperintense cyst (*white arrow*) and a T2 hypointense niveau in the caudal part of the cyst caused by sedimentation of blood in the lying position during examination (*purple arrow*).

reported. Exophytic components, similar to brain stem gliomas, have also been described with spinal cord astrocytomas (see Fig. 15-9A,B).

Primary glioblastoma multiforme of the spinal cord is a rare entity, and only few reports are found in the literature. Like intracranial primary glioblastoma multiforme, the intraspinal counterpart also shows a strong peripheral enhancement, surrounding edema, as well as, in 60% of cases, a leptomeningeal spread, which helps to differentiate it from other intramedullary tumors (Fig. 15-14).

Oligodendroglioma

This neuroepithelial tumor originates from oligodendroglial cells. According to the histologic grading they include oligodendroglioma (WHO grade II) and anaplastic oligodendroglioma (WHO grade III).

Epidemiology

Primary spinal oligodendroglioma is a very rare pathologic entity representing 2% of spinal cord tumors and 1.5% of

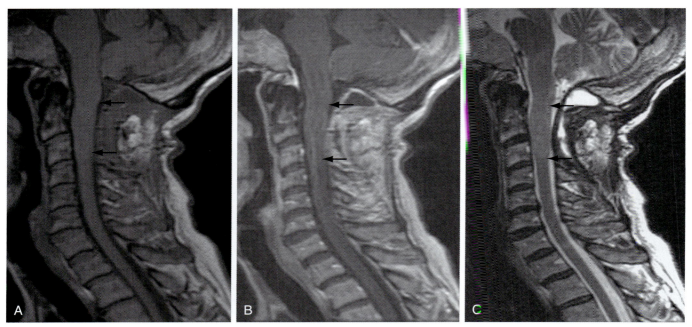

■ **FIGURE 15-13** Intramedullary cervical low-grade astrocytoma. **A,** Sagittal T1W MRI demonstrates an intramedullary, isointense mass at C2-C3 (*black arrows*) with diffuse enlargement of the cord. **B,** Contrast-enhanced sagittal T1W image demonstrates the same mass (*black arrows*) with no enhancement. **C,** Sagittal T2W image demonstrates inhomogeneous isointense/hyperintense mass with poorly defined margins (*black arrows*).

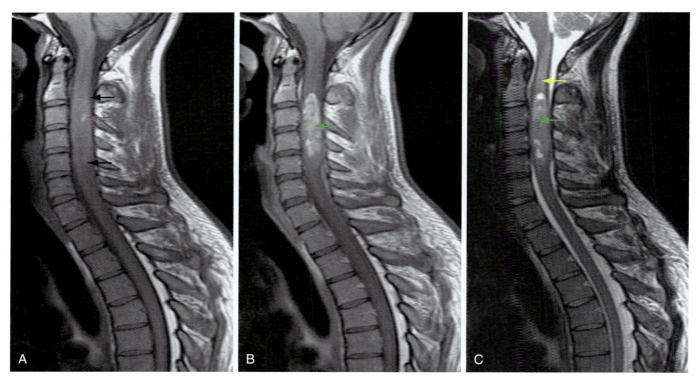

■ **FIGURE 15-14** Intramedullary cervical glioblastoma multiforme. **A,** Sagittal T1W MR image demonstrates an intramedullary mass of the cord at C2 to C5 with mostly isointense signal (*black arrows*) leading to diffuse enlargement of the affected cord. Intratumoral hemorrhage is seen presenting as hyperintense signal (*purple arrow*). **B,** Contrast-enhanced sagittal T1W image demonstrates strong, inhomogeneous enhancement (*green arrow*). **C,** Sagittal T2W image demonstrates mixed signal intensity with predominant isointense/hyperintense signal (*green arrow*) and peritumoral edema (*yellow arrow*).

all oligodendrogliomas. Fewer than 50 cases have been reported in the literature. Among these cases, 60% of patients were older than age 16 years and 40% were younger. A slight male predominance was observed.[8]

Clinical Presentation

Depending on the involved segment, the clinical presentation is one of long-standing back pain and sensorimotor symptoms.

Pathophysiology

Oligodendrogliomas arise from oligodendroglial cells of the neural tissue.

Pathology

Oligodendrogliomas usually appear as soft, well-defined grayish masses. The frequently observed calcification may impart a gritty texture to the tissue.

The tumors appear moderately cellular and are composed of monomorphic cells with round nuclei that are often surrounded by an empty halo ("honeycomb" appearance). A dense network of branching capillaries and microcalcifications are also typical features. If oligodendrogliomas undergo malignant transformation (anaplastic oligodendroglioma, WHO grade III), cell density, mitotic activity, and proliferation are higher and necroses and vascular proliferations are common. A specific immunohistochemical marker for oligodendrogliomas is not available, although a perinuclear staining pattern of microtubule associated protein-2 (MAP2) is typical for these tumors.

The most common site of involvement is the thoracic and cervical spine with much fewer cases in the lumbar area. Cases of holocord involvement are also reported, with all these patients being younger than 16 years of age.[8]

Imaging

CT

On CT there are no typical features to differentiate these tumors from other intramedullary gliomas except for intratumoral calcification, which may suggest the diagnosis of oligodendroglioma.

MRI

Oligodendrogliomas are isointense to spinal cord on T1W images and hyperintense on T2W images and show inhomogeneous, spotty contrast enhancement. Intratumoral hemorrhages, calcification, and associated syringohydromyelia are common findings.[8]

Ganglioglioma

Gangliogliomas are rare tumors composed of a mixture of neoplastic mature neuronal elements and glial elements. According to the predominance of glial or neuronal elements in their histologic composition, various names are used, including ganglioglioma, gangliocytoma, ganglioneuroblastoma, ganglionic neuroma, neuroastrocytoma, ganglionic glioma, neuroglioma, and ganglioneuroma.

Epidemiology

Overall, around 90 cases of spinal intramedullary gangliogliomas have been described in the literature. Gangliogliomas account for 1% of spinal cord tumors and 0.4% to 6.5% of all primary CNS tumors. The mean age at presentation is 19 years of age with a predominance in childhood. There is no gender predilection.

Clinical Presentation

Gangliogliomas are usually considered slow-growing, nonaggressive, benign tumors and, therefore, the clinical course is mostly slowly progressive. Duration of symptoms ranges from 1 month to 5 years. The most common symptom is paraparesis (50%), followed by segmental pain (46%), but gait disturbance, sensory deficit, and sphincter disturbance have also been reported. Scoliosis is often associated.

In general, the symptoms are very mild considering the extent of the tumor as seen on the MRI examination, which often involves several spinal cord segments at the time of diagnosis. In the very rare cases of malignant variant (anaplastic ganglioglioma, WHO grade III), the clinical symptoms are rapidly progressive.

Pathophysiology

The histologic classification of gangliogliomas is based on the relative differentiation of the neuronal component and the presence of glial elements. When composed of mature neuronal components without a glial component, that is, when tumors contain only mature ganglion cells, they are classified as gangliocytomas (WHO grade I). When additional neoplastic astrocytic elements are present, they are classified as gangliogliomas (WHO grade I/II). Less-differentiated types are extremely rare and include the anaplastic ganglioglioma (WHO grade III).

Pathology

Gangliogliomas usually appear as well-circumscribed solid lesions. Cysts and calcifications are seen less frequently than in their intracranial counterparts.

Gangliogliomas are composed of neuronal and glial components. The neuronal component often consists of large, multipolar or multinucleated neurons ("dysplastic" neurons), whereas the glial component may resemble other low-grade glial tumors such as pilocytic astrocytoma, diffuse astrocytoma, or oligodendroglioma (Fig. 15-15).

In immunohistochemistry the neuronal component is usually stained by antibodies for neural proteins such as MAP2, NeuN, neurofilament, or synaptophysin. The glial component usually stains for GFAP.

Gangliogliomas of the spinal cord have a preference for the cervical and thoracic segments. They frequently extend to multiple segments and may involve the entire spinal axis (holocord presentation).

Imaging

CT

Bony remodeling and calcifications can be depicted with CT.

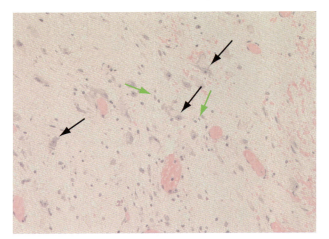

■ **FIGURE 15-15** Multipolar or multinucleated neurons ("dysplastic" neurons) (*black arrows*) accompanied by mostly inconspicuous glial cells (*green arrows*). The glial component of a ganglioglioma may be more prominent than in this case. (H & E stain.)

MRI

Gangliogliomas do not have any specific imaging feature that would help differentiating them from low-grade glial tumors of the spinal cord. They result in fusiform enlargement of the spinal cord and they are eccentrically located (like astrocytomas, preferentially in the cervical cord and thoracic cord, with only few cases reported in the conus medullaris like astrocytomas). The only helpful feature in the characterization might be the mixed signal intensity on T1W images, which is speculated to be the reflection of the dual cellular composition from glial and neuronal elements. On T2W images gangliogliomas are mostly hyperintense (Fig. 15-16), and on contrast-enhanced T1W images there is a mostly absent or a mild patchy enhancement pattern. Calcifications occur much less frequently in spinal gangliogliomas than in intracranial gangliogliomas.[3,9]

Hemangioblastoma

This meningothelial-related tumor has an unknown cell of origin.

Epidemiology

Hemangioblastomas represent the third most frequent intramedullary spinal cord tumor after ependymoma and

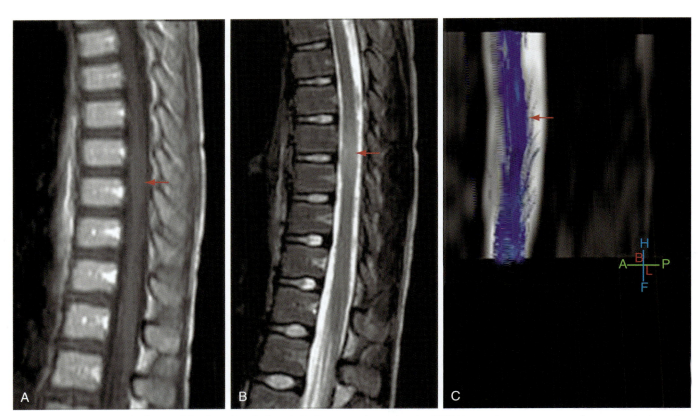

■ **FIGURE 15-16** Ganglioglioma of the thoracic spinal cord. **A,** Contrast-enhanced sagittal T1W image demonstrates no enhancement in the region of the enlarged thoracic cord (*red arrow*). **B,** Sagittal T2W image demonstrates inhomogeneous mild hyperintense signal (*red arrow*). **C,** The diffusion tensor image shows that the longitudinal fibers of the spinal cord are not disrupted through the tumor (*red arrow*).

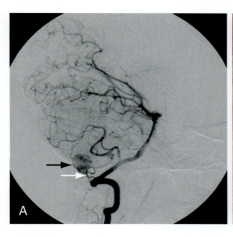

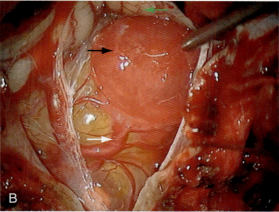

■ **FIGURE 15-17** Hemangioblastoma of the medulla oblongata. The preoperative catheter angiogram (**A**) and the intraoperative photograph (**B**) show the hypervascularized red nodulus of the tumor (*black arrow*) with a feeder meningeal artery of the right vertebral artery (*white arrow*). Observe the compressed cerebellar tonsil on the right side (*green arrow*). (*Intraoperative photograph courtesy of Dr. Evaldas Cesnulis, Neurosurgery, University Hospital of Zürich.*)

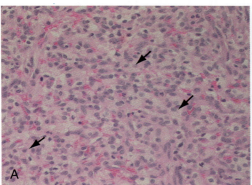

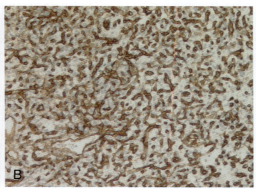

■ **FIGURE 15-18** **A,** Hematoxylin and eosin stain of a hemangioblastoma shows the large and often vacuolated stromal cells (*black arrows*). **B,** Immunohistochemical stain for endothelial marker CD34 shows the "matrix" of abundant vascular cells forming thin-walled vessels.

astrocytoma.[10] They account for up to 1% to 7% of all spinal cord neoplasms and show no gender predilection. The age at presentation is younger than 40 years.

Clinical Presentation

Because of the tumor's preferential location in or near the dorsal columns, sensory deficits are the most common clinical presentation, especially with deficits in proprioception. Back pain and motor dysfunction are also common. The course of symptoms is usually slowly progressive owing to the slow growth of these lesions. The mean duration of symptoms is 38 months. Patients may also present with acute subarachnoidal or intramedullary hemorrhage due to the high vascularity of these tumors, which may lead to spontaneous or chronic microhemorrhages.[10]

Pathophysiology

Hemangioblastoma can occur as a solitary tumor in up to 70% of cases or as multiple lesions as part of the von Hippel-Lindau (VHL) syndrome in up to 30%.[3] VHL is an autosomal dominant disorder characterized by the development of tumors in different organs. Apart from cerebellar and spinal hemangioblastomas, other associated tumors include retinal hemangioblastomas, pheochromocytomas, renal cell carcinomas, renal cysts, pancreatic cystadenomas, and pancreatic neuroendocrine tumors. The incidence of VHL is estimated to be 1:40,000 live births, and nearly 70% of patients with VHL will develop hemangioblastomas of the CNS as part of the syndrome during their life. The VHL syndrome is classified as type 1 when pheochromocytoma is not part of the clinical features and as type 2 when it is present. Type 2 is further classified into subtype A when renal cell carcinoma is present and subtype B when it is absent. *VHL* is a tumor suppressor gene located on chromosome 3p25-26 and is responsible for this disease spectrum on inactivation. Genetic testing for mutations in *VHL* should therefore be considered in patients with hemangioblastomas and other neoplasms of the VHL syndrome.[11]

Pathology

Hemangioblastomas appear as well-circumscribed, highly vascular reddish nodules (Fig. 15-17) and are often found along the wall of large cysts with prominent dilated vessels. These tumors consist of large and often vacuolated stromal cells that lie in a "matrix" of abundant vascular cells forming thin-walled vessels (Fig. 15-18).

On immunohistochemistry, the stromal cells variably express S-100 and neuron-specific enolase while the endothelial cells stain for various endothelial markers (CD31, CD34).

Spinal cord hemangioblastomas present in the thoracic region in up to 50% of cases, followed by the cervical region in up to 40% of cases. This distribution probably

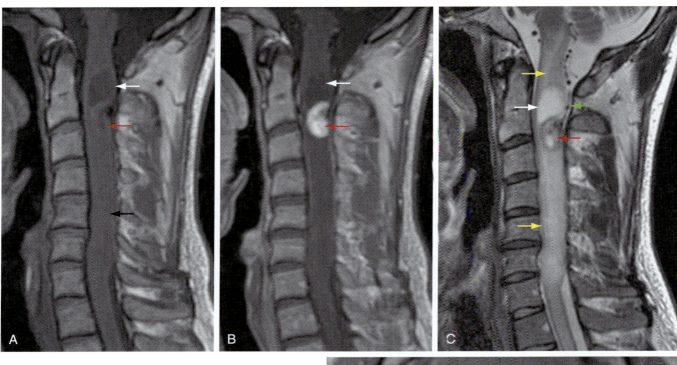

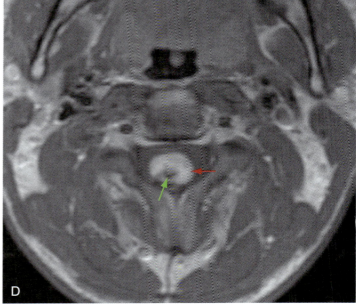

■ **FIGURE 15-19** Intramedullary cervical hemangioblastoma. **A,** Sagittal T1W MRI demonstrates the isointense tumor nodulus (*red arrow*), the well-circumscribed hypointense cyst at C2 segment (*white arrow*), and diffuse enlargement of the spinal cord below the mass reaching the C7 segment (*black arrow*). **B,** Contrast-enhanced sagittal T1W image demonstrates the strong enhancing, well-delineated tumor nodule (*red arrow*) and the hypointense, nonenhancing cyst (*white arrow*). **C,** Sagittal T2W image demonstrates the supplying artery as flow void (*green arrow*), the hyperintense cyst (*white arrow*), the inhomogeneous nodule (*red arrow*), and the diffuse edema of the cord, cranial and caudal from the tumor (*yellow arrows*). **D,** Contrast-enhanced axial T1W image demonstrates the intramedullary location of the mass with strong enhancement of the nodule (*red arrow*) and a central hypointensity (flow void) representing the feeder artery (*green arrow*).

reflects the longest length of the thoracic cord with its 12 segments. Up to 75% of these tumors appear intramedullary, and 25% can involve the intradural or extradural space.

Imaging

CT

CT may reveal the diffuse expansion of the spinal cord and the hypodense cystic lesion.

MRI

The classic MR appearance of hemangioblastoma is a strongly enhancing tumor nodule with tortuous flow voids, representing feeding arteries, in the periphery of a cyst (cyst with a mural nodule) (see Box 15-3). Extensive spinal cord enlargement is common owing to venous congestion and edema (Fig. 15-19).[10] Hemangioblastomas appear isointense/hypointense on T1W images and hyperintense on T2W images. The tumor nodule enhances homogeneously and intensively after intravenous administration of a contrast agent. MR angiography (MRA) is an important noninvasive method for the preoperative evaluation of the tumor, particularly when endovascular embolization is performed before surgery. Contrast-enhanced MRA provides detailed information about the tumor's vascular architecture by demonstrating the dilated and tortuous feeding arteries as well as the perimedullary draining veins (see Analysis and Fig. 15-99, later). The solid nodule of the tumor is mostly small, measuring a few millimeters, but it has the potential to extend over several segments. Hemangioblastomas, particularly when associated with VHL disease, can be multiple (see Box 15-3); and, therefore, it is important that the entire spinal axis is included in the diagnostic MRI protocol. Associated cysts are a common feature of cerebellar hemangioblastomas, but in the spinal cord entirely solid lesions are more frequent.

MRI is an important modality for screening of patients with a positive family history of VHL syndrome.

Special Procedures

Myelography may show the tortuous vessels, although this method is today completely replaced by MRI/MRA.

Catheter spinal angiography is performed for preoperative embolization to reduce intraoperative bleeding and demonstrates the highly vascularized mass and identifies the feeding arteries and the draining veins (see Fig. 15-17; see Box 15-3). With the advent of MRI/MRA, catheter angiography has lost its diagnostic significance and is only indicated if preoperative superselective embolization of the tumor is planned.

Intramedullary Spinal Cord Metastasis

The Greek word "metastasis" means displacement and is applied to describe the spreading or dissemination of neoplastic cells from distant primary tumors.

Epidemiology

Intramedullary metastases are very rare, with a reported incidence of up to 2% in patients with different types of cancer. Metastatic disease of the spinal cord is more often extramedullary in location, arising via cerebrospinal fluid (CSF) seeding from a primary intracranial CNS neoplasm, or more uncommonly is intramedullary from hematogenous spread of other systemic carcinomas. The most common primary sources of intramedullary metastatic disease are lung cancer (61%), breast cancer (11%), melanoma (5%), renal cell carcinoma (4%), colorectal carcinoma (3%), lymphoma (3%), and tumors of unknown origin (5%).[12]

Clinical Presentation

The most common complaints are pain, bowel and bladder dysfunction, and paresthesia. The clinical course is usually rapidly progressive, and in most cases the duration of symptoms is less than 1 month before diagnosis. Survival after diagnosis ranges from weeks to months in most series.

Pathophysiology

Metastatic disease may develop due to vascular (hematogenous) or lymphatic (lymphogenic) spreading or directly via CSF (drop metastasis) with finally seeding of the neoplastic cells into the spinal cord, generating intramedullary metastasis.

Pathology

Metastases are often circumscribed, rounded, gray-white or tan masses. They often show central necrosis or hemorrhages or contain mucous material in the case of adenocarcinoma.

Tumor metastases often resemble their tissue of origin; therefore, they would all be different histologically.

Intramedullary metastasis may occur anywhere along the spinal cord.

Imaging

MRI

In general, intramedullary metastasis results in mild expansion of the spinal cord with high signal intensity on T2W images, representing the tumor but also edema and syrinx (Fig. 15-20). The associated edema is disproportionately extensive compared with the size of the tumor. Accompanying tumorous cysts are rare, as opposed to primary intramedullary tumors. Contrast enhancement is intensive with or without central necrotic areas (Fig. 15-21). There are no typical features for characterizing the different metastatic neoplasms; the only clue is the histologically verified primary tumor.

Other Very Rare Spinal Intramedullary Tumors

Paragangliomas, lipomas, schwannomas, and neurofibromas are discussed in the "intradural extramedullary" section, hematopoietic tumors in the "extradural" section, and germ cell tumors in the chapter on the pediatric spine.

Very rarely, sarcomas may arise in the spinal cord. Depending on the mesenchymal cell of origin they represent specific histologic types such as meningeal sarcoma, hemangiosarcoma, gliosarcoma, granulocytic sarcoma, fibrosarcoma, and Ewing's sarcoma. They do not possess distinct neuroradiologic features, which could help in characterizing them.

Melanocytomas and melanomas, on the other hand, demonstrate typically low signal on T2W images and isointensity/hyperintensity on T1W images, owing to the paramagnetic radicals from melanin pigment. However, this feature is often mistaken for blood decomposition products and these cases are most commonly misdiagnosed as cavernoma or hemorrhagic neuroepithelial (ependymal/glial cell) tumors.

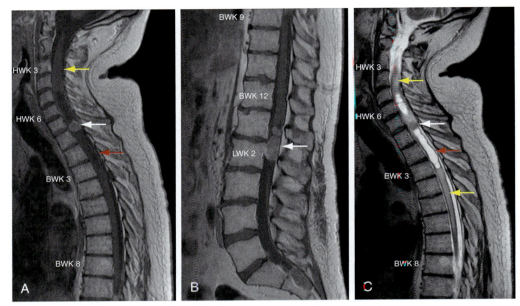

■ **FIGURE 15-20** Intramedullary metastasis. **A,** Contrast-enhanced sagittal T1-weighted image of the cervical and upper thoracic spine shows extensive intramedullary hypointense signal on the cord segments C5-T3 representing edema (*yellow arrow*), syrinx (*red arrow*), and a nodular contrast-enhancing lesion on the segment C7-T1 representing the tumor mass (*white arrow*). **B,** Contrast-enhanced sagittal T1-weighted image of the lower thoracic and lumbosacral spine shows a second contrast-enhancing lesion at the level of the conus medullaris and filum terminale (*white arrow*). **C,** Sagittal T2-weighted MRI shows the isointense signal of the tumor (*white arrow*), the diffuse hyperintensity representing edema (*yellow arrows*), and dilatation of the central canal caudal from the tumor mass, termed syrinx (*red arrow*).

INTRADURAL EXTRAMEDULLARY SPINAL TUMORS

The intradural extramedullary space comprises the anatomic area between the pia mater surrounding the neural tissue with the superficial vessels of the spinal cord and the dural sac extending from the foramen magnum to the S2-S3 vertebral bodies. Approximately 30% of all spinal tumors in adults arise in the intradural extramedullary space (slightly less common in children), and an additional 5% show concomitant intradural and extradural components. Tumors within this space either arise primarily from nerve sheath cells covering the spinal nerve roots (schwannomas and neurofibromas) or from arachnoidal cells of the arachnoidea covering the inner surface of the dura (meningiomas). Less commonly, mesenchymal tumors, mixed neuronal-glial tumors, hematopoietic tumors, and metastases are observed in this space. Several textbooks classify myxopapillary ependymomas in the category of intradural extramedullary spinal tumors owing to their frequent origin from the filum terminale and their primary extramedullary location. They represent a particular histologic subtype of ependymomas and are discussed together with other types of ependymomas in the section dealing with intramedullary tumors. MRI is the modality of choice for imaging of spinal tumors. Hallmark findings for the localization of a mass in the intradural extramedullary space are the focal displacement of the cord away from the mass and the enlargement of the subarachnoid space both caudal and cranial to the tumor (see Fig. 15-1B). Often, but not always, the dural sac itself can be identified as a thin line, hypointense on both T1W and T2W images in the periphery of the tumor, which facilitates the correct localization in the intradural space.

Nerve Sheath Tumors: Schwannoma and Neurofibroma

Schwannomas are benign, encapsulated nerve sheath tumors composed of proliferating Schwann cells. Alternate names for schwannoma are neurinoma and neurilemmoma.

Neurofibromas are benign, unencapsulated tumors of the peripheral nerves composed by proliferating Schwann cells mixed with fibroblasts.

Epidemiology

Nerve sheath tumors (schwannoma + neurofibroma) represent the most common primary neoplasia (30%) in the spine as well as in the intradural extramedullary space (30%).[14] The incidence of spinal nerve sheath tumors is reported to be slightly higher or equal to that of spinal meningiomas.

The peak incidence of nerve sheath tumors is in the fourth to fifth decades, and they affect men and women equally. Schwannomas are much less common in children, representing less than 10% of intraspinal tumors. The presence of multiple schwannomas in a young child should prompt further investigations for NF2, particularly owing to the higher risk of malignant transformation and the predisposition of NF2 to other neoplasms in addition to nerve sheath tumors such as intramedullary ependymomas. Neurofibromas are much less common than schwannomas.

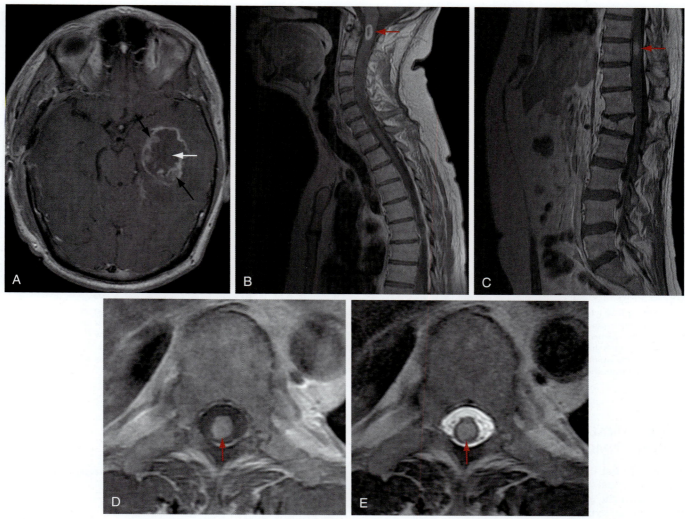

■ **FIGURE 15-21**   Metastatic glioblastoma multiforme. **A,** Contrast-enhanced axial T1W image demonstrates primary tumor of the left temporal lobe with typical peripheral contrast enhancement (*black arrows*) and hypointense necrotic core (*white arrow*). **B,** Contrast-enhanced sagittal T1W MR image of the cervical and upper thoracic spine demonstrates a second mass with peripheral enhancement representing metastasis at the level of the medulla oblongata (*red arrow*). **C,** Contrast-enhanced sagittal T1W MR image of the lower thoracic and lumbar spine demonstrates a second enhancing intramedullary lesion of the segment at T10 (*red arrow*). **D,** Contrast-enhanced axial T1W image confirms the intramedullary location of the thoracic mass (*red arrow*). **E,** Observe in an axial T2W image the hyperintense signal of the mass (*red arrow*).

Clinical Presentation

Symptoms related to the presence of a nerve sheath tumor may precede the diagnosis by more than 2 years because there is usually little functional impairment. The most frequent symptoms, common to all nerve sheath tumors, are pain and radiculopathy.

Malignant transformation of a nerve sheath tumor should be suspected if there is rapid growth or exacerbation of pain.

Pathophysiology

Schwannomas (WHO grade I) are usually solitary lesions and are most commonly sporadic. They arise from a single focus, most commonly in the dorsal sensory roots, and usually develop asymmetrically forming a well-encapsulated, lobulated, firm mass that compresses the adjacent tissue without invading the involved nerve.

Multiple schwannomas occur with NF2, a phacomatosis caused by inactivation or deletion of *NF2* on chromosome 22 that occurs sporadically in 50% of cases and as an autosomal dominant disorder in another 50% of cases. A subgroup of patients with multiple schwannomas in the absence of bilateral vestibular schwannomas (which is pathognomonic of NF2) has also been described. This condition is known as schwannomatosis in the literature, although it is still controversial as to whether it is a distinct clinicopathologic entity or a phenotypic manifestation of NF2.

Neurofibromas (WHO grade I) are commonly associated with neurofibromatosis type 1 (NF1), particularly when multiple, but can also occur sporadically. Neurofibromas associated with NF1 are related to a defect or loss of *NF1* on chromosome 17.

Melanotic schwannoma is differentiated from a typical schwannoma by heavy pigmentation. Psammoma bodies

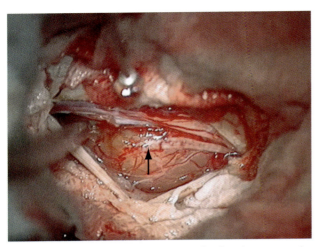

■ **FIGURE 15-22** Intraoperative photograph of a schwannoma shows a well-circumscribed, global lesion attached to (i.e., arising from) a nerve root (*arrow*). (*Courtesy of Prof. Helmut Bertalanffy, Neurosurgery, University Hospital of Zürich.*)

can be visualized in more than 50% of melanotic schwannomas. Half of patients with such "psammomatous melanotic schwannomas" have Carney complex, a dominantly transmitted autosomal disorder consisting of myxomas (cardiac, cutaneous, and mammary), mucocutaneous spotty pigmentation, and pigmented adrenal tumors with endocrine overactivity.[15]

Malignant types of nerve sheath tumors (WHO grade III/IV) are rare (2% to 6% of cases) and arise either de novo from the nerve sheath or as a malignant degeneration of preexisting nerve sheath tumors (more often neurofibromas than schwannomas). Plexiform neurofibromas associated with NF1 show malignant degeneration in 3% to 5% of cases, and 50% to 60% of malignant peripheral nerve sheath tumors (MPNSTs) are associated with NF1. Malignant nerve sheath tumors have a variety of names such as malignant neuroma, malignant schwannoma, nerve sheath fibrosarcoma, and neurofibrosarcoma, reflecting their histologic heterogeneity. Malignant nerve sheath tumors only rarely arise in the CNS but may arise more peripherally and then infiltrate back into the spinal column.

Pathology

Schwannomas arise from the Schwann cells of the nerve axon's myelin sheath. They are usually encapsulated globoid masses (Fig. 15-22) with a cut surface of light tan tissue with yellow patches (see Box 15-4).

Neurofibromas are usually firm, fusiform, and well-circumscribed lesions that are grayish tan on cut surface.

Schwannomas are composed of neoplastic Schwann cells that grow in two distinct growth patterns, either as compact areas with elongated cells and occasional nuclear palisading (Antoni A pattern) or as less cellular regions with indistinct processes (Antoni B pattern). They are usually composed of a variable mix of both patterns but can also be composed exclusively of one of these patterns (Fig. 15-23A). Most tumor cells show a basement membrane along their surface as demonstrated by a reticulin

stain. Vessels in schwannomas are often highly hyalinized (see Fig. 15-23A).

Schwannomas may also demonstrate extensive cystic change (see Fig. 15-23B). A rare subtype of schwannoma is the melanocytic schwannoma (see Fig. 15-23C, D). These tumors resemble schwannomas but additionally contain melanosomes, leading to a brownish coloration of a fraction of tumor cells. They are strongly reactive to various melanoma markers.

Neurofibromas are to a large part composed of small Schwann cells along fewer numbers of intermixed fibroblasts in a matrix of collagen fibers and myxoid material (see Fig. 15-23E). On immunohistochemistry, neurofibromas are invariably stained by antibodies against S-100. Staining for neurofilament often demarcates remnants of infiltrated nerve disrupted by infiltrating tumor cells (see Fig. 15-23F).

Rarely schwannomas and more often neurofibromas may show transformation to an epithelial malignant peripheral nerve sheath tumor (EMPNST) or to an angiosarcoma and then display a high grade of nuclear pleomorphism and cellular density. Mitotic figures are frequently seen (see Fig. 15-23G) and the proliferation index is high (see Fig. 15-23H). On immunohistochemistry, the tumor cells strongly express S-100, and staining for basal lamina (collagen IV) often demonstrates a surface staining of most cells. The staining for S-100 is often weak after transformation to EMPNSTs.

Seventy to 80 percent arise from the nerve roots (most commonly the dorsal sensory nerve roots) before leaving the dural sac and are entirely intradural (Fig. 15-24A). A further 10% to 20% arise as the nerve root leaves the dural sac and therefore display both intradural and extradural components (dumbbell tumors) (see Fig. 15-24B). Entirely extradural schwannomas are less common (<10%) (see Fig. 15-24C, D). Intramedullary schwannomas are very rare (<1%) and are believed to arise from the perivascular nerve sheaths that accompany penetrating spinal cord vessels.

Most commonly affected are the cervical regions, with less frequent involvement of the thoracic and lumbar spine.[14]

Neurofibromas are histologically more complex lesions of proliferated Schwann cells and fibroblasts mixed with acid polysaccharides that enlarge within the nerve itself, spreading apart the axons to produce a fusiform lesion. Brachial or lumbar plexus neurofibromas may extend centrally into the intradural space along multiple nerve roots and may even result in subpial extension.

Imaging

CT

CT is not the primary modality for imaging of spinal tumors and is only indicated in cases when there are contraindications to MRI, in which case a CT myelography should be performed for better anatomic delineation of the lesion in the intradural extramedullary space and its relationship to nerve roots. CT provides additional information related to the consequences of the tumor on the adjacent bony

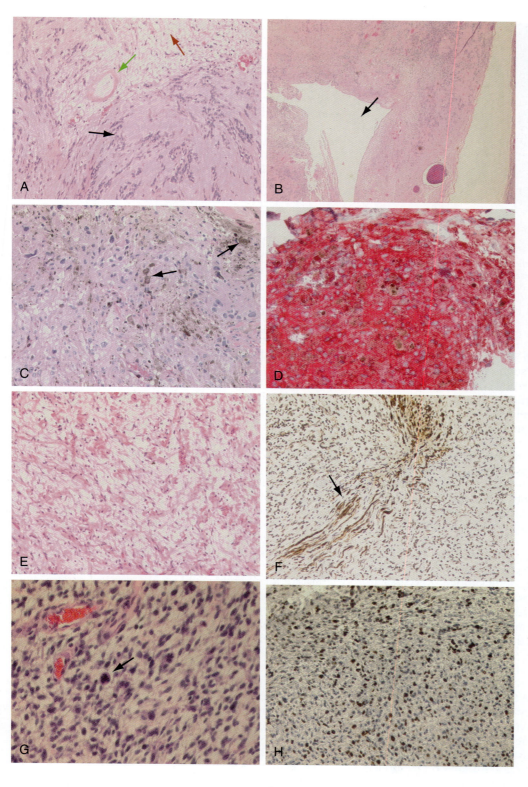

■ **FIGURE 15-23** A to D, Schwannoma. **A**, Neoplastic Schwann cells that grow either as compact areas with elongated cells and occasional nuclear palisading (Antoni A pattern, *black arrow*) or as less cellular regions with indistinct processes (Antoni B pattern, *red arrow*). Vessels are often highly hyalinized (*green arrow*). **B**, Intratumoral cyst (*black arrow*). **C**, Melanocytic schwannoma with the pathognomonic melanosomes leading to a brownish coloration of a fraction of tumor cells (*black arrows*). **D**, Tumor cells are strongly reactive to Melan A with a red immunoreaction product. **E** and **F**, Neurofibroma. **E**, A tumor mainly composed of small spindle-shaped cells (Schwann cells) along with fewer numbers of intermixed fibroblasts in a matrix of collagen fibers and myxoid material. **F**, Remnants of infiltrated nerve disrupted by infiltrating tumor cells (*black arrow*). **G** and **H**, Malignant peripheral nerve sheath tumor. **G**, High-grade nuclear pleomorphism and cellular density. Mitotic figures are frequently seen (*black arrow*). **H**, MIB-1 proliferation index is high (here around 10%). (A-C, E, G: H & E stain; D, F, H: immunohistochemical stain.)

structures. Foraminal enlargement with erosion of the pedicles and thinned laminae and posterior vertebral scalloping are adequately demonstrated on bone window CT images and may provide useful information for the preoperative planning. The tumor itself appears as an isodense or slightly hypodense soft tissue mass displacing the cord.

After contrast agent administration a variable degree of contrast enhancement is observed, ranging from moderate to intense, depending on the consistency of the tumor (see Fig. 15-24). Calcifications and gross hemorrhages are rare. Melanotic schwannomas present as hyperdensity on native CT (see Fig. 15-27).

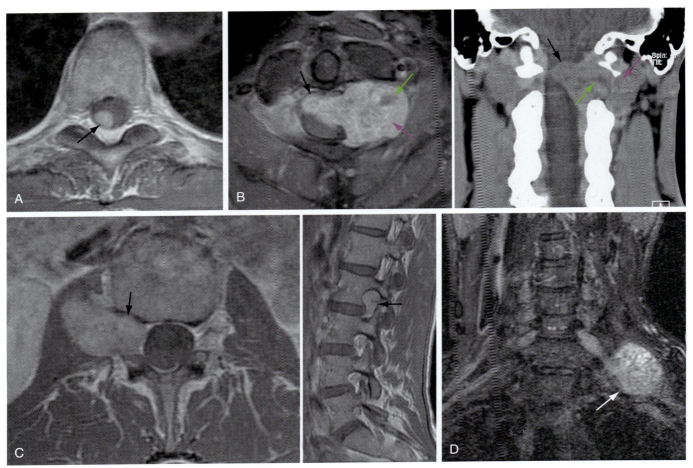

■ **FIGURE 15-24** Possible localizations of a schwannoma. **A,** Axial contrast-enhanced MR image shows an intradural schwannoma (*black arrow*). **B,** Axial contrast-enhanced MR image (*left*) and coronal contrast-enhanced CT (*right*) demonstrate a dumbbell-shaped schwannoma with a smaller intradural (*black arrows*) and a larger extradural (*purple arrows*) compartment. Note the consecutive bony erosions of the adjacent bony structures as well as the cystic degenerative part of the lesion, corresponding to Antoni B pattern (*green arrows*). **C,** Axial (*left*) and sagittal (*right*) contrast-enhanced MR images show an extradural intraforaminal schwannoma enlarging the intervertebral foramen (*black arrows*). **D,** Coronal STIR MR image demonstrates a giant paravertebral schwannoma (*white arrow*).

MRI

MRI provides an excellent delineation of nerve sheath tumors and their location relative to the dural sac, and the cord is depicted accurately in most cases (see Fig. 15-24). Schwannomas and neurofibromas are mostly indistinguishable on imaging, although there are some hints that help in the characterization (see Analysis and Fig. 15-101, later). They appear as solid, circumscribed masses, isointense to slightly hypointense on T1W images and hyperintense on T2W images compared with cord. Schwannomas often demonstrate a heterogeneous signal on T2W images, corresponding to the mixed Antoni A and B pattern (i.e., compact areas and less cellular regions, respectively). A schwannoma may also present predominantly with one or the other pattern (see Analysis and Fig. 15-103, later). On postcontrast T1W images, they show an intense contrast enhancement (Fig. 15-25).

Intraforaminal and extraforaminal lesions can be better delineated on short tau inversion recovery (STIR) images owing to the suppression of the epidural intraforaminal and paraspinal intermuscular fat (see Fig. 15-24D).

Most schwannomas are small (a few millimeters), but they can be large as well. By definition a lesion is called a "giant schwannoma" if it (1) stretches over two vertebral levels or (2) extends extraspinally more than 2.5 cm or (3) extends into the myofascial plains (see Box 15-4; see Fig. 15-24D). These tumors require biopsy because the differential diagnosis includes malignant nerve sheath tumor.[15] Spinal schwannomas may rarely result in hemorrhages in all compartments of the spine (intramedullary, subarachnoidal, subdural, intratumoral bleeding).

Schwannomas may show a cystic morphology; however, nodular thickening of the wall on contrast-enhanced images helps to differentiate them from other cystic lesions of the spine (Fig. 15-26).

A subtype of schwannomas is the melanotic/melanocytic schwannoma, which is characterized by cytoplasmic deposition of melanin pigment. This is also reflected by the hypointensity on T2W images and hyperintensity on T1W images (and hyperdensity on native CT) due to the paramagnetic effect of the melanin (Fig. 15-27). It is difficult to differentiate this tumor from metastatic malignant melanoma by MRI.

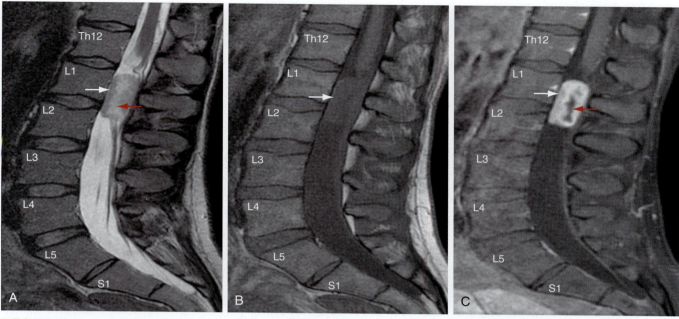

■ **FIGURE 15-25** Sagittal T2W (**A**), T1W (**B**) and contrast-enhanced (**C**) MR images show a typical schwannoma in the region of the cauda equina with a hyperintense signal on T2W, isointense signal on T1W, and a strong contrast enhancement (*white arrows*). Observe the degenerative cystic part of the lesion (*red arrows*).

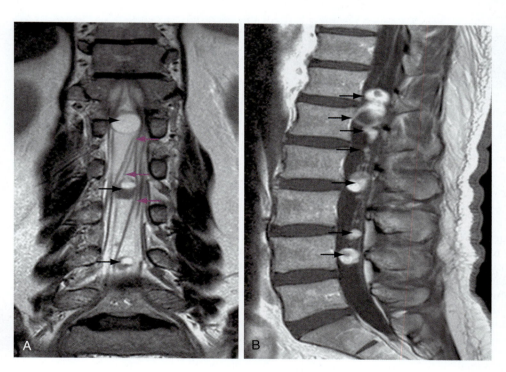

■ **FIGURE 15-26** Coronal T2W (**A**) and sagittal contrast-enhanced (**B**) MR images show multiple cystic lesions with strong contrast enhancement (*black arrows*), which was presumed to be cystic schwannomatosis. No other tumors and no stigmata for neurofibromatosis type 2 or other phacomatoses were present. Note the displacement of the cauda equina nerve roots (*purple arrows*).

Intraosseous schwannoma has been reported in the literature with an extensive bony destruction.[16]

Malignant transformation may be suspected in the presence of a rapidly increasing tumor mass on follow-up examination, ill-defined tumor margins with unclear separation from the cord parenchyma, prominent tumor heterogeneity with central necrosis, and prominent edematous changes in the compressed cord tissue. Malignant transformation is most commonly associated with plexiform neurofibromas and NF1.

Special Procedures

Positron emission tomography (PET) is useful in distinguishing benign from malignant nerve sheath tumors.

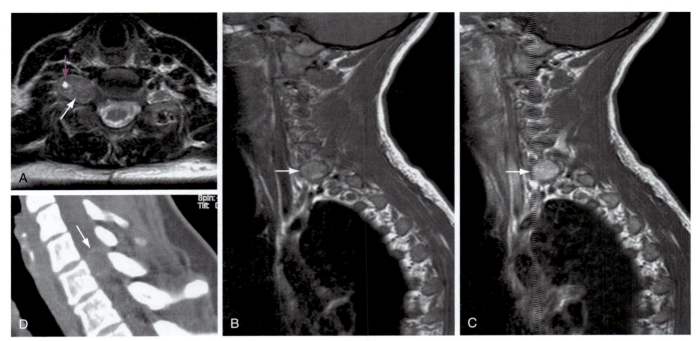

■ FIGURE 15-27   Axial T2W (**A**), sagittal T1W (**B**), sagittal contrast-enhanced (**C**) MR images and sagittal CT (**D**) image demonstrates a melanotic schwannoma (*white arrows*) with the typical signal intensities for melanin pigment: hypointensity on T2W, hyperintensity on T1WI, and hyperdensity on CT. Strong contrast enhancement is typical. Observe the small cystic degeneration on the T2W image (*purple arrow, A*).

Meningioma

Meningioma is a neoplasm arising from cells of the arachnoidea.

Epidemiology

Meningioma is a common tumor among primary spinal neoplasms, accounting for 25% to 46% of cases, and is the second most common tumor (25%) after schwannomas in the subarachnoid space (extramedullary intradural location) in the spine. Ten to 13 percent of all meningiomas arise in the spine.

Females are most often affected (82%), with tumors occurring most frequently in middle-aged and elderly women. Most of the patients are 40 to 80 years old; however, some cases in children have also been reported.

Ossified meningiomas are extremely rare and estimated to be 0.7% to 5.5% of all spinal meningiomas.

Clinical Presentation

The predominant symptom is localized or radicular pain (83%), followed by sensory loss (50%). Paresis is present in 83% of the patients at the time of diagnosis. Bladder or bowel disturbances occur in 36% of cases. Meningiomas are benign, slow-growing tumors; therefore, the duration of symptoms before diagnosis may range from 4 months to 2 years. The very rare anaplastic meningiomas follow an aggressive clinical course with 70% recurrence rate and 30% metastasis rate.

Pathophysiology

Spinal meningiomas arise either from cap cells of the arachnoid membrane (meningothelial cells), hence the name meningotheliomatous meningioma, or from fibroblasts or trabecular cells of the deep arachnoid layers, hence the name fibrous and transitional meningioma.

It has been suggested that the histologic progression and growth of spinal meningiomas depend on genetic changes as well as on sex steroid hormones. Genetic studies showed a loss of one homologue of the long arm of chromosome 22, which is supposed to be the site of a putative tumor suppressor gene.

Almost 99% of all spinal meningiomas are WHO grade I. WHO grade II spinal meningioma has not yet been reported and grade III meningioma occurs only in 1.3% of all spinal meningiomas. WHO grade II and III meningiomas occur far less frequently in the spine than in intracranial locations, which can be explained by different meningeal development in these regions.[17] A dural tail sign is present in 57% to 67% of all meningiomas regardless of intraspinal or intracranial location. It can represent either tumor invasion or hypervascularity with vessel congestion or both. The dural tail sign (either intracranial or intraspinal) is not specific for meningiomas, and it has been identified with other intradural tumors (e.g., metastasis, lymphoma, sarcoidosis). However, spinal schwannoma with dural tail has not yet been reported; therefore, it seems to be a useful feature in distinguishing meningiomas from schwannomas in the spine.

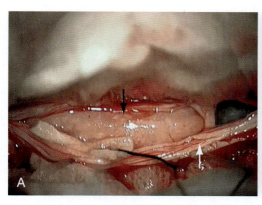
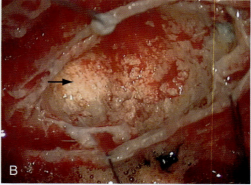

■ **FIGURE 15-28** **A,** Meningioma with a firm surface (*black arrow*). **B,** Meningioma with a rubbery surface (*black arrow*). Both are well-circumscribed lesions. Notice the compressed nerve roots of the cauda equina (*white arrow*). (*Intraoperative photographs:* **A,** *courtesy of Prof. Helmut Bertalanffy, Neurosurgery, University Hospital of Zürich;* **B,** *courtesy of Dr. Réne-Ludwig Bernays, Neurosurgery, University Hospital of Zürich.*)

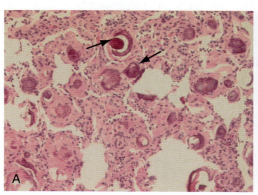
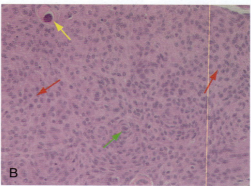

■ **FIGURE 15-29** **A,** Psammomatous meningioma characterized by excessive numbers of psammomatous bodies (*black arrows*). **B,** Meningotheliomatous meningioma shows large pseudosyncytial lobules (*red arrows*), less well-formed whorls (*green arrow*), and only a few psammomatous bodies (*yellow arrow*). (H & E stain.)

Pathology

The adjacent bony structures are much less affected (sclerosis, infiltration) in the spine than intracranially, probably owing to the wider and fat-filled epidural space.

Meningiomas arise from various cells of the arachnoidal layer with potential infiltration of the adjacent dura.

The adjacent nerves are displaced through the tumor.

Meningiomas appear as firm or rubbery (Fig. 15-28), well-demarcated globular masses often with a broad attachment to the dura. The cobblestoned external contour is reflected by the characteristic lobulated cut surface of these lesions.

Meningiomas show a wide range of histologic appearance. The most common benign subtypes are meningotheliomatous (syncytial) and fibrous and transitional meningiomas. Most meningioma subtypes share some histologic features, including indiscernible cellular borders ("pseudosyncytial appearance"), frequent cytoplasmic-nuclear inclusions, whorl formation, a collagen-rich matrix with foci of spindle cells, and the occurrence of calcification in the form of psammoma bodies. The subtypes of meningiomas show a characteristic combination of these features. For example, psammomatous meningioma is characterized by excessive numbers of psammomatous bodies (Fig. 15-29A) while meningotheliomatous meningioma shows large pseudosyncytial lobules, less well-formed whorls, and only a few psammomatous bodies (see Fig. 15-29B). On immunohistochemistry the vast majority of meningiomas stain for EMA.

Because the thoracic spine is the longest segment of the spine, most meningiomas present there (55%-80%); however, the cervical (15%-18%) and the lumbar (2%) spine can be involved as well. The location of meningiomas is completely intradural-extramedullary in 83%-87%, intramedullary in 3%, and extradural in 14% of the cases. Meningiomas are most often located lateral (50%-68%), posterior (18%-31%), and anterior (15%-19%) to the spinal cord.

Imaging

CT

CT reveals the hyperdense calcifications of the lesion as well as the adjacent dura mater (Fig. 15-30D). Osseous sclerosis or infiltration in the spine is rare, as opposed to the intracranial meningiomas.

MRI

Meningiomas are well-circumscribed lesions with a lobular architecture. Characteristic signal intensity of spinal meningiomas is relative homogeneous isointensity or hyperintensity both on T1W and T2W images compared with the spinal cord. These tumors show relatively homogeneous and moderate contrast media enhancement (in contrast to the strong and irregular contrast enhancement of schwannomas (see Analysis and Fig. 15-103, later). Meningiomas are somewhat lobular with a slightly

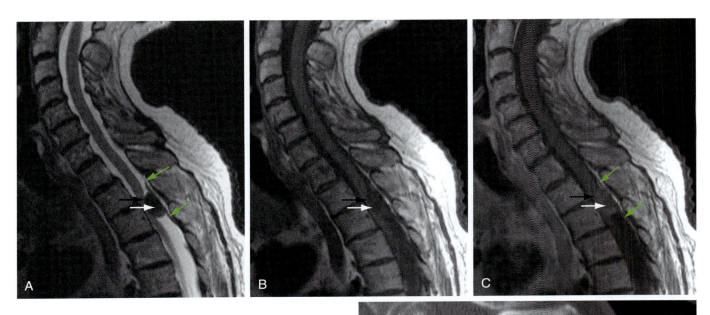

■ FIGURE 15-30 Psammomatous meningioma (*black arrows*) on sagittal T2W (**A**), sagittal T1W (**B**), sagittal contrast-enhanced (**C**) MR images and sagittal CT (**D**). Characteristic is the prominent calcification of the lesion reflected by the hypointense signal both on T2W and T1W imaging and the hyperdensity on the CT image. Note the central hypointensity and hyperdensity consistent with a denser calcification (*white arrows*). The *green arrows* indicate the calcification in the adjacent dura mater. There is mild contrast enhancement.

irregular surface, and they have a broad dural attachment. Although thickening and strong contrast enhancement of the dura adjacent to the tumor ("dural tail sign") is not specific for meningiomas, it occurs in most (57%-67%) of the cases (Fig. 15-31).

Special Procedures

Meningiomas demonstrate a typical angiographic architecture with a strong and long-lasting tumor blush. The capillary blush often is characteristic in persisting through the venous phase of the arteriogram. To reduce bleeding during surgery, superselective embolization and devascularization of the tumor can be performed.

Lipoma

A lipoma is a benign tumor of adipose tissue. Histologic variants include angiolipoma and myolipoma.

Epidemiology

Nondysraphic intradural lipoma is a rare lesion, accounting for 4% of all spinal lipomas. It represents less than 1% of all spinal tumors.

Filum terminale lipoma accounts for 12% of spinal lipomas. It is a relatively common lesion, with an incidence of 4% to 6% in the population.

Spinal lipoma is commonly associated with spinal dysraphism; 84% of all spinal lipomas belong to the lipo/myelo/meningocele group.

Angiolipoma, myolipoma and liposarcoma represent very rare histopathologic entities.

Clinical Presentation

Nondysraphic lipomas become symptomatic in early adulthood, usually in the second decade of life. Compression of the spinal cord produces a slow, progressive deterioration of neurologic function, including spinal pain, dysesthesias, paraparesis and tetraparesis, ataxia, and incontinence, usually followed by rapid progression of the symptoms.[18] Although lipomas are not neoplasms, they have the potential to grow with increasing body fat or in association with metabolic changes, such as in pregnancy.

Pathophysiology

Nondysraphic lipomas are congenital, benign lesions of the adipose tissue. They are considered to be hamartomas

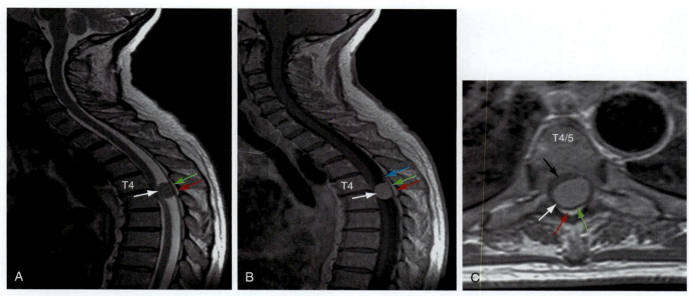

■ FIGURE 15-31   Typical meningioma (*white arrows*) on sagittal T2W (**A**), sagittal (**B**), and axial contrast-enhanced (**C**) MR images present as isointensity on T2W imaging and with homogeneous mediocre contrast enhancement. The spinal cord is compressed anterior and to the right side (*black arrow*). Observe the dura mater (*green arrows*), the dural tail (*blue arrow*), the epidural fat (*red arrows*), and the broad-based attachment of the tumor to the dura mater.

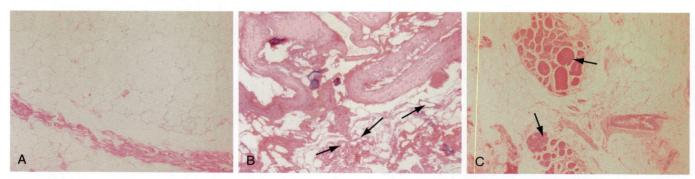

■ FIGURE 15-32   **A,** A lipoma with a typical chicken-wire appearance. **B,** The abundance of blood vessels (especially capillary blood vessels) (*arrows*) leads to the diagnosis of angiolipoma. **C,** The additional presentation of skeletal muscle (*arrows*) or smooth muscle leads to the diagnosis of myolipoma. (H & E stain.)

by development from pluripotent embryonic mesenchymal cells (e.g., meninx primitiva) that may occur during neural tube closure. As a consequence, there is no clear cleavage plane between lipoma and spinal cord, which can make total removal impossible, especially when lipomas incorporate adjacent nerve roots.

Pathology

Lipomas are bright yellow lesions and often adhere to the spinal cord. They may show a delicate encapsulation and septation on cut surface.

Because lipids are lost during histologic preparation in alcohol and xylene, only the empty cells remain for histology. The lesion is practically indistinguishable from mature adipose tissue and presents as a typical chicken-wire appearance (Fig. 15-32A). In some cases the abundance of blood vessels (especially capillary blood vessels) has led

to the designation of angiolipoma; in many cases, however, as in this example, the differentiation of angiolipomas from fat-rich hemangiomas is not possible (see Fig. 15-32B). In some lumbar lipomas with developmental origin, skeletal muscle or smooth muscle may be an additional feature (see Fig. 15-32C). Because the histologic appearance of lipomas is so typical, generally no immunohistochemistry is required for diagnosis.

Among nondysraphic lipomas, the thoracic and cervicothoracic locations are the most common, followed by the cervical spine. Most of the lumbosacral lipomas are associated with a dysraphic state. They are almost always located in a dorsal, juxtamedullary position with anterolateral compression of the spinal cord and encasement of the nerve roots (Fig. 15-33). Most often, they extend over several spinal levels and may reach a significant size before diagnosis.

Filum fibrolipomas are located in the filum terminale. Most angiolipomas arise in the thoracic epidural spine.

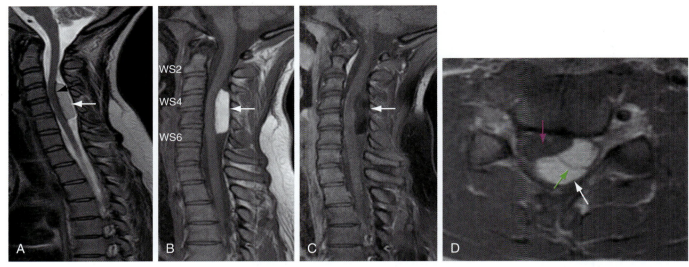

■ **FIGURE 15-33** Intradural lipoma of the cervical spine. Sagittal T2W (**A**), sagittal T1W (**B**), contrast-enhanced fat-saturated sequence (**C**), and axial T1W (**D**) MR images demonstrate a T1/T2 hyperintense, well-circumscribed lesion intradural and extramedullary (*white arrows*) with local widening of the spinal canal and compression of the spinal cord anteriorly and to the right (*purple arrow,* **D**). Observe the chemical shift artifact (*black arrow,* **A**) and the encasement of a dorsal nerve root (*green arrow,* **D**). The fat-saturated sequence with hypointensity of the lesion confirms the diagnosis.

Imaging

Ultrasonography

Lipomas show as echogenic intraspinal masses on ultrasound evaluation.

CT

CT features for lipoma are characteristic: the widened spinal canal is filled out by a lesion with fat density. The spinal cord is compressed anterolaterally. A large lesion may cause spinal block on myelography.

MRI

MRI demonstrates specific patterns that help differentiate lipoma from other primary spinal tumors. Both on T1W and T2W images these tumors show a hyperintense signal with no particular contrast enhancement (see Fig. 15-33). They are well-circumscribed, lobulated masses. An imaging technique with suppression of the fat (hypointense to CSF) confirms the diagnosis.

Filum fibrolipomas demonstrate a hyperintense mass in the region of the filum terminale and can be associated with a low-lying conus and tethered cord (Fig. 15-34).

Myolipoma can be indistinguishable from teratoma or dermoid cyst (Fig. 15-35).

Paraganglioma

Paragangliomas are extra-adrenal pheochromocytomas originating from the chromaffin cells of the autonomic nervous system. They are also called chemodectomas or glomus tumors.

Epidemiology

There is no age or gender predominance. The average age at presentation is 45 to 50 years.

Clinical Presentation

Because paraganglioma is most frequently located in the region of the conus medullaris and cauda equina, common symptoms are back or leg pain, sensory or motor disturbances, and bowel/bladder incontinence. The duration of symptoms ranges from days to years. Most of the spinal paragangliomas are not functional, that is, they do not produce catecholamines.

Pathophysiology

Paragangliomas arise from extra-adrenal neural crest cells. Eighty to 90 percent are in the carotid body or jugular bulb. The spine is an uncommon location. A paraganglionic differentiation of peripheral neuroblasts in the filum terminale is the suggested cause. Intraspinally, only sporadic cases have been reported. In contrast to paragangliomas of the head and neck, there have been no reports of familial cases of cauda equina paragangliomas. However, a germline mutation has been reported in a patient with spinal paraganglioma.[19]

Pathology

Paragangliomas are well-circumscribed, delicately encapsulated soft masses with a red to brown coloration and an occasional calcification of the capsule.

These tumors are composed of uniform round chief cells forming small nests (Zellballen) that are surrounded by a single layer of elongated sustentacular cells. Delicate septa of reticulin fibers and capillaries separate the nests,

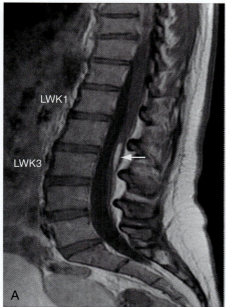

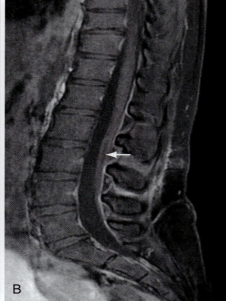

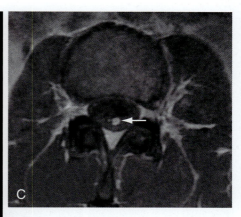

■ **FIGURE 15-34** Fibrolipoma of the filum terminale. Sagittal contrast-enhanced T1W images without (**A**) and with (**B**) fat saturation and axial contrast-enhanced T1W (**C**) MR image show the thickened fatty filum terminale (*white arrows*). Note the normal position of the conus medullaris.

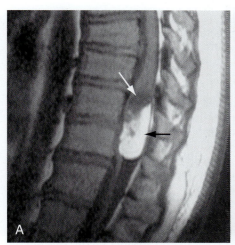

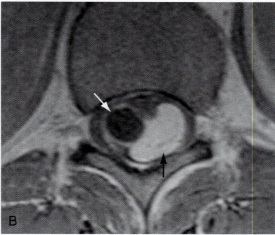

■ **FIGURE 15-35** Myolipoma of the conus medullaris. Sagittal T1W (**A**) and axial contrast-enhanced (**B**) MR images show the lipoid (*black arrows*) as well as a cystic, contrast-enhancing (*white arrows*) compartment. The diagnosis was made by histology, because the tumor is indistinguishable from teratoma or dermoid on imaging.

giving the tumor a lobulated appearance (Fig. 15-36A). In some cases, mature ganglion cells are also seen. On immunohistochemistry, the chief cells show a neuronal differentiation and stain for various neuronal markers such as chromogranin A (see Fig. 15-36B). The sustentacular cells are typically stained by S-100 and GFAP.

Paragangliomas of the spine occur almost exclusively in the region of the cauda equina.

Imaging

CT

CT may depict bony erosion due to large paragangliomas as well as a well-delineated, contrast-enhancing mass.

MRI

Paragangliomas present as a hypointense/isointense signal on T1W images and isointense/hyperintense signal on T2W images. The lesions are well circumscribed and show intense contrast enhancement (Fig. 15-37). Characteristic are the multiple flow voids representing the hypervascularity of the tumor, which gives the typical "salt and pepper" appearance; that is, "salt" represents the contrast enhancement of the tumor and "pepper" reflects the flow voids of the arteries.

Special Procedures

Selective catheter angiography demonstrates tumor blush in the early arterial phase. Angiography is indicated if preoperative embolization is performed.

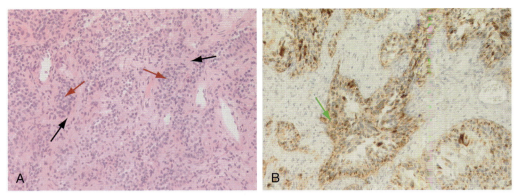

■ **FIGURE 15-36** **A,** Hematoxylin and eosin stain of a paraganglioma shows the uniform, round chief cells forming small nests (Zellballen) (*red arrows*) that are surrounded by a single layer of elongated sustentacular cells that are not easily identified in conventional histology. Delicate septa of reticulin fibers and capillaries separate the nests (*black arrows*), giving the tumor a lobulated appearance. **B,** Immunohistochemistry for chromogranin A marks the chief cells in a brown color (*green arrow*).

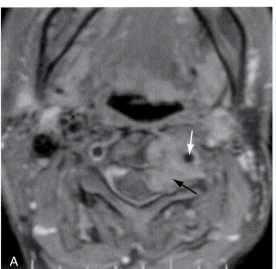
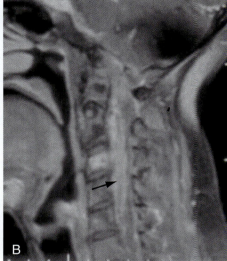

■ **FIGURE 15-37** Axial (**A**) and sagittal contrast-enhanced (**B**) MR images demonstrate a transforaminal and transosseous paraganglioma extension in the intradural space (*black arrows*) with compression of the spinal cord. The vertebral artery is encased but not narrowed (*white arrow*). The patient had multiple paragangliomas: glomus caroticum, vagale, and jugulotympanicum.

Metastasis

Epidemiology

At autopsy, approximately 5% of cancer patients have intradural extramedullary spinal metastasis. They are either drop lesions from intracranial metastasis of breast (36%), lymphoma (28%), or lung (16%) cancer and melanoma[10] or drop lesions from intracranial primary CNS tumors such as medulloblastoma (48%), high-grade glioma (26%), ependymoma (12%), retinoblastoma (5%), pineal tumors (3%), and choroid plexus papilloma (1%). Tumor dissemination from primary CNS tumors occurs more often in younger patients, whereas metastasis from secondary CNS tumors is more common in older patients.

In about 9% of cases, leptomeningeal metastasis is the first presentation of a systemic malignancy.

Clinical Presentation

Patients may be asymptomatic or present with nonspecific symptoms, such as localized spinal pain, radicular syndromes, motor and sensory deficits, and incontinence.

Pathophysiology

Metastasis in the intradural extramedullary space develops from direct dissemination through CSF of cells originating from intracranial primary or secondary neoplasms.

Pathology

As tumor cells are disseminated through CSF, infiltration of the leptomeninges (pia mater and arachnoidea) may occur.

The nerve roots, especially the cauda equina fibers, may be infiltrated, visualized by linear/nodular contrast enhancement along the nerve roots.

The gross pathologic features are strongly dependent on the histologic type of metastasis. As an example, an ependymoma metastasis shows a grayish appearance and a lobulated surface (see Fig. 15-40) and a breast carcinoma metastasis presents as a white mass (see Fig. 15-41C). In the latter situation there may be small groups of atypical epithelial cells surrounded by strands of collagenous tissue (dura mater) (see Fig. 15-41D). The cells

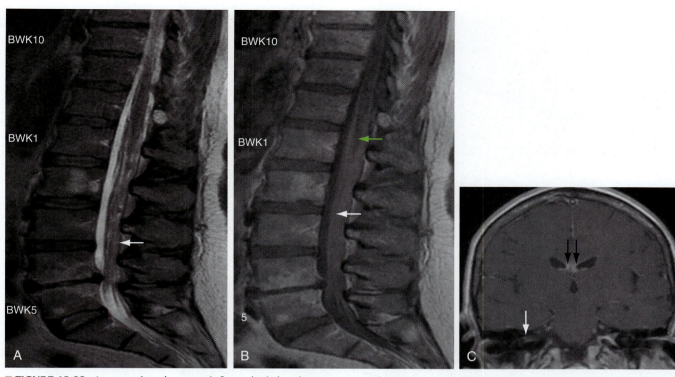

■ **FIGURE 15-38** Leptomeningeal metastasis from a brain lymphoma: sugar-coating pattern. Sagittal T2W (**A**) and sagittal contrast-enhanced (**B**) MR images demonstrate the thickened, strong contrast-enhanced cauda equina fibers (*white arrows*) with clear delineation of the conus medullaris (*green arrow*, **B**). **C**, Coronal contrast-enhanced MRI of the brain shows the lymphoma with involvement of the fornix on both sides (*black arrows*) as well as the branches of the right nervus vestibulocochlearis (*white arrow*).

are strongly positive for cytokeratin 7 and HER2/neu (see Fig. 15-41E).

The most common location of drop metastases is the lumbar and thoracolumbar spine.

Imaging

MRI

Leptomeningeal (intradural extramedullary space) metastases demonstrate three patterns on imaging:

1. Diffuse contrast enhancement along the pia mater of the cord and the nerve roots, hence the name "sugar coating" pattern (Fig. 15-38).
2. Multiple contrast-enhancing nodules in the subarachnoid space (Fig. 15-39).
3. A contrast-enhancing single mass in the subarachnoid space (Figs. 15-40 and 15-41).

Metastases present as isointensity on T1W images and hyperintensity on T2W images and with strong linear, nodular, or mass-like contrast enhancement, according to the dissemination pattern.

EXTRADURAL SPINAL TUMORS

Primary tumors of the spine are uncommon and represent less than 5% of all bone neoplasms, as compared with secondary metastatic disease, multiple myeloma, and lymphoma. A wide variety of benign neoplasms can involve the spine, including endosteoma, osteoid osteoma, osteoblastoma, aneurysmal bone cyst, giant cell tumor, and osteochondroma. Common malignant primary neoplasms are chordoma, chondrosarcoma, Ewing's sarcoma or primitive neuroectodermal tumor (PNET), and osteosarcoma. The most common symptom is pain, which is present in 85% of patients with primary spinal tumors.[20]

Extradural spinal lesions arise from outside the dura mater and may compress the dura with tapered narrowing of the underlying subarachnoid (intradural) space (see Fig. 15-1C). Imaging features of these spinal lesions are often characteristic, and the various available imaging modalities provide useful tools for narrowing the differential diagnosis and for planning further clinical treatment (Table 15-2).

Enostosis

Enostosis refers to asymptomatic focal areas of bony sclerosis. Other terms for this entity are bone island, calcified medullary defect, calcified island, compact island, and osteoma.

Epidemiology

Based on autopsy data, the incidence of enostosis in the spine is 14%. Most commonly it occurs in the pelvis,

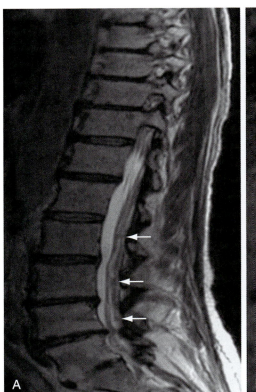
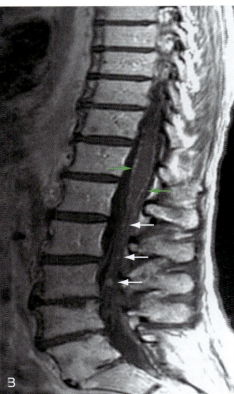

■ **FIGURE 15-39** Leptomeningeal metastasis from a bronchus carcinoma: sugar coating and nodular pattern. Sagittal T2W (**A**) and sagittal contrast-enhanced (**B**) MR images show small, T2 isointense, well-circumscribed nodules with strong contrast enhancement (*white arrows*), as well as linear-nodular pial contrast enhancement (*green arrow,* **B**) along the surface of the conus medullaris.

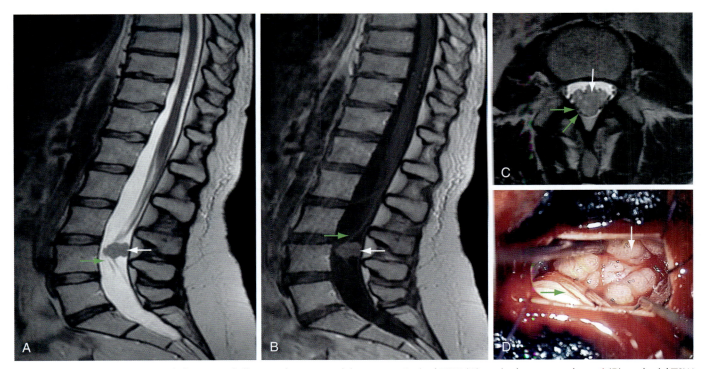

■ **FIGURE 15-40** Drop metastasis from a cerebellar ependymoma: nodular pattern. Sagittal T2W (**A**), sagittal contrast-enhanced (**B**), and axial T2W (**C**) MR images show the T2 hyperintense, homogeneous contrast-enhanced solid lesion between the cauda equina fibers (*white arrows*) with compression of the nerve roots (*green arrows*). On the intraoperative photograph (**D**), observe the lobulated surface and the soft grayish appearance of the lesion, resembling ependymoma (*white arrow*), and the compression of the nerve roots (*green arrow*). *(Intraoperative photograph courtesy of Dr. Richard Marugg, Neurosurgery, University Hospital of Zürich.)*

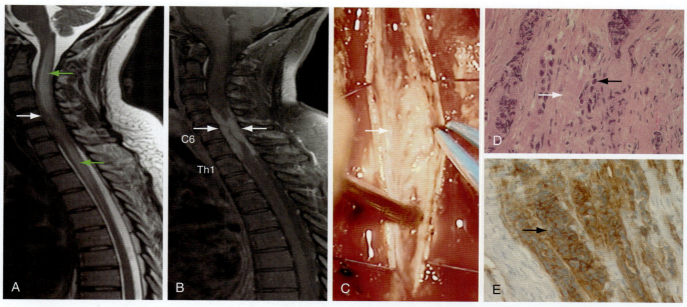

■ **FIGURE 15-41**   Metastasis from breast carcinoma: mass-like pattern. Sagittal T2W (**A**) and sagittal contrast-enhanced (**B**) MR images demonstrate the strong, homogeneous contrast-enhancing infiltrative lesion with a circumferential location around the spinal cord in the intradural extramedullary space (*white arrows*). Observe the prominent spinal cord edema (*green arrows*). **C**, Intraoperative photograph of the same patient demonstrates the white mass (*white arrow*). Hematoxylin and eosin (**D**) and cytokeratin 7 (**E**) stains show the small groups of atypical epithelial cells (*black arrows*) surrounded by strands of collagenous tissue (dura mater) (*white arrow*). (*Intraoperative photograph courtesy of Dr. Richard Marugg, Neurosurgery, University Hospital of Zürich.*)

femur, and ribs. It can be discovered in any age group. Males and females are equally affected.

Clinical Presentation

Enostoses are asymptomatic and discovered incidentally. Rarely they will increase or decrease in size over time.

Pathophysiology

Enostosis is considered a developmental hamartomatous lesion (i.e., normal tissue in abnormal location).

Pathology

Histologically, an enostosis consists of lamellar compact bone. The most frequent spinal location is at the thoracic (T1-T7) and the lumbar (L2 and L3) levels.

Imaging

CT

On CT, enostoses are round or oval, osteoblastic, very dense lesions with an abrupt transition to the surrounding normal bone (Fig. 15-42). They often lie under the cortex and commonly have radiating spicules at the lesion margin, which is also called "brush border." Their size is very variable, ranging from 2 mm to more than 2 cm. No associated soft tissue component is found.

MRI

In MRI, enostoses show low signal intensity on all sequences with normal signal intensities in the surrounding bone marrow (Figs. 15-43 to 15-46). After gadolinium administration no contrast enhancement is shown.

Special Procedures

Bone scintigraphic scan is positive in 33% of cases, most frequently in lesions of more than 2 cm owing to the increased osteoblastic activity (Fig. 15-47).

Osteoid Osteoma

An osteoid osteoma is a benign osteoid-producing tumor less than 2 cm in diameter. There is a small radiolucent tumor nidus with surrounding sclerosis. Intranidal calcification may or may not be present.

Epidemiology

Osteoid osteomas account for 10% to 12% of all benign bone tumors. The patient age at presentation is between 5 and 25 years. The majority of these tumors occur in the second decade of life. There is a male predominance of 2:1 to 3:1.

Clinical Presentation

The clinical symptoms typically include intense pain, which might be worse at night and usually is relieved by salicylates or nonsteroidal anti-inflammatory drugs (NSAIDs). The classic patient history is painful scoliosis

TABLE 15-2. Characteristic Imaging Features of Specific Extradural Spinal Tumors

Lesion	Age/Sex	Location in Vertebra	Imaging Features
Benign			
Enostosis	Any age M = F	Vertebral body	Sclerotic bony island, brush border
Osteoid osteoma	Majority in second decade of life M:F = 2-3:1	Almost all involve neural arch; L > C > T > S	Radiolucent tumor nidus with surrounding sclerosis, <1.5 cm
Osteoblastoma	90% in 2nd-3rd decade M:F 2-2.5:1	Originate in neural arch, often extend into vertebral body C > L = T = S	Expansile mass occurring in posterior elements, may be aggressive, osteolysis
Epidural lipomatosis	Mean age at presentation 43 years, M > F, no racial predilection	Thoracic spine 60%, T6-8; lumbar spine 40%, L4-5, dorsal to spinal cord	Abundant epidural fat in midthoracic and distal lumbar spinal canal compressing thecal sac, "Y" sign; epidural fat ≥7 mm
Aneurysmal bone cyst	Predominantly afflicts children; 60% in those younger than 20 years; slightly more common in females	Arise in neural arch; 75-90% extent into vertebral body; 10-30% in sacrum or spine	Expansile benign neoplasm containing thin-walled blood-filled cavities with fluid-fluid levels
Hemangioma	Peak incidence 4th-6th decade M = F, aggressive lesion more common in women	Vertebral body and posterior elements; may extend epidurally and cause cord compression	Vertebral body vascular tumor, well- circumscribed lesion with coarse vertical trabeculae on axial CT ("white polka dots")
Giant cell tumor	80% 3rd to 5th decade; in spine peak incidence 2nd to 3rd decade; rare before skeletal maturity M:F = 1:2.5 in spine	Centered in vertebral body or sacrum; rarely involves multiple sites; 3% affect spine, 4% the sacrum	Lytic expansile lesion; matrix absent; margin usually not sclerotic; may have cortical breakthrough
Osteochondroma	Peak age 10-30 years M:F = 3:1	Cervical (50%, C2 predilection) > thoracic > lumbar > > sacral spinous/transverse process > vertebral body; <5% occur in spine	Sessile or pedunculated osseous cauliflower lesion with marrow/ cortical continuity with parent vertebra; size 1-10 cm
Malignant			
Chordoma	Peak incidence 5th-6th decade; rare in children M:F = 2:1 spine; no gender predilection if sacrum affected	Sacrococcygeal > spheno-occipital > vertebral body (50% > 35% > 15%) arising from notochord remnants; 2-4% of all primary malignant bone tumors	Heterogeneous destructive mass; hyperintense to discs on T2W images with multiple septa
Osteosarcoma	In spine, peak incidence in 4th decade; age range 8-80 years M = F	4% occur in spine and sacrum; 79% arise in posterior elements; 17% involve two adjacent spinal levels; 84% invade spinal canal	Aggressive lesion forming immature bone; permeative appearance; cortical breakthrough and soft tissue mass
Chondrosarcoma	45 years; age range 20-90 years M:F = 2:1	In spine 3-12%; third most common primary bone tumor	Lytic mass with or without chondroid matrix; cortical disruption and extension into soft tissues; chondroid matrix with rings and arcs is characteristic
Ewing's sarcoma	90% present before 20 years, second smaller peak at 50 years M:F = 2:1	In spine 5%; involves vertebral body and neural arch; sacrum more common site than spine	Permeative lytic lesion centered in vertebral body or sacrum; may originate in soft tissues
Plasmacytoma	Mean age 55 years; affects younger patients than multiple myeloma M > F	Vertebral body most common site of solitary bone plasmacytoma	T1-hypointense marrow with low signal curvilinear areas; a second lesion is found in 33% of patients with solitary bone plasmacytoma
Multiple myeloma	Peak incidence from age 40-80 M:F 3:2 Less common in Asians	Axial skeleton; 87% vertebral fractures between T6 and L4	Multifocal, diffuse, or heterogeneous T1 hypointensity; diffuse osteopenia in 85%; multiple lytic lesions in 80%
Metastases, osteoblastic	Children and adults; gender predilection varies with specific tumor	Lesion destroys posterior cortex and pedicle; bone production exceeds bone destruction	Sclerosis may occur as discrete nodular appearance; ivory vertebra may be present (prostate, multiple myeloma, chordoma, lymphoma)
Metastases, osteolytic	Children and adults; gender predilection varies with specific tumor; middle-aged most often affected	Lesion destroys posterior cortex and pedicle; bone destruction exceeds bone	Lytic, permeative, destructive lesion; epidural tumor extension may cause paralysis

(70%), which should raise the suspicion for this spinal tumor. The diagnosis is made often months or years later, and muscle atrophy is a frequent associated finding.

Osteoid osteomas are most commonly located in long bones, especially in the femur and the tibia, but about 10% occur in the spine. In about 75% of those cases they are localized in the posterior vertebral elements (pedicles, articular facets, laminae), with only 7% being localized in the vertebral body and rarely in the transverse and spinous processes. The lumbar spine is the most common location (59%), followed by the cervical (27%), thoracic (12%), and sacral (2%) spine.[21]

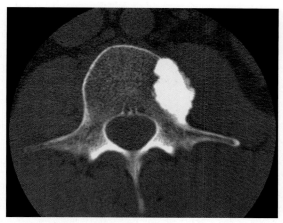

■ **FIGURE 15-42**   Enostosis. CT image shows a focal area of high attenuation with well-defined margins. No soft tissue component is evident.

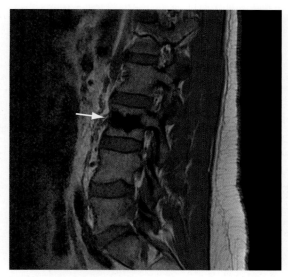

■ **FIGURE 15-43**   Enostosis. Sagittal T1W MR images demonstrate a focal area of low signal (*arrow*) in the L3 vertebral body.

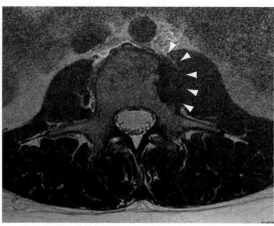

■ **FIGURE 15-44**   Enostosis. Corresponding transverse T2W MR image shows a lesion with low signal intensity and well-defined margins (*arrowheads*).

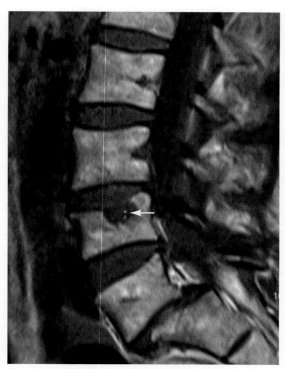

■ **FIGURE 15-45**   Differential diagnosis of enostosis. Sagittal T1W MR image shows Schmorl node adjacent to end plate L4 (*arrow*). A Schmorl node may also enhance.

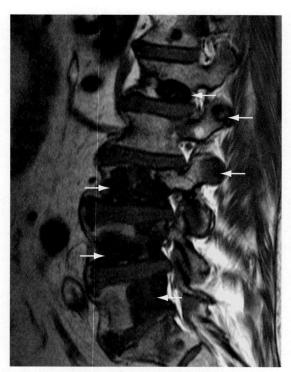

■ **FIGURE 15-46**   Differential diagnosis of enostosis. Sagittal T1W MR image shows prostate metastases (*arrows*). Multiple lesions are present.

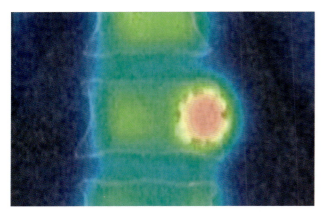

■ **FIGURE 15-47** Coronal SPECT image with ^{99m}Tc-DPD shows increased radiotracer uptake (*red*) in a large enostosis of a lumbar vertebral body. There is normal radiotracer uptake (*green*) in the adjacent bone.

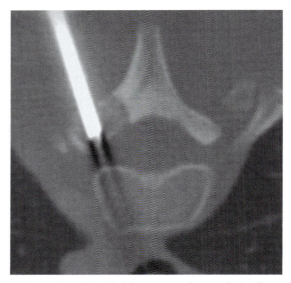

■ **FIGURE 15-49** CT-guided biopsy was done and the diagnosis of osteoid osteoma was confirmed.

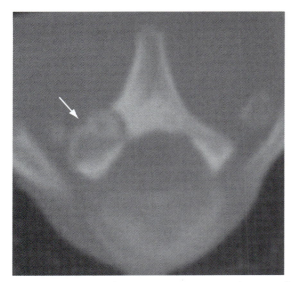

■ **FIGURE 15-48** Osteoid osteoma. Transverse CT shows a sclerotic lesion in the lamina of T2 (*arrow*).

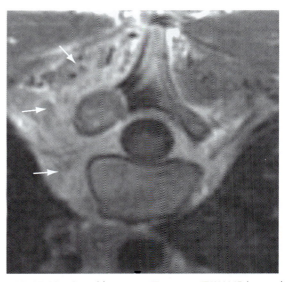

■ **FIGURE 15-50** Osteoid osteoma. Transverse T1W MR image shows, after administration of a contrast agent, a contrast-enhancing reactive zone of paraspinous soft tissues (*arrows*).

Pathophysiology

Histopathologically, an osteoid osteoma consists of a nidus that is less than 2 cm and pink to red, representing vascular fibrous connective tissue, surrounded by organized bony trabeculae and a variable degree of sclerotic bone reaction. It has no potential for malignant transformation.

Imaging

CT

CT is the imaging modality of choice for the diagnosis of these tumors. The classic finding is an oval or round radiolucency, the nidus, which is less than 2 cm in diameter (Figs. 15-48 and 15-49). More than 50% are partially calcified, approximately 20% are completely calcified, and 30% show no calcifications. The nidus is surrounded by bone sclerosis and periosteal new bone formation. If scoliosis

is present, the nidus is localized on the concave side at the deepest portion of the curve.

MRI

MRI findings are generally nonspecific. The nidus has usually low to intermediate signal intensity on T1W images and low to high signal intensity on T2W images (Figs. 15-50 and 15-51). It may show gadolinium enhancement. Small lesions can be obscured owing to the signal changes caused by sclerosis or bone marrow edema. The differential diagnosis includes chronic osteomyelitis (Fig. 15-52), stress fracture, Langerhans histiocytosis, osteoblastoma, enostosis, fibrous dysplasia, melorheostosis, and Ewing's sarcoma.

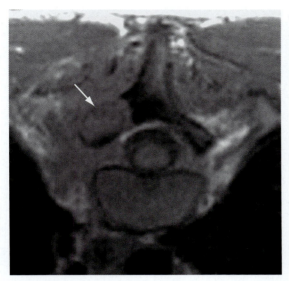

■ FIGURE 15-51 Transverse T1W MR image shows osteoid osteoma (*arrow*). The osseous lesion is centered in the lamina.

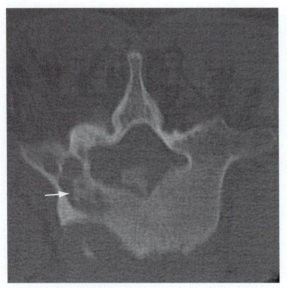

■ FIGURE 15-52 Differential diagnosis for osteoid osteoma. Transverse CT shows osteomyelitis proven by biopsy. Sequestrum shows irregular shape that can mimic the nidus of osteoid osteoma (*arrow*).

Special Procedures

Bone scintigraphy demonstrates an increased radionuclide uptake by the nidus.

Osteoblastoma

An osteoblastoma is an osteolytic lesion more than 2 cm in diameter with a fibrovascular nidus and sclerotic ring. It is a benign tumor, producing osteoid. Osteoblastoma may behave aggressively. It can also be referred to as a giant osteoid osteoma.

Epidemiology

This tumor is rare, accounting for 1% of all bone tumors. Most patients are younger than 30 years of age (90%), and the male-to-female ratio is 2 to 2.5:1.

Clinical Presentation

The clinical symptoms are nonspecific: patients complain about a dull aching pain that is usually associated with soft tissue swelling at the site of the tumor. As opposed to osteoid osteomas, the pain does not show nocturnal exacerbations and is not relieved by salicylates. Scoliosis may occur, and neurologic deficits (paresthesia, paraparesis, paraplegia) are present in about 40% of cases. The natural history of osteoblastomas is slow growth as opposed to the relative stability of osteoid osteomas. Rarely, malignant transformation to osteosarcoma is observed.

Osteoblastomas are more aggressive than osteoid osteomas, having a higher recurrence rate: 10% to 15% for the less aggressive lesions and more than 50% for the more aggressive lesions. Hence, the surgical excision should be wide and en bloc.

Pathology

Histologically, osteoblastoma and osteoid osteoma are indistinguishable (interconnecting trabecular bone and fibrovascular stroma), and they are considered as variants of the same benign process. Only the size is used as a differential criterion in which a lesion with a nidus greater than 2 cm is classified as osteoblastoma. These tumors hardly ever undergo malignant transformation.

Thirty to 40 percent of all osteoblastomas occur in the spine (cervical > lumbar = thoracic = sacral), typically affecting the posterior elements (55%). They originate in the neural arch and often extend to the vertebral body. The long bones are affected in 30%, with predilection for the femur and tibia. In the remaining cases the skull and facial bones (15%), hands and feet (14%), and ribs (4%) are involved.

Imaging

CT

The radiologic appearance of spinal osteoblastomas is variable: (1) they may look similar to osteoid osteomas and are composed of a radiolucent center and a surrounding sclerotic band but they are more than 2 cm in diameter; (2) they can appear more expansile with a prominent sclerotic rim and with multiple small calcifications (this is the most common appearance of spinal osteoblastomas); and (3) they can have an aggressive appearance with even more expansile pattern, matrix calcifications, bone destruction, and paravertebral extension. This last type may be indistinguishable from aneurysmal bone cyst or bone metastasis (Figs. 15-53 and 15-54).

CT is the diagnostic examination of choice, but MRI depicts better the surrounding soft tissue involvement. CT shows the nidus, the multifocal (as opposed to central in osteoid osteomas) matrix calcification, the sclerotic

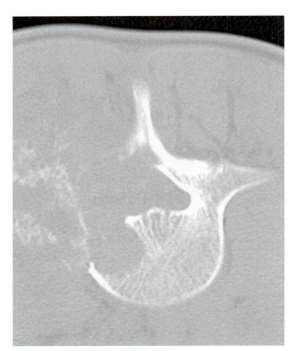

■ **FIGURE 15-53** Differential diagnosis for osteoblastoma: Transverse CT shows an aneurysmal bone cyst presenting as an expansile lesion of the posterior elements.

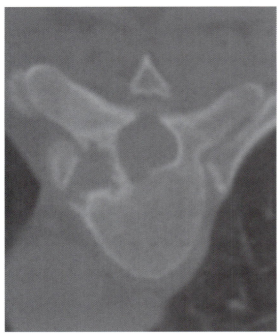

■ **FIGURE 15-54** Differential diagnosis for osteoblastoma: Transverse CT shows a metastasis (melanoma) with destroyed cortex and additional involvement of the posterior elements and/or vertebral body.

margin, the expansile bone remodeling, or a thin osseous shell around its margins.

MRI

MRI findings are generally nonspecific. The nidus has usually low to intermediate signal intensity on T1W

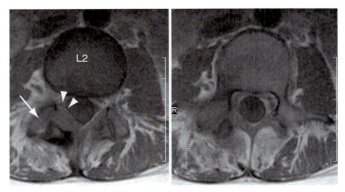

■ **FIGURE 15-55** Osteoblastoma. T1W transverse consecutive MR images of L2 show intraspinal and extraspinal soft tissue mass (*arrowheads*) including the right lamina (*arrow*).

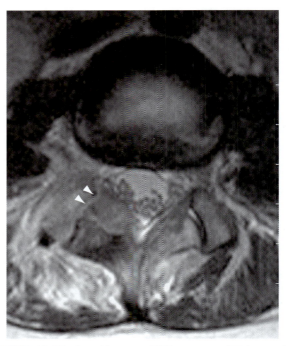

■ **FIGURE 15-56** Osteoblastoma. T2W transverse MR image shows typical heterogeneous signal intensity (*arrowheads*). The bony matrix is of low signal.

images and low to high signal intensity on T2W images (Figs. 15-55 to 15-57).

Special Procedures

Osteoblastomas exhibit marked radionuclide uptake in bone scintigraphy.

Epidural Lipomatosis

Excessive accumulation of intraspinal fat causing compression of the dural sac is called epidural lipomatosis or spinal epidural lipomatosis.

Epidemiology

The mean age at presentation is 43 years. Males are affected more often than females. There is no racial predilection.

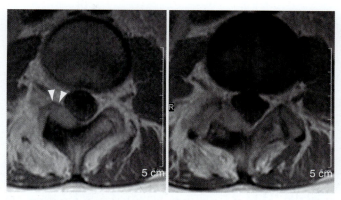

■ **FIGURE 15-57** Osteoblastoma. T1W transverse consecutive MR images of L2 show contrast enhancement in a soft tissue mass (*arrowheads*) and fatty infiltration of the erector spinal muscles.

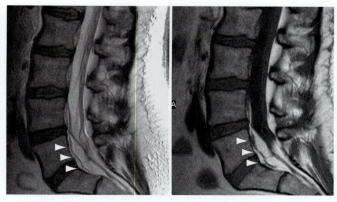

■ **FIGURE 15-58** Epidural lipomatosis. T2W and T1W sagittal MR images show increased extradural fat in the lumbar spinal canal (*arrowheads*), compressing the thecal sac.

The thoracic spine is affected in 60%, the lumbar spine in 40%.

Clinical Presentation

Eighty-five percent of patients present with weakness, and about 60% present with back pain. More than 80% of patients show postsurgical pain relief. The prognosis is better with presurgical low-dose corticosteroid administration and idiopathic spinal epidural lipomatosis. The etiology is long-term exogenous steroid administration or excessive endogenous steroid production.

Pathophysiology

Long-term exogenous steroid administration or excessive endogenous steroid production can be responsible for the development of spinal epidural lipomatosis. Epidural lipomatosis is considered when the epidural fat measures more than 7 mm in the anteroposterior length in the thoracic spine and is associated with mass effect on the thecal sac and the nerve roots.[22]

Pathology

Spinal epidural lipomatosis consists of adipose tissue external to the thecal sac without any capsule. The hyperplastic epidural fat is found most often in the midthoracic and distal lumbar spinal canal compressing the thecal sac.

Imaging

CT

There is increased fat density in the spinal canal, usually posterior to the dural sac, associated with cord compression without associated contrast enhancement or bony erosions.

MRI

The homogeneous mass is hyperintense/hypointense on fat-suppressed T1W imaging, of intermediate signal inten-

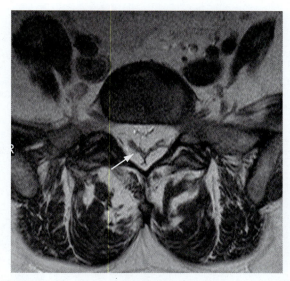

■ **FIGURE 15-59** Transverse T2W MR image shows excessive epidural lipomatosis presenting the "Y" sign (*arrow*).

sity on T2W imaging, and hypointense on STIR sequence, without contrast enhancement (Figs. 15-58 to 15-62). Prominent epidural veins can be distinguished, especially in the lumbar spine, as linear signal voids on T1W and T2W images within the prominent epidural fatty tissue. On the transverse images a typical "Y"-shaped configuration of the dural sac is present ("Y" sign), explained by meningovertebral ligaments, which anchor the outer surface of the dura mater to the osteofibrous walls of the lumbar canal.

Aneurysmal Bone Cyst

An aneurysmal bone cyst is an expansile benign neoplasm containing thin-walled, blood-filled cavities.

Epidemiology

These lesions predominantly afflict children; 60% occur in patients younger than age 20 years. They are slightly more

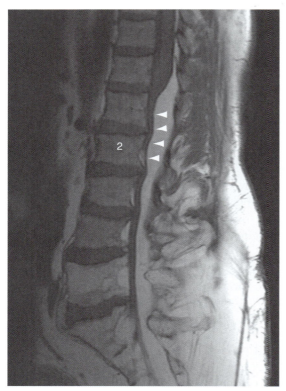

■ **FIGURE 15-60** Epidural lipomatosis. T1W sagittal MR image shows a prominent scalloping of the vertebrae L2-L5. The spinal cord is displaced and compressed (*arrowheads*).

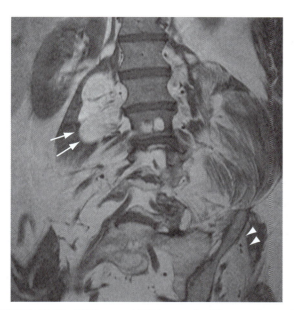

■ **FIGURE 15-61** T1W coronal MR image of a 30-year-old man demonstrates an idiopathic diffuse epidural, paraspinal, and subcutaneous lipomatosis. Note the fatty infiltration of the psoas muscle (*arrows*) and fatty infiltration of the gluteal muscles (*arrowheads*).

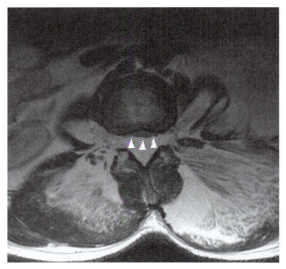

■ **FIGURE 15-62** T2W axial MR image shows diffuse fatty mass in the spinal canal. The spinal cord is compressed and dislocated (*arrowheads*). The spinal canal is enlarged, and epidural lipomatosis is present.

common in females, and a familial incidence has been reported.

Clinical Presentation

Back pain is most severe at night. There may be an association with scoliosis, and other focal neurologic symptoms may result from root or cord compression. The recurrence rate is 20% to 30%.

Pathophysiology

There are three theories regarding their pathophysiology: (1) as a consequence of trauma and local circulatory disturbances; (2) as an underlying tumor-inducing vascular process; and (3) de novo genesis as a primary neoplasm with cytogenic abnormalities.

Pathology

Macroscopically, an aneurysmal bone cyst looks like a spongy red mass composed of multiple blood-filled spaces. Its expansile appearance reflects containment of tumor by appositional periosteal new bone.

Microscopically, the cyst may consist of a dense cellular composition containing plump stromal cells, multinuclear giant cells, and thin-walled blood vessels or a preponderance of fibrous tissue with enlarged vascular spaces.[23]

Ten to 30 percent of all aneurysmal bones cysts occur in the spine. Typically they arise in the neural arch, and 75% to 90% extend to the vertebral body.

Imaging

Radiography

Conventional radiographs show an expansile remodeling of the bone, absent pedicle sign (expansion of the pedicle results in loss of pedicle contour on anteroposterior radiographs), cortical thinning, and focal cortical destruction.

CT

A balloon-like expansile remodeling of the bone is associated with cortical thinning ("eggshell cortex"), focal cortical destruction (Fig. 15-63), fluid-fluid levels caused by hemorrhage, and blood product sedimentation. Bony septa may be present as well as solid components showing diffuse contrast enhancement.

MRI

On MRI the typical appearance is one of a lobulated mass with cystic spaces on both T1W and T2W images, which may contain hemorrhagic products surrounded by a hypointense rim of periosteum. Part or all of the mass may be solid. The epidural extension is well seen on all sequences. On postcontrast T1W images enhancement may be present in the periphery, in the septa between the cystic spaces, as well as in the solid portions of the lesion (Fig. 15-64).

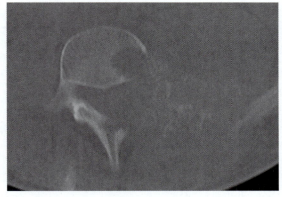

■ **FIGURE 15-63** Aneurysmal bone cyst. Transverse CT shows a sharply lytic lesion in a vertebral body with extension into the epidural space.

Special Procedures

On bone scintigraphy, a typical "donut sign" (rim of activity around a photopenic region) is present related to the hypervascularity of the lesion with more prominent vessels in the periphery.

Hemangioma

This vascular tumor of the vertebral body may extend epidurally and cause cord compression. Hemangiomas are common and usually benign. They can be called vertebral hemangiomas or intraosseous, extraosseous, or compressive hemangiomas.

Epidemiology

Hemangiomas are the most common spinal axis tumors and are present in 11% of spines at autopsy.[24] Peak incidence is during the fourth to sixth decades. There is a male predilection, but aggressive lesions are more common in women.

Clinical Presentation

A hemangioma is often an incidental finding on spinal imaging but may extend epidurally and cause symptoms from nerve root or spinal cord compression. It may rarely cause an acute fracture of the vertebral body, presenting as acute onset of pain and rarely also as epidural hemorrhage.

Pathophysiology

Hemangiomas are usually incidental lesions. The etiology is developmental.

Pathology

A hemangioma consists of vascular/fatty stroma with sparse thick trabeculae. It is slow growing and of capillary, cavernous, or venous origin. The cavernous type heman-

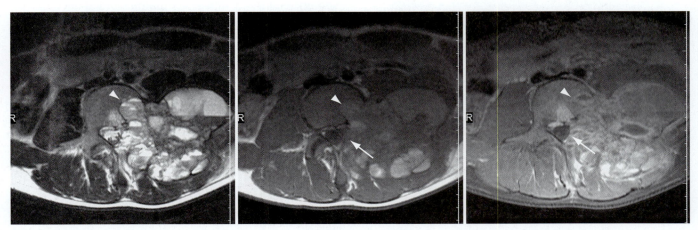

■ **FIGURE 15-64** T2W, T1W, and T1W postcontrast transverse MR images at the level of T2 demonstrate the extension of the aneurysmal bone cyst into the vertebral body (*arrowheads*) and the spinal canal (*arrows*). Multiple fluid-fluid levels are present.

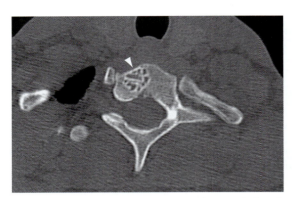

■ **FIGURE 15-65** Hemangioma. Transverse CT shows typical corduroy pattern (*arrowhead*) of thickened trabeculae and intervening low attenuation fat ("white polka dots").

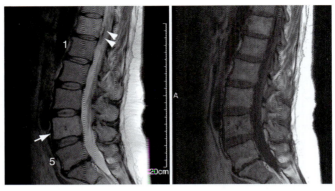

■ **FIGURE 15-66** Sagittal T2W and T1W MR images showing hemangiomas in vertebrae T12 and L4. Typical hyperintense signal on T2W image (left, *arrow*) is shown. Epidural extension is shown at T12 (*arrowheads*).

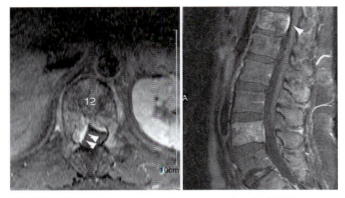

■ **FIGURE 15-67** Hemangioma. Transverse and sagittal T1W postcontrast MR images show the epidural extent (*arrowheads*) and the intense contrast enhancement. Cord compression is present on the sagittal image at left (*arrowhead*)

giomas are most common. Aggressive lesions containing less fat and more vascular stroma are uncommon.

These benign lesions show mature, thin-walled, endothelium-lined capillary and cavernous sinuses interspersed among sparse, osseous trabeculae and fatty stroma.

In 25% to 30% of cases multiple hemangiomas are present. The thoracic spine is the most commonly affected region, followed by the lumbar spine, cervical spine, and sacrum, respectively. Thoracic lesions (between T3 and T9) are more often aggressive. They are mostly localized in the vertebral bodies and uncommonly involve the posterior elements (10%-15%).

Imaging

Radiography

Conventional radiographs show a vertebral body lesion with coarse vertical trabeculae resembling corduroy or a honeycomb. These represent reinforcement of remaining trabeculae—a reaction to the stress redistribution caused by destruction of other trabeculae.

CT

Hypodense, well-circumscribed lesions are centered in the vertebral body with a spotted appearance on transverse images ("white polka dots") representing the remaining thickened trabeculae (Fig. 15-65). Aggressive lesions show prominent contrast enhancement.

MRI

A benign hemangioma presents as a T1W hyperintense and T2W hyperintense lesion with intense contrast enhancement (Figs. 15-66 to 15-68).

Aggressive hemangiomas show T1W isointense or hypointense and T2W hyperintense signal with intense contrast enhancement. Pathologic fracture or epidural extension with a characteristic "curtain sign" (see Fig. 15-67) is common.

MRA shows the angioarchitecture of the hypervascular tumor and may be requested for follow-up after embolization (Fig. 15-69).

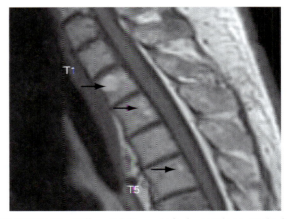

■ **FIGURE 15-68** Differential diagnosis for hemangioma: Sagittal T1W MR image with multiple round lesions representing focal fatty marrow (*arrows*).

Special Procedures

Angiography is unnecessary unless preoperative or palliative embolization is considered.

Giant Cell Tumor

A giant cell tumor is a locally aggressive tumor that presents as a lytic expansile lesion in a vertebral body or the sacrum and is composed of osteoclast-like giant cells.

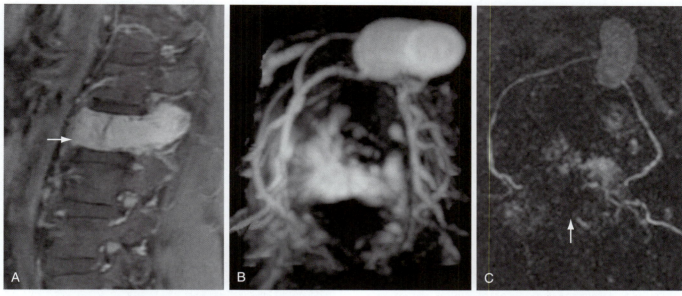

Preembolization   Postembolization

■ **FIGURE 15-69**   Hemangioma. **A,** Sagittal contrast-enhanced T1W MR image shows the highly vascularized tumor in the vertebral body and pediculus (*arrow*). Contrast-enhanced fast angiography before (**B**) and after (**C**) embolization demonstrates the devascularization of the tumor (*arrows*).

Epidemiology

Giant cell tumors represent 5% of all primary bone tumors. They are the sixth most common primary bone tumors but only 2.7% are located in the spine. Eighty percent of all giant cell tumors present during the third to fifth decades. Of the tumors located in the spine, the peak incidence is from the second to third decades. These tumors are rare before skeletal maturity. The male-to-female ratio is 1 : 2.5.[25]

Clinical Presentation

Back pain of insidious onset that is greatest at night and the clinical consequences after pathologic fractures (30%) are the most common symptoms.

Pathophysiology

Locally aggressive, these tumors have a 12% to 50% recurrence rate. They can undergo sarcomatous transformation after radiation therapy or spontaneously. Primary malignant giant cell tumor is rare but has a poor prognosis, with lung, liver, and bone metastasis.

Pathology

A soft, tan, well-demarcated tumor is seen on gross evaluation. In 10% to 15% of patients there is an aneurysmal bone cyst component.

Multinucleated osteoclastic giant cells and spindle cell stroma are evident on histologic examination. Reactive osteoid, hemorrhage, necrosis, or hemosiderin may also be present.

Giant cell tumors are the most frequent benign tumors involving the sacrum. The other regions of the spine are less often affected.

Imaging

Radiography

Conventional radiographs show a lytic, expansile lesion in the vertebral body or sacrum with margins that usually are not sclerotic and an absent matrix. Cortical breakthrough may be present.

CT

CT demonstrates the same features as conventional radiography. Fluid-fluid attenuation regions are evident if an aneurysmal bone cyst component is present.

MRI

There is a low to intermediate signal on T1W imaging, an intermediate to high signal on T2W imaging, and heterogeneous enhancement on T1W postcontrast imaging; and areas of necrosis may be present.

Special Procedures

Bone scintigraphy may be positive in all three phases.

Chordoma

A chordoma is a malignant tumor arising from the embryonic remnants of the notochord. Histologic identification of physaliphorous ("bubble bearing" vacuolated) cells confirms the diagnosis.

Epidemiology

Chordomas represent 2% to 4% of all primary malignant bone tumors. Peak incidence is in the fifth to sixth decades;

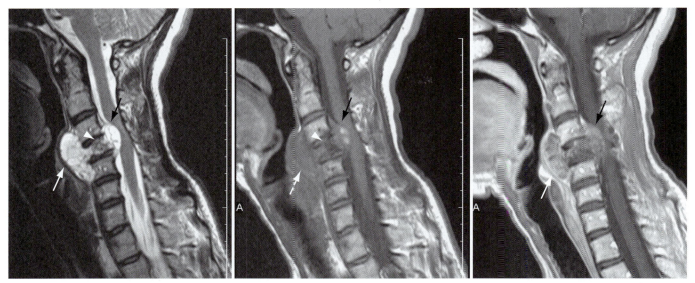

■ **FIGURE 15-70** Chordoma. T2W MR image (*left*) shows hyperintense mass involving the C4 vertebral body (*arrowheads*) with extensive epidural and prevertebral extension (*white arrows*) and cord compression (*black arrows*). T1W MR image (*middle*) shows heterogeneous signal, and postcontrast T1W MR image (*right*) demonstrates inhomogeneous contrast enhancement of the tumor mass.

it is rarely seen also in patients younger than age 30 years.[26] The male-to-female ratio is 2:1 when it occurs in the spine. No gender predilection is observed in sacral chordoma. Chordomas are rare in African-Americans.

Clinical Presentation

Chordoma remains asymptomatic for a long time which explains its often very large size at the time of clinical presentation and diagnosis. The main symptom is pain, particularly while sitting. There are signs of compression of nerve roots with radiculopathy as well as rectum or bladder symptoms from constipation and tenesmus.

Pathophysiology

Tumor arises from the notochord remnants. Losses on chromosomal arms 3p and 1p (50% and 44%) and gains on 7q (69%), 5q (38%), and 12q (38%) indicate a genetic etiology. Local recurrence is common (90%), and distant metastases are more rare (5%-40% in bone, lymph node, liver, and lung). The 5-year survival is 67% to 84%.

Pathology

A lobulated, grayish gelatinous mass is present on gross examination. Three different types are described: (1) typical lobules of myxoid matrix with sheets and cords of clear cells with intracytoplasmic vacuoles (physaliphorous cells); (2) chondroid with hyaline cartilage; and (3) a dedifferentiated type with sarcomatous elements.

The tumor involves the sacrococcygeal region in 50%, the spheno-occipital region in 35%, and the vertebral bodies in 15% of the cases.

Imaging

Radiography

A midline lobular soft tissue mass with osseous destruction can extend into the disc or involve two or more vertebral segments. Bony destruction and calcification are present in 70% of cases. Conventional radiographs show a lucent lesion with sclerosis appearing as a destructive heterogeneous mass.

CT

CT shows a lytic destructive lesion, a hypodense soft tissue mass, and amorphous bulging of the cortex. Intratumoral calcifications in the sacrum are seen in more than 70% of cases and in 30% they occur in the vertebrae. There is moderate inhomogeneous contrast enhancement.

MRI

Chordoma presents on T1W images as heterogeneous hypointense to isointense signal intensity compared with bone marrow and on T2W images as hyperintense signal intensity compared with CSF. Intervertebral discs have a variable, but usually moderate contrast enhancement. The tumor may have septations or destroyed intratumoral bony trabeculae (Figs. 15-70 to 15-73).

Special Procedures

Bone scintigraphy shows decreased intratumoral uptake.

Osteochondroma

A cartilage-covered osseous excrescence in continuity with parent bone is an osteochondroma. Alternative

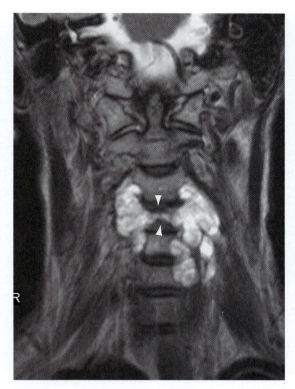

■ **FIGURE 15-71**   Chordoma. T2W coronal image also shows the hyper-intense signal of extensive tumor mass prevertebral and paravertebral to C3-C6 with involvement of the C4 body (*arrowheads*).

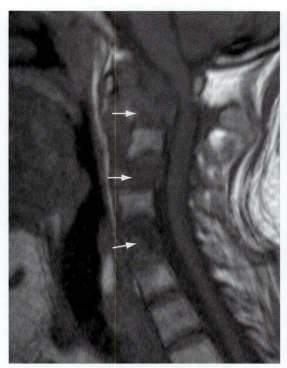

■ **FIGURE 15-73**   Differential diagnosis for chordoma. Sagittal T1W MR image shows multiple metastases in a patient with breast cancer.

names include hereditary multiple exostosis, diaphyseal aclasis, hereditary deforming chondroplasia, multiple osteochondromatosis, multiple cartilaginous exostosis, dyschondroplasia, and Ehrenfried's disease.[27]

Epidemiology

Osteochondroma is the most common benign bone tumor (30%-45%), encompassing 9% of all bone tumors. Only 3% of all osteochondromas and 7% of all hereditary multiple exostoses occur in the spine. Incidence of solitary osteochondroma is unknown; the incidence of hereditary multiple exostosis is 1 : 50,000 to 1 : 100,000. The peak age at onset is 10 to 30 years, with a male-to-female ratio of 3 : 1. Patients with hereditary multiple exostosis are usually diagnosed by age 5 years.

Clinical Presentation

Osteochondroma is most often an asymptomatic incidental finding; sometimes a palpable mass with or without pain is present. Spinal cord compression, radiculopathy, dysphagia, hoarseness, and scoliosis are rare complications. Markers for possible malignant transformations are growth of the lesion or new pain and a cartilage cap larger than 1.5 cm in adults evident on imaging.

Pathophysiology

Hereditary multiple exostosis is an autosomal dominant disease. Inactivation of one *EXT* gene on chromosomes 8, 11, and 19 (tumor suppressor sites) gives rise to exostosis; subsequent inactivation of a second *EXT* gene causes

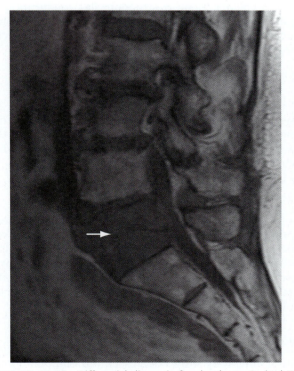

■ **FIGURE 15-72**   Differential diagnosis for chordoma: Sagittal T1W MR image shows lymphoma (*arrow*).

malignant transformation. Malignant transformation occurs in less than 1% of cases in solitary lesions and 3% to 5% of cases of hereditary multiple exostosis.

Pathology

The lesion presents as a cortical and medullary cavity contiguous with the parent bone. A cartilage cap may be present or entirely absent.

Osteochondromas occur most often in the metaphysis of long tubular bones (85%). In the vertebral column the main location is the posterior elements, especially the spinous process. Vertebral body involvement is unusual. The thoracic and lumbar spine is the most often affected region.

Imaging

Radiography

Imaging shows a cartilage-covered osseous excrescence in continuity with the parent bone—a sessile or pedunculated osseous "cauliflower" lesion. On conventional radiographs the lesion presents as a sessile or pedunculated osseous protuberance. The cartilage cap is only visible if extensively mineralized.

Ultrasonography

A hypoechoic nonmineralized cartilage cap can be seen on ultrasound evaluation.

CT

CT shows a sessile or pedunculated osseous protuberance with heterogeneous contrast enhancement. A chondroid matrix may be present as well (Fig. 15-74).

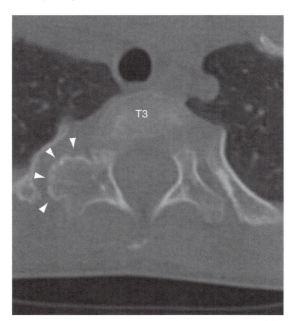

■ **FIGURE 15-74** Transverse bone CT demonstrates a T3 osteochondroma in the right transverse process (*arrowheads*). The lesion is typically in continuity with a parent vertebra.

MRI

On T1W imaging the lesion is centrally hyperintense, surrounded by a hypointense cortex. On T2W imaging it is centrally isointense to hyperintense and surrounded by a hypointense cortex. After contrast agent administration T1W imaging shows septal and peripheral enhancement of the cartilage cap.

Special Procedures

Scintigraphy is variable, showing uptake by metabolically active osteochondromas and no uptake in quiescent osteochondromas.

Osteosarcoma

An osteosarcoma is a malignant tumor containing immature matrix and osteoid material produced directly by the malignant cells. It is also called an osteogenic sarcoma.

Epidemiology

Osteosarcoma is the second most common primary bone tumor. Of all osteosarcomas, 0.6% to 3.2% occur in spine. Spinal localization has a peak incidence in the fourth decade; the age range is 8 to 80 years. There is no gender predilection.

Clinical Presentation

Pain is greatest at night, and patients present with increased serum levels of alkaline phosphatase. Pulmonary, bone, and liver metastases are common. Osteosarcoma may be associated with Paget's disease and with previous radiation therapy. An unusual association of osteosarcoma is its presentation as a second tumor approximately 10 years after detection of retinoblastoma.[28] Median survival time is 23 months, and survival rates are lower in patients with sacral tumors.

Pathophysiology

This malignant tumor produces osteoid directly from neoplastic cells. To establish the diagnosis it is necessary to identify osteoid formed from sarcomatous tissue. Osteosarcomas developing in association with retinoblastoma are associated with alterations of the *RB* genes.

Pathology

A heterogeneous mass is present with ossified and nonossified components. Necroses are common.

Osteosarcoma is a pluripotential neoplasm consisting of malignant cells producing osteoid. Classic osteosarcomas show a high degree of anaplasia and high mitotic rate. The tumor cells may be spindle shaped or round.

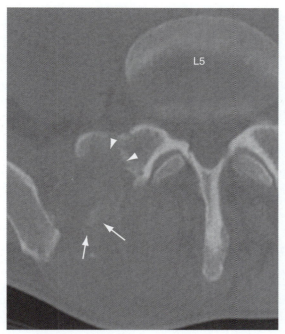

■ **FIGURE 15-75** Osteosarcoma. Transverse bone CT shows bone destruction of the posterior elements of L5 (*arrowheads*). Ossifications (*arrows*) and soft tissue mass are also present.

Imaging

Radiography

On conventional radiographs the lesion presents predominantly as osteosclerotic but most often it has a mixed osteosclerotic/osteolytic appearance. An ivory vertebral body may be recognized with loss of vertebral height, permeative appearance, cortical breakthrough, and soft tissue mass.

CT

CT depicts moth-eaten bone destruction with a wide zone of transition and associated soft tissue mass (Figs. 15-75 and 15-76).

MRI

T1W imaging shows low signal in mineralized tumors, and T2W imaging shows low signal in mineralized tumors and high signal in nonmineralized tumors. In telangiectatic osteosarcoma, a soft tissue mass and fluid-fluid levels are characteristic. There is inhomogeneous contrast enhancement on T1W imaging after administration of a contrast agent (Fig. 15-77).

Special Procedures

Bone scintigraphy shows increased uptake in all three phases.

Chondrosarcoma

A malignant tumor of connective tissue, chondrosarcoma is characterized by formation of chondroid matrix by tumor cells.

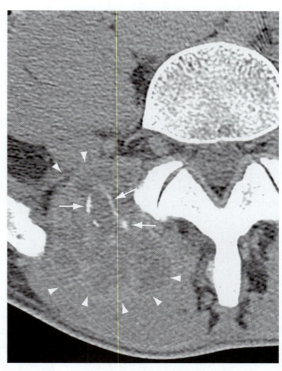

■ **FIGURE 15-76** Transverse CT shows soft tissue mass (*arrowheads*) adjacent to the right L5 vertebra. Ossifications are present (*arrows*).

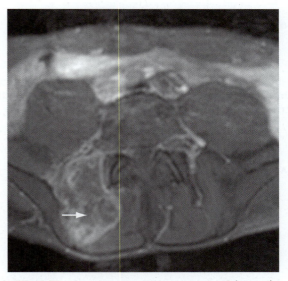

■ **FIGURE 15-77** Osteosarcoma. T1W transverse MR image shows an inhomogeneously contrast-enhancing soft tissue mass adjacent to L5/S1 on the right side (*arrow*). Its appearance is similar to that of other sarcomas.

Epidemiology

Chondrosarcoma is the third most common primary malignant bone tumor, encompassing 10% to 25% of all primary bone sarcomas. Three to 12 percent of all chondrosarcomas are located in spine. The mean age at presentation is 45 years (range: 20-90 years), and the male-female ratio is 2:1.

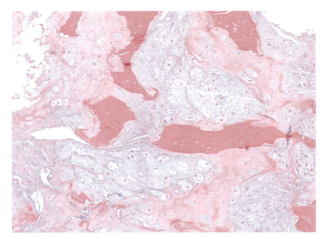

■ **FIGURE 15-78** Chondrosarcoma infiltrating the bone with destructive growth pattern. (H & E, original magnification ×50.)

Clinical Presentation

Dull aching pain and swelling, a palpable mass, and neurologic symptoms due to nerve root or spinal cord compression may be present. The 5-year survival rate for grade I tumors is 90%; for grade II tumors, 81%; and for grade III tumors, 29%. The overall 5-year survival rate is 48% to 60%. Metastases occur in 66% of patients with grade III tumors.

Pathophysiology

Chondrosarcomas are composed of hyaline cartilage within myxoid matrix and exhibit increased cellularity, nuclear atypia, and permeation of bony trabeculae. Accumulation of TP53 protein may indicate a poor prognosis. These tumors can present as primary chondrosarcomas or as malignant transformation of osteochondromas or enchondromas.

Pathology

A chondrosarcoma is a lobulated tumor composed of translucent hyaline nodules, focal areas of extensive enchondral ossification, hemorrhage and necrosis.

Histologically, mature hyaline cartilage and/or myxoid stroma and irregularly shaped lobules of cartilage are seen, which may be separated by fibrous bands. The chondrocytes are arranged in clusters (Fig. 15-78). On immunohistochemistry the tumor is positive for P-100 protein and vimentin.

Only 2% to 4% of chondrosarcomas arise in the spine, with an equal distribution.

Imaging

Radiography

On conventional radiographs one can see a lytic mass with or without a chondroid matrix and bone destruction with punctate as well as flocculent calcifications ("rings and arcs and nodules"), which represent mineralization of the cartilaginous matrix.

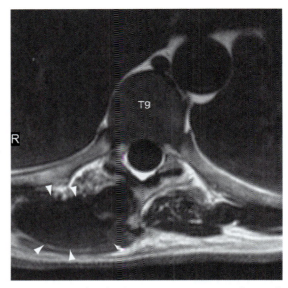

■ **FIGURE 15-79** Chondrosarcoma. T1W transverse image shows a large soft tissue mass with hypointense signal in the right paravertebral region (*arrowheads*), without intraspinal extension.

CT

CT depicts a lytic mass, cortical disruption, and extension into the soft tissues. The chondroid matrix shows the "rings and arcs and nodules" type of calcification. The nonmineralized portions of tumor are hypodense to muscle from the high water content of hyaline cartilage.

MRI

T1W images are necessary to better outline the intramedullary extent of the soft tissue mass, which appears of low to intermediate signal intensity, contrasting to the hyperintense signal intensity of the bone marrow. T2W images show the high signal intensity of cartilage and the low signal intensity of the mineralized portions.

After administration of a contrast agent T1W imaging demonstrates enhancement of the septa with a "rings and arcs" pattern and lack of enhancement in the cartilaginous, necrotic and cystic mucoid tissue portions of the tumor (Figs. 15-79 to 15-81).

Special Procedures

Bone scintigraphy shows an increased uptake of radiotracer.

Ewing's Sarcoma

Ewing's sarcoma is a small round cell sarcoma of bone. It is also known as Ewing's tumor.

Epidemiology

Ewing's sarcoma represents the sixth most common malignant bone tumor. Of all Ewing's sarcomas, 90% present before the age of 20 years. A second smaller peak is observed in patients at age 50 years. The male-to-female ratio is 2:1.

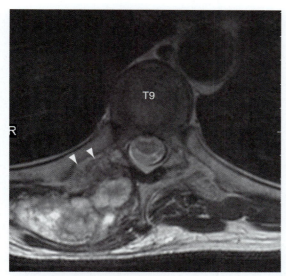

■ FIGURE 15-80 Chondrosarcoma. T1W postcontrast transverse MR image shows inhomogeneous contrast enhancement and infiltration of the transverse process of T9 (*arrowheads*).

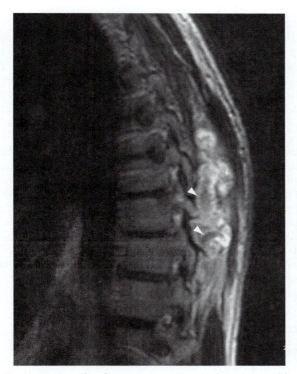

■ FIGURE 15-81 Chondrosarcoma. T1W sagittal MR image with contrast enhancement shows soft tissue mass extending over multiple levels. Nonenhancing areas (*arrowheads*) represent necrosis, cartilage, or cystic mucoid tissue.

Clinical Presentation

The nonspecific nature of pain is the most common presentation. An elevated erythrocyte sedimentation rate may simulate an osteomyelitis, and fever and leukocytosis may occur. Pathologic fracture of the vertebral body with vertebra plana may cause epidural compression and myelopathy. Metastases are present in 30% at the time of initial diagnosis, more often in lungs, regional lymph nodes, and other bones. There is a significant risk for a second bone malignancy. Spinal Ewing's sarcomas have worse prognoses than peripheral ones because of the increased difficulty in surgical resection.

Pathophysiology

Ewing's sarcoma represents a prototype of nonhematologic small round cell tumor. PNET is a closely related tumor. There is a reciprocal translocation between the *EWS* gene on chromosome 22 and *ETS*-like genes on chromosome 11.

Pathology

Ewing's sarcoma is a grayish white, poorly demarcated tumor that contains areas of hemorrhage, necroses, and cysts. It can originate in bones or in soft tissues.

Histologically, these tumors are composed of small round cells that are in solid sheets or divided into irregular masses by fibrous strands. There is scant cytoplasm and a single oval or round nucleus.

The spine is the site of origin in 4% to 18% of all Ewing's sarcomas,[29] and the lumbosacral spine is the most common site. These tumors arise typically in the vertebral bodies.

Imaging

Radiography

On conventional radiographs the tumor is typically centered in the vertebral body or sacrum with permeative/motheaten destruction and a wide zone of transition.

CT

On CT, a permeative lytic lesion is seen with an associated, heterogeneously enhancing soft tissue mass. No ossification in the associated soft tissue mass is observed. Fracture may result in vertebra plana.

MRI

T1W imaging shows an intermediate to low signal intensity that is hypointense to surrounding bone marrow. On T2W images there is intermediate to high signal intensity, and on T1W postcontrast images there is moderate enhancement as well as areas of necrosis (Figs. 15-82 to 15-84).

Special Procedures

Bone scintigraphy may show increased uptake in all three phases.

Lymphoma

Lymphoma is a lymphoreticular neoplasm with a variety of specific disease locations and cellular differentiations (epidural, intradural extramedullary, intradural intramedullary, osseous, leptomeningitic).

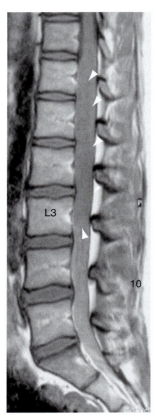

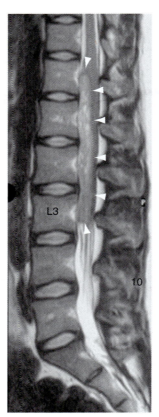

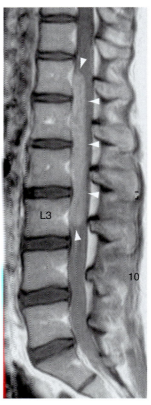

■ **FIGURE 15-82** T1W sagittal MR image shows Ewing's sarcoma of the spine to be of hypointense signal intensity (*arrowheads*) when compared with surrounding bone marrow.

■ **FIGURE 15-83** Ewing's sarcoma. T2W sagittal MR image shows an intermediate to high signal intensity (*arrowheads*).

■ **FIGURE 15-84** Ewing's sarcoma. T1W sagittal MR image after contrast agent administration shows moderate contrast enhancement of the soft tissue mass (*arrowheads*).

Epidemiology

Non-Hodgkin's lymphoma occurs more often than Hodgkin's disease; 80% to 90% are B-cell lymphomas. Lymphoma represents the most common malignancy of the epidural space. Primary epidural lymphomas comprise 1% to 7% of all non-Hodgkin's lymphomas, and primary osseous lymphomas represent 3% to 4% of all malignant bone tumors. The peak age at onset of lymphoma is the fourth to seventh decade, and there is a slight male predominance.

Clinical Presentation

The most common presenting symptom is back pain. The best prognosis is observed in primary osseous lymphoma in which the 5- to 10-year survival rate is about 90%.

Pathophysiology

The exact etiology is unknown. Risk factors are chemical exposure to pesticides, fertilizers, or solvents; infection with Epstein-Barr virus; or a family history of non-Hodgkin's lymphoma.

Pathology

Lymphoma varies from a well-circumscribed mass to a poorly marginated infiltrative disease. The tumor is often gray to yellow and of a firm to friable consistency. Some lesions also may be centrally necrotic.

The tumor most often consists of cells with large pleomorphic nuclei and a high nuclear-cytoplasmic ratio. In the periphery of the tumor mass the tumor cells typically demonstrate an angiocentric infiltration pattern forming collars around blood vessels. The invasion of parenchyma is either in the form of compact aggregates or in a diffuse fashion. Large geographic necrosis is often seen in the tumor center.

On immunohistochemistry, lymphomas are stained by the leukocyte common antigen (LCA/CD45) and because most represent B-cell lymphomas they also stain for B-cell markers such as CD20 (Fig 15-85).

Imaging

Radiography

Conventional radiographs in osseous lymphoma may show bone destruction, an ivory vertebral body, or vertebra plana.

CT

On CT the epidural lymphoma appears as a homogeneous dense mass with or without bone destruction, with intense epidural homogeneous enhancement.

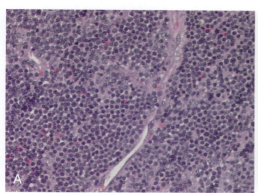

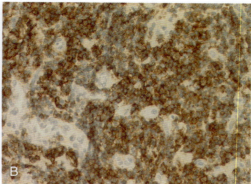

■ FIGURE 15-85 A, Hematoxylin and eosin stain of a lymphoma shows the cells with large pleomorphic nuclei and a high nuclear-cytoplasmic ratio. **B,** The cells of a B-cell lymphoma are stained in immunohistochemistry CD20.

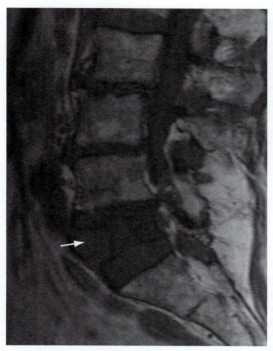

■ FIGURE 15-86 Lymphoma. T1W sagittal MR image shows hypointense signal of the lesion compared with normal marrow (*arrow*).

MRI

Epidural lesions have an isointense homogeneous signal intensity on T1W images, whereas bony lesions appear hypointense to normal bone marrow owing to replacement of the fatty marrow by cellular elements. On T2W imaging, lymphoma appears isointense/hyperintense compared with the spinal cord. Diffuse uniform enhancement is typical (Figs. 15-86 and 15-87).

Dynamic contrast-enhanced MRI shows bone marrow enhancement in a patient with lymphoproliferative disease, with an accuracy of 99%.

Special Procedures

Bone scintigraphy shows increased uptake. Gallium-67 scintigraphy has high sensitivity and specificity for the diagnosis of bone lymphoma.

Plasmacytoma

A plasmacytoma is a solitary monoclonal plasma cell tumor of bone or soft tissue, with no evidence of multiple myeloma elsewhere. This entity is also known as a solitary bone plasmacytoma, a solitary plasmacytoma, a solitary myeloma, or a solitary plasma cell tumor.

Epidemiology

Mean age at presentation is 55 years (younger than for multiple myeloma).

Clinical Presentation

These tumors can be asymptomatic. Pain is the most common symptom. Pathologic fracture can cause cord compression and myelopathy. In solitary bone plasmacytoma with indolent course the median survival is 10 years. Laboratory investigation shows low levels of serum/urine monoclonal proteins.

Pathophysiology

The marrow is infiltrated with neoplastic plasma cells. Genetic findings are unknown.

Pathology

There is gray-purple fatty marrow replacement. A collection of neoplastic plasma cells is seen with eccentric, round, pleomorphic nuclei with "clock face" chromatin and basophilic cytoplasm.

Imaging

Radiography

Conventional radiographs show a lytic multicystic lesion. Compression fracture is common.

CT

On CT there is a lytic, destructive vertebral body lesion. Compression fracture can occur with or without a soft tissue mass. Osteosclerosis is present in 3%.

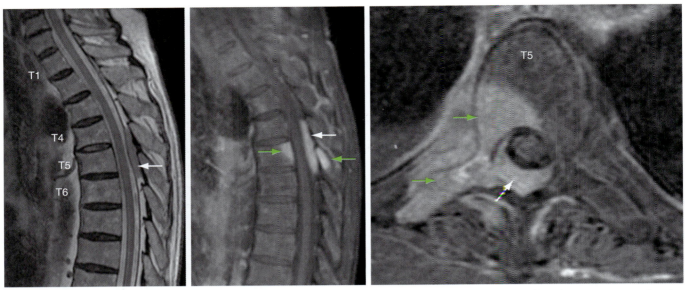

■ **FIGURE 15-87** T2W (*left*), T1W sagittal (*middle*), and axial (*right*) MR images after contrast application show a hyperintense, contrast-enhancing epidural lesion (*white arrows*), as well as intraosseous extension into vertebra T5 (*green arrows*) in a patient with non-Hodgkin's lymphoma.

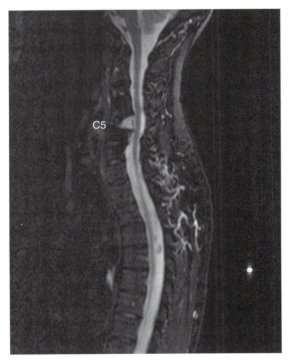

■ **FIGURE 15-88** Plasmacytoma. T2W fat-saturated sagittal MR image shows collapse of C5 vertebra with posterior bony epidural extension and slight cord compression. There is no associated soft tissue mass.

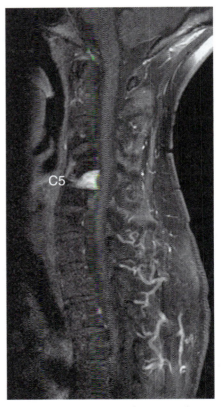

■ **FIGURE 15-89** Plasmacytoma. T1W fat-saturated postcontrast sagittal MR image shows moderate contrast enhancement of the C5 vertebral body. Mild posterior extension effaces the ventral thecal sac.

MRI

T1W imaging shows a solitary vertebral body lesion with hypointense marrow with low-signal curvilinear areas. T2W imaging shows a heterogeneous signal and focal hyperintensities compared with fat and also curvilinear areas of signal void. After administration of a contrast agent, T1W imaging shows mild to moderate enhancement (Figs. 15-88 to 15-90).

Special Procedures

Bone scintigraphy depicts intense uptake but can be normal in the early stage of disease.

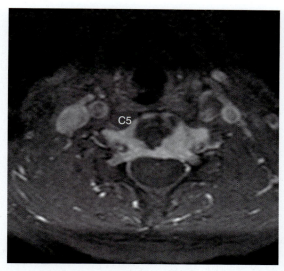

■ FIGURE 15-90   T1W fat-saturated postcontrast transverse MR image shows the contrast-enhancing plasmacytoma in the C5 vertebra.

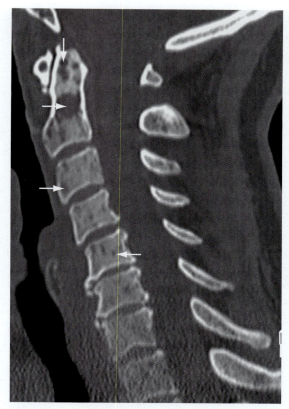

■ FIGURE 15-91   Sagittal CT scan shows multifocal lytic lesion (*arrows*) in a patient with multiple myeloma.

Multiple Myeloma

Multiple myeloma is characterized by multifocal malignant proliferation of monoclonal plasma cells within the bone marrow.

Epidemiology

The incidence of this common primary bone tumor is 3 to 4 per 100,000 per year. The peak age at onset is 60 to 70 years, and there is a male-to-female ratio of 3 : 2.

Clinical Presentation

Bone pain is present in 75%, with 20% of patients asymptomatic at presentation. Pathologic fractures (50%-70%), spinal cord compression (10%-15%), renal failure, monoclonal gammopathy, or Bence Jones proteinuria can be found. Diffuse osteopenia occurs in 85% of cases. Median survival rate with chemotherapy is 3 to 5 years, and in 5% complete remission can be achieved.

Pathophysiology

Replacement of fatty bone marrow due to neoplastic plasma cells leads to accelerated osteoclastic bone resorption and to inhibited osteoblastic bone formation. The etiology is unknown. Risk factors include ionizing radiation, autoimmune disease, and human immunodeficiency virus infection.

Pathology

Multiple myeloma is a well-circumscribed, gray-red soft tumor that replaces cancellous bone. There are aggregates of neoplastic plasma cells with eccentric, round hyperchromatic nuclei with "cartwheel" chromatin that replace normal bone marrow.

Imaging

Radiography

Conventional radiographs show well-circumscribed, punched-out lesions, sometimes with surrounding sclerosis, a soft tissue mass adjacent to bone destruction, and often compression fractures.

CT

On CT there are multifocal lytic lesions, which might be accompanied by vertebral destruction and fractures, cortical disruption, and an extraosseous soft tissue mass (Fig. 15-91).

MRI

MRI may be normal or may show multiple patchy areas of heterogeneous low to intermediate signal intensity on T1W images compared with normal marrow. On T2W and STIR images the lesions are hyperintense. On postcontrast imaging diffuse contrast enhancement of the lesions is seen (Fig. 15-92).

Special Procedures

Bone scintigraphy is typically negative. On positron emission tomography, lesions of multiple myeloma appear metabolically active.

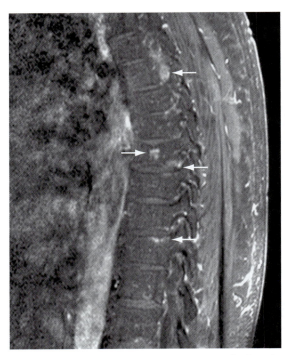

■ FIGURE 15-92 T1W fat-saturated postcontrast sagittal MR image of the thoracic spine shows multiple, small, enhancing vertebral myelomatous lesions (*arrows*).

Osteoblastic Metastases

There may be metastatic extension of a primary tumor to the spine with bone destruction. These metastases can also be referred to as sclerotic or osteosclerotic metastases.

Epidemiology

Vertebral metastases are present in 10% to 40% of patients with systemic cancer. Both children and adults are affected, but the average age of patients with epidural metastasis ranges from 53 to 58 years. The gender predilection varies with the specific primary tumor. Ninety percent of prostate cancer metastases involve the spine.

Clinical Presentation

Pain is the leading complaint. Compression fractures are common. There is an epidural component that may cause myelopathy or radiculopathy. Myelopathy caused by epidural metastasis is seen in 5% of adults with systemic cancer. Spinal metastases are the most common cause for epidural cord compression.

Pathophysiology

The bone marrow is initially infiltrated, followed by trabecular and subsequently cortical destruction. Hematogenous dissemination is more common than perineural, lymphatic, or CSF spread. Osteosclerotic primary lesions include prostate, carcinoid, bladder, nasopharynx cancer, and medulloblastoma. Mixed lytic and blastic metastases are more often caused by lung, breast, cervix, and ovarian primary carcinomas.

Pathology

Gross appearance is of softened, eroded bone with or without an adjacent soft tissue mass. The histology varies with the histology of the primary tumor.

The most common location of epidural metastasis is the thoracic spine, followed by the lumbosacral and the cervical regions. The lesions preferentially destroy the posterior cortex of the vertebral body and the pedicle.

Imaging

Radiography

On conventional radiographs the lesions appear as multiple dense foci scattered throughout the vertebral bodies.

CT

On CT, sclerotic lesions are well or ill defined. The posterior vertebral body is involved in almost all cases; in 80% the anterior body is involved, and in 60% the pedicle is involved. An "ivory" vertebra may be present. Enhancement is not detectable due to sclerosis.

MRI

On T1W imaging the signal intensity is different from normal marrow. Hypointense solitary or multiple lesions may be seen. The intervertebral discs are generally spared. On T2W imaging sclerotic metastases appear hypointense. After contrast agent administration T1W imaging shows variable enhancement depending on the degree of sclerosis (Figs. 15-93 to 15-95).

A patient with a known primary lesion presenting with acute myelopathy is an absolute indication for emergency MRI to detect the sites (or sites) of compression and the extent of the epidural tumor for planning further treatment.

Special Procedures

Bone SPECT is superior to planar imaging for the detection of bone metastases. Diffuse increased uptake ("superscan") is seen with prostate cancer.

Osteolytic Metastases

Metastasis can occur from a primary tumor to the spine. Bone destruction exceeds bone production. These lesions also can be called lytic osseous metastases.

Epidemiology

Osteolytic spine metastases are found in 5% to 10% of all cancer patients; vertebral metastases occur in 10% to 40% of patients with systemic cancer. Epidural spinal cord

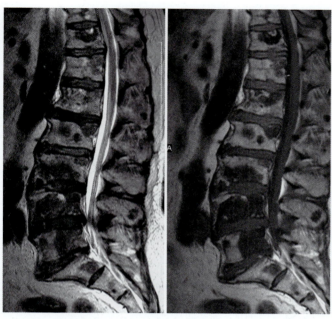

■ **FIGURE 15-93** T2W and T1W sagittal MR images show multiple blastic osseous metastatic lesions in the vertebral bodies with low signal intensity in a patient with prostate cancer.

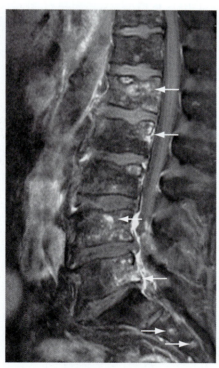

■ **FIGURE 15-94** T1W sagittal postcontrast image in the same patient as in Figure 15-93 shows a variable contrast enhancement related to the degree of sclerosis (*arrows*).

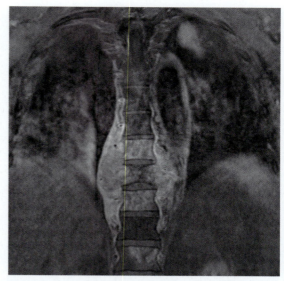

■ **FIGURE 15-95** T1W coronal MR image after contrast agent administration shows the epidural and paravertebral extent of the metastatic disease in a patient with prostate cancer.

Clinical Presentation

Pain is present, and an epidural component may cause myelopathy and radiculopathy. Compression fractures are often found.

Pathophysiology

The marrow is initially infiltrated, followed by trabecular and, subsequently, cortical destruction. Bone resorption and bone formation are often present at variable degrees. Hematogenous dissemination is more common than perineural, lymphatic, or CSF spread. In 15% to 25% of cases a primary lesion is unknown.

Pathology

The gross appearance is of softened, eroded bone with or without an adjacent soft tissue mass. The histology of the metastases varies with the histology of the primary tumor.

Imaging

Radiography

Conventional radiographs require 50% to 70% of bone destruction to be visible and more than 1 cm diameter of the osteolytic lesion. Useful diagnostic findings are an absent pedicle and destroyed posterior cortical line.

CT

On CT, single or multiple, lytic, permeative, destructive lesion(s) are seen involving the posterior vertebral body in almost all cases, the anterior body in 80% of cases, and the pedicle in 60% of cases (Fig. 15-96). Enhancement is often not detectable.

compression is seen in 5% of adults with systemic cancer. Any age group may be involved, and gender varies with the specific type of primary tumor. The most common primary tumors producing lytic skeletal metastases include those of the breast, lung, kidney, and thyroid and melanoma.

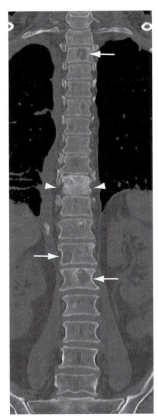

■ **FIGURE 15-96** Coronal bone CT shows multiple blastic (*arrowheads*) and lytic (*arrows*) metastatic lesions in a patient with mesothelioma of the pleura.

MRI

On T1W imaging there are solitary or multiple lesions with hypointense signal intensity as compared with normal marrow; the intervertebral discs are generally spared. On T2W imaging there is hyperintense to normal marrow on STIR sequences. After contrast agent administration diffuse enhancement is evident on fat-saturated T1W images.

Special Procedures

Bone SPECT is superior to planar imaging. The uptake represents regions of bone production, not directly the tumor.

ANALYSIS

The most common intramedullary tumors of the spinal cord are ependymoma, glioma, and hemangioblastoma, accounting for up to 60%, 30%, and 6% of all intramedullary tumors, respectively. The differentiation of these tumors from other diseases of the spine (e.g., congestive myelopathy by dural arteriovenous fistula [DAVF], spinal cord infarct, or multiple sclerosis) may be challenging on imaging. However, some characteristics can be observed as follows: On the axial plain radiograph ependymoma is mostly centrally located and exhibits a concentric growth pattern, whereas gliomas are rather eccentric (Fig. 15-97). Hemangioblastomas are also eccentric, but the presence of flow void is characteristic. Flow void is also typical in congestive myelopathy by DAVF, but the edema

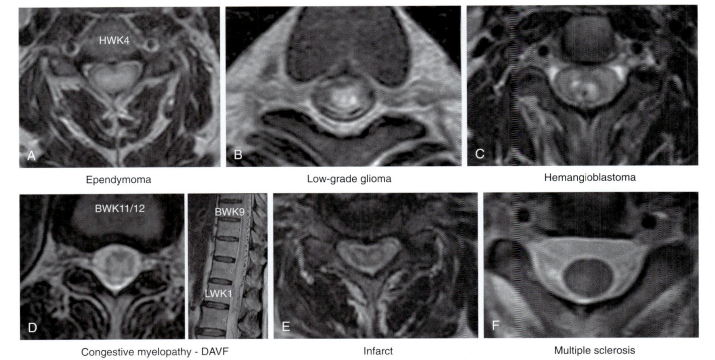

■ **FIGURE 15-97** A to F, Characteristics of differentiation among ependymoma, glioma, and hemangioblastoma, as well as DAVF, infarct, and multiple sclerosis on imaging.

is central and there is no tumorous mass. Spinal cord infarcts present as a characteristic "snake bite" morphology in the ventral columns of the gray matter. Plaques in multiple sclerosis are typically in the posterior and lateral funiculi.

Low-grade gliomas most commonly result in mild enlargement of the spinal cord as opposed to cavernomas, which may cause a more focal and pronounced expansion. Important distinctive features are the more circumscribed morphology, the hemosiderin ring on the T2W

image around the lesion, as well as the patchy hyperintensities on the T1W image (Fig. 15-98) representing methemoglobin in the cavernous hemangioma.

Hemangioblastoma as well as arteriovenous malformations of the spinal cord characteristically present as dilated, tortuous feeding arteries and draining veins. However, differentiation is straightforward because hemangioblastomas have a tumorous nodule (Fig. 15-99) whereas arteriovenous malformations have an arteriovenous nidus between arteries and veins.

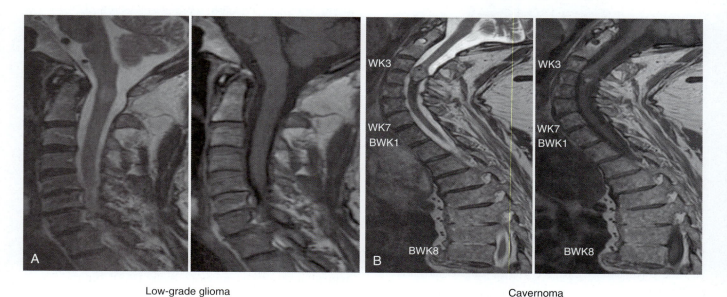

Low-grade glioma   Cavernoma

■ **FIGURE 15-98**   **A** and **B,** Low-grade gliomas resulting in mild enlargement of the spinal cord are distinct from cavernomas, which may cause a more focal and pronounced expansion. Note the more circumscribed morphology, the hemosiderin ring on the T2W image around the lesion, as well as the patchy hyperintensities on the T1W image in cavernomas.

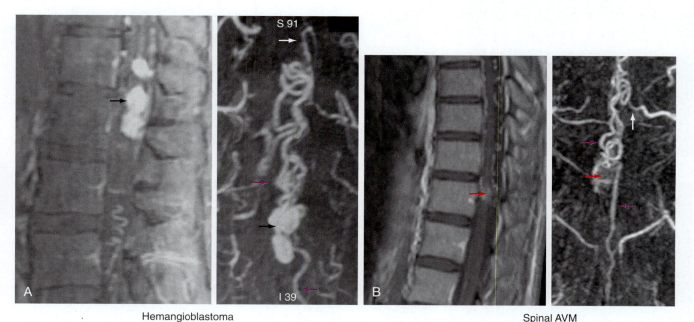

Hemangioblastoma   Spinal AVM

■ **FIGURE 15-99**   **A** and **B,** Differentiation of hemangioblastoma and arteriovenous malformation of the spinal cord in imaging is straightforward because hemangioblastomas have a tumorous nodule (*black arrows*), whereas an arteriovenous malformation has an arteriovenous nidus (*red arrows*) between feeding arteries (*white arrows*) and draining veins (*purple arrows*). (**A**, right, from Binkert CA, Kolias SS, Valavanis A: Spinal cord vascular disease: Characterization with three-dimensional contrast-enhanced angiography. Am J Neuroradiol 20:1785-1793, 1999.)

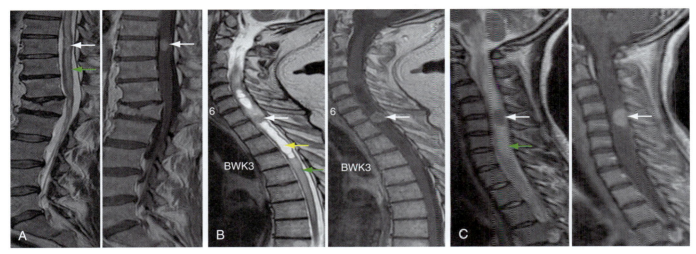

GBM metastasis   Plexus ca. metastasis   Toxoplasmosis

■ **FIGURE 15-100** A to C, Differentiation among non-neoplastic lesions in imaging. The known intracranial glioblastoma multiforme and the known plexus-carcinoma in the first two patients and the known HIV infection in the third patient suggest the diagnosis of a glioblastoma multiforme metastasis, plexus-carcinoma metastasis, and an opportunistic infection (*white arrows*), respectively. However, the presence of the prominent syrinx (*yellow arrow*) is suggestive of a neoplastic disease. Observe the edema (*green arrows*) in all cases.

A non-neoplastic etiology of a spinal lesion always has to be considered and evaluated carefully. Sometimes only the anamnesis is helpful in the differential diagnosis. A known intracranial glioblastoma multiforme or plexus-carcinoma or human immunodeficiency virus infection (Fig. 15-100) can suggest the diagnosis of a glioblastoma multiforme metastasis, plexus-carcinoma metastasis, or an opportunistic infection, respectively. However, the presence of the prominent syrinx is suggestive of a neoplastic disease. Edema is also present.

Schwannomas and neurofibromas (Fig. 15-101) are often indistinguishable when referring to their signal intensities on T1W and T2W images. The following neuroradiologic features may provide hints in the differentiation between the two entities:

- Schwannomas are most commonly lobulated masses located eccentric to the nerve root, displacing it to the contralesional side (*purple arrow* on Fig. 15-101F), whereas neurofibromas encase the nerve root itself and therefore are more smoothly circumscribed with a fusiform appearance.
- Schwannomas are more often heterogeneous on T2W imaging and on postcontrast T1W imaging, owing to cystic or fatty degeneration or intratumoral hemorrhage (*red arrow* on Fig. 15-101A), whereas neurofibromas mostly show homogeneous signal (*white arrows* on Fig. 15-101D).

Other characteristics of these lesions may additionally help in their differentiation:

- Solitary schwannomas are much more common than spinal neurofibromas.
- Schwannomas are more often solitary and when multiple often associated with NF1, whereas in NF1 almost all nerve root tumors are neurofibromas.
- Spinal neurofibromas are very rare outside NF1.

- A large paraspinal mass extending intradurally through the spinal foramina at one or multiple segments is most probably a plexiform neurofibroma.

In the case of multiple schwannomas and multiple neurofibromas the presence of bilateral vestibular schwannomas suggests the diagnosis of schwannoma with association of NF2 whereas the presence of subcutaneous neurofibromas (*black arrows* on Fig. 15-101D,E) suggests the diagnosis of neurofibroma with association of NF1.

Multiple schwannomas or schwannomatosis in the lumbar spine needs to be differentiated from other lesions that give rise to thickening of the cauda equina fibers and to multiple enhancing nodules such as drop metastasis, lymphoma, or sarcoidosis. However, the only clue can be the knowledge of the underlying illness or associated lesions (Fig. 15-102).

Concerning the neuroradiologic distinction between spinal schwannomas and meningiomas, there are some features that are more characteristic for one than for the other. Typical schwannomas (Fig. 15-103A, B) present as a rather regular shape with smooth margin but with more heterogeneous signal intensity on T2W images (compare A to E on Fig. 15-103) and as a stronger, irregular contrast-enhancement than meningiomas (compare B with F on Fig. 15-103). The difference in the intensity of contrast enhancement between the two can be explained by the fact that the open gap junctions between the epithelial cells of the blood vessels in schwannomas are shorter and straight and thus more permeable to gadolinium molecules than in meningiomas.

However, schwannomas with Antoni A pattern (more cellular type—homogeneous signal intensity and contrast enhancement) (see Fig. 15-103C, D) may strongly resemble meningiomas (compare C with E and D with F on Fig. 15-103). In these cases, elderly age, female gender, thoracic localization, and presence of a dural tail sign (*red arrow* on Fig. 15-103F) support the diagnosis of a menin-

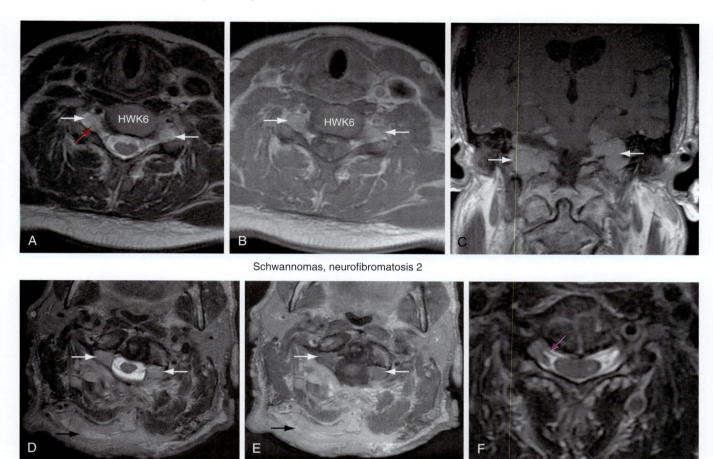

Schwannomas, neurofibromatosis 2

Neurofibromas, neurofibromatosis 1

■ **FIGURE 15-101** A to F, Schwannomas and neurofibromas (*white arrows*) are often indistinguishable when referring to their signal intensities on T1W and T2W MR images, although there are some neuroradiologic features that may provide hints in the differentiation between the two entities (see text for more details).

gioma. Tumor localization clearly along a nerve root with foraminal extension favors schwannoma.

The differential diagnoses of a number of entities are summarized in the following list:

- *Enostosis:* A solitary osteoblastic metastasis may be difficult to differentiate from a growing enostosis especially with radionuclide uptake, which can be confusing. However, the normal adjacent trabecular bone and the typical "brush border" pattern can support the diagnosis of enostosis. Operation is not necessary. Other differential diagnoses are Schmorl node, osteoid osteoma, and osteopoikilosis (see Figs. 15-45 and 15-46).
- *Osteoid osteoma:* Osteoblastoma, enostosis, lymphoma, osteomyelitis, reactive (degenerative) sclerosis and especially sequestrum in the case of osteomyelitis or a focal abscess can mimic the nidus of osteoid osteoma; however, osteomyelitis usually involves the vertebral body and CT usually shows end plate destruction or destruction of the facet joint (see Fig. 15-52).
- *Osteoblastoma:* Osteoid osteoma, eosinophilic granuloma, aneurysmal bone cyst, giant cell tumor, infection, and osteosarcoma are included in the differential diagnosis. An aneurysmal bone cyst component of oste-

oblastoma is present in 10% to 15% of osteoblastomas. Peritumoral edema may obscure the lesion and mimic malignancy or infection on MRI. Typically, an expansile mass occurring in the posterior elements is present (see Figs. 15-53 and 15-54).

- *Epidural lipomatosis:* Subacute epidural hematoma, spinal angiolipoma, and epidural metastasis or abscess may mimic this condition. Subacute epidural hematoma remains hyperintense on fat-suppressed MR sequences and manifests as an acute onset of symptoms. Spinal angiolipoma, epidural metastases, and epidural abscess show diffuse contrast enhancement.
- *Aneurysmal bone cyst:* Osteoblastoma, giant cell tumor, and telangiectatic osteogenic sarcoma need to be differentiated. These entities are present in patients of nearly the same age and all present as "absent pedicle sign" on conventional radiographs (expansion in pedicle results in loss of pedicle contour on anteroposterior radiographs). Giant cell tumor and osteoblastoma may be associated with aneurysmal bone cyst. Osteogenic sarcoma presents as more prominent permeative bone destruction and a wider transition zone. Other differential diagnoses include metastases and plasmacytoma.

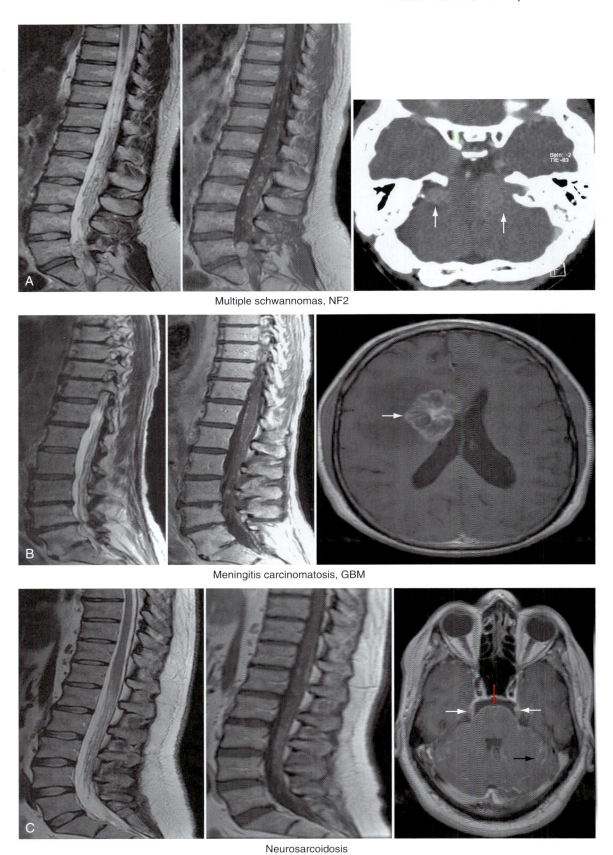

Multiple schwannomas, NF2

Meningitis carcinomatosis, GBM

Neurosarcoidosis

■ **FIGURE 15-102** **A,** Multiple schwannomas of the cauda equina fibers by neurofibromatosis type 2 as demonstrated on an axial brain CT showing the bilateral acoustic schwannomas (*arrows*). **B,** Meningitis gliomatosa of the cauda equina fibers by metastatic dissemination from a brain glioblastoma multiforme (*arrow*). **C,** Leptomeningeal dissemination of neurosarcoidosis with thick leptomeningeal contrast enhancement of the cerebellar foliae (*black arrow*), surface of the pons (*red arrow*), as well as the trigeminal nerves on both sides (*white arrows*).

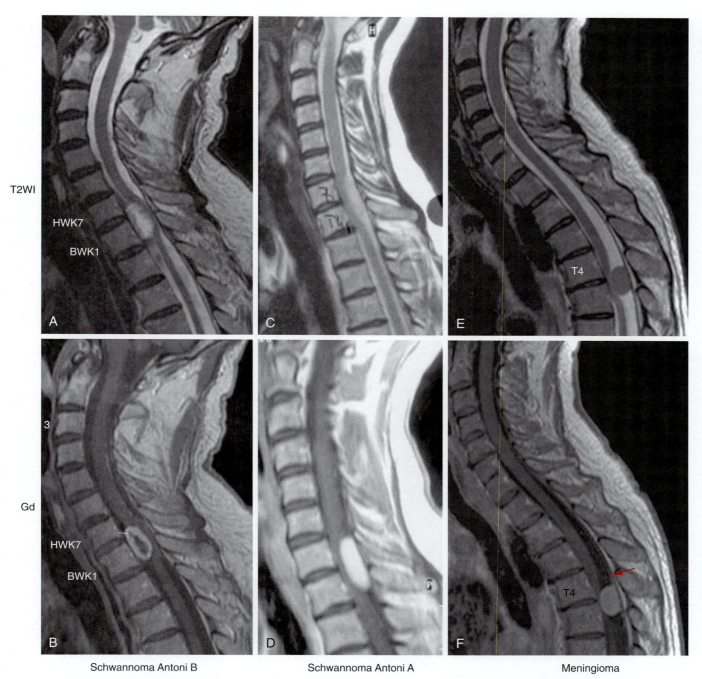

T2WI

HWK7

BWK1

A

C

E

T4

3

Gd

HWK7

BWK1

B

D

F

T4

Schwannoma Antoni B   Schwannoma Antoni A   Meningioma

■ **FIGURE 15-103** Characterization of differentiation among schwannoma type Antoni A (**A** and **B**), type Antoni B (**C** and **D**), and meningioma (**E** and **F**). (See text for more details.)

- *Hemangioma:* STIR sequences will show marked lesion hypointensity that is difficult to demarcate from the fatty marrow; however, hemangiomas typically retain some high signal owing to the vascular components of the lesion. Degenerative end plate disease type II will involve adjacent end plates. Paget's disease will not show epidural extension. Vertebral metastases characteristically extend into the pedicles.

- *Giant cell tumor:* Aneurysmal bone cyst can coexist with giant cell tumor arising most commonly in the arch but can extend into the vertebral body. Chordoma arises in the midline and can have a large soft tissue

component. Metastases are usually in older patients and often multiple.

- *Osteochondroma:* In chondrosarcomas the peak age is older than in osteochondroma and a lytic destructive lesion with a soft tissue mass is present. Osteoblastoma and aneurysmal bone cyst are both expansile lesions, with the latter multicystic with fluid-fluid levels.

- *Chordoma:* Chondrosarcoma presents as similar MR characteristics but shows typical chondroid matrix with rings and arcs. Giant cell tumor shows a more heterogeneous MR signal with blood products and a low T2 signal. Sacrococcygeal teratoma is seen more commonly in the pediatric population (chordomas are rare in patients < age 30 years). Metastases and multiple myeloma and lymphoma are often multifocal diseases (see Figs. 15-72 and 15-73).

● *Osteosarcoma:* Sclerotic metastases of prostate, breast, or gastrointestinal tract are often multiple and do not extend beyond the borders of the bone. The aggressive form of osteoblastoma can mimic osteosarcoma on imaging. Fluid-fluid levels are similar to those of telangiectatic osteosarcoma. Osteomyelitis is occasionally sclerotic but usually involves two contiguous vertebrae and the intervening disc space.

● *Chondrosarcoma:* Chondroblastoma may be indistinguishable from clear cell chondrosarcoma. Osteosarcoma presents as an osteoid matrix and no chondroid matrix, and the patients are usually younger. In myositis ossificans a history of trauma is present. In lymphoma or metastatic disease a soft tissue mass is present and often multiple sites are involved.

● *Ewing's sarcoma:* Primitive neuroectodermal tumor (PNET) is clinically and radiologically identical to Ewing's sarcoma. Also, Langerhans cell histiocytosis may have the same radiologic appearance but may form discrete geographic lytic lesions. Other small round cell tumors such as lymphoma, leukemia, or myeloma have the same radiologic appearance but involve the vertebral body more than the vertebral arch. Patients can show an elevated erythrocyte sedimentation rate, which may simulate an osteomyelitis.

● *Lymphoma:* All epidural diseases that mimic epidural lymphoma such as hematoma, abscess, or metastases need to be differentiated. Hematoma presents as a heterogeneous signal, and abscess commonly shows a contrast-enhancing rim and a central hypointensity on T1W images. Osseous lymphoma mimics metastatic disease and eosinophilic granuloma, which presents as vertebra plana and usually occurs in younger patients.

● *Plasmacytoma:* Multiple myeloma needs to be distinguished. A second lesion is found in 33% of patients with solitary bone plasmacytoma. Metastases also may not be distinguishable from solitary bone plasmacytoma but do not involve the adjacent vertebral bodies or the disc. Benign osteoporotic compression fractures show signal intensity like normal bone marrow. Aggressive hemangiomas can mimic solitary bone plasmacytoma, and Paget's disease shows vertebral body expansion with thickened trabeculae.

● *Multiple myeloma:* In metastases the pedicle is involved earlier than in multiple myeloma and no monoclonal gammopathy or Bence Jones proteinuria is present. In osteoporosis no endosteal scalloping on plain radiography is present. Hypoplastic marrow shows no postgadolinium enhancement.

● *Osteoblastic metastases:* Hemangioma typically shows hyperintensity on T1W imaging. Renal osteodystrophy has a "rugger jersey" appearance on conventional radiographs, and no paravertebral/epidural mass is present. In patients with Paget's disease, thickened trabeculae are present. In solitary bone plasmacytoma, multiple myeloma, or leukemia a diffuse marrow involvement is more common than in metastases.

● *Osteolytic metastases:* In solitary bone plasmacytoma, multiple myeloma or leukemia a diffuse marrow involvement is more common than in metastases. These metastases may be difficult to differentiate from an acute osteoporotic fracture; however, diffusion-weighted imaging sequences may be helpful. Patients with osteoporotic fractures show an intact pedicle and cortex, and no soft tissue involvement is present.

BOX 15-1   Ependymoma

PATIENT HISTORY

A 62-year-old woman presented with a chief complaint of progressive pain in the shoulders and neck for 2 years. Initially the pain was restricted to the left shoulder and then progressed to involve the right shoulder and neck. The patient had a subtotal resection of the thyroid gland 10 years earlier owing to struma multinodosa. Otherwise, her past medical history was free of disease. MRI was performed 1 year after onset of the symptoms in another institution and showed only degenerative changes of the cervical spine. In the past months new onset of hypesthesia of the arms and hands led to a new consultation. Carpal tunnel syndrome was suspected and ruled out with neurophysiologic studies.

TECHNIQUE

Axial and sagittal T2W, sagittal T1W, and axial and sagittal T1W contrast-enhanced sequences (gadolinium, 0.1 mmol/kg) were obtained of the cervical spine.

FINDINGS

There is an intramedullary tumor on cord segment C3-4 (Fig. 15-104).

COMMENT

The patient was admitted to the neurosurgical department for operative treatment. Preoperative neurologic examination was normal except for hypesthesia of the arms and hands without a clear dermatome pattern. The patient underwent a laminectomy of C3-C4 and the tumor was resected (see Fig. 15-104E). Histopathologic examination confirmed the diagnosis of a cellular ependymoma (WHO grade II). Postoperative neurologic examination revealed ataxia and disturbance of fine motor skills, especially of the left hand. Postoperative MRI showed no residual tumor (see Fig. 15-104F-G). The patient underwent rehabilitation and 3 months later showed evidence on follow-up examination of a full recovery.

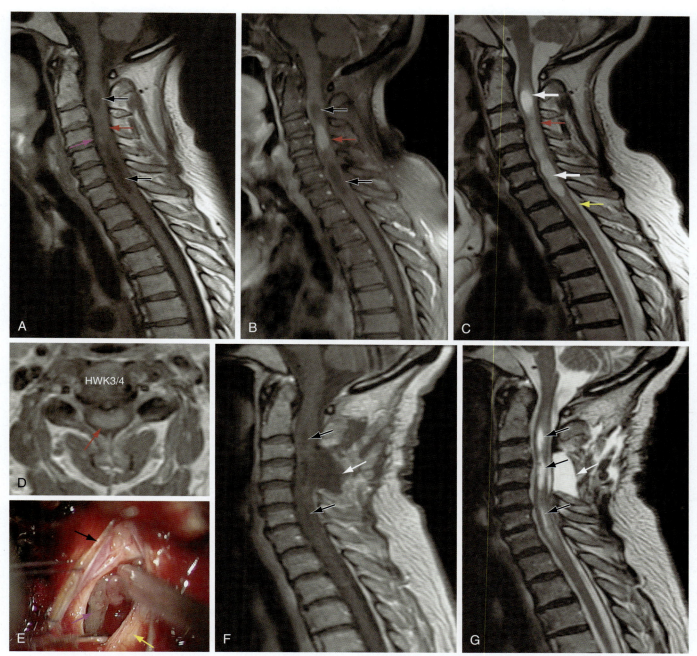

■ **FIGURE 15-104** Intramedullary ependymoma. **A,** Sagittal T1W MRI demonstrated hypointense signal on the cervical cord at segments C2-C7 (*black arrows*), an isointense signal component at the segment C3-C4 representing the tumor mass (*red arrow*), and a minor hyperintense signal component most likely representing blood products (*purple arrow*). Observe as well the diffuse enlargement of the cervical cord. **B,** Contrast-enhanced sagittal T1W MR image demonstrated hypointense signal (*black arrows*) cranial and caudal of a homogeneous enhancing tumor at C3-C4 (*red arrow*). **C,** Sagittal T2W MR image demonstrated a relatively well-circumscribed inhomogeneous hyperintense mass that represents the tumor (*red arrow*) as well as a strong hyperintense signal on the cranial and caudal cord caused by a cranial and caudal syrinx (*white arrows*). Also note the diffuse hyperintensity under the syrinx caused by edema (*yellow arrow*). **D,** Contrast-enhanced axial T1W image demonstrates the intramedullary central location of the mass with homogeneous contrast enhancement (*red arrow*). The intramedullary tumor was suspected to be an ependymoma owing to its MRI features. **E,** Intraoperative photograph shows the macroscopic view of the tumor. Note the retracted dura mater (*black arrow*), the opened spinal cord (*yellow arrow*), and the intramedullary tumor, clearly distinguishable from the healthy cord (*purple arrow*). **F** and **G,** Postoperative MRI of the cervical spine. Contrast-enhanced sagittal T1W (**F**) and T2W (**G**) MR images show no residual tumor. Only the syrinx is present, but it is decreased in size because of the removal of the tumor (*black arrows*). Also note the postoperative changes by laminectomy at the C3-4 level, including the hypointense cerebrospinal fluid collection (*white arrows*). (*Intraoperative photograph courtesy of Dr. René-Ludwig Bernays, Neurosurgery, University Hospital, Zürich.*)

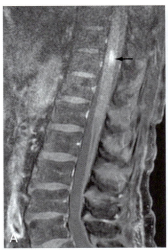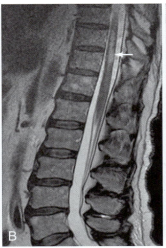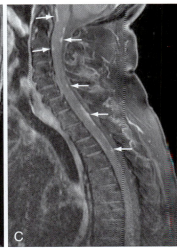

■ **FIGURE 15-105** Glioblastoma multiforme metastasis. **A,** Fat-saturated, contrast-enhanced sagittal T1W MR image of the thoracolumbar spine shows enhancement of spinal intramedullary metastasis at the level of T10 (*black arrow*). **B,** Sagittal T2W MR image shows the mass and the perifocal edema with T2 hyperintense signal (*white arrow*). **C,** Contrast-enhanced sagittal T1W image of the cervicothoracic spine shows leptomeningeal enhancement indicating subarachnoidal dissemination of the tumor (*white arrows*).

BOX 15-2   Glioblastoma Multiforme Metastasis

PATIENT HISTORY

A 68-year-old man presented with complex partial seizures in the form of uncinate seizures (unpleasant odor). MRI of the brain led to the possible diagnosis of a glioblastoma multiforme of the temporal lobe. The patient underwent subtotal resection of the tumor and combined radiochemotherapy. Almost 2 months after initial diagnosis the patient complained of progressive difficulty to stand up and walk. On neurologic examination a paraparesis and a stiff neck supposedly due to meningeal irritation were documented.

TECHNIQUE

Fat-saturated, contrast-enhanced sagittal T1W and sagittal T2W images of the thoracolumbar spine were obtained along with a contrast-enhanced sagittal T1W image of the cervicothoracic spine.

FINDINGS

Tumor dissemination is intraparenchymal, frontal, and cerebellar and there is metastatic disease of the spinal cord and of the intraspinal meninges (Fig. 15-105).

COMMENT

The patient was admitted to the hospital due to disease progression. Therapy with dexamethasone led to an improvement of the neurologic status. Because of other medical problems, including known cardiovascular disease and stroke, a nonoperative treatment was preferred. The patient underwent two cycles of chemotherapy.

BOX 15-3   Hemangioblastoma

PATIENT HISTORY

A 15-year-old girl presented with amaurosis fugax. Diagnostic imaging led to the finding of a retinal hemangioma and two additional tumors located in the foramen magnum and the cervical spinal cord (Fig. 15-106A, B). Because of initial MRI findings the diagnosis of multifocal hemangioma in association with von Hippel-Lindau syndrome was suspected and was genetically confirmed. The patient was treated first in the ophthalmology department owing to the retinal hemorrhage that led to the amaurosis fugax. Because of lack of additional neurologic symptoms no further treatment of the additional hemangioblastomas was initially indicated.

The patient presented for follow-up after 15 months. Clinically, only a minimal hypesthesia of the dermatome C8 on the left side was documented with no other neurologic deficit.

TECHNIQUE

Contrast-enhanced sagittal T1W and T2W MR images were obtained.

FINDINGS

In control MRI of the spinal cord a progression of the hemangiomas in the foramen magnum and cervical cord is observed (see Fig. 15-106C, D).

COMMENT

Because of the growth of the hemangioblastomas and the new symptom the patient was admitted for neurosurgical therapy and underwent a suboccipital craniotomy, a laminectomy at C1, and a hemilaminectomy at C2-3. The foramen magnum lesions were removed, and the cyst at C2-C4 was drained (see Fig. 15-106E, F). Postoperatively only a minimal rest hypesthesia of the dermatome C8 on the left was observed. Three months later the patient complained of a new recurring mild paresthesia of the right hand. Control MRI showed a new cyst formation at the level of C2-C4 (see Fig. 15-106G, H). Further therapy is not yet planned.

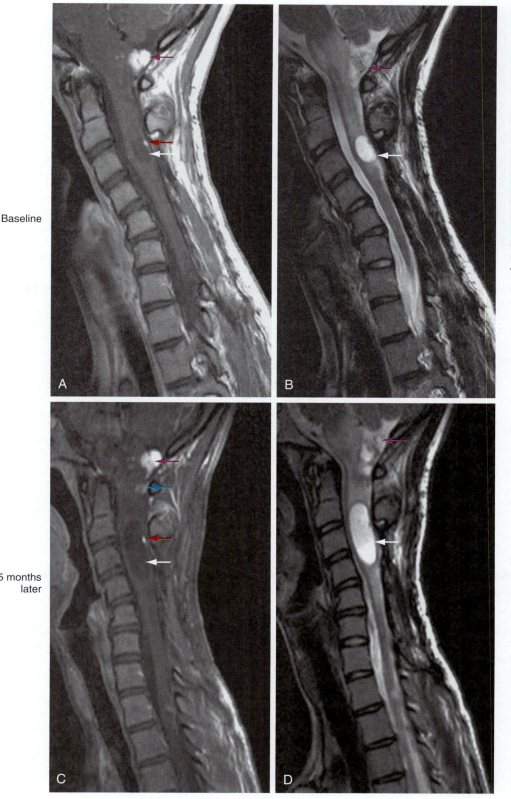

Baseline

15 months later

■ **FIGURE 15-106** Multifocal presentation of hemangioblastomas and course of disease. Baseline contrast-enhanced sagittal T1W (**A**) and T2W (**B**) MR images demonstrate a cystic lesion of the intramedullary segment C3 (*white arrow*) with a small enhancing part (*red arrow*) and a second mass in the foramen magnum with a strong enhancing component (*purple arrow*). Follow-up MRI after 15 months. Contrast-enhanced sagittal T1W (**C**) and T2W (**D**) MR images demonstrate growth of the intramedullary cyst at C2-C3 (*white arrow*) with known small enhancing component (*red arrow*) and the second lesion in the foramen magnum with strong enhancing mass (*purple arrow*) and a new area of enhancement suspected to correspond to disease progression (*blue arrow*).

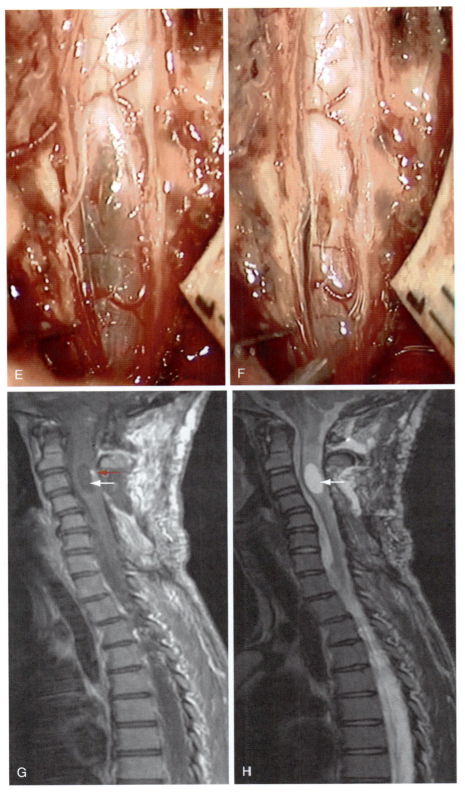

■ **FIGURE 15-106, cont'd** Intraoperative photographs show the cyst before (**E**) and after (**F**) drainage. Follow-up MRI after 3 months. Contrast-enhanced sagittal T1W (**G**) and T2W (**H**) MR images demonstrate a recurrent cyst at C2-C3 (*white arrow*) with the enhancing nodulus (*red arrow*). (**E** *and* **F** *courtesy of Dr. Evaldas Cesnulis, Neurosurgery, University Hospital Zürich.*)

BOX 15-4   Schwannoma

PATIENT HISTORY

A 36-year-old woman presented with a 6-month history of paresis of the left foot followed by the leg, which was slowly progressive. Since 1 month before admission she had bladder incontinence.

TECHNIQUE

Axial and sagittal T2W, sagittal T1W, and axial and sagittal T1W contrast-enhanced sequences (gadolinium 0.1 mmol/kg) of the spine were obtained.

FINDINGS

A possible diagnosis is thoracic intraspinal schwannoma (Fig. 15-107). Patient underwent hemilaminectomy at T1-4 and total resection of the tumor. Postoperatively, a great improvement of the symptoms was documented. Postoperative control MRI showed no evidence of tumor.

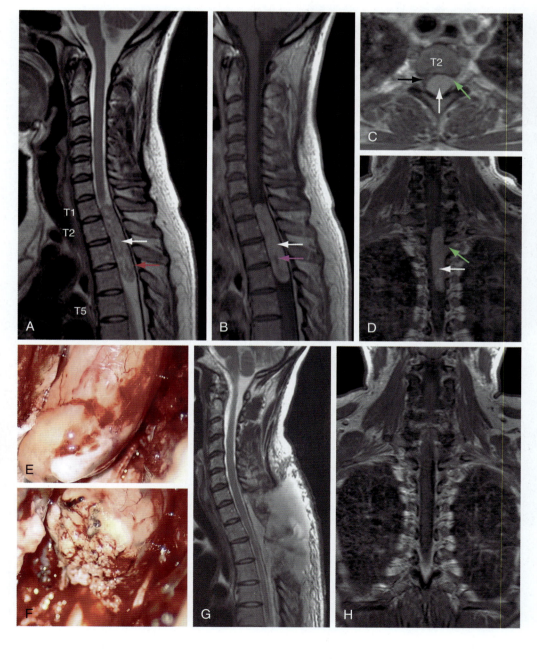

■ **FIGURE 15-107** Intraspinal schwannoma. Sagittal T2 (**A**), sagittal T1 contrast-enhanced (**B**), axial T1 contrast-enhanced (**C**), and coronal T1 contrast-enhanced (**D**) images of the cervicothoracic spine show the sausage-like intradural extramedullary tumor (*white arrows*). The dura mater is indicated with the red arrow on **A**. Except for the small cyst on **B** (*purple arrow*) note the strong homogeneous contrast enhancement. The spinal cord is compressed to the right anteriorly (*black arrow* on **C**). Observe the intraforaminal extension of the tumor (*green arrow* on **C** and **D**). Intraoperative photo (**E**) shows the encapsulated glossy tumor with a greasy cut surface of light tan tissue with yellow patches (**F**). Postoperative sagittal T2 MRI (**G**) and coronal T1 contrast-enhanced (**H**) images demonstrate the unfolded spinal cord and no rest tumor. (**E** and **F**, *Courtesy of Dr. Evaldas Cesnulis, Neurosurgery, University Hospital Zürich.*)

BOX 15-5   Osteosarcoma

PATIENT HISTORY

A 14-year-old girl came to the outpatient clinic with persistent pain in the right shoulder after gymnastics training in school. MRI of the right shoulder (Fig. 15-108) shows the primary tumor. A biopsy confirmed the diagnosis of an osteosarcoma (Enneking IIb) in the right humerus. Chemotherapy was immediately started (Euramos scheme).

Operation was performed 2 months later. An intraoperative tumor presented a close contact to the brachial plexus, and the long head of biceps tendon was surrounded by tumor. The tumor was extending intramedullary about 14 cm distal to the tip of the humerus. Two years later the patient presented again with pain in the right thigh and an MRI examination was performed.

TECHNIQUE

A coronal T1W postcontrast MR image was obtained.

FINDINGS

Metastasis in the ischiocrural muscles is present. Histology confirmed the diagnosis of metastasis from a high-grade osteosarcoma (Fig. 15-109).

COMMENT

One year later, the patient, now age 17 years, presented with a 2-week history of back pain especially at night with no other neurologic symptoms. MRI of the thoracolumbar spine showed an epidural mass with homogeneous contrast enhancement. The T10 vertebra was infiltrated by a metastasis from the osteosarcoma (Figs. 15-110 and 15-111). Decompression and tumor reduction was performed, and histology showed a highly cellular malignant neoplasm with tumor osteoid corresponding to metastasis of a high-grade osteosarcoma (Fig. 15-112).

Three weeks after decompression, a postoperative MRI was performed and showed a progression of the epidural and paravertebral mass. The T10 vertebra was infiltrated by the tumor. Postoperative changes with blood products are present retrospinal in the soft tissues (Fig. 15-113). Additionally, a CT of the lung was performed and multiple lung metastases were present (Fig. 15-114).

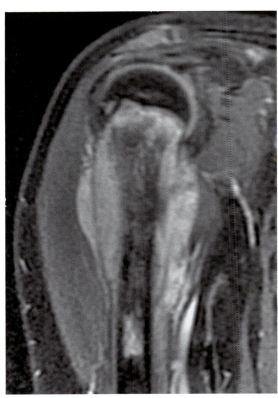

■ **FIGURE 15-108**   T1W coronal postcontrast image shows a primary osteosarcoma (Enneking IIb) in the right humerus diagnosed about 2¹/₂ years earlier.

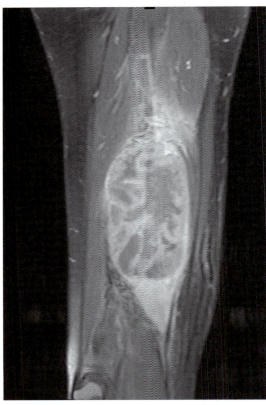

■ **FIGURE 15-109**   A soft tissue metastasis in the right thigh in this patient is shown on a T1W coronal postcontrast MR image.

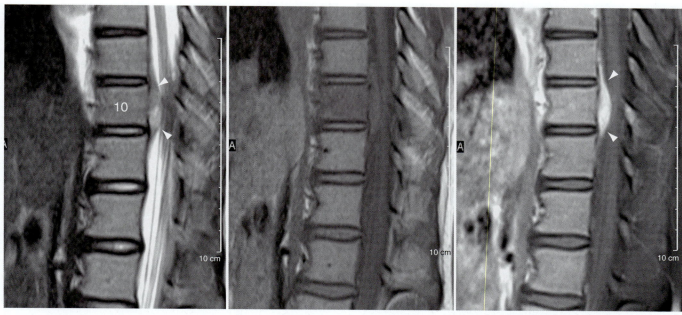

■ **FIGURE 15-110**   T2W, T1W, and T1W postcontrast MR images show an epidural mass with homogeneous contrast enhancement (*arrowheads*) in a 17-year-old girl with a known primary osteosarcoma of the right humerus. The T10 vertebra is infiltrated by metastasis from the osteosarcoma.

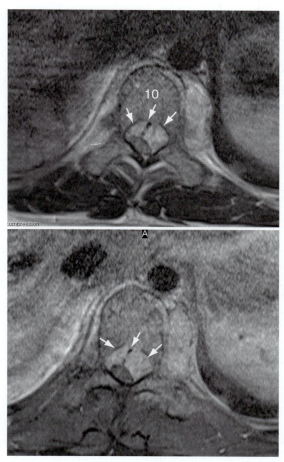

■ **FIGURE 15-111**   Transverse T2W and postcontrast T1W MR images show an extensive epidural mass (*arrowheads*) with compression of the spinal cord. A decompressive operation was performed.

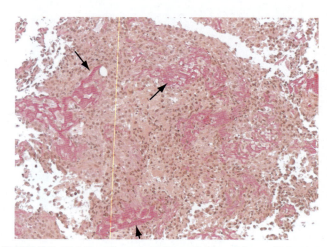

■ **FIGURE 15-112**   Microscopically, a highly cellular malignant neoplasm with tumor osteoid (*arrows*) corresponds to metastasis of a high-grade osteosarcoma. (Elastica van Gieson stain; original magnification ×100.)

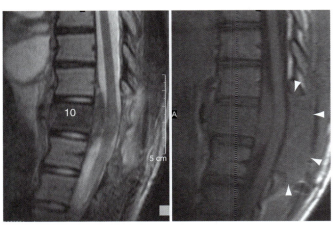

FIGURE 15-113 On T2W and T1W MR images 3 weeks after decompression, the epidural and paravertebral mass has progressed when compared with Figure 15-110. Vertebra T10 is infiltrated by tumor. Postoperative changes with blood are present in the retrospinal soft tissues (*arrowheads*).

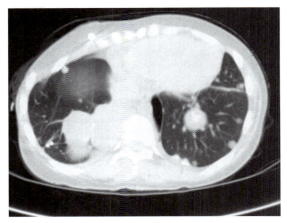

FIGURE 15-114 CT was performed for detection of lung metastases and shows multiple lung lesions. Additionally, a small pneumothorax on the left side is present after port-A-Cath implantation.

KEY POINTS: DIFFERENTIAL DIAGNOSIS

- In the case of intramedullary tumor, consider primary tumor versus metastasis based on the medical history and age of the patient. Always remember that intramedullary metastases are very rare.
- In the case of a primary intramedullary tumor of the cervical or thoracic spine, consider ependymoma (60%) > astrocytoma (30%) > hemangioblastoma (up to 6%) > other tumors.
  - If tumor is more central, concentric, and well-delineated, consider ependymoma.
  - If tumor is asymmetric and infiltrative with indistinct margins, consider astrocytoma.
  - If tumor shows flow voids, consider hemangioblastoma, and, rarely, paraganglioma.
- In the case of a primary tumor of the conus medullaris or filum terminale, consider myxopapillary ependymoma > glioma > paraganglioma.
- Reactive (polar) cyst (without contrast enhancement) is more often associated with ependymoma.
- Tumorous cyst (with contrast enhancement) is more often associated with astrocytoma.
- Cap sign (hemosiderin cap) and peripheral hemorrhages are suggestive of ependymoma.
- A diffuse homogeneous tumor extending over multiple segments with minimal or no contrast enhancement in a young patient with mild clinical symptoms is most probably a ganglioglioma.
- Always remember that a single contrast-enhancing lesion with edema in the spinal cord may not necessarily be of neoplastic etiology. It may also be an acute demyelinating lesion. Examining the brain (multiple sclerosis, acute disseminated encephalomyelitis) or the optic nerves (Devic's disease) may provide the correct diagnosis.
- Compression of the cord away from the lesion with enlargement of the subarachnoid space ipsilaterally is the imaging hallmark of an intradural extramedullary lesion.

- The most common tumors in the intradural extramedullary space are nerve sheath tumors (young adults). The second most common are meningiomas (elderly women).
- A tumor intimately associated with the nerve roots suggests a schwannoma or neurofibroma.
- The majority of schwannomas arise from a dorsal nerve root, whereas ventral nerve root tumors are most commonly neurofibromas.
- Multiple lesions in and around the cord and in the cauda equina should be differentiated from leptomeningeal metastatic disease (look for a primary neoplasm). These may indicate NF1 (neurofibroma) or NF2 (schwannoma or meningioma).
- A broad dural attachment and dural enhancement (dural tail) on the postcontrast images is more typical for a meningioma and very untypical for schwannoma.
- Presence of multiple lesions in the intradural extramedullary space should prompt genetic counseling for neurofibromatosis.
- A round-to-oval intradural lesion with mild, homogeneous contrast enhancement, eventually with calcification, in an elderly woman suggests meningioma.
- A hyperintense lesion on both T1W and T2W MR images with hypointensity on a fat-suppression sequence is diagnostic of lipoma. Lipoma subtypes (angiolipoma, myolipoma) with nonlipomatous, solid compartments are difficult to differentiate from teratoma or dermoid.
- Well-delineated, hypervascularized lesions with strong contrast enhancement in the region of the cauda equina are suggestive of paraganglioma. Myxopapillary ependymoma and schwannoma are less vascularized and do not show flow voids. Hemangioblastoma may present as flow voids but is less frequent in this location. Meningioma is also rare in this location and often presents as a dural tail. Metastasis may be indistinguishable.
- *Enostosis*: no pain, brush border of the sclerotic island, abrupt transition to the normal bone, any bone may be involved.

KEY POINTS: DIFFERENTIAL DIAGNOSIS—cont'd

- *Osteoid osteoma:* pain worsens at night and is relieved by salicylates; it is an osteolytic lesion that is less than 2 cm with a sclerotic ring.
- *Osteoblastoma:* pain is nonspecific; it is an osteolytic lesion that is greater than 2 cm with a sclerotic ring. It may be aggressive.
- *Epidural lipomatosis:* neurologic deficits such as weakness and back pain occur because of excessive intraspinal fat compressing the thecal sac. Fat-saturated sequences are helpful in the diagnosis.
- *Aneurysmal bone cyst:* back pain is most severe at night; pathologic fractures occur. Patients are young, and 75% to 90% of tumors extend into the vertebral body. An expansile, multiloculated neural arch mass is seen with fluid-fluid levels often containing hemorrhagic components.
- *Hemangioma:* well-circumscribed lesion with coarse vertical trabeculae on axial CT ("white polka dots"). Aggressive lesions are more common in women. This tumor may extend epidurally and cause vertebral fracture or cord compression.
- *Giant cell tumor:* locally aggressive tumor presents as lytic expansile lesion in vertebral body or sacrum. Back pain of insidious onset is greatest at night. Pathologic fractures occur in 30%. This tumor is rare before skeletal maturity.
- *Osteochondroma:* cartilage-covered osseous excrescence in continuity with parent bone—"cauliflower" lesion; less than 5% are located in the spine, and spinal cord compression is a rare complication.
- *Chordoma:* mass is hyperintense to the disc on T2W MR images with multiple septa. Histologic identification of physaliphorous cells confirms the diagnosis. This tumor remains asymptomatic for a long time. Clinical symptoms are pain, particularly while sitting; distant metastases are uncommon, but secondary sites may be involved.
- *Osteosarcoma:* aggressive lesion forming immature bone. It may be associated with Paget's disease and previous radiation therapy. Pain is greatest at night; patients present with increased serum levels of alkaline phosphatase. Pulmonary metastases are common and pneumothorax may occur.
- *Chondrosarcoma:* lytic mass with or without chondroid matrix, cortical disruption, and extension into soft tissues. Clinically there is pain, swelling, and a palpable mass. Chondroid matrix mineralization of "rings and arcs" is characteristic, and malignant degeneration of osteochondroma or enchondroma is possible.
- *Ewing's sarcoma:* permeative lytic lesion centered in the vertebral body or sacrum with moth-eaten destruction and a wide zone of transition. It may also originate in soft tissues. Clinically, localized pain is present; an elevated erythrocyte sedimentation rate may simulate osteomyelitis.
- *Lymphoma:* lymphoreticular neoplasm with variety of specific localizations (epidural, osseous, leptomeningitic, intramedullary). The most common presenting symptom is back pain. Imaging shows an enhancing epidural mass with or without vertebral involvement.
- *Plasmacytoma:* There is T1 hypointensity to marrow with low-signal curvilinear areas. Most patients with a solitary bone plasmacytoma represent the early stage of multiple myeloma. A vertebral body is the most common site of a solitary bone plasmacytoma.
- *Multiple myeloma:* There is multifocal, diffuse, or heterogeneous T1 hypointensity. Diffuse osteopenia occurs in 85%, multiple lytic lesions in 80%, and vertebral fractures between T6 and L4 in 87%. It is the most common primary tumor of bone. Bone pain is present in 75%, and well-circumscribed, punched-out lesions are seen on conventional radiographs.
- *Osteoblastic metastases:* Can be solitary or multiple lesions. Sclerosis may occur as a discrete nodular appearance. Lesions destroy preferentially the posterior cortex and pedicle. Osteosclerotic primary tumors are prostate cancer, carcinoid, bladder cancer, nasopharyngeal cancer, or medulloblastoma. Mixed lytic and blastic primary tumors occur in the lung, breast, cervix, and ovaries.
- *Osteolytic metastases:* Lesions destroy preferentially the posterior cortex and pedicle. There is a round focus with bone destruction. Primary lesions that most often cause lytic metastases include tumors of the breast, lung, kidney, and thyroid and melanoma. The spine is the most frequent site of skeletal metastases.

SUGGESTED READINGS

Abul-Kasim K, Thurnher MM, McKeever P, Sundgren PC. Intradural spinal tumors: Current classification and MRI features. Neuroradiology 2008; 50:301-314.

Beall DP, Googe DJ, Emery RL, et al. Extramedullary intradural spinal tumors: A pictorial review. Curr Probl Diagn Radiol 2007; 36: 185-198.

Bloomer CW, Ackerman A, Bhatia RG. Imaging for spine tumors and new applications. Top Magn Reson Imaging 2006; 17:69-87.

Drevelegas A, Chourmouzi D, Boulogianni G, Sofroniadis I. Imaging of primary bone tumors of the spine. Eur Radiol 2003; 13:1859-1871.

Gitelis S, Schajowicz F. Osteoid osteoma and osteoblastoma. Orthop Clin North Am 1989; 20:313-325.

Knoeller SM, Uhl M, Gahr N, et al. Differential diagnosis of primary malignant bone tumors in the spine and sacrum: The radiological and clinical spectrum. Neoplasma 2008; 55:16-22.

Murphey MD, Andrews CL, Flemming DJ, et al. Primary tumors of the spine: Radiologic pathologic correlation. RadioGraphics 1996; 16: 1131-1158.

Parsa AT, Lee J, Parney IF, et al. Spinal cord and intradural-extraparenchymal spinal tumors: Current best care practices and strategies. J Neurooncol 2004; 69:291-318.

Sansur CA, Pouratian N, Dumont AS, et al. Spinal-cord neoplasms: Primary tumors of the bony spine and adjacent soft tissues. Lancet Oncol 2007; 8:137-147.

Smith JK, Lury K, Castillo M. Imaging of spinal and spinal cord tumors. Semin Roentgenol 2006; 41:274-293.

Solero CL, Fornari M, Giombini S, et al. Spinal meningiomas: Review of 174 operated cases. Neurosurgery 1989; 25:153-160.

Traul DE, Shaffrey ME, Schiff D. Spinal-cord neoplasms: Intradural neoplasms. Lancet Oncol 2007; 8:35-45.

Waldron JS, Cha S. Radiographic features of intramedullary spinal cord tumors. Neurosurg Clin North Am 2006; 17:13-19.

REFERENCES

1. Abul-Kasim K, Thurnher MM, McKeever P, Sundgren PC. Intradural spinal tumors: Current classification and MRI features. Neuroradiology 2008; 50:301-314.
2. Rennie AT, et al. Intramedullary tumours in patients with neurofibromatosis type 2: MRI features associated with a favourable prognosis. Clin Radiol 2008; 63:193-200.
3. Koeller KK, Rosenblum RS, Morrison AL. Neoplasms of the spinal cord and filum terminale: Radiologic-pathologic correlation. RadioGraphics 2000; 20:1721-1749.
4. Evans DG, et al. Management of the patient and family with neurofibromatosis 2: A consensus conference statement. Br J Neurosurg 2005; 19:5-12.
5. Henson JW. Spinal cord gliomas. Curr Opin Neurol 2001; 14:679-682.
6. Ng C, et al. Spinal cord glioblastoma multiforme induced by radiation after treatment for Hodgkin disease: Case report. J Neurosurg Spine 2007; 6:364-367.
7. Maher EA, et al. Malignant glioma: Genetics and biology of a grave matter. Genes Dev 2001; 15:1311-1333.
8. Fountas KN, Karampelas I, Nikolakakos LG, et al. Primary spinal cord oligodendroglioma: Case report and review of the literature. Childs Nerv Syst 2005; 21:171-175.
9. Satyarthee GD, Mehta VS, Vaishya S. Ganglioglioma of the spinal cord: Report of two cases and review of literature. J Clin Neurosci 2004; 11:199-203.
10. Miller DJ, McCutcheon IE. Hemangioblastomas and other uncommon intramedullary tumors. J Neurooncol 2000; 47:253-270.
11. Shuin T, et al. Von Hippel-Lindau disease: Molecular pathological basis, clinical criteria, genetic testing, clinical features of tumors and treatment. Jpn J Clin Oncol 2006; 36:337-343.
12. Findlay JM, Bernstein M, Vanderlinden RG, Resch L. Microsurgical resection of solitary intramedullary spinal cord metastases. Neurosurgery 1987; 21:911-915.
13. Denaro L, Pallini R, Di Muro L, et al. Primary hemorrhagic intramedullary melanoma: Case report with emphasis on the difficult preoperative diagnosis. J Neurosurg Sci 2007; 51:181-183.
14. Jinnai T, Koyama T. Clinical characteristics of spinal nerve sheath tumors: Analysis of 149 cases. Neurosurgery. 2005; 56:510-515.
15. Carrasco CA, Rojas-Salazar D, Chiorino R, et al. Melanotic non-psammomatous trigeminal schwannoma as the first manifestation of Carney complex: Case report. Neurosurgery 2006; 59:E1334-E1335.
16. Parmar HA, Ibrahim M, Castillo M, Mukherji SK. Pictorial essay: diverse imaging features of spinal schwannomas. Comput Assist Tomogr 2007; 31:329-334.
17. Sade B, Chahlavi A, Krishnaney A, et al. World Health Organization Grades II and III meningiomas are rare in the cranial base and spine. Neurosurgery 2007; 61:1194-1198.
18. Klekamp J, Fusco M, Samii M. Thoracic intradural extramedullary lipomas: Report of three cases and review of the literature. Acta Neurochir (Wien) 2001; 143:767-773; discussion 773-774.
19. Masuoka J, Brandner S, Paulus W, et al. Germline SDHD mutation in paraganglioma of the spinal cord. Oncogene 2001; 20:5084-5086.
20. Weinstein JN. Surgical approach to spine tumor. Orthopedics 1989; 12:897-905.
21. Ozaki T, Liljenqvist U, Hillmann A, et al. Osteoid osteoma and osteoblastoma of the spine: Experiences with 22 patients. Clin Orthop Relat Res 2002; (397):394-402.
22. Fassett DR, et al. Spinal epidural lipomatosis: A review of its causes and recommodations for treatment. Neurosurg Focus 2004; 16(4):article 11.
23. Saccomanni B. Aneurysmal bone cyst of spine: A review of literature. Arch Orthop Trauma Surg 2008; 128:1145-1147.
24. Ross JS, et al. Vertebral hemangiomas: MR imaging. Radiology 1987; 165:165-169.
25. Kwon JW, et al. MRI findings of giant cell tumors of the spine. AJR Am J Roentgenol 2007; 189:246-250.
26. Gerber S, et al. Imaging of sacral tumors. Skeletal Radiol 2008; 37:277-289.
27. Giudicissi-Filho M, de Holanda CV, Borba LA, et al. Cervical spinal cord compression due to an osteochondroma in hereditary multiple exostosis: Case report and review of literature. Surg Neurol 2006; 66(Suppl 3):S7-S11.
28. Bloem JL. Osseous lesions. Radiol Clin North Am 1993; 31:261-278.
29. Eggli KD, et al. Ewing sarcoma. Radiol Clin North Am 1993; 31:325-337.

PART
NINE

Metabolic Conditions

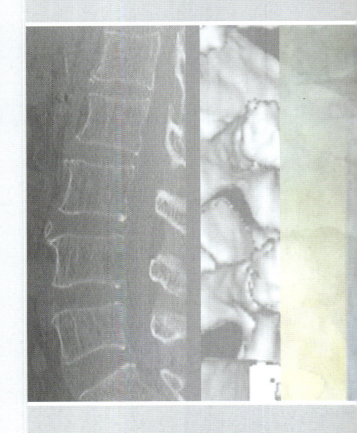

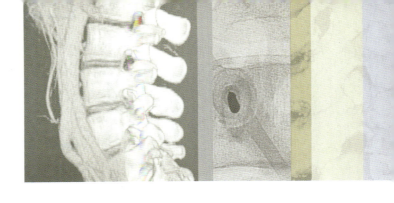

CHAPTER 16

Metabolic Conditions Affecting the Spinal Column

Maria Vittoria Spampinato

The skeletal manifestations of metabolic disease are a heterogeneous group of conditions resulting from endocrinopathy, vitamin deficiency, renal tubular dysfunction, and disorders of endogenous metabolism. As a group, they are characterized by altered function of the osteoblasts and osteoclasts or abnormal rates of mineralization. Consequently, there are pathologic changes in the bone mass, the collagen framework of the bone, the degree of bone mineralization, and the level of osteoclastic and osteoblastic activity.

The two most common metabolic conditions affecting the spinal column are osteoporosis and renal osteodystrophy. Crystal deposition diseases typically involve the appendicular skeleton more than the spinal column. Endocrinopathies are associated with remodeling of the axial and appendicular skeleton secondary to the systemic effects of the hormonal imbalances.

Paget's disease, although not a metabolic bone disorder, is also characterized by abnormal function of osteoclasts and osteoblasts resulting in bone remodeling.

OSTEOPOROSIS

The term *osteoporosis* signifies decreased volume of normal bone, predisposing a person to an increased risk of fractures. Osteoporosis arises as a multifactorial disorder of bone mineral homeostasis that reduces bone mineral density, compromises bone strength, and leads to increased risk of fractures, particularly in the elderly. Osteoporosis is to be distinguished from *osteopenia*, which signifies reduced bone mass and *osteomalacia*, which signifies abnormal increase in unmineralized osteoid.

Epidemiology

Osteoporosis affects one in four women and one in eight men older than age 50 years: 10 million individuals in the United States are affected.[1] Both men and women experience age-dependent decline in bone mineral density (BMD) starting in midlife. However, in women bone loss occurs more rapidly right after menopause.

Primary generalized osteoporosis is classified into perimenopausal and senile osteoporosis.[2] The two major risk factors for osteoporosis are female gender and increased age. Other significant risk factors are estrogen deficiency, late menarche, early menopause, white race, low body mass index, family history of osteoporosis, and smoking. Senile osteoporosis is seen in both males and females after age 70 years.

Secondary osteoporosis occurs in many medical conditions that interfere with bone homeostasis, including genetic, endocrine, gastrointestinal, hematologic, connective tissue disorders, and nutritional deficiencies. In males, 30% to 60% of osteoporosis is secondary osteoporosis, mainly from hypogonadism, use of glucocorticoids, or alcohol abuse.

Clinical Presentation

Senile and postmenopausal osteoporosis may be asymptomatic. Back pain may be associated with loss in the height of the vertebral bodies and increased kyphosis. The weakened vertebrae may fracture after minimal trauma.

Pathophysiology

Bone mass increases throughout childhood and adolescence until the third decade of life. Adequate nutrition, exposure to sex hormones at puberty, physical activity, and individual genetic factors determine the peak bone mass attained early in life. Postmenopausal osteoporosis affects mainly the trabecular bone, leading to vertebral and wrist fractures. In senile osteoporosis both cortical and trabecular bone density are decreased.[3] The bone is

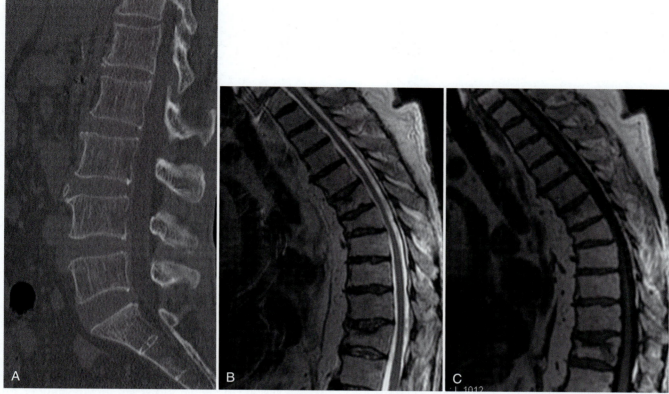

■ **FIGURE 16-1**   Osteoporosis. **A,** Sagittal CT image of the lumbar spine demonstrates decreased bone density with accentuation of primary vertical bony trabeculae. In a different patient, sagittal T2W (**B**) and T1W (**C**) images of the lumbar spine show wedge-shaped vertebrae in the mid and low thoracic spine, multiple end plate deformities, and Schmorl's nodes.

lost because the resorption associated with endogenous metabolism is not counterbalanced by normal osteoblastic activity. Sex hormones have an anabolic effect on skeletal metabolism, whereas glucocorticoid adrenocortical hormones have a catabolic action on skeletal metabolism. Metabolically, postmenopausal status and senescence are characterized by both relative hypoestrogenism and hypercortisolism, leading to bone loss.

Hyperparathyroidism causes a distinctive replacement of lamellar bone with woven bone and fibrous tissue.

Pathology

The spinal column is composed predominantly of trabecular bone, so osteoporosis affects the spine early on. Macroscopically, decreased numbers of bone trabeculae are observed within normal-appearing bone marrow.

The histopathologic appearance of osteoporosis is designated "smooth bone atrophy" and is characterized by thin, sparse bone trabeculae with smooth surfaces situated within enlarged intertrabecular marrow spaces.

Imaging

Radiography

The diagnosis of spinal osteoporosis is based on changes in bone radiolucency, trabecular pattern, and shape of the

vertebral bodies (Fig. 16-1). Accentuation of the vertical trabecular pattern, resorption of horizontal trabeculae, and depression of the superior margin of the vertebral body are noted, with overall decreased number and thinning of the trabeculae. Vertebral wedging, compression fractures, biconcave deformities of the vertebral bodies ("fish-mouth vertebrae"), and Schmorl's nodes can be observed.

Quantitative Measurements for Assessment of Bone Mass

BMD is used to quantify bone strength. BMD corresponds to the bone mineral content divided by the area or volume of bone, depending on the technique used to measure it. A T-score is defined as the number of standard deviations above or below the average BMD value for young healthy white women. The Z-score represents the number of standard deviations above or below the average BMD value for age- and sex-matched controls. According to the World Health Organization, osteoporosis is present when the T-score is 2.5 standard deviations below the mean for young white adult women.[4] T-scores were based originally on assessment of BMD at the hip by dual-energy x-ray absorptiometry (DEXA). However, they have been extended to include diagnostic thresholds at other skeletal sites and for other technologies, such as peripheral DEXA, quantitative CT (QCT), and quantitative ultrasonography (QUS).[5]

MRI

MR spectroscopy and MR perfusion have been used to measure vertebral bone marrow fat content and bone marrow perfusion in elderly men.[1] Vertebral bone marrow fat content is significantly increased in patients with osteoporosis or osteopenia compared with matched controls. Bone marrow perfusion is significantly decreased in osteoporotic patients compared with both osteopenic and normal subjects.

High-resolution bone MRI successfully displays the trabecular structure of peripheral joints. However, present MR-based quantitative measurements, such as trabecular bone volume fraction and trabecular thickness, likely overestimate trabecular volume and thickness owing to partial volume effects.[6]

GOUT

Gout is a metabolic arthropathy caused by deposition of monosodium urate crystals in the articular cartilage, subchondral bone, synovium, and capsular and periarticular soft tissues of one or more joints.

Epidemiology

Gout typically affects the distal joints of the appendicular skeleton and rarely involves the spine. The initial attack of gout commonly occurs in the fifth decade of life in men but can occur in postmenopausal women (M : F = 20 : 1).[7] The prevalence of spinal gout is not known. Patients affected by spinal gout are mostly men 33 to 76 years of age.[8] Eighty-two percent of patients with spinal gout have chronic polyarticular tophaceous gout and hyperuricemia with a mean duration of disease of 14 years. However, spinal involvement can be the first manifestation of the disease.[9]

Clinical Presentation

Acute gouty arthritis presents as recurrent episodes of monoarticular or oligoarticular pain, tenderness, and swelling. The initial attack typically occurs in the first metatarsophalangeal joint. Chronic gouty arthritis develops in less than 50% of patients with recurrent acute gout. About 73% of patients with spinal gout have neurologic symptoms, including neck or back pain, fever, cord compression, and radiculopathies. In patients with acute or progressive myelopathy, spinal gout should be suspected when there is a past history of gout or a current history of active gouty arthritis (synovitis of the elbows, knees, and first metatarsophalangeal joints). In contrast, the correct diagnosis can be challenging when spinal involvement is the only manifestation of gout. Acute attacks are treated with nonsteroidal anti-inflammatory agents, intravenous colchicine, or systemic or intra-articular corticosteroids. Long-term management of spinal gout is with allopurinol.

Pathophysiology

In humans, the end product of purine metabolism is uric acid. Hyperuricemia can result from several metabolic

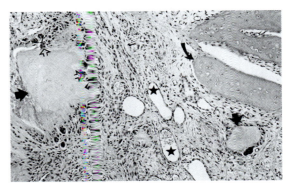

■ **FIGURE 16-2** Gout. Histologic section of a surgically resected specimen. Two tophaceous deposits (*thick black arrows*) surrounded by histiocytes and multinucleated giant cells (*open arrows*) are embedded in a chronic inflammatory stroma. Vascular channels (*stars*) and cancellous bone fragments (*curved arrow*) without lamellar organization are present. Note pseudopalisadic disposition of histiocytes surrounding tophi (*small double arrowhead*). (*From Laprez TP, et al. Gout in the cervical spine: MR pattern mimicking diskovertebral infection. AJNR Am J Neuroradiol 1996; 17:151-153.*)

abnormalities, including (1) increased activity of phosphoribosylpyrophosphate synthetase, which is involved in the conversion of purine nucleotides into uric acid; (2) deficiency of glucose-6-phosphatase; (3) deficiency of hypoxanthine-guanine phosphoribosyltransferase; and (4) renal disease with decreased tubular secretion of urate. Uric acid salts, particularly monosodium urate crystals, form in the presence of elevated concentration of uric acid. Deposition of monosodium urate crystals in the synovia produces arthritis of the peripheral joints. Chronic gouty arthritis is characterized by deposits of monosodium urate called tophi in subjects with long-standing gout or a high body load of urate. Involvement of the cervical, thoracic, and lumbar spine and the sacroiliac joint has been reported.[10]

Pathology

Macroscopically, tophi appear as chalky white material deposited in the cartilage, vertebral bodies, facet joints, and intervertebral discs.

In chronic tophaceous gout, urate deposition can occur in the articular cartilage, subchondral bone, synovium, and capsular and periarticular soft tissues. When gout is a consideration, biopsy material must be sent for pathologic analysis in 100% alcohol because formalin dissolves urate crystals.[10] Histologic evaluation of tophaceous deposits shows a matrix containing urate crystals embedded in a chronic granulomatous stroma (Fig. 16-2). Examination of the specimen with negatively polarized light reveals negatively birefringent crystals, which are diagnostic of tophaceous gout.

Imaging

Radiography

In spinal gout, spine radiographs can be normal or show nonspecific findings that mimic degenerative disc disease.[11] Spinal gout may present as an erosive arthritis centered at

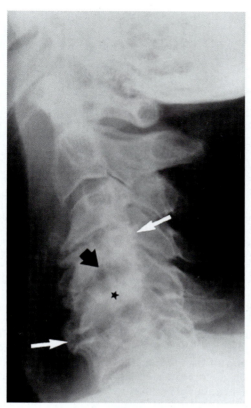

■ **FIGURE 16-3** Gout. Lateral view radiograph of the cervical spine shows atypical discovertebral changes from C3 to C6. Deep erosions of several end plates (*black arrow*) are associated with hyperostosis (*star*) and prominent marginal osteophytosis (*white arrows*).

the level of the disc, with disc space narrowing, end plate erosions (caused by urate crystal deposits), and secondary proliferative bone changes, such as hyperostosis and marginal osteophytosis (Fig. 16-3). Joint subluxations, spinal deformities, pathologic fractures, and erosions of the odontoid and of the facet joints can also occur.

CT

CT has limited utility in spinal gout. CT better delineates the erosions of the vertebral end plates and facet joints that are frequently seen in spinal gout.[10] On CT, tophi may resemble calcifications, because monosodium urate deposits have high attenuation values (170 ± 30 HU), similar to calcium.

MRI

On MRI, the involved discs and end plates appear inhomogeneous and often show low T2 signal due to fibrous tissue and crystal deposition.[11] The affected intervertebral discs, adjacent end plates, facet joints, posterior elements, and epidural space may show abnormal contrast enhancement due to the vascularized reactive tissue within the lesions (Fig. 16-4).[10] Gouty tophi can extend posteriorly from the intervertebral disc and end plates into the epidural space and mimic epidural abscess.[12] However, gouty tophi have low signal intensity on T2-weighted imaging (T2W), which may help to differentiate spinal gout from

discovertebral infection.[11] Spinal gout can mimic other conditions, including epidural abscess, discovertebral infection, facet joint infection, metastases, dialysis-related spondyloarthropathy, and calcified tumors.[7,11,12] At the atlantoaxial joint, gout may erode the odontoid process and resemble rheumatoid arthritis. For these reasons, the imaging diagnosis of spinal gout can be challenging.

CALCIUM PYROPHOSPHATE DIHYDRATE AND CALCIUM HYDROXYAPATITE CRYSTAL DEPOSITION DISEASES

Calcium pyrophosphate dihydrate (CPPD) crystal deposition disease is a disorder characterized by accumulation of CPPD crystals in or around the joints. These depositions may cause pseudogout with recurrent acute attacks of arthritis affecting one or more joints.

Calcium hydroxyapatite (HA) crystal deposition disease (HADD) is characterized by para-articular deposition of HA crystals, leading to calcification of tendons, bursae, ligaments, and peritendinous tissues.

Epidemiology

CPPD crystal deposition disease is a common condition affecting middle-aged and elderly patients, with a slight female prevalence.[13] Three forms of CPPD crystal deposition disease are known: sporadic, familial, and secondary (associated with other metabolic diseases such as hemochromatosis, hyperparathyroidism, hypothyroidism, and Wilson's disease).[13] Spinal manifestations of CPPD crystal deposition disease are not uncommon and in certain cases can be the only manifestation of the disease. Japanese patients manifest spinal involvement in CPPD crystal deposition disease more commonly than do other ethnic populations.[13]

HADD is usually monoarticular and presents between the ages of 40 and 70 years.

Clinical Presentation

CPPD crystal deposition disease presents a variable clinical picture, ranging from acute arthritis to chronic progressive arthritis, with or without acute exacerbations. Pseudogout attacks can occur spontaneously or be triggered by direct trauma, medical conditions, or surgery. CPPD crystal deposition disease affects the thoracic and lumbar spines more than the cervical spine. Spinal involvement may cause no symptoms or only minimal back pain. In patients with large calcific deposits in the spine there may be an insidious myelopathy or myeloradiculopathy. The acute back pain can be accompanied by fever, joint pain, constitutional symptoms, and elevated erythrocyte sedimentation rate. Therapy for CPPD crystal deposition disease is directed at the relief of symptoms, because there is no specific medical therapy to dissolve the crystals or prevent new crystal formation.

Patients with HADD present with swelling, pain and decreased mobility of the affected joints, and occasionally fever. Treatment of HADD is symptomatic.

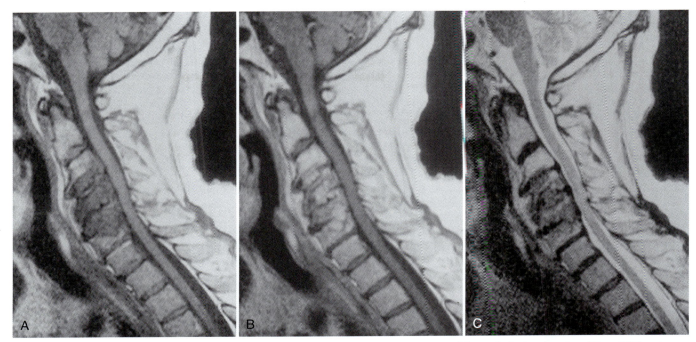

■ FIGURE 16-4 Sagittal unenhanced T1W (**A**), postcontrast T1W (**B**), and T2W (**C**) MR images of the cervical spine show large T1 and T2 hypointense areas within the C4, C5, and C6 vertebral bodies, with foci of enhancement within the disc spaces and the contiguous end plates, without changes in the adjacent epidural and prevertebral spaces. Abnormal T2 signal of the spinal cord is seen at the C5-6 level. *(From Duprez TP, et al. Gout in the cervical spine: MR pattern mimicking diskovertebral infection. AJNR Am J Neuroradiol 1996; 17:151-153.)*

Pathophysiology

The pathophysiology of CPPD deposition is still unclear. CPPD crystals accumulate in the intervertebral discs, intraspinal and extraspinal ligaments, median atlantoaxial joint, facet joints, and sacroiliac joints, among other sites.[14] Within the disc, the crystals may deposit in the annulus fibrosus, nucleus pulposus, or both. Acute and chronic CPPD deposition induces destructive lesions of vertebral bodies and discs that may be confused with infectious discitis or neuropathic disease. Facet disease can lead to destructive arthropathy and spondylolisthesis. CPPD can accumulate in the ligamentum flavum and posterior longitudinal ligament, causing myelopathy and spinal canal stenosis in very severe cases. Accumulation of CPPD crystals in the transverse and alar ligaments about the dens causes the "crowned dens syndrome" with cord compression, bone erosion, fracture, and atlanto-odontoid subluxation.

HADD is thought to be secondary to deposition of HA crystals in the soft tissues either after microtrauma or secondary to a metabolic disorder. The condition becomes symptomatic when calcific deposits rupture into adjacent bursae or soft tissues. Phagocytosis of the crystals by macrophages and neutrophils then activates an inflammatory response, causing calcific periarthritis.

Pathology

Grossly, the CPPD crystals appear as chalky white deposits of crystals. Spinal specimens show that disc calcifications are more common in the thoracic and lumbar spine than in the cervical spine, often involve the annulus fibrosus, and rarely involve the nucleus pulposus. The crystal deposits appear as calcifications in the facet joints, ligaments, and, in one specimen, the transverse ligament of the atlas and synovium of the atlantodental joint.[14]

Histology shows amorphous calcifications in the context of chronic inflammatory and fibrous tissue. The CPPD crystals are rhomboid or rod shaped and are positively birefringent with polarized-light microscopy (Fig. 16-5).

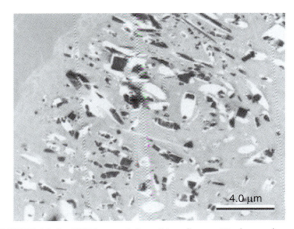

■ FIGURE 16-5 CPPD crystal deposition disease. Nucleus pulposus of a disc specimen with CPPD deposit showing the crystal shape, rhomboid shape in cross section, and rod shape (unstained, osmicated section). *(From Lee RS, Kayser MV, Ali SY. Calcium phosphate microcrystal deposition in the human intervertebral disc. J Anat 2006; 208:13-19.)*

Imaging

Radiography

Plain radiographs show densities at the margins of the intervertebral disc spaces consistent with calcification of the outer fibers of the annulus fibrosus. These resemble the early syndesmophytes of ankylosing spondylitis. Disc space narrowing and significant vertebral sclerosis are additional nonspecific features of CPPD crystal deposition disease. The calcifications may not be dense enough to be detected on conventional radiographs. They may be difficult to distinguish from adjacent osteophytes in spines affected by degenerative disc and joint disease.

HADD of the spine is characterized by calcification of the longus colli muscle, in particular of the superior lateral portion of the muscle near to C2. The calcification can be accompanied by soft tissue swelling. Calcifications of the ligamentum flavum, interspinous bursae, facet joints, and infraoccipital region can also occur.

CT

CT typically shows linear calcifications of the intervertebral discs, calcifications of the ligamenta flava and facet joints, and additional perivertebral calcific deposits (Fig. 16-6). The calcifications of the ligamenta flava are usually nodular or ovoid and are contiguous with the lamina. The dura mater can also contain calcific deposits.

MRI

CPPD crystal deposits in the ligamentum flavum and discs demonstrate low T1 and T2 signal intensity. The ossified ligamenta flava appear as ovoid or nodular hypointense masses, which, if large, may compromise the spinal canal and compress the spinal cord.[13] Tumorous deposits of CPPD crystals in the ligamenta flava may mimic bone tumors.[16] In the cervical spine, CPPD crystal deposits may form a periodontoid mass indistinguishable from

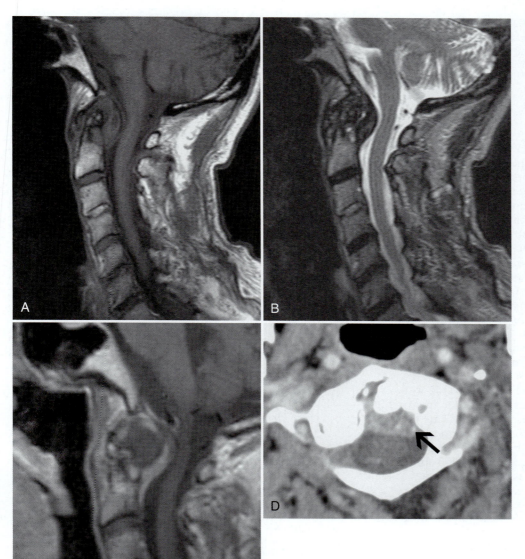

■ **FIGURE 16-6** CPPD crystal deposition disease. Sagittal T1W (**A**) and T2W (**B**) MR images of the cervical spine reveal a hypointense periodontoid mass, secondary to CPPD deposition in the synovia of the median atlas-odontoid joint, the transverse ligament, the posterior longitudinal ligament, and its cephalad continuation with the tectorial membrane. There is diffuse abnormal low signal in the dens. **C,** Sagittal post-gadolinium T1W MR image through the upper cervical spine demonstrates peripheral enhancement of the soft tissue mass and enhancement of the immediately adjacent bone. **D,** Axial CT shows thickening of the posterior longitudinal ligament and transverse ligament with amorphous calcifications (*arrow*). (*Courtesy of Dr. Z. Rumboldt.*)

rheumatoid arthritis (Fig. 16-6), compressive ossifications of the ligamenta flava below the axis, or both.[15]

PAGET'S DISEASE

Paget's disease is a chronic disorder of the adult skeleton characterized by bone remodeling. It is also called osteitis deformans.

Epidemiology

Paget's disease affects 3% to 4% of the population older than 40 years and up to 10% to 11% older than age 80 years. The prevalence is slightly higher in males and in individuals of English descent.[17] Monostotic disease occurs in 10% to 35% of cases, more commonly in the axial skeleton. Polyostotic disease is more frequent (65%-90%) and more commonly involves the lower extremities. The spine is involved in 30% to 75% of Paget's disease cases, as a single vertebra, multiple vertebrae, or all of the vertebrae.

Clinical Presentation

Symptoms of spinal involvement include pain, tenderness, increased warmth, kyphosis of the spine, and decreased range of motion. Bone enlargement can narrow the neural foramina and cause radiculopathies. Complications of Paget's disease include fractures, scoliosis, arthritis, and neurologic symptoms. Sarcomatous transformation occurs in 1% of cases overall, more in polyostotic disease (5%-10%). Secondary sarcomatous transformation is rarer in the spine than in the hip, pelvis, and shoulder and usually manifests as severe pain at the site of previous paucisymptomatic disease. The sarcoma types include osteosarcoma, malignant fibrous histiocytoma/fibrosarcoma, and chondrosarcoma.

Paget's disease characteristically evolves through three phases: (1) a lytic phase that is usually asymptomatic; (2) a mixed phase characterized by bone remodeling, bone resorption and production, elevation of alkaline phosphatase, and fractures; and (3) a late phase characterized by further bone remodeling, bone weakening, overall decreased osteoblastic and osteoclastic activity, and late complications such as neoplasms.[17] Serum levels of calcium and phosphate are normal in most cases, but secondary hyperparathyroidism develops in 10% of cases due to hypercalcemia. During the lytic phase, serum levels of hydroxyproline are typically elevated. In the mixed and blastic phases of the disease the serum alkaline phosphatase value is often elevated. Patients with Paget's disease may be treated with oral bisphosphonates, alone or in combination with calcitonin, to inhibit bone resorption and alleviate pain.[18]

Pathophysiology

The pathophysiology of Paget's disease has not been defined. A viral etiology has been proposed, because intranuclear inclusion bodies and multinucleate osteoclasts are observed in histologic specimens of Paget's disease, similar to findings in paramyxovirus infection.[19] A genetic com-

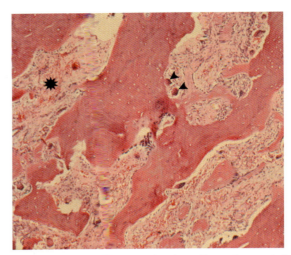

■ **FIGURE 16-7** Paget's disease: active phase. Photomicrograph (hematoxylin-eosin stain) shows fibrovascular tissue replacing the marrow cavity (*asterisk*) and osteoclastic activity (*arrowheads*). (*Courtesy of Dr. T. Rumboldt.*)

ponent of Paget's disease has also been proposed, because Ashkenazi Jews with HLA-DR2 have a high prevalence of this disease. Other possible causes include a metabolic disorder of parathyroid hormone, a connective tissue disorder, and an autoimmune or vascular disorder.

Pathology

Grossly, the bones in Paget's disease are widened with thickened trabeculae resembling pumice stone. The trabeculae are more brittle than normal despite their increased thickness. Increased vascularity is noted in the late phases of the disease.[19]

The three stages of Paget disease represent a continuum rather than discrete entities.[17] In the lytic or incipient-active phase, osteoclasts predominate and cause bone resorption. In the mixed or active phase, osteoclastic bone resorption and osteoblastic activity coexist. In the late mixed phase, osteoblastic activity predominates. In the blastic or inactive phase, osteoblastic activity declines and the activity of both osteoclasts and osteoblasts is minimal.

During the lytic and early mixed phases of the disease fibrovascular tissue replaces the fatty bone marrow (Fig. 16-7). During the late mixed phase there is a progressive increase in fatty marrow deposition, with an ultimate increase in marrow fat deposition versus the normal yellow bone marrow of the inactive phase.

Imaging

Radiography

On plain radiographs, the vertebrae exhibit an accentuated, coarse, trabecular pattern, especially in the vertical weight-bearing trabeculae. The anterior border of the vertebral bodies becomes flattened and squared. In the mixed phase, the cortex is thickened along *all* the vertebral margins, giving the pathognomonic "picture frame" appearance.[20] In renal osteodystrophy only the superior

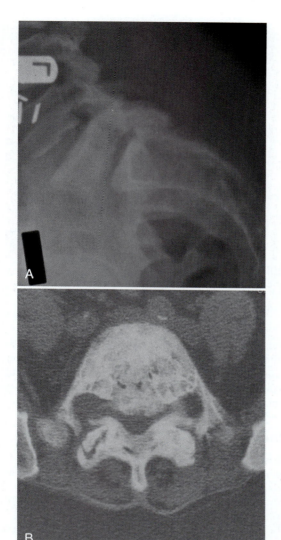

■ **FIGURE 16-8** Paget's disease. **A,** Plain film of the lumbosacral spine shows enlargement and sclerotic appearance of L5. **B,** Axial CT image demonstrates diffuse bone sclerosis of the vertebral body and posterior elements of L5. *(Courtesy of Dr. T. Pope.)*

and inferior end plates are thickened. During the blastic phase, diffuse sclerosis of the affected vertebral body can create a highly dense "ivory" vertebra (Fig. 16-8).[20] Differential diagnoses of the blastic phase of vertebral Paget's disease include osteoblastic metastatic disease, lymphoma, chordoma, and, possibly, tuberculosis. The typical enlargement and sclerosis of the affected vertebral body and similar involvement of the posterior elements differentiate Paget's vertebrae from other conditions. Cortical erosions, aggressive osteolysis, and soft tissue masses are features suggestive of sarcomatous transformation. Sarcomas associated with Paget's disease are usually osteolytic owing to a high degree of dedifferentiation. Periosteal reaction is rarely present because of the rapidity of bone destruction.

CT

CT demonstrates the typical remodeling of pagetic bone, with cortical and trabecular thickening. CT is superior to plain films for demonstrating the abnormal trabecular architecture, the loss of joint cartilage, and the joint space narrowing that indicate pagetic facet arthopathy.[21] Simple Paget's disease does not show cortical destruction or soft tissue mass, and CT demonstration of these findings suggests sarcomatous transformation.

MRI

MRI is useful for assessing the presence and complications of Paget's disease.[18] The signal intensity of the bone marrow has three different patterns. These patterns parallel but do not precisely conform to the three histologic stages described earlier. In the lytic and early mixed active phases the bone marrow signal is heterogeneous on T2W imaging (more pronounced on short tau inversion recovery [STIR] images). The bone marrow is isointense to the muscle on T1 weighting (T1W) with multiple intermixed foci of high T1 signal. This "speckled" appearance on T1W images mirrors the fibrovascular marrow replacement seen at pathology in the active phases of the disease. The late mixed active phase is characterized by maintained high signal intensity from fatty bone marrow on T1W and T2W images and by low signal on STIR images. In the blastic inactive phase of Paget's disease, the bone marrow eventually demonstrates low signal intensity on all pulse sequences, consistent with sclerosis. After gadolinium administration, contrast enhancement can be seen in the active phases of the disease, both at the level of the cortex and with a "speckled" appearance in the intramedullary compartment.

Sarcomatous degeneration of the cortex appears as a replacement of the normal "speckled" high signal of the bone marrow by enhancing and necrotic tumor that is isointense on T1W images and hyperintense on T2W images, accompanied by epidural or paravertebral soft tissue masses.[18,20]

Nuclear Medicine

Bone scintigraphy is a sensitive but nonspecific examination for Paget's disease. It is potentially helpful for staging polyostotic disease. Hyperemia and osteoblastic activity cause increased metabolic uptake in all phases of Paget's disease. Early in Paget's disease, increased radionuclide uptake can be seen even before an obvious area of lucency becomes evident on plain films. Late in the disease, activity tends to decrease.

ACROMEGALY

Acromegaly is an endocrine disorder characterized by growth hormone hypersecretion. It is also referred to as Marie's disease.

Epidemiology

Acromegaly affects men and women equally and most commonly presents in the third and fourth decades of life.

Clinical Presentation

Typical clinical traits of acromegaly are coarse facial features, large mandible ("lantern jaw"), poor dental occlusion with separation of the teeth, prominence of the forehead, deepening of the voice, enlargement of the tongue, and thickening of the skin. Additional features include splanchnomegaly, diabetes mellitus, and increased cortisol production by the adrenal glands. Patients may present with signs and symptoms of a pituitary mass rather than with the clinical picture of acromegaly. Common signs and symptoms of spinal involvement are backache, painful kyphosis of the thoracic spine, and, at times, signs of spinal cord compression.

Pathophysiology

Hypersecretion of growth hormone can result from a focal adenoma of the anterior pituitary gland, diffuse hyperplasia of the adenohypophysis, or nonpituitary sources. In immature patients, hypersecretion of growth hormone causes excessive disproportionate growth of the immature skeleton, resulting in pituitary gigantism. In the adult patient with a mature skeleton, hypersecretion of growth hormone may reactivate endochondral bone formation at osteocartilaginous junctions (e.g., costochondral junctions), cause periosteal new bone formation, and stimulate growth of soft tissue. The bones and soft tissues widen, especially in the hands, feet, and lower jaw.

Acromegaly reactivates endochondral ossification, gradually induces formation of new periosteal bone, especially in the skull and vertebrae, and stimulates the formation and thickening of subligamentous bone at tendon insertions.

Imaging

Radiography

In the spine, acromegaly affects the thoracic and lumbar regions predominantly. The vertebral bodies appear increased in their anteroposterior and transverse diameters (Fig. 16-9) due to subperiosteal bone deposition (platyspondyly). The intervertebral discs are typically increased in height, unless there is secondary disc degeneration.[22] Degenerative disc disease, hypertrophic changes of the facet joints, prominent osteophytes like those seen in diffuse idiopathic skeletal hyperostosis, thoracic kyphosis, and scalloping of the posterior margins of the vertebral bodies are additional manifestations of acromegaly. Overgrowth of soft tissues and bone can cause spinal canal stenosis.

PARATHYROID DISORDERS

Hyperparathyroidism is a pathologic condition characterized by increased parathyroid hormone (PTH) secretion.

Hypoparathyroidism results from deficient production of PTH or from resistance to the action of the hormone produced.

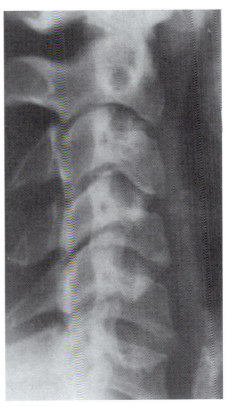

■ **FIGURE 16-9** Acromegaly. Lateral view of the cervical spine reveals increased anteroposterior diameter and posterior scalloping of the vertebrae. There is also increased disc height. *(From Efird TA, Genant HK, Wilson CB. Pituitary gigantism with cervical spinal stenosis. AJR Am J Roentgenol 1980; 134:171-173.)*

Epidemiology

In primary hyperparathyroidism, the abnormal production of PTH may result from a parathyroid adenoma (80%-90% of cases), parathyroid hyperplasia (10%-15% of cases), or parathyroid carcinoma (<2% of cases).[23] Secondary hyperparathyroidism results from increased PTH that is produced in response to chronic hypocalcemia, usually owing to chronic renal insufficiency. In long-standing secondary hyperparathyroidism, the parathyroid glands come to function independently, a condition called tertiary hyperparathyroidism. The incidence of primary hyperparathyroidism is 25 to 50 cases per 100,000 people per year and is higher in individuals older than 60 years of age. Women are affected two to four times more often than men.

Hypoparathyroidism can result from excision of the parathyroid gland, from iatrogenic trauma during thyroid surgery, or from unknown cause (idiopathic form). Pseudohypoparathyroidism and pseudopseudohypoparathyroidism are characterized by end organ unresponsiveness to parathyroid hormone. Pseudohypoparathyroidism is more common in women than men and is transmitted as an X-linked dominant trait. This condition is usually diagnosed in the second decade of life.

Clinical Presentation

The symptoms of primary hyperparathyroidism can be nonspecific.[23] Weakness, joint pain, lethargy, and even cognitive impairment can occur in older patients with undiagnosed hypercalcemia. Primary hyperparathyroidism can also present with recurrent nephrolithiasis, bone pain, or recurrent fractures. Laboratory tests disclose elevated serum calcium levels, with increased serum alkaline phosphatase, serum PTH, and renal adenosine monophosphate levels.

Hypoparathyroidism presents as hypocalcemia, hyperphosphatemia, and calcifications of the basal ganglia and soft tissue. Pseudohypoparathyroidism manifests chemically as hypocalcemia and hyperphosphatemia and clinically as characteristic short stature, mental retardation, strabismus, obesity, round face, and brachydactyly (leading to the short 4th metacarpal sign). Pseudopseudohypoparathyroidism presents as the same somatotype but with normal serum calcium levels.

Pathophysiology

PTH and vitamin D keep serum calcium levels within a narrow physiologic range controlled by a negative feedback mechanism. PTH increases serum calcium levels via bone resorption, increased distal renal tubular calcium reabsorption, decreased phosphorus reabsorption, and stimulation of vitamin D to increase the absorption of calcium and phosphorus in the gut. In primary hyperparathyroidism there is inappropriately increased PTH production. In secondary hyperparathyroidism, PTH production is an appropriate response to hypocalcemia.

Pathology

In advanced cases, hyperparathyroidism displays subperiosteal resorption of bone with thinning of the cortex. The trabeculae are distorted, and there may be cysts, brown tumors, fractures, and deformities.

Bone specimens of hyperparathyroid patients reveal osteitis fibrosa cystica, with replacement of bone marrow by fibrovascular tissue. Histologically brown tumors contain a fibrous matrix, spindle-shaped stromal cells, and multinucleated osteoclasts.

Imaging

Radiography

Bone resorption becomes radiographically evident only when 30% to 50% of the bone has been lost.[24] The most common radiographic findings of hyperparathyroidism are generalized osteopenia (71.8%) and juxta-articular osteopenia (84.3%). Plain radiographs of the spine may reveal (1) subchondral bone resorption at the sacroiliac joints and discovertebral junction, with formation of end plate erosions or Schmorl's nodes (2) resorption of the secondary trabeculae with accentuation of the primary weight-bearing trabeculae and thinning of the bony cortex; and (3) single or multiple lytic, expansile lesions, without matrix production, representing brown tumors (Fig. 16-10).

Generalized or localized osteosclerosis and soft tissue calcifications are the most common radiographic findings of hypoparathyroidism and pseudohypoparathyroidism. In rare cases, abnormalities of the spine similar to ankylosing

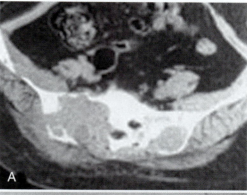
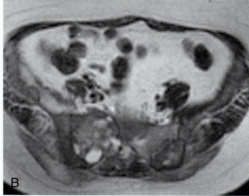

■ **FIGURE 16-10** Brown tumor. **A,** Axial CT of the pelvis shows a large soft tissue mass within the right sacrum. **B,** Axial T2W image of the sacrum demonstrates heterogeneous signal intensity of the sacral mass. *(From Hoshi M, et al. A case of multiple skeletal lesions of brown tumors, mimicking carcinoma metastases. Arch Orthop Trauma Surg 2007; 128:149-154.)*

spondylitis or diffuse idiopathic skeletal hyperostosis have been described, with calcification of the anterior and posterior longitudinal ligaments and associated osteophytes.

THYROID DISORDERS

Thyroid disorders include hypothyroidism, cretinism, myxedema, hyperthyroidism, and thyrotoxicosis.

Epidemiology

Sporadic congenital hypothyroidism has a prevalence of 1 per 4000 people. The musculoskeletal manifestations of congenital hypothyroidism are not commonly observed because most countries mandate screening for thyroid-stimulating hormone or thyroxine at birth. The prevalence of hypothyroidism is 2% to 5% worldwide. Hypothyroidism can be primary or secondary to pituitary disorders. The prevalence of thyrotoxicosis is 3% in women and 0.3% in men in countries where iodine deficiency is not endemic. Toxic diffuse goiter (Graves' disease) and toxic nodular goiter are the more common forms of thyrotoxicosis.

Clinical Presentation

Clinical manifestations of thyrotoxicosis include weight loss, tachycardia, weakness, nervousness, and hypersensitivity to heat. In adults, hyperthyroidism increases bone turnover, leading to diffuse osteoporosis in elderly patients. Clinically detectable osteoporosis is rare in patients younger than 50 years of age. In children, the main musculoskeletal effect of hyperthyroidism is accelerated skeletal maturation. Severe hyperthyroidism beginning early in life may induce premature closure of the cranial sutures and epiphyses of the hands and feet.[25]

In infants, hypothyroidism results in cretinism. In children it causes juvenile myxedema. If left untreated, both cretinism and myxedema cause delayed skeletal maturation, retarded bone age, short stature, obesity, and mental retardation. In adults, hypothyroidism does not affect the skeleton appreciably. The bone turnover rate is slower than normal and the total bone mass can be normal or slightly increased, but there is no clinical consequence to these.

Pathophysiology

Thyroid hormone is essential for postnatal development. In the absence of normal thyroid hormone, bone and dental maturation almost stop. There is delayed development and growth of centers of ossification, retarded bone growth at the epiphyseal plates, and persistence of these structures beyond the normal time of closure. Excessive thyroid hormone levels activate both osteoclasts and osteoblasts, increase the rate of new bone remodeling cycles, and cause a net decrease of bone mass.

In hyperthyroidism, the bone shows increased metabolic activity with increased numbers of remodeling sites containing metabolically active osteoblasts and osteoclasts. As a result, there is a negative mineral balance.[26] The increased metabolic activity is more pronounced in the cortex than in the trabecular bone.

Imaging

Radiography

In elderly hyperthyroid patients plain radiographs may demonstrate osteopenia, compression fractures of the spine, and accentuation of the thoracic kyphosis. These findings are more pronounced in the thoracic and lumbar spine. The radiographic findings may appear and progress quickly and then stabilize or improve when the thyrotoxicosis is treated medically.

Adult hypothyroid patients show no significant abnormality on radiographs of the spine. Newborns with hypothyroidism exhibit immature bone maturation with absence of the distal femoral and proximal tibial epiphyses. Infantile hypothyroidism shows spinal immaturity with short, wedge-shaped vertebrae at the thoracolumbar junction (bullet-shaped vertebrae) and relatively large intervertebral discs.

CUSHING'S DISEASE

Cushing's disease is a clinical syndrome resulting from exposure to excessive amounts of glucocorticoids.

Epidemiology

Cushing's disease can develop from endogenous or exogenous hypercortisolism. Endogenous Cushing's disease most commonly results from adrenal hyperplasia (about 75% of cases) and from adrenal adenoma, adrenal carcinoma, pituitary adenoma, neuroblastoma, ectopic adrenal tissue, and adrenocorticotropic hormone (ACTH)-producing tumors in the remaining cases. The disease is more common in women between the ages of 20 and 60 years.

Clinical Presentation

Central obesity, easy bruisability, growth of fat pads on the back of the neck (buffalo hump), insomnia, infertility, amenorrhea, and psychological disturbances are common clinical features. Other signs include persistent hypertension, insulin resistance that can lead to diabetes mellitus, hirsutism, and purple striae along the abdomen and axillae. Cushing's syndrome due to excess ACTH may also induce hyperpigmentation of the skin.

Pathophysiology

The major musculoskeletal manifestations of Cushing's disease are osteoporosis, osteonecrosis, delayed skeletal maturation, muscle atrophy, and accumulation of fat in the trunks of adults and in the trunks and extremities of children. Osteoporosis is the result of increased bone resorption and decreased bone deposition and can be severe in Cushing's disease. Osteonecrosis is more frequently observed in exogenous than endogenous hypercortisolism.

Imaging

Radiography

Osteopenia, biconcave deformities of vertebral bodies (fish-mouth vertebrae), compression fractures, and accentuation of the thoracic kyphosis are nonspecific findings often seen in patients with Cushing's disease. Occasionally, excess formation of callus at the fractured end plates may cause an increased density of the superior and inferior end plates.

RENAL OSTEODYSTROPHY

Renal osteodystrophy includes a group of secondary musculoskeletal abnormalities that result from the disordered calcium and phosphate metabolism caused by chronic renal insufficiency.

Epidemiology

End-stage renal disease develops in 0.01% of the United States population each year. Musculoskeletal manifestations are becoming increasingly common, because hemodialysis and renal transplant allow patients with chronic renal failure to survive longer.

Clinical Presentation

Renal osteodystrophy comprises several musculoskeletal abnormalities, including secondary hyperparathyroidism, osteosclerosis, osteoporosis, osteomalacia, and rickets. Spinal complications of long-term hemodialysis and renal transplant include destructive spondyloarthropathy, crystal deposition disease (CPPD crystal deposition disease, calcium HA deposition), aluminum toxicity (causing osteomalacia), and spondylodiscitis. Osteopenia increases the risk of fractures after minor trauma or even spontaneously. Vertebral fractures occur in 5% to 25% of patients on hemodialysis. Destructive spondyloarthropathy affects mostly the cervical and lumbar spine and presents as mild to moderate pain or as instability due to facet and ligamentous involvement. In children, chronic renal insufficiency may lead to rickets with general delay in bone age, scoliosis, and epiphyseal displacement.

Pathophysiology

Impairment of the renal parenchyma leads to chronic renal insufficiency with increased serum phosphate levels and low levels of the active form of vitamin D (1,25-dihydroxyvitamin D).[27] These cause chronic hypocalcemia, which induces secondary hyperparathyroidism.[27] The etiology of osteosclerosis is unclear. The increased bone density seen in chronic renal insufficiency may be due to the increased osteoblastic activity induced by PTH or to an increased production of mineralized osteoid. Osteosclerosis can be generalized but more often affects the axial skeleton. Bone loss results from bone resorption,

osteomalacia, and osteoporosis, which result from chronic metabolic acidosis, hyperparathyroidism, hypocalcemia, and/or poor nutritional status. In children with chronic renal insufficiency, osteomalacia and rickets are secondary to deficient production of the active form of vitamin D, hypocalcemia, inhibitors of calcification present in the uremic state, aluminum toxicity (a complication of long-term hemodialysis), and liver dysfunction. Destructive spondyloarthropathy seems to be strongly associated with hemodialysis-related amyloid deposition in the intervertebral discs.[28] Brown tumors have been described in secondary hyperparathyroidism, although they are more common in primary hyperparathyroidism.

Pathology

Gross bone specimens may reveal thickened, disorganized, or thinned bone trabeculae.

The histologic features depend on the prevailing manifestation of renal osteodystrophy but include bone resorption, scarring, and new bone formation of the vertebral spongiosa.

Imaging

Radiography

Osteosclerosis of the spine is a common finding in secondary hyperparathyroidism. It typically involves the end plates and spares the central portion of the vertebrae, resulting in the so-called "rugger jersey" appearance (Fig. 16-11). The sacroiliac joints are frequently affected and show widening of the joint space, subchondral erosions, and osteosclerosis

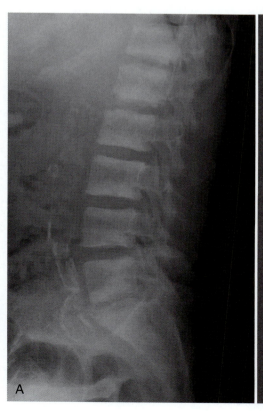
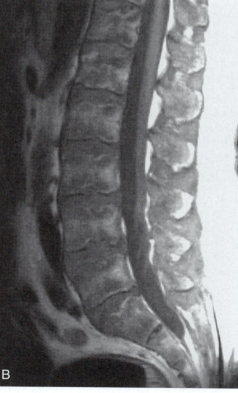

■ **FIGURE 16-11** Renal osteodystrophy. **A,** Lateral view of the spine reveals "rugger jersey" appearance with sclerosis of the end plates and intervening normal bone density. Vascular calcifications are also noted. **B,** Sagittal T1W MR image shows heterogeneous signal intensity of the bone marrow, with predominantly low signal intensity adjacent to the end plates, consistent with osteosclerosis. *(Courtesy of Dr. M. Castillo.)*

(Fig. 16-12).[27] In cases with predominant osteopenia there are pathologic fractures and spinal deformities. The vertebral bodies may often show vertical striations, because the vertical weight-bearing trabeculae are preserved whereas the transverse trabeculae are resorbed.

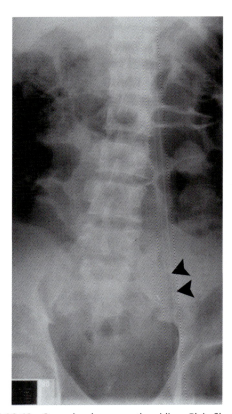

■ **FIGURE 16-12** Secondary hyperparathyroidism. Plain film of the lumbosacral spine reveals bilateral widening and erosion of the sacroiliac joints (*arrowheads*). *(Courtesy of Dr. W. Conway.)*

Destructive spondyloarthropathy is characterized by severe narrowing of the disc spaces, erosions and cysts in the adjacent end plates, but minimal osteophyte formation (Fig. 16-13).[29] Early in the disease the erosions are confined to the anterosuperior and anteroinferior corners of the vertebral bodies.[28] The lower cervical spine is affected most frequently, but destructive spondyloarthropathy can also affect the craniocervical junction.

Radiographic findings of rickets include concave deformities of multiple vertebral end plates, scoliosis, and basilar invagination.

MRI

In destructive spondyloarthropathy, the affected intervertebral discs and end plates typically show low signal intensity on T1W and T2W images (see Fig. 16-13). In rare cases, there is high signal in the discs and end plates on T2W imaging and enhancement after gadolinium administration, mimicking the appearance of spondylodiscitis.[28] Other possible differential diagnoses include CPPD crystal deposition disease, neuropathic osteoarthropathy, and severe degenerative disc disease. In destructive spondyloarthropathy there is no paraspinal extension of the disease despite the presence of pronounced discovertebral erosions. Imaging features of destructive spondyloarthropathy of the craniocervical junction include erosions of the dens, periodontoid soft tissue masses, and basilar invagination.[28]

RICKETS AND OSTEOMALACIA

Metabolic bone diseases are characterized by incomplete mineralization of normal osteoid tissue. Osteomalacia signifies abnormal increase in unmineralized osteoid.

Rickets and osteomalacia are two manifestations of the same pathologic process.[3] Rickets reflects abnormal organization and mineralization of the growth plate, so it is

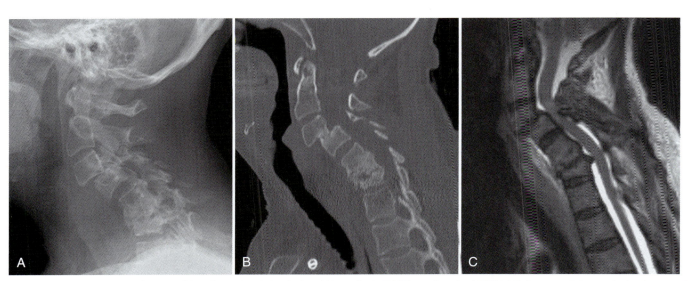

■ **FIGURE 16-13** Destructive spondyloarthropathy. Lateral view (**A**), sagittal CT (**B**), and sagittal T2W (**C**) images of the cervical spine reveal C3-C4 subluxation, severe narrowing of the intervertebral disc spaces, erosions, and destruction of the vertebral end plates at the C3-4, C5-6, and C6-7 levels. *(Courtesy of Dr. M. Castillo.)*

seen in young patients before the growth plate closes. Osteomalacia reflects inadequate or delayed mineralization of osteoid into mature cortical and trabecular bone.

Epidemiology

In the early 1900s, rickets was a common condition among young children in large cities.[30] Since the pharmaceutical synthesis of vitamin D, vitamin D–deficient rickets has nearly disappeared. Potentially, rickets might still be seen in infants exclusively breast fed by vitamin D–deficient mothers.

Over 50 pathologic conditions can present as rickets, osteomalacia, or both. These diseases can be categorized into three groups:

1. Abnormalities of vitamin D metabolism, including malnutrition, neonatal rickets, malabsorption, liver disease, anticonvulsant therapy, renal osteodystrophy, and parathyroid disorders
2. Disturbances of calcium and phosphorus metabolism secondary to renal tubular loss of phosphate (X-linked hypophosphatemia, Fanconi's syndrome, tumor associated)
3. Idiopathic, without detectable abnormalities of vitamin D, calcium, and phosphorus metabolism, including axial osteomalacia, hypophosphatasia, and metaphyseal chondrodysplasia

Clinical Presentation

Rickets can present as poor muscle development and tone, impaired growth, and skeletal deformities (pigeon chest, bow legs, and deformities of the spine). In the adult population, the symptoms of osteomalacia are nonspecific: bone pain and tenderness, muscle weakness, susceptibility to bone fractures, and decreased vertebral height due to compression fractures.

Pathophysiology

Endogenous vitamin D is synthesized in the skin and converted to 25-hydroxyvitamin D in the liver. The 25-hydroxyvitamin D is then converted to the active hormone 1,25-dihydroxyvitamin D (calcitriol) in the kidney. Calcitriol increases the concentrations of calcium and phosphate in extracellular fluid, so the osteoid becomes mineralized.[22] When calcitriol levels are low, hypocalcemia develops and stimulates secretion of PTH. Increased secretion of PTH returns calcium levels to the normal range, but the phosphate level usually decreases. Alkaline phosphatase, produced by very active differentiated osteoblasts, is released into the extracellular fluid, elevating the serum levels.

Rickets and osteomalacia represent two manifestations of the same pathologic process.[30] Rickets is secondary to abnormal organization and mineralization of the growth plate. Therefore, it is seen in young patients before the

growth plate closes. Osteomalacia results from an inadequate or delayed mineralization of osteoid into mature cortical and trabecular bone. Individuals who are affected by this condition before their skeleton is mature demonstrate rickets at the growth plates and osteomalacia in the cortical and trabecular bone.

Pathology

In osteomalacia the cortical bone shows increased number and widening of the haversian canals, which are lined with unmineralized osteoid (also called osteoid seams). Trabeculae appear thin and decreased in number. Osteitis fibrosa cystica due to secondary hyperparathyroidism can be superimposed on osteomalacia.

In rickets the zones of maturation of the growth plate are abnormal, with a disorganized increase in the number of cells and loss of the usual columnar pattern, leading to an increase in length and width of the growth plate.[30]

Imaging
Radiography

Radiographic features of rickets include growth retardation and osteopenia. In infants, the skull may be deformed. In early childhood the long bones are deformed, with typical bowing of the arms and legs. The most striking abnormalities are seen at the growth plates of the distal femur, proximal tibia, costochondral junctions of middle ribs, and distal ends of radius and ulna. These regions show enlargement of the growth plate and demineralization and disorganization of the adjacent metaphysis. In older children, abnormalities of the spine become more obvious due to the effects of weight bearing. Scoliosis is common. The intervertebral discs may expand, causing a biconcave appearance of the vertebrae (fish-mouth vertebrae).

Most adult patients with osteomalacia are affected by renal osteodystrophy. In this patient population radiographic signs of secondary hyperparathyroidism ("rugger jersey" spine) predominate.[22] When osteomalacia is the prevalent pathologic abnormality, the trabeculae become coarsened with poorly defined margins due to the presence of surrounding unmineralized osteoid. When osteoporosis is predominant there is thinning and accentuation of the vertebral trabeculae. In adults, osteomalacia typically manifests as Looser transformation zones. Looser zones are pseudofractures formed by lines of unmineralized bone at sites of mechanical stress in the long bones, pelvis, ribs, and scapulae.

ANALYSIS

Osteoporosis and osteomalacia are both characterized by osteopenia and decrease in number of bony trabeculae. In osteoporosis the trabeculae appear thin (Fig. 16-14), while in osteomalacia they are more prominent and coarse.

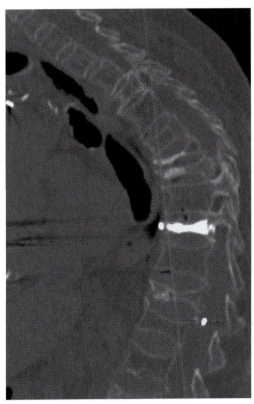

■ **FIGURE 16-14** Osteoporosis. Diffuse decreased bone density, with multiple compression fractures and biconcave deformities of the vertebral bodies ("fish-mouth vertebrae") are seen. High-density material consistent with methyl methacrylate from prior vertebroplasty is also noted.

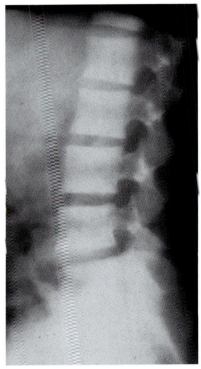

■ **FIGURE 16-15** Renal osteodystrophy. "Rugger jersey" appearance of the spine with sclerosis of the end plates and intervening normal bone density. *(Courtesy of Dr. T. Pope.)*

Paget and renal osteodystrophy are both characterized by sclerotic changes of the vertebral bodies, with an ivory vertebra or "picture frame appearance" in Paget's disease and a "rugger jersey" appearance in renal osteodystrophy (Fig. 16-15).

Spinal gout, pseudogout, and destructive spondyloarthropathy seen in patients treated with hemodialysis can mimic the appearance of spondylodiscitis (see Box 16-1); however, the affected end plates and intervertebral discs have generally low signal intensity on T1W and T2W images (Fig. 16-16).

The diagnosis of endocrinologic disorders is usually based on clinical and laboratory findings and not primarily on radiographic findings. Imaging of the spine demonstrates nonspecific osteopenia in some disorders (Cushing's disease, hyperthyroidism, and hyperparathyroidism) or subtle increase of the bone mass (hypoparathyroidism).

Acromegaly and Paget's disease are both characterized by enlargement of the affected vertebrae. In Paget's disease the skeletal involvement is either monostotic or polyostotic, whereas acromegaly is a systemic disease, with remodeling of the entire skeleton. Furthermore, Paget's disease is characterized by typical changes in bone marrow signal that are well documented on MRI and that reflect the different histologic stages of the disease.

BOX 16-1   CT Findings in Destructive Spondyloarthropathy

PATIENT HISTORY

A 55-year-old man with end-stage renal disease and a 5-year history of hemodialysis presented with neck pain.

TECHNIQUE

Helical CT images of the cervical spine were obtained at 2-mm collimation without intravenous administration of a contrast agent. Coronal and sagittal reformatted images were also obtained.

FINDINGS

There is destruction of most of the C5 vertebral body and of the superior aspect of the C6 vertebral body with diffuse bone sclerosis. There is retropulsion of the posterior wall of C5, with moderate stenosis of the spinal canal at this level. An osteophyte is evident arising from the anterior superior aspect of C6. The craniocervical junction appears normal (Fig. 16-17).

IMPRESSION

Destructive changes of the C5 and C6 vertebral bodies are seen, with bone sclerosis and no obvious soft tissue masses. The differential diagnosis includes destructive spondyloarthropathy secondary to amyloid deposition in long-term hemodialysis and spondylodiscitis. An MRI of the cervical spine with gadolinium is recommended for further evaluation.

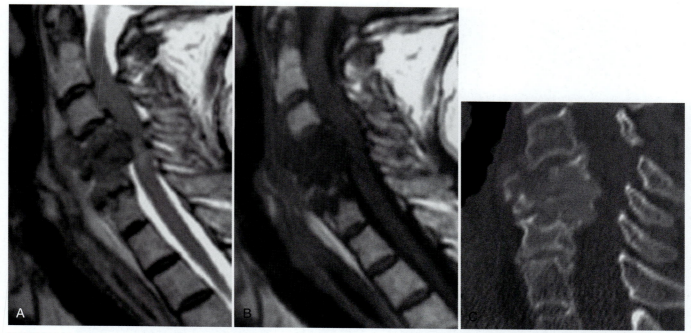

■ **FIGURE 16-16**   Gout. **A** and **B**, MR sagittal images of the cervical spine demonstrate abnormal tissue, hypointense on T1W and T2W images, replacing the discs and vertebral bone marrow at the level of C4-5, causing compression of the spinal cord. **C**, CT sagittal image shows C4-C5 vertebral body erosions with overhanging edges. The abnormal tissue replacing the normal trabecular bone appears hyperdense on CT and is consistent with tophus. *(From Dharmadhikari R, Dildey P, Hide IG. A rare cause of spinal cord compression: imaging appearances of gout of the cervical spine. Skeletal Radiol 2006; 35:942-945.)*

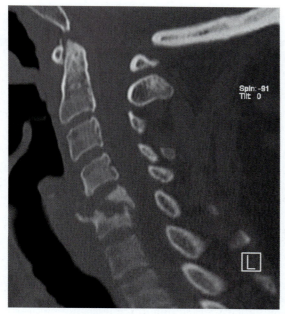

■ **FIGURE 16-17**   Helical CT image of the cervical spine in a 55-year-old man with end-stage renal disease and a 5-year history of hemodialysis. *(Courtesy of Dr. M. Castillo.)*

KEY POINTS: DIFFERENTIAL DIAGNOSIS

■ CPPD crystal deposition disease is a cause of compressive myelopathy in middle-aged and elderly patients. Excised ossified ligamenta flava should be analyzed with polarized-light spectroscopy to identify CPPD crystals.

■ Destructive spondyloarthropathy, CPPD crystal deposition disease, and gout of the discs and end plates can be differentiated from spondylodiscitis based on their MRI appearance. In these metabolic disorders, on T2W images the abnormal discs have overall low signal intensity whereas the infected discs usually have high signal intensity.

■ In primary hyperparathyroidism of the spine, osteopenia is the most prominent feature, whereas in secondary hyperparathyroidism, bone sclerosis ("rugger-jersey" spine) is more common.

SUGGESTED READINGS

Chew FS. Radiologic manifestations in the musculoskeletal system of miscellaneous endocrine disorders. Radiol Clin North Am 1991; 29:135-147.

Marcove RC, Arlen M, Jaffe HL. Metabolic diseases: disorders of endogenous metabolism. In Atlas of Bone Pathology. Philadelphia, JB Lippincott, 1992, pp 60-114.

Murphey MD, Sartoris DJ, Quale JL, et al. Musculoskeletal manifestations of chronic renal insufficiency. RadioGraphics 1993; 13:357-379.

Osteoporosis prevention, diagnosis, and therapy. NIH Consensus Statement 2000; 17:1-45.

Resnick D. Osteoporosis. In: Bone and Joint Imaging, 2nd ed. Philadelphia, WB Saunders, 1996, pp 491-510.

Resnick D. Parathyroid disorders and renal osteodystrophy. In: Bone and Joint Imaging, 2nd ed. Philadelphia, WB Saunders, 1996, pp 552-571.

Resnick D. Pituitary disorders. In: Bone and Joint Imaging, 2nd ed. Philadelphia, WB Saunders, 1996, pp 537-545.

Smith SE, Murphey MD, Motamedi K, et al. From the archives of the AFIP. Radiologic spectrum of Paget disease of bone and its complications with pathologic correlation. RadioGraphics 2002; 22:1191-1216.

Steinbach LS. Calcium pyrophosphate dihydrate and calcium hydroxyapatite crystal deposition diseases: imaging perspectives. Radiol Clin North Am 2004; 42:185-205, vii.

REFERENCES

1. Griffith JF, Yeung DK, Antonio GE, et al. Vertebral bone mineral density, marrow perfusion, and fat content in healthy men and men with osteoporosis: dynamic contrast-enhanced MR imaging and MR spectroscopy. Radiology 2005; 236:945-951.
2. Riggs BL, Melton LJ 3rd. Involutional osteoporosis. N Engl J Med 1986; 314:1676-1686.
3. Gillespy T 3rd, Gillespy MP. Osteoporosis. Radiol Clin North Am 1991; 29:77-84.
4. Osteoporosis prevention, diagnosis, and therapy. NIH Consensus Statement 2000; 17:1-45.
5. Cummings SR, Bates D, Black DM. Clinical use of bone densitometry: scientific review. JAMA 2002; 288:1889-1897.
6. Kazakia GJ, Majumdar S. New imaging technologies in the diagnosis of osteoporosis. Rev Endocr Metab Disord 2006; 7:67-74.
7. Dharmadhikari R, Dildey P, Hide IG. A rare cause of spinal cord compression: imaging appearances of gout of the cervical spine. Skeletal Radiol 2006; 35:942-945.
8. Hausch R, Wilkerson M, Singh E, et al. Tophaceous gout of the thoracic spine presenting as back pain and fever. J Clin Rheumatol 1999; 5:335-341.
9. Justiniano M, Colmegna I, Cuchacovich R, Espinoza LR. Spondyloarthritis as a presentation of gouty arthritis. J Rheumatol 2007; 34:1157-1158.
10. Barrett K, Miller ML, Wilson JT. Tophaceous gout of the spine mimicking epidural infection: case report and review of the literature. Neurosurgery 2001; 48:1170-1172; discussion 1172-1173.
11. Duprez TP, Malghem J, Vande Berg BC, et al. Gout in the cervical spine: MR pattern mimicking diskovertebral infection. AJNR Am J Neuroradiol 1996; 17:151-153.
12. Bonaldi VM, Duong H, Starr MR, et al. Tophaceous gout of the lumbar spine mimicking an epidural abscess: MR features. AJNR Am J Neuroradiol 1996; 17:1949-1952.
13. Muthukumar N, Karuppaswamy U. Tumoral calcium pyrophosphate dihydrate deposition disease of the ligamentum flavum. Neurosurgery 2003; 53:103-108; discussion 108-109.
14. Resnick D, Pineda C. Vertebral involvement in calcium pyrophosphate dihydrate crystal deposition disease: radiographic-pathological correlation. Radiology 1984; 153:55-60.
15. Lin SH, Hsieh ET, Wu TY, Chang CW. Cervical myelopathy induced by pseudogout in ligamentum flavum and retro-odontoid mass: a case report. Spinal Cord 2006; 44:692-694.
16. Kinoshita T, Maruoka S, Yamazaki T, Sakamoto K. Tophaceous pseudogout of the cervical spine: MR imaging and bone scintigraphy findings. Eur J Radiol 1998; 27:271-273.
17. Mirra JM, Brien EW, Tehranzadeh J. Paget's disease of bone: review with emphasis on radiologic features: I. Skeletal Radiol 1995; 24:163-171.
18. Boutin RD, Spitz DJ, Newman JS, et al. Complications in Paget disease at MR imaging. Radiology 1998; 209:641-651.
19. Mirra JM, Ficci P, Gold RH. Bone Tumors: Clinical, Radiologic, and Pathologic Correlations. Philadelphia, Lea & Febiger, 1989, vol 2, p 1831.
20. Mirra JM, Brien EW, Tehranzadeh J. Paget's disease of bone: review with emphasis on radiologic features: II. Skeletal Radiol 1995; 24:173-184.
21. Zlatkin MB, Lander PH, Hadjipavlou AG, Levine JS. Paget disease of the spine: CT with clinical correlation. Radiology 1986; 160:155-159.
22. Resnick D. Rickets and Osteomalacia. Bone and Joint Imaging 2nd ed. Philadelphia, WB Saunders, 1996, pp 491-524.
23. Hayes CW, Conway WF. Hyperparathyroidism. Radiol Clin North Am 1991; 29:85-96.
24. Richardson ML, Pozzi-Mucelli RS, Kanter AS, et al. Bone mineral changes in primary hyperparathyroidism. Skeletal Radiol 1986; 15:85-95.
25. Riggs W Jr, Wilroy RS Jr, Etteldorf JN. Neonatal hyperthyroidism with accelerated skeletal maturation, craniosynostosis, and brachydactyly. Radiology 1972; 105:621-625.
26. Rosenberg AE. The pathology of metabolic bone disease. Radiol Clin North Am 1991; 29:19-36.
27. Jevtic V. Imaging of renal osteodystrophy. Eur J Radiol 2003; 46:85-95.
28. Leone A, Sundaram M, Cerase A, et al. Destructive spondyloarthropathy of the cervical spine in long-term hemodialyzed patients: a five-year clinical radiological prospective study. Skeletal Radiol 2001; 30:431-441.
29. Kuntz D, Naveau B, Bardin T, et al. Destructive spondylarthropathy in hemodialyzed patients: a new syndrome. Arthritis Rheum 1984; 27:369-375.
30. Pitt MJ. Rickets and osteomalacia are still around. Radiol Clin North Am 1991; 29:97-118.

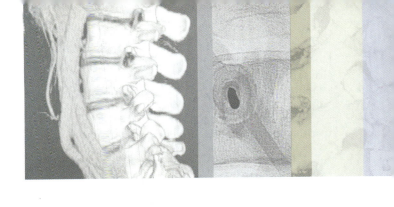

17

Metabolic Conditions Affecting the Spinal Cord

Maria Vittoria Spampinato

Metabolic disorders of the spinal cord are less common than metabolic disorders of the brain and peripheral nerves. Such metabolic myelopathies can be secondary to nutritional deficiencies, especially vitamin B_{12} deficiency, or to systemic metabolic disorders.

VITAMIN B_{12} DEFICIENCY

Subacute combined degeneration (SCD) of the spinal cord is a symmetric spongy vacuolation and degeneration of myelin that results from deficiency of vitamin B_{12}. It affects the dorsal and lateral columns of the cervicothoracic spinal cord symmetrically, leading to symmetric paresthesias, stiffness, and gait unsteadiness and is worse in the lower than the upper extremities.

Epidemiology

The prevalence of vitamin B_{12} deficiency is estimated at 4.8% to 12% in the elderly population living in the community and up to 30% to 40% among hospitalized elderly people.[1] SCD is most commonly diagnosed between the fifth and eighth decades of life.[3] Subclinical myelopathy occurs in up to 40% of patients with pernicious anemia. About one fourth of the patients with SCD have no known hematologic abnormalities.

Dietary deficiency of vitamin B_{12} may result from insufficient ingestion of vitamin B_{12} in strict vegetarians (vegans). Malabsorption of ingested vitamin B_{12} may occur in patients with insufficient production of intrinsic factor (pernicious anemia); hypochlorhydria (partial/complete gastrectomy); insufficient absorption of vitamin B_{12} (ileal resection, multiple causes of intestinal malabsorption including celiac disease, chronic pancreatic insufficiency, Crohn's disease); or intestinal competition for the ingested vitamin B_{12} (bacterial overgrowth in blind-loop syndrome, infestation with the fish tapeworm *Diphyllobothrium latum*).[2] SCD of the spinal cord can be also caused by nitrous oxide abuse, copper deficiency, folate deficiency, human immunodeficiency virus (HIV) infection, and rare inherited defects of methylation.

Clinical Presentation

Vitamin B_{12} deficiency causes megaloblastic anemia, glossitis, gastrointestinal disturbances, SCD of the spinal cord, and peripheral neuropathy. The clinical presentation of SCD reflects (1) dysfunction of the dorsal columns (disturbed vibration sense, disturbed position sense, and ataxia), (2) dysfunction of the lateral corticospinal tracts (hyperreflexia, spasticity, and extensor plantar responses), and (3) dysfunction of the spinothalamic tracts (sensory loss). Early symptoms of SCD consist of symmetric paresthesias, which are first distal, then also proximal; stiffness; and gait unsteadiness. Progression leads to spastic paraparesis, ataxia, and anesthesia of the lower limbs and trunk. The upper extremities are typically less affected.

The diagnosis of vitamin B_{12} deficiency is confirmed by demonstrating low serum levels of vitamin B_{12} or, if the vitamin B_{12} level is borderline, elevated levels of homocysteine and methylmalonic acid. Hematologic changes are not reliable markers for vitamin B_{12} deficiency. Pernicious anemia is confirmed by the Schilling test or by the presence of anti–intrinsic factor antibodies. The treatment of vitamin B_{12} deficiency consists of monthly intramuscular injections of vitamin B_{12}. After supplementation with vitamin B_{12}, patients may show clinical and radiologic improvement. Reversal of symptoms, however, is inversely proportional to symptom duration and severity.[4]

Pathophysiology

SCD of the spinal cord is thought to result from defective methylation of myelin basic protein and other central nervous system proteins. Both vitamin B_{12} and folate are important coenzymes in the production of methionine, which acts as a methyl-group donor in the synthesis of myelin basic protein.[2]

Vitamin B_{12} is mostly found in animal food (meat, dairy products, and yeasts). It is released during gastric digestion and must bind to intrinsic factor, a glycoprotein produced by the gastric parietal cells, in order to be absorbed in the distal ileum and stored in the liver.[1] Pernicious anemia is an immune-mediated process that destroys the gastric parietal cells, so less intrinsic factor is available. Conditions such as gastric surgery or gastric reconstruction, intestinal bacterial overgrowth, and gastric atrophy (possibly secondary to *Helicobacter pylori* infection) cause hypochlorhydria and inability to release vitamin B_{12} from food. Other causes of malabsorption of vitamin B_{12} are surgical resection of the terminal ileum and a variety of disorders that result in damage to the last 80 cm of the small bowel mucosa (e.g., Crohn's disease, lymphoma, tuberculosis, Whipple's disease, and celiac disease).

Pathology

In chronic SCD, the spinal cord may appear atrophic with discoloration of the posterior and lateral columns, especially in the lower cervical and thoracic regions.

Early findings of SCD include spongy vacuolation and degeneration of myelin, most commonly in the thoracic region. Initially, there is symmetric involvement of the posterior columns (fasciculi gracilis and cuneatus) and later the lateral columns (corticospinal and spinocerebellar tracts) (Fig. 17-1). Perivascular demyelination and inflammation may cause breakdown of the blood-brain barrier. Chronically, astrocytic gliosis, axonal degeneration, and macrophage infiltration of the posterior spinal cord are observed. In severe cases the anterior columns are also involved. Extension to the medulla has been reported.

Imaging

CT

CT of the spine is often normal. Mild cord swelling can be seen in some cases.

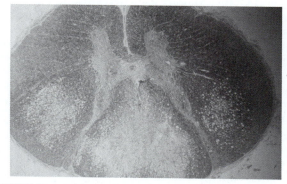

■ **FIGURE 17-1** Vitamin B_{12} deficiency. Degeneration of the myelin of the posterior and lateral columns. *(Courtesy of Dr. T. Rumboldt.)*

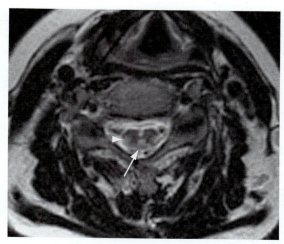

■ **FIGURE 17-2** Vitamin B_{12} deficiency. Axial T2W MR image of the cervical spine demonstrates abnormal symmetric increased signal in the posterior (*arrow*) and lateral columns (*arrowhead*) of the cervical spinal cord. *(Courtesy of Dr. M. Castillo.)*

MRI

T2-weighted (T2W) images demonstrate increased signal intensity of the dorsal and possibly lateral columns of the spinal cord (Fig. 17-2). There may be mild contrast enhancement, or not. Axial MR images display the symmetric involvement of the dorsal (and/or lateral) columns as increased T2 signal in an "inverted V" or "inverted rabbit ears" configuration. Sagittal sequences show continuous lengths of increased T2 signal running vertically for long distances along the dorsal surface of the thoracic or cervicothoracic cords. This is a helpful sign. In SCD a continuous area of abnormal signal extends over several vertebral bodies, whereas in multiple sclerosis and other demyelinating disorders the cord lesions are often multiple not single and each segment is typically shorter than two vertebral bodies. The lateral columns may not show signal abnormalities, even when there is clinical evidence they are affected.

On follow-up MRI, the T2 signal abnormalities of the posterior columns may appear decreased when vitamin B_{12} treatment is initiated promptly.[2]

NITROUS OXIDE TOXICITY

Nitrous oxide toxicity is a myelopathy that develops in patients with clinically silent or borderline vitamin B_{12} toxicity, who are then exposed to nitrous oxide anesthesia.

Epidemiology

Nitrous oxide is an inhaled gas used as an anesthetic in dentistry and as a propellant in the food industry (e.g., in whipped cream dispensers). Myelopathy may develop 2 to 6 weeks after nitrous oxide anesthesia. Most patients are found to have a subclinical or undiagnosed vitamin B_{12} deficiency.[5,6] Several cases of nitrous oxide neurotoxicity have been described after abuse of nitrous oxide by health care providers or occupational exposure, even in subjects with normal vitamin B_{12} levels.[7]

Clinical Presentation

The signs and symptoms of toxic nitrous oxide myelopathy are analogous to those seen in SCD of the spinal cord secondary to vitamin B_{12} deficiency. Signs of involvement of the posterior columns include loss of position and vibration sense, ataxia, and broad-based gait. Dysfunction of the corticospinal tracts may manifest as weakness, spasticity, hyperreflexia, clonus, incontinence, and extensor plantar response.[7] There may also be mental status changes, emotional instability, and, in some cases, psychosis with intellectual deterioration.[8]

Pathophysiology

Vitamin B_{12} is active in a reduced state of oxygenation. Nitrous oxide irreversibly oxidizes the cobalt ion of cobalamin (vitamin B_{12}). Oxidation of the cobalt ion inhibits the formation of a complex between methylcobalamin and methionine synthase, which is necessary for the methylation of myelin sheath phospholipids and myelin formation. The conversion of methylmalonyl-coenzyme A to succinyl-coenzyme A is also inhibited, so methylmalonate and propionate accumulate. This leads to production and incorporation of abnormal fatty acids into the myelin sheath.[7] In normal subjects, new methionine synthase/vitamin complexes are usually produced, so no manifestations of vitamin B_{12} deficiency ensue. In subjects with subclinical vitamin B_{12} deficiency, however, exposure to nitrous oxide may cause neurologic symptoms.

Nitrous oxide toxicity is treated with vitamin B_{12} and possibly methionine supplementation. The symptoms may then improve, especially if the condition is diagnosed and treated early. Patients may also improve in the absence of vitamin B_{12} supplementation.[7]

Pathology

The gross pathologic features and the histologic findings are those of SCD of the spinal cord.

Imaging

MRI

The MRI features of nitrous oxide toxicity in the spinal cord resemble those of SCD secondary to vitamin B_{12} deficiency, with symmetrically increased T2 signal in the posterior columns and sometimes of the lateral columns (Fig. 17-3A), possibly with enhancement of the posterior columns after gadolinium administration (see Fig. 17-3B).[9]

COPPER DEFICIENCY MYELOPATHY

Acquired myeloneuropathy can occur in patients with copper deficiency.

Epidemiology

Acquired dietary copper deficiency is exceedingly rare in humans because copper is universally available and the

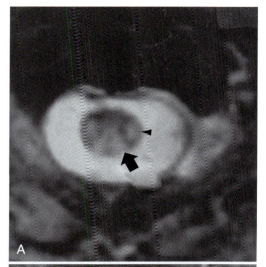

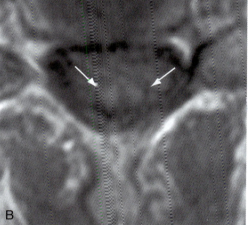

■ FIGURE 17-3 Nitrous oxide toxicity. **A,** Axial T2W MR image of the spinal cord reveals abnormal increased signal in the posterior (*arrow*) and lateral columns (*arrowhead*). **B,** Axial post-gadolinium T1W MR image shows abnormal contrast enhancement of the posterior columns (*arrows*). (*A from Beltramello A, Puppini G, Cereni R, et al. Subacute combined degeneration of the spinal cord after nitrous oxide anaesthesia: role of magnetic resonance imaging. J Neurol Neurosurg Psychiatry 1998; 64:563-564; B from Naidich MJ, Ho SU. Case 87: Subacute combined degeneration. Radiology 2005; 237:101-105.*)

human daily requirement is low.[10] In ruminants, copper deficiency causes a progressive ataxic myelopathy known as swayback.[11] In humans, copper deficiency can occur in patients maintained on parenteral or enteral feedings deficient in copper, in premature and malnourished infants, in patients with nephrotic syndrome, gastrectomy, malabsorption, or ingestion of copper-chelating agents, as a complication of penicillamine therapy, and secondary to excessive zinc ingestion.[12]

Copper deficiency may also be seen in Menkes' disease, an X-linked inherited disorder of copper metabolism characterized by deficient copper absorption and transport. Menkes' disease typically develops in infancy (estimated incidence: 1 : 30,000-250,000).

Another cause of copper deficiency is idiopathic acquired copper deficiency. This condition may represent a copper transport defect, abnormalities of metallochaperones (cytosolic proteins involved in intracellular copper management), or abnormalities of the Menkes protein.[10]

Clinical Presentation

Patients with copper deficiency present with an ataxic gait. Sensory examination shows loss of proprioception and vibration in the distal lower limbs and loss of perception of pinprick and touch in a stocking distribution. Lower limb weakness and spasticity have been described.[13] Abnormal findings are usually subtle or absent in the upper limbs.[13] Associated hematologic findings are anemia, neutropenia, sideroblastosis, and myelodysplastic syndrome.[10] Serum copper and ceruloplasmin levels are usually markedly decreased. Treatment with oral copper supplementation (2 mg/day) typically prevents further neurologic deterioration in patients with acquired copper deficiency and in some cases leads to clinical improvement.[13]

Pathophysiology

Copper absorption takes place in the stomach and proximal duodenum. The absorbed copper is an essential trace metal involved as a cofactor in multiple enzymatic processes crucial to the function of the central nervous system, including cytochrome-*c* oxidase, copper-zinc superoxide dismutase, tyrosinase, and dopamine-β-hydroxylase.[14] Copper is required for the normal function of the vascular and skeletal systems and in hematopoiesis.

Zinc therapy is used for treatment of Wilson's disease to reduce body copper stores. Increased intake of zinc induces higher concentrations of metallothionein in the enterocytes of the proximal small bowel. Copper has a higher affinity for metallothionein than zinc and remains in the enterocytes instead of being absorbed.

Pathology

Pathologic studies in animals have shown early edematous changes followed by cavitation or gelatinous lesions of the cerebral white matter, chromatolysis, necrosis, and demyelination of the white matter of the spinal cord and brain stem.[11]

Imaging

MRI

Imaging features of copper deficiency myelopathy consist of high T2 signal in the dorsal columns and central spinal cord (Fig. 17-4). Exclusive involvement of the central spinal cord has also been described.[12] No abnormal enhancement of the cord has been reported in copper deficiency myelopathy. In a series of 11 patients, the cervical cord was involved in 10, the thoracic spinal cord in 6, and both in 5.[12] Mild spinal cord atrophy can be seen in copper deficiency myelopathy. After increase in serum copper levels, the signal abnormalities in the dorsal columns may improve.[12]

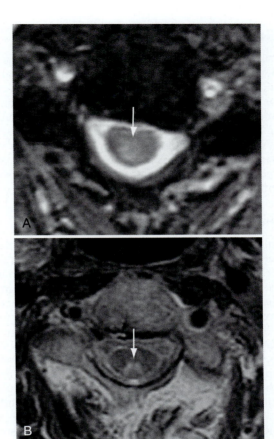

■ **FIGURE 17-4** Copper deficiency myelopathy. **A,** Axial T2W MR image of the cervical spinal cord demonstrates symmetric signal abnormalities involving the central and dorsal cord (*arrow*). **B,** In a different case, only the dorsal columns appear involved (*arrow*). (*From Kumar N. Imaging features of copper deficiency myelopathy: a study of 25 cases. Neuroradiology 2006; 48:78-83.*)

MYELOPATHY IN SYSTEMIC METABOLIC DISORDERS

The spinal cord can be involved in diabetes mellitus and chronic liver disease and is known as diabetic myelopathy or hepatic or portosystemic myelopathy.

Epidemiology

The prevalence of diabetic myelopathy is currently unknown. Research studies on diabetic neurologic impairment have focused mainly on the peripheral nervous system, although involvement of the central nervous system, especially the spinal cord, has been described.[15-17]

Progressive myelopathy is an uncommon complication of chronic liver disease with portal hypertension.[18] It is observed less frequently than hepatic encephalopathy. The two conditions can coexist.[19]

Clinical Presentation

Patients with diabetic myelopathy usually present with leg weakness, abnormal gait, sensory peripheral neuropathies, abnormal joint position sense in their lower extremities, ataxia, and brisk deep tendon reflexes.[20] The combination of posterior column involvement and pyramidal signs is comparable to the clinical picture seen in SCD of the spinal cord.

The clinical presentation of hepatic myelopathy consists of walking difficulties, tremor, increased muscle tone, spastic paraparesis, brisk deep tendon reflexes, and extensor plantar responses, without significant sensory involvement or sphincteric disturbances.[18] Hepatic myelopathy is a diagnosis of exclusion, after conditions such as spinal cord infarction, spinal cord compression, intramedullary masses, HIV and human T-lymphotropic virus (HTLV) type 1 infections, and other metabolic disorders have been ruled out. Hepatic myelopathy is not reversible, although some clinical improvement has been described after liver transplantation.[21]

Pathophysiology

The pathophysiology of the spinal cord involvement in diabetes mellitus is not well known. A combination of progressive angiopathy, metabolic disturbances, and genetic predisposition is most likely responsible for this neurologic syndrome. The spinal cord may show volume loss in diabetics even in the absence of clinical signs of myelopathy.[15,17]

In patients with spontaneous or surgically created portosystemic shunts, ammonia and other neurotoxic compounds may bypass the liver and cause both encephalopathy and myelopathy.[19]

Pathology

The most common pathologic findings of diabetic myelopathy are demyelination of the posterior and lateral columns and microinfarctions, mainly of the spinal cord white matter, secondary to arteriolosclerosis of the intrinsic vessels of the spinal cord.[20]

Patients with hepatic myelopathy show selective demyelination of the corticospinal tracts,[22] first in the cervical region and eventually in the distal spinal cord as well. Concomitant abnormalities of the posterior columns, spinothalamic tracts, or spinocerebellar tracts are probably secondary to alcohol abuse.[19]

Imaging

MRI

The imaging features of hepatic and diabetic myelopathy have not been evaluated systematically. MRI has shown mild atrophy or no abnormality of the spinal cord in the few cases of hepatic myelopathy reported in the literature.[18,19] Spinal cord abnormalities are present in up to 41% of autopsies in diabetic patients.[20] They may be associated with diabetic peripheral neuropathy, even when there are no clinical signs of myelopathy.[15] The cervical MRI of a single young man with diabetes mellitus type 1 and cervical myelopathy showed increased T2 signal of the posterior columns (Fig. 17-5).[16] Extensive work-up

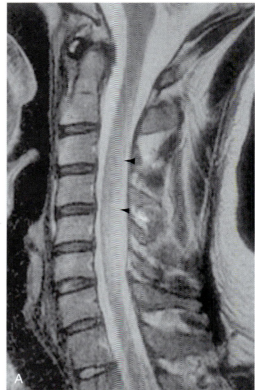

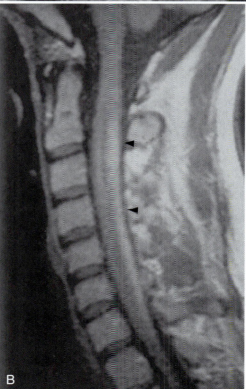

■ **FIGURE 17-5** Diabetic myelopathy. **A,** Sagittal T2W MR image of the cervical spine shows increased T2 signal of the posterior spinal cord (*arrowheads*). **B,** Sagittal post-gadolinium MR image demonstrates abnormal enhancement of the posterior columns (*arrowheads*). *(From Prick JJW, Prevo RL, Hoogenraad TU. Transient myelopathy of the cervical posterior columns in a young man with recently diagnosed diabetes mellitus. Clin Neurol Neurosurg 2001; 103:234-237.)*

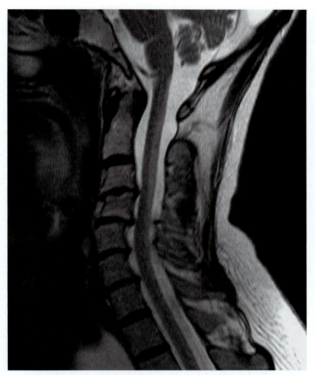

■ FIGURE 17-6   Vitamin B$_{12}$ deficiency. Sagittal T2W MR image of the cervical spine shows increased signal in the posterior columns extending over multiple vertebral segments. *(Courtesy of Dr. M. Castillo.)*

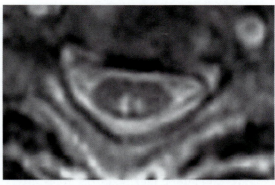

■ FIGURE 17-7   HIV vacuolar myelopathy. Axial T2W MR image of the cervical spine shows T2 signal abnormality in the dorsal aspect of the spinal cord. Differential diagnosis includes subacute combined degeneration of the spinal cord. *(From Thurnher MM, Cartes-Zumelzu F, Mueller-Mang C. Demyelinating and infectious diseases of the spinal cord. Neuroimaging Clin North Am 2007; 17:37-55.)*

showed no other metabolic disturbances, infections, or nutritional deficiencies. The symptoms and MRI abnormalities resolved completely over several months.

ANALYSIS

The differential diagnosis of myelopathy includes neoplasms, demyelinating diseases, SCD of the spinal cord, infectious etiologies (HIV vacuolar myelopathy, HTLV-1 and herpes simplex virus infection), spinal cord infarct, inflammatory conditions (e.g., sarcoidosis), and paraneoplastic syndrome, among other conditions. SCD secondary to vitamin B$_{12}$ deficiency is a treatable condition, and full recovery can be achieved with an early diagnosis and treatment. SCD secondary to nitrous oxide toxicity must also be considered in the differential diagnosis in patients with postsurgical myelopathy. Copper deficiency, tabes dorsalis, and HIV-related vacuolar myelopathy have similar imaging appearances and need to be ruled out with the appropriate laboratory tests. Metabolic conditions affecting the spinal cord affect mostly the white matter tracts. The presence of symmetric signal abnormalities confined to the posterior columns and, in some cases, also to the lateral columns over multiple vertebral segments is suggestive of SCD and in general of a metabolic etiology of the myelopathy (Figs. 17-6 to 17-10 and Box 17-1).

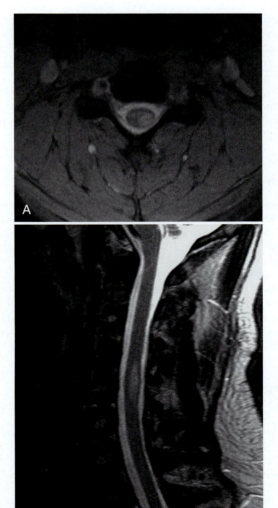

■ FIGURE 17-8   Multiple sclerosis. Axial (**A**) and sagittal (**B**) T2W MR images of the cervical spine show abnormal signal involving the lateral and posterior aspects of the spinal cord, extending longitudinally for less than two vertebral bodies.

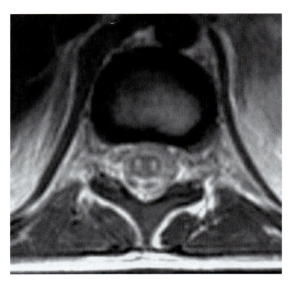

■ **FIGURE 17-9** Spinal cord infarct in a child. Axial T2W MR image of the thoracic spine demonstrates abnormal signal of the gray matter of the spinal cord. *(Courtesy of Dr. Z. Rumboldt.)*

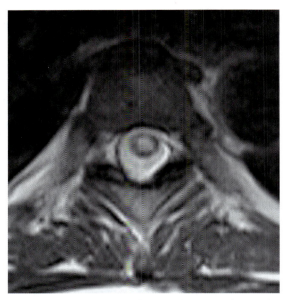

■ **FIGURE 17-10** Transverse myelitis. Axial T2W MR image of the thoracic spine reveals high T2 signal involving more than two thirds of the spinal cord cross-sectional area. *(Courtesy of Dr. Z. Rumboldt.)*

BOX 17-1   MRI Evaluation in a Patient with Myelopathy

PATIENT HISTORY

A 60-year-old man presented with ataxia and paresthesias of the upper and lower extremities.

TECHNIQUE

Multiplanar, multisequence MRI of the cervical and thoracic spine was obtained before and after the intravenous administration of 20 ml of gadolinium chelate.

FINDINGS

There is bilateral, symmetric, high T2 signal of the dorsal columns of the cervical spinal cord, extending over multiple segments (see Fig. 17-6). After gadolinium administration there is no abnormal contrast enhancement of the dorsal spinal cord.

There are no epidural or intradural masses. There is no compression of the spinal cord. The vertebrae of the cervical and thoracic spine demonstrate normal height, alignment, and signal intensity.

IMPRESSION

Signal abnormalities of the dorsal columns of the spinal cord are seen. The differential diagnosis includes subacute combined degeneration of the spinal cord, HIV vacuolar myelopathy, and other demyelinating disorders.

KEY POINTS: DIFFERENTIAL DIAGNOSIS

- Myelopathies secondary to vitamin B_{12} deficiency, nitrous oxide toxicity, copper deficiency, HIV vacuolar myelopathy, and demyelinating disease may have similar imaging appearances.
- Serum levels of vitamin B_{12}, homocysteine, methylmalonic acid, copper, ceruloplasmin; 24-hour urine copper excretion; and serologic tests for Lyme disease, syphilis, HIV, and herpes simplex virus should be part of the work-up of patients with myelopathy of undetermined origin.
- The use of nitrous oxide should be avoided in patients with increased mean corpuscular volume, anemia of unknown cause, or known vitamin B_{12} deficiency.
- In patients with neurologic symptoms weeks after exposure to nitrous oxide, consider cobalamin deficiency as a possible cause.

SUGGESTED READINGS

Bassi SS, Bulundwe KK, Greeff GP, et al. MRI of the spinal cord in myelopathy complicating vitamin B12 deficiency: two additional cases and a review of the literature. Neuroradiology 1999; 41:271-274.

Healton EB, Savage DG, Brust JC, et al. Neurologic aspects of cobalamin deficiency. Medicine (Baltimore) 1991; 70:229-245.

Kumar N. Copper deficiency myelopathy (human swayback). Mayo Clin Proc 2006; 81:1371-1384.

Lindenbaum J, Healton EB, Savage DG, et al. Neuropsychiatric disorders caused by cobalamin deficiency in the absence of anemia or macrocytosis. N Engl J Med 1988; 318:1720-1728.

Thurnher MM, Cartes-Zumelzu F, Mueller-Mang C. Demyelinating and infectious diseases of the spinal cord. Neuroimaging Clin North Am 2007; 17:37-55.

Weir DG, Scott JM. The biochemical basis of the neuropathy in cobalamin deficiency. Baillieres Clin Haematol 1995; 8:479-497.

REFERENCES

1. Andres E, Loukili NH, Noel E, et al. Vitamin B_{12} (cobalamin) deficiency in elderly patients. Can Med Assoc J 2004; 171:251-259.

2. Timms SR, Cure JK, Kurent JE. Subacute combined degeneration of the spinal cord: MR findings. AJNR Am J Neuroradiol 1993; 14:1224-1227.

3. Hemmer B, Glocker FX, Schumacher M, et al. Subacute combined degeneration: clinical, electrophysiological, and magnetic resonance imaging findings. J Neurol Neurosurg Psychiatry 1998; 65:822-827.

4. Ravina B, Loevner LA, Bank W. MR findings in subacute combined degeneration of the spinal cord: a case of reversible cervical myelopathy. AJR Am J Roentgenol 2000; 174:863-865.

5. Ilniczky S, Jelencsik I, Kenez J, Szirmai I. MR findings in subacute combined degeneration of the spinal cord caused by nitrous oxide anesthesia—two cases. Eur J Neurol 2002; 9:101-104.

6. Hadzic A, Glab K, Sanborn KV, Thys DM. Severe neurologic deficit after nitrous oxide anesthesia. Anesthesiology 1995; 83:863-866.

7. Pema PJ, Horak HA, Wyatt RH. Myelopathy caused by nitrous oxide toxicity. AJNR Am J Neuroradiol 1998; 19:894-896.

8. Beltramello A, Puppini G, Cerini R, et al. Subacute combined degeneration of the spinal cord after nitrous oxide anaesthesia: role of magnetic resonance imaging. J Neurol Neurosurg Psychiatry 1998; 64:563-564.

9. Naidich MJ, Ho SU. Case 87: Subacute combined degeneration. Radiology 2005; 237:101-105.

10. Kumar N, Crum B, Petersen RC, et al. Copper deficiency myelopathy. Arch Neurol 2004; 61:762-766.

11. Barlow RM. Further observations on swayback: I. Transitional pathology. J Comp Pathol 1963; 73:51-60.

12. Kumar N, Ahlskog JE, Klein CJ, Port JD. Imaging features of copper deficiency myelopathy: a study of 25 cases. Neuroradiology 2006; 48:78-83.

13. Kumar N, Gross JB Jr, Ahlskog JE. Copper deficiency myelopathy produces a clinical picture like subacute combined degeneration. Neurology 2004; 63:33-39.

14. Goodman BP, Chong BW, Patel AC, et al. Copper deficiency myeloneuropathy resembling B_{12} deficiency: partial resolution of MR imaging findings with copper supplementation. AJNR Am J Neuroradiol 2006; 27:2112-2114.

15. Selvarajah D, Wilkinson ID, Emery CJ, et al. Early involvement of the spinal cord in diabetic peripheral neuropathy. Diabetes Care 2006; 29:2664-2669.

16. Prick JJ, Prevo RL, Hoogenraad TU. Transient myelopathy of the cervical posterior columns in a young man with recently diagnosed diabetes mellitus. Clin Neurol Neurosurg 2001; 103:234-237.

17. Eaton SE, Harris ND, Rajbhandari SM, et al. Spinal cord involvement in diabetic peripheral neuropathy. Lancet 2001; 358:35-36.

18. Utku U, Asil T, Balci K, et al. Hepatic myelopathy with spastic paraparesis. Clin Neurol Neurosurg 2005; 107:514-516.

19. Campellone JV, Lacomis D, Giuliani MJ, Kroboth FJ. Hepatic myelopathy: case report with review of the literature. Clin Neurol Neurosurg 1996; 98:242-246.

20. Giladi N, Turezkite T, Harel D. Myelopathy as a complication of diabetes mellitus. Isr J Med Sci 1991; 27:316-319.

21. Troisi R, Debruyne J, de Hemptinne B. Improvement of hepatic myelopathy after liver transplantation. N Engl J Med 1999; 340:151.

22. Kott E, Bechar M, Bornstein B, Sandbank U. Demyelination of the posterior and anterior columns of the spinal cord in association with metabolic disturbances. Isr J Med Sci 1971; 7:577-580.

PART TEN

Spinal Infection

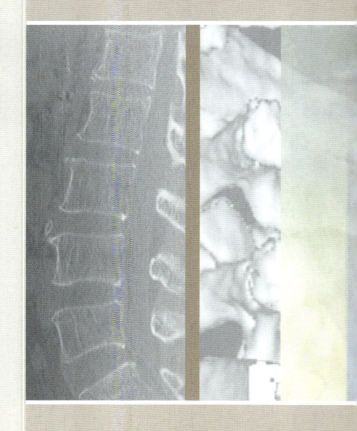

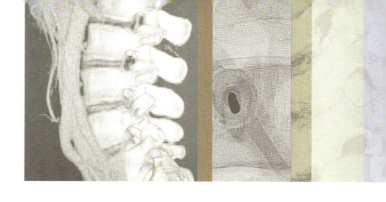

CHAPTER 18

Infections of the Spinal Column

E. Turgut Tali and Serap Gultekin

Spinal infection frequently injures the vertebral bodies, intervertebral discs, paraspinal soft tissues, epidural space, meninges, and spinal cord. Clinically, it is notoriously difficult to differentiate spinal infection from degenerative processes, noninfective inflammatory disorders, and spinal neoplasms. Spinal infections are a common cause of morbidity and mortality, especially in immunocompromised patients.

Epidural and intradural extramedullary infections are most often caused by pyrogens. Intramedullary infections are usually caused by viral agents. Infections in each spinal compartment present distinct imaging features, permitting differential diagnosis on the basis of characteristic imaging patterns.

PYOGENIC DISCITIS-OSTEOMYELITIS

Pyogenic discitis-osteomyelitis is infection of the vertebral bones and the adjacent discs. It is also referred to as discitis and vertebral osteomyelitis or as pyogenic spondylitis.

Epidemiology

Vertebral osteomyelitis presently accounts for 2% to 4% of all pyogenic bone infection. Its incidence appears to be increasing, possibly because of the increasing age of the population, increased intravenous drug abuse, AIDS, reactivation of latent infections, overuse of antibiotics, drug-resistant pathogens, new pathogens, worsening of socioeconomic conditions, and biologic war/terrorism. Other predisposing factors include malnutrition, immune compromise, chronic steroid use, diabetes mellitus, malignancy, chronic alcoholism, renal failure, implantation of intravascular devices, and recent spinal surgery.

Males are affected more frequently than females in a ratio of 1.5 to 3:1. Discitis is more common in children especially before age 4 years.[1] After childhood, spinal infection shows a bimodal age distribution with a smaller peak in the second decade and a dominant peak in the fifth decade.

Clinical Presentation

The neurologic deficits depend on the site and extent of infection, the type and virulence of the causative agent, and the host's ability to contain or resist the infection. The onset of symptoms may be indolent, with only back pain, malaise, and discomfort. There may be a history of recent infection elsewhere in the body. The patient may complain of back pain persisting over months to years, malaise, fever, anorexia, muscular spasm, stiffness, rigidity, weakness, fatigue, dysphagia, weight loss, and night sweats. Typically, motion aggravates the pain of spinal infection and rest ameliorates it. Children may show irritability and refuse to walk, sit, or stand.

Physical examination often discloses local tenderness, subcutaneous flank mass, and spinal deformity, such as increased thoracic kyphosis. Neurologic examination reveals signs of nerve root compression, including radiculopathy, signs of meningeal irritation, and neurologic deficits, such as lower extremity weakness, loss of reflexes, and paraplegia. Collapse of the vertebral body and/or epidural inflammatory tissue may compress neural structures and their blood supply, leading to impaired cord function or infarction. Cervical spondylitis can extend anteriorly and progress to retropharyngeal abscess and mediastinitis, with esophageal dysfunction. Thoracic spondylitis can cause mediastinitis, empyema, and pericarditis. Lumbar spondylitis can cause peritonitis and subdiaphragmatic abscess. Cardiac and respiratory signs and symptoms vary according to the severity of the involvement.

Untreated infection may result in permanent spinal deformity with wedging of the vertebral bodies, angular kyphosis (gibbus), and scoliosis. Severe infection may cause permanent neurologic deficits, particularly paraplegia and tetraplegia. Extension of the infection to the psoas musculature may lead to transient or permanent hip contractures.

Chronic spinal infection may present a more confusing clinical picture. The pain is less severe. The onset of paresis of the extremities is gradual, with signs and symptoms of cord and/or cauda compression but no fever. Generally, pain is less severe.

Laboratory findings also vary with the grade of infection and the specific infective agent but typically include elevated erythrocyte sedimentation rate (ESR), white blood cell (WBC) count, and C-reactive protein (CRP) levels. Cultures of blood and biopsy specimens are frequently negative.

Pathophysiology

Bacterial, fungal, and parasitic organisms can cause spinal infections. *Staphylococcus aureus* accounts for approximately 60% and *Enterobacter* species about 30% of spinal infections. Other organisms are found most commonly in specific types of patients: *Salmonella* (in sickle cell disease), *Klebsiella* and *Pseudomonas* (in intravenous drug abusers), *Streptococcus* (in patients with endocarditis and colonic polyposis), and *Serratia*. *S. aureus* is known to produce several proteolytic enzymes, including hyaluronidase, which is postulated to cause lysis of the disc.[2] The source for the spinal infection may be concurrent urinary tract, pulmonary, pelvic, or cutaneous infection; contamination from a dirty intravenous needle; or, less frequently, inflammatory bowel diseases, septic abortion, cellulitis, fasciitis, subcutaneous abscess, or pyomyositis. More than 65% of cases of pyogenic spinal infection have an identifiable primary site of infection.

Hematogenous Dissemination

Arterial Route

Hematogenous spread occurs more frequently via the arteries than the veins. The arterial network of ascending arteries, descending arteries, and anastomosing branches, which neighbor the vertebrae, give rise to minute branches that penetrate the cortex and ramify within it. The richest nutrient arteriolar network is located in the subchondral region of the vertebral body, which is the equivalent of the metaphysis of a long bone. Hematogenous organisms arrive in the vertebrae via end-arteriolar arcades in the subchondral plate adjacent to the disc, particularly in the anterior part of the subchondral plate. They disrupt the overlying cortical bone, extend to disc, extend to the opposite vertebral body, and even extend to the subligamentous paravertebral and epidural spaces in adults.[3]

In adults, the intervertebral disc is avascular. However, secondary vascularization may occur with degenerative disc disease, because vascularized granulation tissue grows into the radial tears of older patients. Direct hematogenous spread of infection to the disc may then become possible in these cases. In children younger than the age of 4 years, vascular channels do extend directly into the discs. In these young children, bacteremia may cause direct hematogenous inoculation of the disc with subsequent bacterial discitis.

Venous Route

Valveless veins leave the vertebral body through the central dorsal nutrient foramen and drain into the extradural venous plexus. The extradural venous plexus is interconnected with the valveless paravertebral venous plexus of Batson. Elevated intra-abdominal pressure allows retrograde hematogenous spread of infection from the pelvis and abdominal organs to the vertebral column. The venous route of dissemination to the vertebral bone is of particular importance in infections of the urinary tract and other pelvic organs.

Nonhematogenous Dissemination

Nonhematogenous inoculations are major routes of discitis in adults.

Direct Extension

Nonhematogenous inoculation of the spine may arise secondary to penetrating trauma, direct extension from contiguous infection, or interventional procedures such as biopsy, chemo/mechanical nucleolysis, laser ablations, pain-relieving procedures, sympathectomy, spinal anesthesia, discography, surgical interventions, and spinal instrumentation. Facet injections with corticosteroids for diagnosis or treatment of pain may cause or exacerbate infection of the posterior elements, including the posterior paraspinal soft tissue, the facet joints, the spinous process, and even the pedicles. In the absence of direct iatrogenic inoculation of these elements, however, infection of the posterior spinal elements is uncommon. In the absence of direct inoculation, infection of the laminae and pedicles should raise suspicion of tuberculous spondylitis.

Spread through the Cerebrospinal Fluid

Spinal infection may also arise from extension of infection from the central nervous system (CNS) through the cerebrospinal fluid (CSF) and by CSF leaks.

Pathology

Suppuration may be seen in the paraspinal soft tissues. Meningitis may be present. The infection may spread to, or from, the neural tissue. Suppurative infection may involve the subarachnoid space.

The virulence of an organism may be determined by major bacterial factors such as surface protein receptors, capsular polysaccharides, and toxins. The organism may produce enzymes such as proteolytic enzymes that assist it to invade the disc by lysis of the annulus. With pyogenic bacteria, the initial local response is acute inflammation, producing an exudate containing polymorphonuclear leukocytes (neutrophils) and fibrin. Because bone and disc cannot expand to relieve pressure by swelling, continuing exudation raises the tissue pressure. The result is destruction of bone, with inflammatory exudate, cellular debris, and vascular proliferation.

Imaging

Plain Radiography

The sensitivity and specificity of plain radiographs are very low. They usually lack the ability to show early findings, and negative results do not exclude the presence of infection. Radiographs typically remain normal for 2 to 3 weeks after the onset of infection. The earliest radiographic sign is loss of definition and irregularity of the vertebral end plate, usually starting anterosuperiorly. In the period from 2 to 8 weeks, the intravertebral disc may show an initial increase in height (rarely observed), followed by loss of disc height (seen commonly). Gradually progressive osteolysis causes poor definition of the end plates. Erosions of the cortical end plates on both sides of a narrowed intervertebral disc with associated paraspinal mass are the hallmarks of pyogenic infection.

After approximately 10 weeks, plain radiographs may show reactive sclerosis, new bone formation with osteophytosis, kyphotic deformity, scoliosis, spondylolisthesis, and bony ankylosis. Plain radiographs may also show signs of infection in the soft tissue surrounding the spondylitis, including increase in the retropharyngeal space due to cervical spondylitis, displacement of the parietal pleura due to thoracic spondylitis, and indistinct margins of the psoas muscle due to lumbar spondylitis.

CT

CT has high sensitivity for spondylitis but lacks specificity. It is not the primary modality for diagnosis of early spondylitis and disc space infection or for follow-up of spondylitis. CT may miss epidural involvement due to beam-hardening artifacts, especially in the cervicothoracic region. This limitation can be overcome by performing CT myelograms after the intrathecal injection of a contrast agent. However, performing spinal taps in patients with pyogenic infection may lead to intradural spread of infection. If myelography must be done, the spinal tap should be performed at a site distant from the source of infection, for example, via a lateral C1-C2 tap for the evaluation of lumbar spinal infection.

CT provides excellent depiction of fine bone detail and displays well any associated changes in the paraspinal soft tissue. It is useful for showing osteopenia, soft tissue calcification, cortical bone erosion, permeative bone destruction, lytic fragmentation, bony sclerosis, paraspinal soft tissue infiltration with obliteration of fat planes, compromise of the spinal canal, and gas within the disc, bone, and soft tissue. Hypodensity of the disc and vertebral body are major findings of the infection. Sagittal reformatted and 3D images demonstrate reduced disc height, but spiral (helical) CT with thin slices and multiplanar reconstructions are needed to avoid artifacts from partial volume averaging. CT is very useful for guiding percutaneous biopsies, drainage of fluid collections, irrigation of spaces with antibiotics, and so on (Fig. 18-1). For CT-guided aspirations and biopsies, the target for the

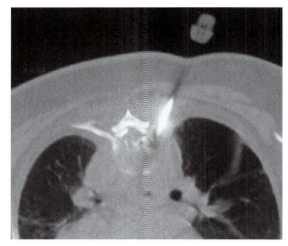

■ **FIGURE 18-1** CT-guided biopsy. CT-guided percutaneous biopsy of a pyogenic spondylodiscitis with extensive bone destruction and a large paravertebral abscess.

needle should be the focus of active abnormal contrast enhancement.

MRI

MRI is sensitive, specific, and accurate (96%, 94%, and 92%, respectively), equal to the results of combined nuclear medicine studies. Therefore, MRI is the modality of choice for assessing of possible spondylitis. Early on, infection causes an exudate containing WBC and fibrin within vertebral marrow. The extracellular water content increases, and tissue pressure rises. This inflammatory reaction, consequent ischemia, and reactive bone marrow stimulation appear to be responsible for the abnormal T1 and T2 signal intensity seen with infection (Fig. 18-2). Morphologic alterations, such as loss of definition of the end plates of a single vertebra, become more marked in time (Fig. 18-3). The infection may extend underneath the anterior and posterior longitudinal ligaments or into the disc, leading to signal alteration on precontrast T1-weighted (T1W) and T2-weighted (T2W) MR images and to contrast enhancement or postcontrast T1W images. Initially, infection of the disc space commonly appears as nonanatomic T2 signal in the intervertebral disc, loss of the low signal equatorial band (the "intranuclear cleft"), and reduction of disc height (see Fig. 18-2). Thereafter, the infection may cause discontinuity of the adjacent bony end plates and progressive destruction of the vertebral bodies, plus frank disc destruction and soft tissue infiltration (Figs. 18-3 and 18-4). The infection can extend posteriorly into the epidural space and/or laterally into the paraspinal tissue (Figs. 18-4 and 18-5). These extensions can be much better defined on the postcontrast images. Infection may cause engorgement of epidural basivertebral veins by direct extension of the inflammatory process, by mechanical obstruction to venous drainage, or by both. However, simple enhancement of the epidural venous plexus should not be confused with epidural infection.

Contrast enhancement increases the conspicuity of the lesion, the specificity of diagnosis, and observer confidence in the diagnosis. Contrast-enhanced studies

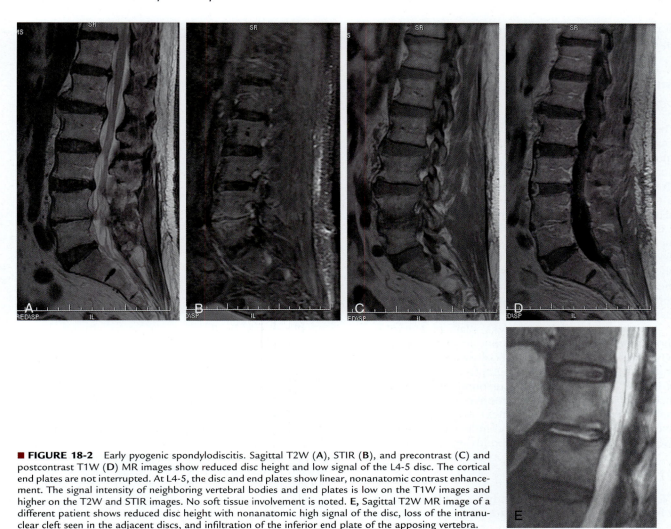

■ **FIGURE 18-2** Early pyogenic spondylodiscitis. Sagittal T2W (**A**), STIR (**B**), and precontrast (**C**) and postcontrast T1W (**D**) MR images show reduced disc height and low signal of the L4-5 disc. The cortical end plates are not interrupted. At L4-5, the disc and end plates show linear, nonanatomic contrast enhancement. The signal intensity of neighboring vertebral bodies and end plates is low on the T1W images and higher on the T2W and STIR images. No soft tissue involvement is noted. **E**, Sagittal T2W MR image of a different patient shows reduced disc height with nonanatomic high signal of the disc, loss of the intranuclear cleft seen in the adjacent discs, and infiltration of the inferior end plate of the apposing vertebra.

facilitate treatment planning and monitoring of spinal infection. Contrast enhancement is an early sign of acute inflammation and may persist for weeks or months in subtle infections. Fat-suppression MRI techniques increase lesion conspicuity on contrast-enhanced studies. Measurement of percentage contrast enhancement has been shown to be a reliable method to quantify diffuse bone marrow changes. Measurement of contrast enhancement is also helpful to differentiate among the disc, the body, and the edema, the phlegmon, or the abscess (see Fig. 18-4). Such differentiation significantly aids treatment planning because surgical drainage is indicated for an abscess whereas conservative therapy is proper for phlegmon. When serial images show that contrast enhancement no longer occurs, active inflammation can be excluded.

Pseudosparing of the end plates is described as a potential pitfall of MRI diagnosis of spondylitis. If the MR images of the spine are obtained with the frequency encoding in the superoinferior direction, increased conspicuity ("pseudosparing") of the discs may complicate diagnosis. Pseudosparing can be seen when the normal chemical shift artifact seen in healthy end plates is lost as a result of replacement of the lipid-rich yellow bone marrow with

water-based infiltrate. Phase encoding (rather than frequency encoding) is strongly preferred for the craniocaudal direction to reduce normal chemical shift artifact, to prevent pseudosparing, and to reduce pulsation artifacts caused by abdominal vessels.[4]

Diffusion-weighted spinal imaging (DWI) has been shown to help differentiate long-standing infection from Modic type I degeneration and metastases.[5,6] Apparent diffusion coefficient (ADC) values are more reliable than qualitative evaluations. Further studies with larger patient groups are needed for more accurate conclusions on this subject. Current research is evaluating magnetic resonance spectroscopy (MRS) for the differential diagnosis of the spinal pathology, but MRS is not presently in widespread use.

Vertebrae

Within the vertebral bodies, low signal areas probably result from replacement of fat cells by stimulated proliferating bone marrow cells that form white blood cells (WBCs). These areas are seen more reliably on spin-echo

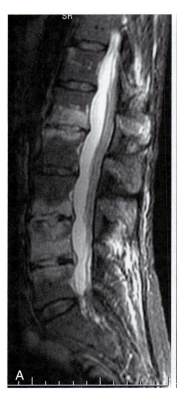 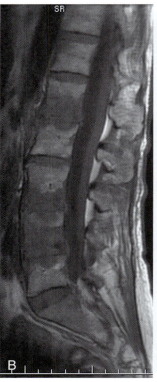 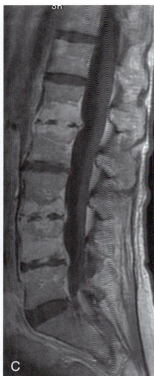

FIGURE 18-3 Pyogenic spondylodiscitis. Sagittal T2W (**A**) and precontrast (**B**) and postcontrast T1W (**C**) MR images show confluent signal alterations of the L1-5 vertebral bodies. Note the T1 hypointensity and T2 hyperintensity in the portions of the L1-L5 vertebrae adjacent to the intervertebral discs, in the anterosuperior portion of T12, and in the entire L4 vertebra. The end plates show interruption of cortical continuity. There is clear but mild extension to the epidural space. On the sagittal T2W image (**A**) the discs show reduced height, nonanatomic high signal, and loss of the intranuclear cleft. The discs and neighboring vertebral bodies show marked nonanatomic contrast enhancement.

T1W images, which are preferable to gradient-echo T1W images. Bone marrow edema may be more difficult to appreciate on T1W images in children and young patients with red marrow and in patients with Modic type III end plate degeneration.

Infections of the vertebral body and disc typically cause high signal on T2W MR images (see Fig. 18-2). In early infectious diseases, this high T2 signal may be obscured by fast spin-echo T2W imaging, owing to the normally bright T2 signal of marrow. Later in the disease, when trabecular sclerosis obliterates the marrow space, and in patients with Modic III degeneration, the decreased T2 signal intensity of sclerosis may mask the increased signal changes of an infectious process. Fat-suppressed T2W and short tau inversion recovery (STIR) techniques increase the conspicuity of infected areas and have slightly higher sensitivity than T2W alone for detecting areas of involvement but also are less specific (see Figs. 18-2 to 18-5). In addition, STIR sequences do not depict fine anatomic detail and are sensitive to patient and CSF motion. Bone marrow edema can also be evaluated by using opposed-phase gradient-recalled-echo sequences. Normal marrow exhibits low signal intensity with signal subtraction of the water and fat-bound proton components, whereas edema exhibits high signal intensity. Use of this sequence does not add more information than the routine sequences for the differential diagnosis of a vertebral pathologic process. For pathology of the intervertebral disc, gradient-recalled-echo sequences may provide images of a quality similar to conventional sequences and their use may save time. Contrast-enhanced series show areas of vertebral infection well and are very helpful in the differential diagnosis.

With advanced infection, T2W MR images display end plate erosions as interruptions of the cortical continuity

and destruction of the vertebral body (see Figs. 18-3 to 18-5). Postcontrast T1W imaging helps to differentiate the disc from the vertebral body. Gas within the vertebral body (intravertebral vacuum clefts) appears as dramatically reduced signal intensity on T1W and T2W images and is pathognomonic of dead bone tissue.

Reactive bone changes, new bone formation, osteophytosis, sclerosis, vertebral body height changes, kyphosis, scoliosis, spondylolisthesis, and ankylosis can all be seen during the late/healing stage of the infective process. Sclerosis is more common in pyogenic spondylitis than in tuberculous spondylitis but is common enough in both that it cannot be used for differential diagnosis.[7]

In infants, spondylitis may present as progressive dissolution of involved vertebral bodies without loss of disc height. Years later, the kyphotic deformity from this infection may mimic congenital kyphosis.

Discs

The normal disc signal and morphology change phasically owing to diurnal variation in disc hydration. These phasic changes must be appreciated and not misinterpreted as a pathologic process. After the second decade, about 94% of normal discs show an equatorial band (intranuclear cleft) of low T2 signal that extends as a line across the equator of the disc. With disc infection, adults typically show reduced disc signal on T1W imaging and increased disc signal on T2W imaging. There is frequently distortion or loss of the normal equatorial band (intranuclear cleft). In children, infection may involve the disc primarily. Acutely, there may be increase in the disc height, followed shortly by decreased disc height (see Fig. 18-2). Unlike in adults, infected discs in children show decreased (not

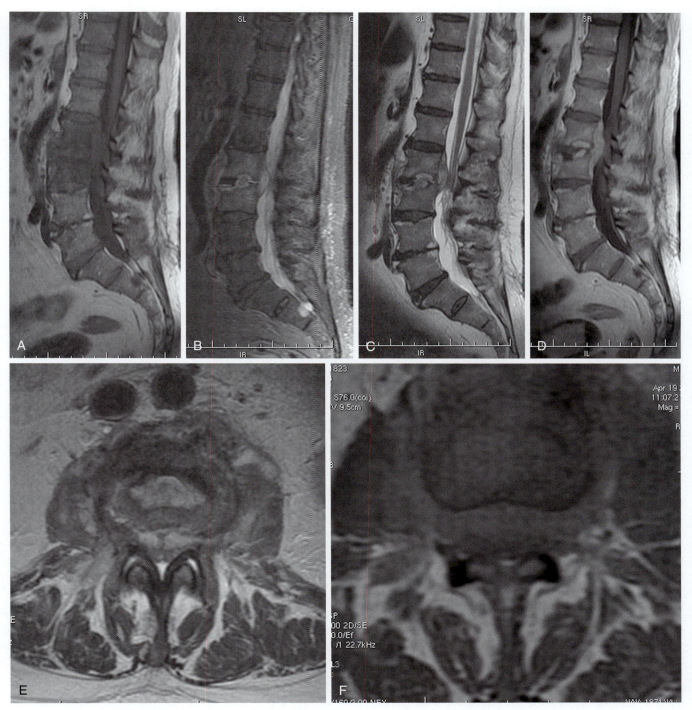

■ FIGURE 18-4 Spondylitis with epidural phlegmon. Sagittal STIR (**A**), T2W (**B**), precontrast (**C**) and postcontrast T1W (**D**), axial T2W (**E**), and T1W (**F**) MR images show diffuse signal abnormalities in the vertebral bodies adjacent to the L2-3 disc with hypointensity on the T1W images and hyperintensity on the T2W images and STIR sequence. The apposing end plates show erosion and destruction. The disc signal is low on T1W images and high on T2W images. There is marked enhancement of the active infection and mild enhancement of the spondylitis. Homogeneous signal and contrast enhancement within the epidural space strongly suggest concurrent epidural phlegmon. Right-sided paraspinal soft tissue involvement is also noted.

increased) signal intensity on T2W imaging. Both children and adults show marked heterogeneous nonanatomic contrast enhancement of the infected disc on postcontrast T1W imaging. Increased signal due to inflammatory disc degeneration should be differentiated from infection. Infected discs show nonanatomic contrast enhancement. Degenerated discs may show "anatomic" peripheral, linear, and/or nodular enhancement due to ingrowth of blood vessels that penetrate the peripheral annulus. In advanced infection the disc is destroyed and cannot be demonstrated. Granulation tissue and osteoid may form new bone that bridges across the annulus. Disc and vertebral changes on T1W images and disc signal alterations on T2W images are reliable findings of infection.

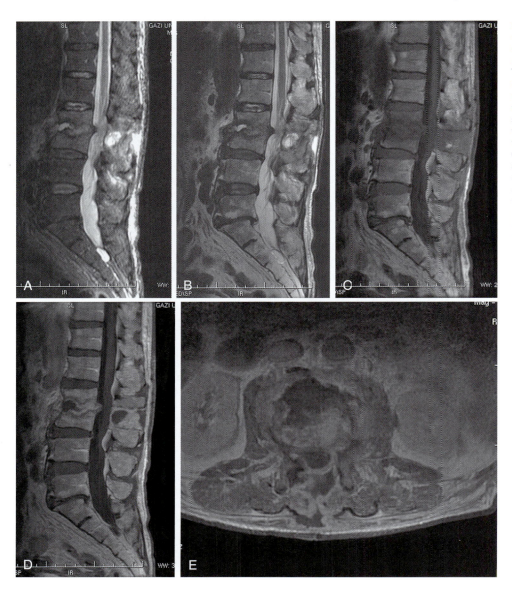

■ **FIGURE 18-5** Late stage spondylitis with paraspinal abscess. Sagittal STIR (A), T2W (B), precontrast (C) and postcontrast T1W (D) and axial postcontrast T1W (E) MR images demonstrate diffuse signal alteration of the vertebral bodies neighboring L3-4 disc space with hypointensity on T1W images and hyperintensity on T2W and STIR images. Erosion of the end plates with destruction and posterior fusion are evident. Anterior half of the disc signal is low on T1W imaging and high on T2W imaging with absence of the intranuclear cleft. Absence of enhancement of the anterior half of the disc space suggests abscess formation whereas enhancement of adjacent vertebral bodies is seen. Extension of infection to the posterior elements, epidural space, and also paravertebral soft tissue is clearly seen on axial images. The axial postcontrast image demonstrates a paravertebral abscess with ring-like enhancement.

Paraspinal Soft Tissues

Spondylitis is reported to extend to the epidural space in 32% of cases. Routine MRI sequences may not show epidural extension adequately, because the abnormal epidural signal may be isointense with and merge into the high signal of CSF. Proton density–weighted (PDW) and fluid-attenuated inversion recovery (FLAIR) images show higher signal in proteinaceous exudates than in CSF, helping to distinguish the inflamed tissue from CSF. Detection of epidural phlegmon and abscess and differentiation from CSF collections is important for treatment planning. Phlegmon typically enhances as a solid inhomogeneous blush, whereas abscess and necrosis appear as peripherally enhancing masses with a hypointense liquefactive center on postcontrast T1W imaging.

Infected paravertebral soft tissues show varying signal and contrast enhancement (see Fig. 18-5). In the acute phase, paraspinal phlegmon appears as ill-defined areas that are hypointense on T1W imaging and hyperintense on T2W imaging, reflecting the extracellular paraspinal edema. There is little mass effect. The necrotic center of a paraspinal abscess is hyperintense on T2W imaging and isointense to hypointense on T1W imaging. The abscess capsule is isointense to hyperintense on T1W imaging and very hypointense on T2W imaging (see Fig. 18-5). Contrast enhancement helps to delineate the full extent of soft tissue infection and usually identifies the abscesses as ring-enhancing lesions.

A specific entity—Griesel's syndrome—is characterized by atlantoaxial subluxation, synovial effusion, and inflammation/infection of neighboring soft tissues. Griesel's syndrome is caused by septic emboli transported from infections of the nasopharynx, tonsils, alveoli of the jaw, and lymph nodes to the spine via connections between the pharyngovertebral veins and the periodontoidal venous plexus and suboccipital epidural sinuses.[8] Pyogenic osteomyelitis of the C1 and C2 vertebrae is rare but clinically significant. Cervical instability may result from inflammatory softening or lysis of the bone at the insertions of the transverse ligament. The outcome of the treatment is influenced by the type of infection and by the degree of neurologic compromise before treatment.

The clinical features of spinal infections can be subtle and misleading. Delays in diagnosis can lead to increased morbidity and mortality, so early diagnosis and treatment are essential. However, successful differentiation of infection from degenerative disease, noninfective inflammatory lesions, spinal neoplasm, and other diseases remains difficult, despite advanced techniques for spinal imaging. Imaging criteria sensitive for identifying spondylitis include evidence of paraspinal or epidural inflammatory tissue, contrast enhancement of the disc, erosion and destruction of the vertebral end plates, and abnormal signal on T1W and T2W imaging.[9]

In summary, MRI findings of pyogenic spondylitis and discitis include the following (see also Box 18-1):

- Decreased signal intensity on T1W images and increased signal intensity on T2W images, with abnormal contrast enhancement
- Irregularity, erosion, and destruction of end plates of vertebral bodies with interruption of the normal signal void of the cortical end plates
- Reduced disc height, loss of intranuclear cleft on T2W images, disc protrusion, and nonanatomic contrast enhancement
- Paravertebral soft tissue infiltration/abscess, which appears hyperintense on T2W imaging and hypointense on T1W imaging and shows homogeneous or ring-like enhancement
- Epidural extension with contrast enhancement (phlegmon: homogeneous; abscess: ring enhancement)
- Late/healing stage of the infective process: reactive bone changes, new bone formation, osteophytosis, sclerosis, altered height of the vertebral body, kyphosis, scoliosis, spondylolisthesis, ankylosis, and bony bridges across the annulus

There is an increasing move away from open surgical intervention toward conservative therapy, percutaneous abscess drainage, or both. It is critical to monitor treatment response, particularly in the immunodeficient patient. In children, discitis may be treated with antimicrobial therapy and bed rest.

MRI is very helpful for monitoring the success of treatment, because successful therapy is associated with the following:

- Reduction in paravertebral soft tissue swelling (perhaps the earliest sign of successful therapy)
- Appearance of a high signal rim at the edge of the lesion (mean, 15 weeks);
- Higher signal of the involved marrow on T1W and fast spin-echo T2W images than noninvolved marrow (the reconstituted marrow is predominantly fatty and appears to be of higher signal intensity than normal marrow and degeneration of hematopoietic marrow is

---

BOX 18-1 MRI for Evaluation of Spondylitis

PATIENT HISTORY

A 45-year-old woman with persistent lower back pain of 6 months' duration was admitted to the hospital. She also had malaise, fatigue, and rigidity. Elevated sedimentation rate and white blood cell count were remarkable laboratory findings. Neurologic examination showed radicular symptoms.

TECHNIQUE

MRI examination of lumbar spine with contrast administration was performed. Pre- and postcontrast axial and sagittal T1W, axial and sagittal T2W, and STIR sagittal images were obtained.

FINDINGS

There is normal height and alignment of the vertebral bodies. Confluent change in signal intensity of the L4 vertebral body is seen with hypointensity on T1W imaging, hyperintensity on T2W imaging, and contrast enhancement of the area. The vertebral end plates show interruption of the cortical continuity, erosion, and destruction. Homogeneous signal intensity and contrast enhancement in the epidural space suggest epidural phlegmon. Abnormal soft tissue rim enhancement at the right anterior aspect of the L4 vertebral body suggests soft tissue abscess. Decreased height of the L4-5 disc, nonanatomic high T2 signal within it, loss of its equatorial band (intranuclear cleft), and contrast enhancement are also noted. The differential diagnosis includes pyogenic spondylitis and other spinal inflammatory diseases.

The remaining vertebral marrow signal is normal. The remaining intervertebral discs are normal in height and hydration. There is no evidence of disc herniation, spinal stenosis, or nerve root compression. The spinal cord is normal in size, signal, and caliber.

IMPRESSION

Diagnosis is L4 spondylitis with epidural and paravertebral soft tissue extensions.

---

probably caused by obliteration of the intramedullary vessels, preventing repopulation with red marrow cells)
- Lower signal within the marrow on both T1W and T2W images (may be a reflection of reactive sclerosis and fibrosis due to healing)
- Decrease of high marrow signal on STIR, PDW, and T2W images
- Decrease in the high disc signal on STIR and T2W imaging, even though the disc remains narrowed
- Reappearance of the equatorial band (intranuclear cleft) (a good indicator of resolution of inflammation)
- New bone formation bridging the disc space
- Resolution of canal compromise
- Progressive reduction in contrast enhancement. (Increasing or persisting contrast enhancement with clinical improvement and increasing destruction does not necessarily indicate treatment failure.)

KEY POINTS: PYOGENIC DISCITIS-OSTEOMYELITIS

- "Good disc bad news, bad disc good news" highlights that the destructive vertebral bone lesion associated with a well-preserved disc space with sharp end plates favors a diagnosis of neoplastic infiltration whereas the destructive bony lesion associated with a poorly defined vertebral bone end plate with or without loss of disc height suggests infection with a better prognosis.
- Exudative pleural effusions may be a manifestation of vertebral osteomyelitis of the thoracic spine. The majority of the effusions have been found to be sterile. Thus, in a patient with pleural effusion of unknown cause, the possibility of vertebral osteomyelitis should be considered, possibly more so in diabetics.[10]

Degenerative End Plate Changes

- Type I degenerative osteoarthritis resembles early pyogenic spondylitis.
- Lack of associated abnormally increased disc signal on T2W imaging (even reduced disc signal), lack of soft tissue involvement, and linear mild contrast enhancement of the disc are the main differentiating findings.
- There may be gas within the severely degenerated discs.
- Schmorl's nodules may be present.
- Cortical continuity of the vertebral end plate is generally intact in the remaining end plate, and there may be signal change of the adjacent vertebral marrow.

Erosive Intervertebral Osteochondrosis

- Inflammatory disc degeneration shows as high signal intensity on T2W imaging. Gas within the disc may also be seen. Focal areas of annular enhancement can be seen with no central enhancement.
- Edema of the vertebral bone marrow adjacent to the disc space uncommonly reaches the middle part and almost never extends to the opposite end plate.
- Erosion of the adjacent end plates occurs with no major destruction.
- No paravertebral/epidural involvement occurs.
- There is minimal or no osteophytosis.
- Dense sclerosis with bone erosions can be seen.

Dialysis Arthropathy

- Decrease of disc height and erosion of the subchondral bone occur at anterior superior and inferior margins.
- Amyloid deposition has a signal intensity similar to that of muscle.
- A clinical history of dialysis for more than 3 years and absence of paravertebral soft tissue infiltration are helpful differential points.

Pseudarthrosis

- Nonunion occurs, resembling destruction, end plate erosions, and sclerosis.

Spinal Metastases

- In the initial stage with no disc space involvement, it is very difficult to differentiate the infection from neoplastic involvement.
- A well-preserved disc space with sharp end plates favors a diagnosis of neoplastic infiltration (in rare instances, metastatic involvement of the disc has been reported).

- Consecutive vertebral involvement is more frequent in spondylitis than in tumoral infiltration.
- The intact vertebral end plate favors the diagnosis of tumor.
- Both infections and tumors may show skip lesions.
- Soft tissue involvement is a diffuse pattern in infections but usually well defined in tumors.
- Signal characteristics were not reliable signs for distinguishing tumors from infection because both of them demonstrated low signal intensity on T1W imaging and high signal intensity on T2W imaging.

Rheumatoid Arthritis

- Signal alterations in the active stage of rheumatoid arthritis can mimic spondylitis.
- Joint effusions, interapophyseal joint erosions, and erosion of the spinous process occur.

Avascular Necrosis

- This is rare.
- Intervertebral vacuum clefts can be seen.

Charcot Spine

- The disease is characterized by destructive process of the vertebral bodies, with end plate and facet joint erosions.
- Joint disorganization is noted.
- Vacuum into the disc and enhancement and decreased disc space are observed.
- There is paraspinal soft tissue swelling.
- Osteophyte formation and sclerosis occur.

Ankylosing Spondylitis

- Vascularized inflammatory tissue of the annulus and longitudinal ligaments shows increased signal on T2W imaging and enhancement.
- Erosions (Romanus lesions) and even destruction of entire discovertebral junction occur in advanced cases.
- End plate and vertebral enhancement can be seen adjacent to the disc space and ligaments.
- Associated sclerosis (subchondral bone formation) neighboring the erosions, syndesmophytes, apophyseal joint fusions, and osseous fusions occur.
- Calcification and ossification of the thickened ligaments occur.
- Sacroiliitis is pathognomonic.
- Disc bulging can also be seen.

Chronic Recurrent Multifocal Osteomyelitis

- This is characterized by relapses and remissions that are unresponsive to treatment; it mimics spondylitis.

Neuropathic Arthropathy

- Disc bulging, disorganization, dislocation, destruction of the vertebras, and spondylolisthesis are seen.
- Soft tissue masses and osseous debris are noted.
- There is rim enhancement of the discs and diffuse enhancement of the vertebral body.
- Spinal cord injury and syrinx are associated.

Lymphoma
Multiple-Solitary Myeloma

PYOGENIC EPIDURAL/SUBDURAL ABSCESS

This is defined as infection of the spinal extradural and subdural spaces with abscess formation. It is also called spinal epidural/subdural empyema.

Epidemiology

Once considered rare, spinal *epidural* empyema is now seen with increasing prevalence. Spinal *subdural* infection remains very rare compared with spinal epidural abscess (SEA), with fewer than 50 cases reported in the literature. Diabetes mellitus, intravenous drug abuse, chronic renal failure, excessive alcohol ingestion, immunodeficiency, and local steroid injections are major risk factors for developing these infections. No genetic or racial predilection has been identified. SEA is seen at all ages but is most frequent in the sixth and seventh decades. Patients may show acute deterioration due to mechanical compression or ischemic compromise of the spinal cord, prior local administration of corticosteroids for pain control, or direct infection of the spinal cord. Surgery is indicated when there is neural/cord compression, progressive neurologic deficit, or persistent severe pain.

Clinical Presentation

Clinical diagnosis is challenging. Symptoms of acute infection include back pain, fever, or both, with or without neurologic (mostly sensory) deficits. The precise nature of any neurologic signs depends on the level of infection. Chronic infections, especially tuberculosis, may not manifest as fever or other clinical signs of infection. Instead, patients with chronic infection present widely varying symptoms ranging from mild back pain to paraplegia. A progressive form of subdural empyema shows sudden onset with rapid progression over 2 to 5 days, leading to marked paralysis, loss of bowel and bladder control, and respiratory distress secondary to denervation of the intercostal muscles and diaphragm. Without treatment, patients with SEA usually show a progressive course from pain to weakness of voluntary muscles and sphincters to paralysis.

Pathophysiology

The major routes of infection are hematogenous spread from extraspinal sources (most common), direct inoculation, and contiguous spread. *S. aureus* is the most common agent (57%-73% of reported cases). The sites most frequently involved are the lower thoracic and lumbar regions.[11] Spinal epidural collections are almost always located at the posterior aspect of the spinal canal. Anterior collections are most frequent with vertebral osteomyelitis. SEA associated with spondylitis typically extends over a limited number of adjoining segments. SEA not associated with vertebral osteomyelitis tends to be more extensive and multifocal. Very long segment SEA often spirals around the spinal canal to lie posterior in some segments and anterior in others.

Pathology

Osteomyelitis may be observed. Meningitis and myelitis may be associated. Frank pus is located in the subdural or epidural space. Leukocytes, cellular debris, vascular proliferation, and granulation tissue are detected on histologic study.

Imaging

Radiography

Plain radiographs provide little benefit for early detection of spinal epidural infection. When spondylodiscitis is associated, it may be evident.

CT

CT may help to demonstrate epidural and paraspinal extensions and associated bone lesions in detail. Myelography with an intrathecal contrast agent may delineate the site(s) of the collections and their relationship to the spinal cord, but the spinal tap needed to perform myelography may spread the infection to previously uninfected sites and is not recommended when infection is suggested.

MRI

Spinal Epidural Abscess

MRI is the imaging modality of choice for spinal epidural infections even for the initial stages. It is reported to be 95% sensitive for the diagnosis of spinal epidural infections and abscess.[12] MRI provides rapid and accurate localization of the lesion(s), defines their extent, and helps in planning and monitoring their treatment.

Typical MRI features of SEA include a soft tissue mass within the epidural space encroaching on the thecal sac, spinal cord, and/or spinal nerve roots (Fig. 18-6). Sagittal views best assess the craniocaudal extent of the lesion and the presence of any skip lesions. Axial views display the lateral extensions of the infection and confirm the severity of any compression of intraspinal structures. The MRI signal depends on the content of the lesion. Frequently, T1W and T2W imaging shows a long-segment, homogeneous or inhomogeneous, isointense/hyperintense epidural mass with hypointense, thickened, displaced dura (see Fig. 18-6). An SEA associated with discitis and osteomyelitis most frequently lies anteriorly in continuity with the infected spinal column. An SEA not related to discitis and osteomyelitis most frequently lies posterior or, if very long segment, spiral circumferentially as it extends along the length of the dural sac. T2W and contrast-enhanced T1W imaging both may show compromise of the spinal cord. It is very important to differentiate spinal epidural phlegmon from abscess. SEA typically requires urgent surgical decompression, whereas phlegmon may be better treated conservatively. Abscesses typically have one or more pockets with liquid component and pus, so they appear inhomogeneous on routine imaging, show restricted diffusion, and demonstrate enhancement on contrast-enhanced images. Pockets of gas may indicate infection

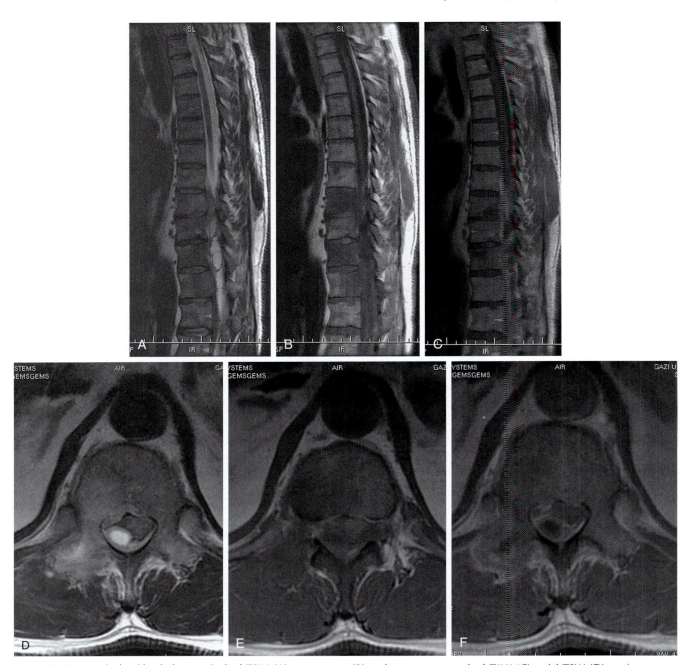

■ **FIGURE 18-6** Spinal epidural abscess. Sagittal T2W (**A**), precontrast (**B**) and postcontrast sagittal T1W (**C**), axial T2W (**D**), and precontrast (**E**) and postcontrast (**F**) axial T1W images demonstrate spinal epidural infection and abscess from T8 to L1 with concomitant spondylitis. The dural sac is displaced to the left by encasing, mainly anterior, epidural infection and posterior epidural abscess. The dura is seen as a thick black line separating the intradural structures from the epidural infection on the axial images. Epidural abscess is seen as a high signal lesion with a surrounding low signal capsule on T2W imaging and as a low signal lesion with a high signal capsule on T1W imaging. Ring-like enhancement of the irregular abscess capsule and right paravertebral infection with developing abscess are also seen on postcontrast axial images. Sagittal images demonstrate the adhesions and loculations of the abscess through L1 with linear/ring-like contrast enhancement. Signal alteration and contrast enhancement patterns of the T9, T11, and T12 vertebrae suggest spondylitis.

with gas-forming organisms. Phlegmon frequently has no liquid component or pus, so it demonstrates no pockets and nearly uniform enhancement (see Fig. 18-6). SEA can occasionally manifest as tiny locules within the posterior epidural space and therefore can easily be confused with pulsatile CSF flow, especially in the thoracic spine. The application of proton density, FLAIR, and gradient-echo sequences and use of intravenous contrast medium may help to differentiate these two processes.

Spinal Dural Empyema

MRI typically shows a thin, elongated and ring-enhancing fluid collection within the subdural space. The dura covering the collection is thickened. The underlying subarachnoid space is narrowed or obliterated. The cross-sectional axial images are most useful for confirming the subdural location of the collection and any associated cord displacement. On occasion, both SEA and SDE are present in the same patient.

KEY POINTS: PYOGENIC EPIDURAL-SUBDURAL ABSCESS

Spinal Epidural Abscess
- The infection lies along the periphery of the spinal canal and often extends outside the canal into the neural foramina.
- Subdural collections remain confined within the spinal canal.

Epidural Metastases
- Epidural tumor frequently presents as a well-circumscribed soft tissue mass contiguous with a vertebral lesion. The involved vertebral body is often expanded.
- Abscesses and metastases both show contrast enhancement. Rim enhancement favors a diagnosis of abscess. Diffuse enhancement may signify either disease.

Epidural Hematoma
- Epidural hematomas may extend over several vertebral segments, simulating abscesses. Heterogeneous signal intensities due to blood degradation products may suggest hemorrhage rather than abscess.
- Hematomas do not show significant contrast enhancement.
- Without appropriate history, however, it may be difficult to distinguish a hematoma from an abscess.

Extruded Disc
- An extruded disc frequently is associated with loss of height in the adjacent disc and disc degeneration.
- The disc usually has a more focal appearance, is most often isointense/hypointense on T2W imaging, and may show mild peripheral contrast enhancement.

Non-Hodgkin Lymphoma
- This tumor may mimic epidural abscess or phlegmon with enhancement.

Spinal Subdural Infection/Abscesses
- The major differential diagnoses of spinal subdural abscesses are spinal epidural abscess, subdural hematoma, and spinal meningitis. The key points in the differential diagnosis include the clinical history, location within the spinal canal, MR signal intensities, and the pattern of contrast enhancement. Spinal meningitis shows smooth or nodular leptomeningeal enhancement, whereas subdural hematomas do not demonstrate contrast enhancement. Spinal epidural abscesses are frequently associated with spondylodiscitis, whereas spinal subdural abscesses are not. A hypointense medial rim representing inflamed dura is seen with epidural infection but not with subdural empyema.

NOCARDIAL BACTERIAL SPONDYLITIS

This infection of the spine and adjacent soft tissue is caused by microorganisms of the genus *Nocardia* and is referred to as nocardiosis.

Epidemiology

Nocardiosis is a rare opportunistic infection associated with significant morbidity and mortality in immunocompromised patients.

Clinical Presentation

Immunocompetent patients classically display infections of the soft tissues, whereas immunosuppressed or immunocompromised patients suffer infections of the brain and lungs, particularly abscesses. There are no differentiating signs or symptoms specific for spinal nocardial infections.

Pathophysiology

Although frequently discussed in the context of fungal infections, *Nocardia* is actually an atypical gram-positive, rod-shaped bacterium. *N. asteroides* is the most common pathogen among this group. The main portal of entry is the respiratory tract, from which bacteria may disseminate hematogenously to the CNS and other tissues. CNS involvement occurs in 26% to 42% of patients. Spinal involvement is extremely rare but has been reported in all segments of the spinal axis. Spinal nocardiosis generally manifests as spondylodiscitis.[13] Nocardial infections often involve the disc space, whereas fungal spondylitis typically spares the disc space. Nocardial spinal cord abscesses are very rare, with few cases reported in the literature.[14]

Imaging

Radiography

Nocardial vertebral osteomyelitis manifests as destruction of the vertebral body and secondary disc space involvement.

CT

CT may help to define the bony pathology. Diagnostic material can be obtained from spinal lesions by CT-guided needle biopsy.

MRI

There is no pathognomonic feature to distinguish between nocardial and pyogenic spondylitis. Nocardial spinal cord abscesses (Fig. 18-7) closely resemble other abscesses with swelling of the cord, high signal intensity in the affected area, and ring enhancement.

KEY POINT: NOCARDIAL SPONDYLITIS

- Nocardiosis is similar to pyogenic spondylitis because both involve the disc space in contrast to other causes of fungal spondylitis.

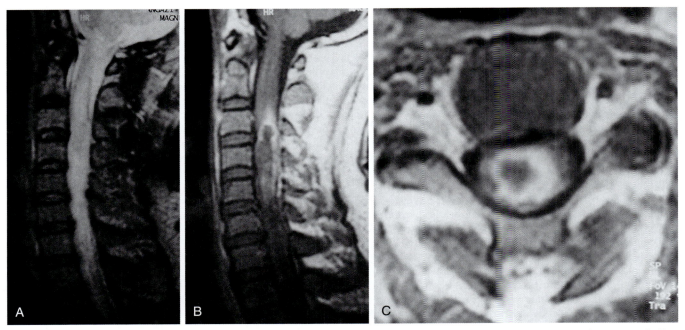

■ FIGURE 18-7 Nocardial abscess of the spinal cord. T2W sagittal (**A**), postcontrast T1W sagittal (**B**), and axial (**C**) MR images demonstrate fusiform enlargement of the cervical spinal cord. Intramedullary lesion is heterogeneously hypointense posterior to the C3-4 disc space. Ring enhancement of the lesion is evident with a thick and irregular capsule extending from the C2-3 to C5-6 disc spaces. *(Courtesy of R. Durmaz and A. Aslantas, Turkey.)*

TUBERCULOUS SPONDYLITIS

This type of spondylitis is caused by tuberculous infection of the spine and adjacent soft tissue. It is known as Pott's disease.

Epidemiology

The incidence of tuberculosis has increased in recent years. The prevalence will rise with increasing numbers of cases of AIDS. Tuberculosis of the spine accounts for 1% of all tuberculous infections and 25% to 60% of all bone and joint infections caused by tuberculosis. The diagnosis remains difficult because the tuberculosis is indolent. Tuberculous infection generally affects adults in the fourth and fifth decades, whereas the peak incidence of pyogenic spondylitis is seen in the sixth to the seventh decades. Skip lesions and posterior element involvement are common differentiating findings of tuberculous spondylitis and tumors. Multidrug-resistant tuberculosis has a higher prevalence particularly in AIDS patients who present with rapid progression and a higher mortality rate (approximately 50%).

Clinical Presentation

Tuberculous infections are indolent with a gradual onset of symptoms over months to years. Spinal pain and local tenderness, night sweats, anorexia, cachexia, and weight loss may be the presenting symptoms. Dysphagia, stiffness, hoarseness, torticollis, and cervical lymphadenopathy are the manifestations of cervical tuberculosis. However, the signs and symptoms of tuberculous spondylitis vary too widely to permit reliable clinical diagnosis.

The erythrocyte sedimentation rate is elevated in more than 80% of patients. The clinical presentation of tuberculosis may be quite different in AIDS patients from that observed in immunocompetent patients. HIV-infected patients with tuberculosis respond well to antituberculous medications in most cases.

Pathophysiology

Tuberculous spondylitis is usually the result of hematogenous seeding of the vertebral body rather than direct extension from a contiguous paraspinal infection. About 10% of patients show concomitant pulmonary tuberculosis. Infection usually originates in the anterior subchondral bone adjacent to the vertebral end plates. The infection then spreads craniad and caudad underneath the longitudinal ligaments, especially the anterior longitudinal ligament, to involve variable numbers of adjacent vertebral bodies and discs. The intervertebral disc is maintained longer and is destroyed more slowly in tuberculous spondylitis than in pyogenic spondylitis. This may be due to a relative lack of proteolytic enzymes in tuberculosis. When both neighboring vertebral bodies are involved, the disc may lose its source of nutrition and become involved secondarily. Bony fragments may migrate into surrounding structures, including the spinal canal and perivertebral soft tissues. Large paraspinal abscesses may extend through the hip, pelvis, and lower limb and reach maximum size within 2 months. The lesions may calcify. Compression fractures with gibbus deformity, ankylosis, and scoliosis are also common in untreated cases. Reactive new bone formation may simulate an "ivory vertebra" if abundant new bone forms during the healing process. Healing may progress for up to 14 months.

Pathology

There is usually extensive destruction, which may be associated with collapse of the affected vertebral bodies and intervertebral discs.

Tuberculous meningitis is characterized by a gelatinous subarachnoid exudate. The changes in the spinal cord reflect a combination of focal compression by epidural inflammatory tissue or vertebral kyphosis, ischemia, and secondary tract degeneration. Compression of the anterior spinal artery may produce a typical watershed infarct involving the upper and mid portions of the thoracic cord. Intramedullary abscess may develop.

Gross examination usually shows edematous tissue, frequently studded with small grayish nodules, sometimes with opaque white centers (granulomas). These granulomas can coalesce into larger areas of caseation (or cheesy) necrosis.

The typical tubercle consists of a central necrotic area surrounded by epithelioid histiocytes. Scattered among these histiocytes are Langerhans type giant cells. At the periphery, a rim of mixed chronic inflammatory cells is present. The center of the tubercle usually shows caseous necrosis in which acid-fast bacilli can be demonstrated by Ziehl-Neelsen or Kinyoun stains.

Imaging

Lower thoracic and lumbar vertebrae are affected most frequently. Cervical vertebrae and sacrum are affected less often. Tuberculosis typically affects the anterior portions of the spine primarily and extends to the posterior elements (mostly laminae) secondarily by spread of infection from the vertebral body. As a rule, multiple vertebral bodies are involved. Skip lesions occur in up to 4% of cases. Involvement of a single, isolated vertebral body, involvement of the posterior elements only, and involvement of the sacrum are atypical for tuberculous spondylitis. Lesions at these sites may be difficult to differentiate from metastases.

Radiography

Initially, plain films demonstrate osteoporosis. Bone destruction, loss of disc height, and soft tissue mass appear later. The soft tissue mass typically calcifies. Reactive sclerosis, vertebral body collapse, and vertebral body fusion are findings of advanced disease. Destruction of the anterior face of the vertebral body with preservation of the posterior elements often causes a gibbus deformity (see Fig. 18-16).[15] Such a gibbus deformity, with shortening of the length of the thoracic spine, may give the ribs a "spider" appearance. Infection limited to a single vertebral body may also lead to vertebral collapse and vertebra plana.[16] Paraspinal abscess formation may be detected on plain radiographs as areas of a fusiform soft tissue mass extending around both sides of the spine. With healing, paravertebral abscesses may calcify as amorphous/teardrop calcifications. Ivory vertebra may result from reossification of the bone as a healing response to osteonecrosis.

CT

In the early stages of infection, areas of erosion or osseous destruction may be subtle and better demonstrated by reformatted sagittal and coronal CT images.[16] In more chronic disease, CT typically shows extensive destruction at the vertebral end plates with well-defined osteolytic, subperiosteal lesions, and sclerotic margins. There may be fragmentation, bone sequestration, and large paravertebral abscesses. Epidural infection is common. In contradistinction to pyogenic spondylitis, the cortical definition of the affected vertebrae is invariably lost. Gas-fluid and fat-fluid levels may arise from necrosis of marrow fat, bone, and disc. The vertebral body is eventually destroyed by erosions caused by the disease and by necrosis from obstruction of the vascular supply to the bone. In a patient with spondylodiscitis, demonstration of a calcified paraspinal mass and thick irregular rim enhancement is nearly pathognomonic for tuberculosis. Percutaneous biopsy and drainage of the abscess can be done by a CT-guided procedure (Fig. 18-8).

MRI

MRI displays signal abnormalities early in the course of tuberculous spondylitis. Compared with pyogenic spondylitis, tuberculous spondylitis more frequently causes loss of definition and destruction of apposing vertebral

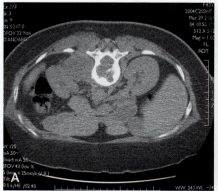
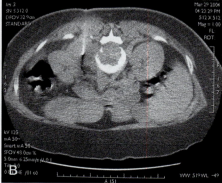
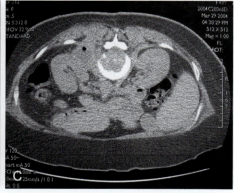

■ **FIGURE 18-8**   CT-guided biopsy and drainage in tuberculous spondylitis. Axial noncontrast CT image (**A**) shows extensive vertebral body destruction and a left paravertebral abscess formation. CT-guided biopsy and drainage (**B**) was performed. An air bubble marks the position of the drained abscess cavity that also shows decrease in size after the procedure (**C**).

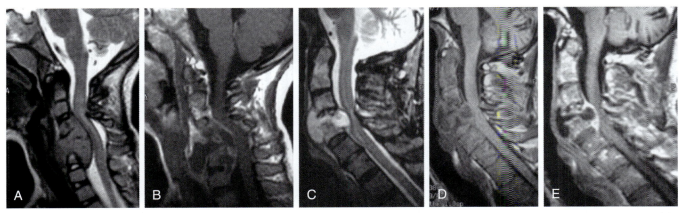

■ **FIGURE 18-9** Tuberculous spondylodiscitis. Sagittal T2W (**A**) and sagittal postcontrast T1W (**B**) MR images reveal a hypointense mass involving the C4-C6 vertebrae and C4-5 and C5-6 discs. The lesion displaces the cord posteriorly, compresses it, and causes spinal cord edema extending from C2 to C6. The C5 vertebral body is completely destroyed and cannot be differentiated from the adjacent discs and vertebrae. The abscess shows ring enhancement. Sagittal T2W (**C**) and sagittal precontrast (**D**) and postcontrast T1W (**E**) MR images in another patient demonstrate tubercular involvement of contiguous vertebral bodies and discs from C2 to C7 with compression of the spinal cord and cord edema. The infection totally destroys the C4 vertebra and forms a mass that extends both anterior and posterior to the vertebra. The postcontrast T1W (E) shows heterogeneous hypointensity of the involved vertebrae, complete involvement of the C4-5 disc, partial involvement of the C3-4 disc, and multiple abscesses at the C4 level. There is sparing of the C3 and C5 vertebral bodies and of the C2-3 and C5-6 discs.

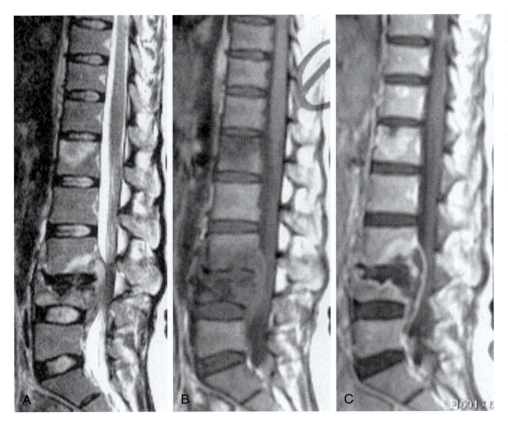

■ **FIGURE 18-10** Tuberculous spondylodiscitis with skip lesions and epidural abscess. Sagittal T2W (**A**) and precontrast (**B**) and postcontrast T1W (**C**) MR images demonstrate L3-4 spondylodiscitis with L1 involvement (skip lesion). There is marked erosion and destruction at the superior end plates of L4 and milder change at L1. The peripherally enhancing tuberculous abscess extends out of the disc space into the epidural space to compress the thecal sac. Contrast enhancement is evident at the T12, L1, L3 and L4 vertebrae. The T12-L1 disc space is spared.

end plates with sparing of the intervening disc, vertebral collapse, marked epidural encroachment, epidural infection, and intraosseous vertebral abscess with ring enhancement (Figs. 18-9 to 18-16). Other typical findings of tuberculous spondylitis include bony fragmentation, subligamentous spread of infection, anterior vertebral osteolysis/wedging, gibbus deformity, intersegmental fusions, involvement of more than two vertebral bodies, and skip areas between sites of infection (Figs. 18-9 to 18-16). The large paraspinal soft tissue masses/abscesses of tuberculosis usually show well-defined borders, whereas paraspinal pyogenic masses usually display ill-defined signal alterations and ill-defined contrast enhancement (see Figs. 18-11 and 18-12). Fistulas develop more commonly with tuberculous spondylitis than pyogenic spondylitis. MRI will also display any concurrent cord displacement or compression by epidural tuberculosis and any associated pleural effusions (see Fig. 18-16).

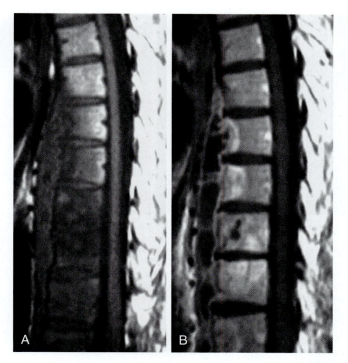

■ **FIGURE 18-11** Tuberculous spondylitis extension underneath the anterior longitudinal ligament. Sagittal precontrast (**A**) and postcontrast (**B**) T1W MR images demonstrate typical anterior multilevel tubercular involvement with extension underneath the anterior longitudinal ligament. Postcontrast image clearly demonstrates vertebral involvements with erosions, spared discs, and multiple ring-enhanced abscesses displacing the ligament anteriorly.

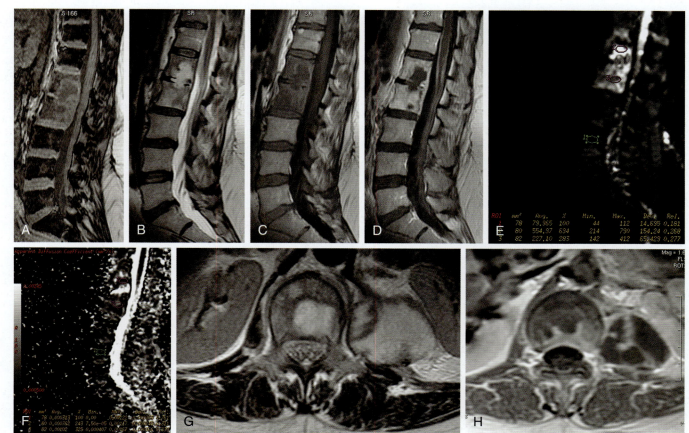

■ **FIGURE 18-12**   Tuberculous spondylodiscitis with paraspinal abscess and meningoarachnoiditis. Sagittal STIR (**A**), T2W (**B**), precontrast (**C**) and postcontrast T1W (**D**), DWI (**E**), ADC map (**F**), axial T2W (**G**), and postcontrast T1W (**H**) images show L1-L2 diffuse tubercular spondylodiscitis with intravertebral and paraspinal abscess. Signal alteration of the entire L1 and L2 vertebral body and intervertebral disc is seen as a low signal on T1W imaging, with high signal on T2W and STIR images. There is also minimal epidural extension. Centrally and caudally located abscesses do not enhance, whereas entire infected vertebral bodies and disc do. Meningeal involvement is evident with linear contrast enhancement and thickening of the cauda. Axial images clearly demonstrate left large paraspinal abscess with thin capsule and internal septations. DWI and ADC map show high signal of both abscess and the infected areas of the vertebrae and disc. The ADC values of the infected areas show at least twofold increase compared with that of the normal vertebra.

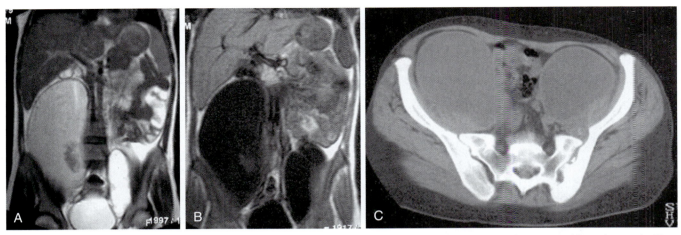

■ **FIGURE 18-13** Large paraspinal tubercular abscesses. Coronal T2W (**A**), T1W (**B**), and axial CT (**C**) images demonstrate bilateral paraspinal large cold abscesses extending to the pelvis.

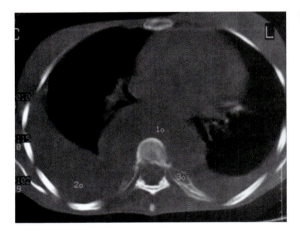

■ **FIGURE 18-14** Tuberculous paravertebral abscess and pleural effusion. Axial non-contrast CT demonstrates a large paravertebral abscess, bilateral pleural effusions (larger on the right), bilateral rib destruction, and slight irregularity of the posterior cortex of the vertebral body.

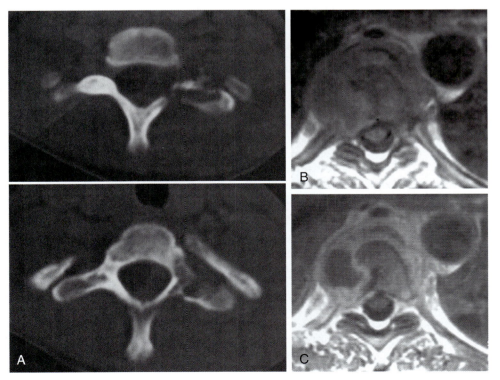

■ **FIGURE 18-15** Tuberculous spondylitis with posterior involvement. Two axial CT images (**A**) demonstrate posterior epidural extension that displaces the dural sac to the right and involvement of the transverse process. Precontrast (**B**) and postcontrast (**C**) axial T1W MR images show right proximal rib and pedicle involvement.

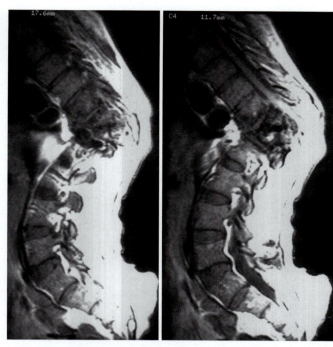

■ FIGURE 18-16 Tuberculous spondylitis and gibbus deformity. Two sagittal T1W images show complete collapse of the T11 and T12 vertebral bodies, resulting in gibbus deformity.

Sites infected by tuberculosis usually display low signal intensity on T1W images and high signal intensity on T2W and STIR images. Contrast enhancement is usually heterogeneous or ring-like and may reveal involvement of the ligaments, epidural space, and meninges (see Figs. 18-10 to 18-13).

MRI is very useful for monitoring the success of therapy.[17] The earliest sign of healing is a reduction in the extent of inflammatory soft tissue. A progressive increase in signal intensity on T1W imaging correlates well with resolving symptoms. Although reduction and then disappearance of contrast enhancement are useful signs of recovery, persistent or increasing enhancement are not necessarily indications of either deterioration or treatment failure.[18]

KEY POINTS: TUBERCULOUS SPONDYLITIS

Pyogenic Spondylitis
- Infection is usually located in the lumbar vertebrae, and the peak age at onset is in the sixth to seventh decades.
- Contrast-enhanced studies are the most important techniques for differential diagnosis.
- The most distinctive MRI findings in tuberculous spondylitis are mainly a pattern of bone destruction with relative disc preservation, focal and heterogeneous contrast enhancement, abnormal signal intensity in paraspinal areas, and an intraosseous abscess with rim enhancement of the vertebral body.
- The most distinctive MRI findings of pyogenic spondylitis are a pattern of discitis with some peridiscal bone destruction, diffuse and homogeneous contrast enhancement of the vertebral body, and peridiscal rim enhancement.[19]

Fungal Spondylitis
- Fungal spondylitis may mimic tuberculosis and could be difficult to differentiate.
- Vertebral deformity and paraspinal involvement are less common and extensive than tuberculous spondylitis.
- Disc space may be spared.
- Posterior elements may be involved as in tuberculous spondylitis.

Spinal Tumors
- Solitary tuberculous involvement may be difficult to differentiate from metastasis or lymphoma, plasmacytoma in adults, and eosinophilic granuloma in children.
- Metastasis in adults usually affects the posterior aspects, the pedicle. If there is sclerosis of a pedicle, differential diagnostic considerations include osteoid osteoma, osteoblastoma, and Brodie's abscess.
- The disc space is preserved and pathologic fractures are often associated.
- Adequate biopsy and bacteriologic and histopathologic examination are essential for the diagnosis.

BRUCELLA SPONDYLITIS

Infection of the spine and adjacent soft tissue can be caused by a gram-negative bacilli belonging to the genus *Brucella*. This is referred to as brucellosis.

Epidemiology

Brucellosis is an important zoonotic infection that occurs commonly among dairy workers, farmers, slaughterhouse workers, and veterinarians especially in developing countries, where it is endemic. Bone involvement of brucellosis has an incidence of 2% to 70% according to different authors, with 2% to 30% of spinal involvement.[20] Men older than 50 years of age are frequently affected.

Clinical Presentation

The clinical manifestations are generally nonspecific and may cause diagnostic difficulty. Brucellosis may begin insidiously as weakness and fatigue, back pain, fever, or malaise. There may be symptoms of nerve root compression, actual herniation of the intervertebral disc, paraplegia, or tetraplegia. Microscopic abscess formation may cause varying degrees of debility. *Brucella* infections may remain active for years, with repeated treatment failures and relapses.

Pathophysiology

Brucella is transmitted from animals to humans via the digestive tract, by direct contact with infected tissues, or by the respiratory system. The most common site of primary infection is the musculoskeletal system. Spinal involvement is generally seen in the subacute and chronic phases of brucellosis. Brucellar spondylitis results from hematogenous dissemination and mostly begins at the superior end plate. From there it may spread to the whole vertebra, disc space, and adjacent vertebra, depending on the virulence of the organism and the immune status of

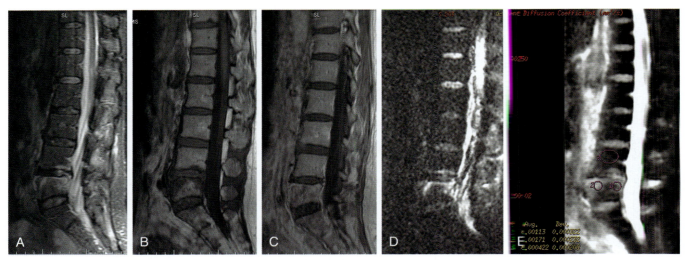

■ **FIGURE 18-17** *Brucella* spondylodiscitis, early form. Sagittal STIR (**A**) and precontrast (**B**) and postcontrast (**C**) sagittal T1W MR images demonstrate abnormal bone marrow signal at the superior end plate of L5 and the inferior end plate of L4 with low signal on T1W images and high signal on the STIR sequence. No signal abnormality or morphologic change is seen on T1W imaging. No contrast enhancement is seen at the L4-5 disc. However, high signal is observed at the posterior aspect of the L4-5 disc, suggesting early phase infection. Sagittal DWI (**D**) and ADC map (**E**) show increased signal of the affected areas. The ADC values of the infected area are at least threefold higher than normal.

the host.[21] Radiculitis and localized neuritis may also occur. Subacute and chronic meningitis with myelitis or myelopathy may develop simultaneously. *Brucella* species are difficult to culture and isolate.

Pathology

After entry by any route, the *Brucella* organisms spread to the reticuloendothelial system, multiply in the histiocytes, and cause generalized histiocytic hyperplasia. In contrast to tuberculosis, brucellosis shows noncaseous granulomas associated with lymphocytic and mononuclear inflammatory cell infiltrates. Healed vertebrae may show dense sclerosis.

Imaging

Radiography

Brucella most frequently affects the lower lumbar spine, especially the L4 vertebra. Brucellar spondylitis may assume a focal or diffuse form. Focal brucellosis limits itself at the anterior portion of an end plate. Diffuse brucellosis may involve the entire vertebral body, extend to the adjacent disc, cross the disc to the apposing end plate and vertebra, and pass into the epidural space.

Early brucellar spondylitis is characterized by osteoporosis of the affected vertebral body. Approximately 3 months after inoculation, plain radiographs show erosion of the anterior aspect of the superior end plate at the discovertebral junction. Posterior elements are rarely involved. The vertebral body is usually morphologically intact. Up to 18% of cases show small collections of air entrapped between the disc and the affected superior end plate ("peripheral vacuum phenomenon"), a characteristic feature likely due to long-standing ischemia and avascular necrosis of the disc adjacent to the infected end plate.[20] As a rule, there is no central caseation or necrosis.

Advanced brucellar spondylitis may destroy the entire vertebral body and cause herniation of the intervertebral disc. Despite the extensive lesion, vertebral collapse and scoliosis are rare. *Brucella* may cause complete ankylosis of the vertebral bodies, which then helps to stabilize the spine. The ankylosed vertebrae tend to keep their morphology, so they may be mistaken for malsegmented vertebrae, which almost always show anterior scalloping.

CT

The bony changes seen on plain radiographs are detected more clearly with CT and best appreciated on 2D- and 3D-reformatted images.

MRI

The affected bone and soft tissues show low signal intensity on T1W images and high signal intensity on T2W images (Fig. 18-17). The focal form of brucellar spondylitis appears as focal areas of abnormal signal intensity, usually localized to the anterosuperior aspect of a vertebra at the discovertebral junction (see Fig. 18-17). Diffuse brucellar spondylitis shows abnormal signal intensity extending diffusely through the adjacent vertebra and the intervening disc (Fig. 18-18). Diffuse reactive bone marrow changes mimic diffuse neoplastic diseases or myeloproliferative pathologic processes. Bone healing starts almost simultaneously with the inflammatory process, and the process of bone healing frequently spills over the edge of the vertebra in the form of an anterior osteophyte, the "parrot's beak" (Fig. 18-19).

Disc space involvement initially manifests as increased signal intensity on T2W imaging. The enlarged, circular disc bulge may mimic a herniated disc (Fig. 18-20). Late findings include moderately reduced disc height and contrast enhancement. The infection commonly extends to the epidural space. The paraspinal soft tissues may show

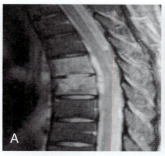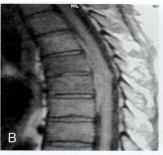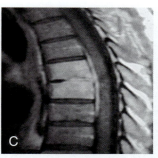

■ **FIGURE 18-18** *Brucella* spondylodiscitis, diffuse form. Sagittal T2W (**A**) and precontrast (**B**) and postcontrast (**C**) sagittal T1W MR images demonstrate diffuse signal abnormality and enhancement of the T8-T9 vertebrae and intervening disc. However, the affected bodies and disc maintain their normal morphology and show no erosions or destruction. Signal alteration and homogeneous contrast enhancement of the epidural space signify epidural phlegmon.

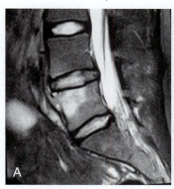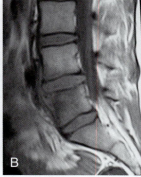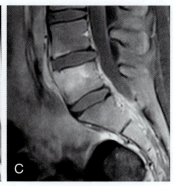

■ **FIGURE 18-19** *Brucella* spondylodiscitis, "parrot's beak" appearance. Sagittal STIR (**A**) and precontrast (**B**) and postcontrast (**C**) sagittal T1W MR images show abnormal bone marrow signal intensity at the anterosuperior aspect of L5 and at the anterior aspect of the inferior end plate of L4, with sparing of the intervening disc. These areas are hypointense on T1W images, are hyperintense on STIR sequence, and show enhancement at the areas of signal alteration. Formation of anterior osteophytes at L4 and L5 cause a "parrot's beak" appearance.

minimal increase in their signal intensity. The adjoining muscle fat planes may be obliterated, presumably by edema and/or granulation tissue. Paraspinal abscess is reported to complicate brucellar spondylitis in approximately 12%, whereas it may occur in up to approximately 50% of cases of tuberculous spondylitis.[20] Brucellar spondylitis may also show imaging features of radiculitis, arachnoiditis, and neuritis.[22] Especially in lumbar brucellosis, the peritoneum adjacent to the involved vertebra may be thickened and periaortic lymph nodes may be enlarged.

**KEY POINTS: *BRUCELLA*
SPONDYLITIS**

- Tuberculous spondylitis, *Salmonella* spondylitis, other pyogenic spondylitis, herniated disc, and metastatic lesions should be considered in the differential diagnosis.
- Proliferative changes are not seen in tuberculous spondylitis. Marked destruction, soft tissue involvement, vertebral body collapse, gibbus deformity, dorsolumbar involvement, and less pain are the main differentiating findings of tuberculous spondylitis.
- Pyogenic spondylitis is usually more acute than brucellar spondylitis.
- The disc is usually spared in the metastatic disease.
- Disc herniations generally do not show high signal intensity on T2W images and do not enhance.

FUNGAL INFECTION

Fungal infection can occur in the spine and adjacent soft tissue.

Epidemiology

Although the incidence of fungal infections has risen markedly in recent years, fungal infections of the spine are relatively uncommon.

Clinical Presentation

Fungal spondylitis shows clinical features that are very similar to those of the other spondylitides. Fungal spondylitis should be suspected at first in immunocompromised/immunosuppressed patients, in patients with AIDS, and in patients receiving long-term corticosteroid and/or cytotoxic therapy. Fungal spondylitis may also be difficult to distinguish from spinal metastases. In such cases, the clinical and histopathologic findings become critical.

Pathophysiology

The fungi that affect humans are classified into two categories: opportunistic fungi and pathogenic fungi. Opportunistic fungi such as *Aspergillus*, *Candida*, and *Mucor* species rarely cause disease in healthy persons but do so

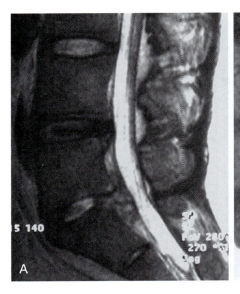 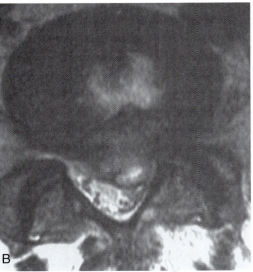

■ FIGURE 18-20 *Brucella* discitis mimicking disc herniation with free fragment. Sagittal (**A**) and axial (**B**) T2W MR images show increased signal within the L5-S1 disc. The subligamentous tissue posterior to S1 shows a heterogeneous fragmentary appearance in continuity with the L5-S1 disc. Operation for possible sequestered disc and subsequent histopathology revealed *Brucella* discitis.

not uncommonly in immunocompromised hosts. Pathogenic fungi such as *Blastomyces dermatitis, Coccidioides immitis,* and *Histoplasma capsulatum* can produce spinal infections (5%-10%) in healthy persons as well as those who are immunocompromised. The spinal involvement is usually the result of hematogenous or direct spread of organisms from an initial pulmonary focus of infection.[23] Fungal infections produce diverse inflammatory reactions ranging from chronic inflammation to suppuration with granuloma formation. Fungi can also produce calcification, infarction (*Aspergillus*), hypersensitivity syndromes, and antibody production.

Pathology

The leptomeninges may be involved and appear thickened and opacified. Some fungi (e.g., *Aspergillus*) take the form of branching hyphae. In these, the prominent microscopic features are infiltration of blood vessels by fungal hyphae, vascular thrombosis, hemorrhage, and variable inflammatory infiltrates.

Other organisms appear as single budding yeast forms (e.g., *Candida, Blastomyces, Coccidioides, Cryptococcus, Histoplasma*). *Candida* may also form pseudohyphae. Small granulomas may be discernible. Because fungal lesions closely resemble those of other granulomatous diseases, correct diagnosis of fungal type and differentiation from tuberculosis depend on identifying the organisms by staining or culture.

Imaging

Radiography

The radiographic features of mycotic spinal infections resemble those of tuberculosis. These include involvement of the anterior vertebral body, relative sparing of the disc, and development of large paraspinal abscesses. Fungal infections may invade the posterior elements and adjacent ribs less often and less frequently form draining sinuses. Certain patterns do occur more commonly with specific fungal infections. For instance, paravertebral soft tissue swelling with involvement of the posterior elements is more common in late coccidioidomycosis. Collapse and gibbus deformity tend to be seen more commonly with infection with *Blastomyces. Cryptococcus* may form lytic lesions within vertebral bodies, which may show discrete margins and surrounding abscess formations that resemble those seen with coccidioidomycosis or the cystic form of tuberculosis. *Cryptococcus* may also appear as a permeative lesion of a single vertebra with collapse. The degree of bone involvement often is more advanced than suggested by the patient's symptoms.[24]

CT

CT defines the extent of disease and may help with the differential diagnosis. In contrast to pyogenic spondylitis, fungal infections often spare the disc. Fungal spondylitis may form cavities and sequestra within the vertebrae, whereas tumors commonly show more complete bone destruction.[24]

MRI

In fungal spondylitis, T2W imaging may show only faint or absent signal abnormalities. Contrast enhancement may be very mild or absent, owing to the poor inflammatory reaction of immunocompromised patients.[25] The disc may not show hyperintensity on T2W imaging. The equatorial band (intranuclear cleft) may be preserved.

Aspergillus infections commonly affect more than one spinal site. Imaging features of *Aspergillus* spondylitis include anterior or posterior bulging of the disc with protrusion of the annulus fibrosus, enhancement of the anterior and posterior longitudinal ligaments, and enhancement of the subligamentous space with minimal or absent enhancement of the disc. There may be collapse of the vertebral body with retropulsion of the bone into the spinal canal, overt spinal instability, or both. *Aspergillus* infec-

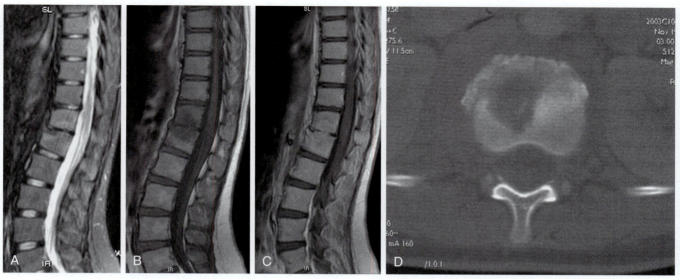

■ FIGURE 18-21 *Candida* spondylodiscitis. Sagittal T2W (**A**) and precontrast (**B**) and postcontrast (**C**) sagittal T1W MR images demonstrate signal alteration of T12-L1 spondylodiscitis. The superior end plate of L1 shows anterior erosion and destruction. The disc appears hypointense on both T1W and T2W MR images (which can also be seen with fungal discitis) but displays enhancement consistent with discitis. Axial bone algorithm CT image (**D**) confirms the erosion of the vertebral body.

tions may extend into the spinal canal to cause fungal epidural abscess or direct fungal involvement of the spinal cord. *Aspergillus* also causes a necrotizing arteritis that often leads to vascular thrombosis, infarction, and vessel rupture. Destruction of the vertebral body may mimic tuberculous spondylitis.

Candidal spondylitis (1%-2%) may occur simultaneously with, or as a late manifestation of, hematogenously disseminated candidiasis (Fig. 18-21).[26] Vertebral and paravertebral involvement may manifest as macroabscesses or as a mass mimicking a granuloma without disc involvement.[27] *Candida albicans* may cause intramedullary abscesses.

Spinal blastomycosis usually affects the anterior aspect of the vertebral body initially. Imaging features of spinal blastomycosis include osteolytic lesions with minimal reactive bone change, skip lesions, vertebral collapse, spinal cord abscess or granulomas, meningitis cord compression, and paravertebral abscess. Blastomycosis may mimic tuberculous spondylitis clinically and radiologically. On occasion, blastomycotic involvement of adjacent ribs, unusual in tuberculous spondylitis, may help to differentiate the two conditions.

Cryptococcal spondylitis most commonly affects the lumbar spine and usually causes sharply marginated destructive lesions with mild or absent perilesional sclerosis and little or no periosteal reaction (Fig. 18-22).[23]

Coccidioidomycosis usually affects multiple vertebrae with preservation of the intervening disc spaces. It causes destructive lesions of the vertebral bodies with sclerotic margins (older lesions), vertebra plana, involvement of posterior elements, and extensive paraspinal masses.

CYSTICERCOSIS

This parasitic infection of the spine and adjacent soft tissue is caused by systemic infestation of the larval form of pig tapeworm *Taenia solium*. It is also called spinal neurocysticercosis.

KEY POINTS: FUNGAL INFECTION

- The most important differential diagnosis is between tuberculous spondylitis and any of the fungal spondylitides and pyogenic spondylitis.
- Imaging features that favor a diagnosis of fungal spondylitis over tuberculous spondylitis include sparing of the disc space, involvement of adjacent ribs, more limited paraspinal involvement, and relatively less vertebral deformity.
- Imaging features that favor a diagnosis of fungal spondylitis over pyogenic spondylitis include sparing of the intervertebral discs, preservation of the equatorial band (intranuclear cleft), and absence of disc hyperintensity on T2W imaging.

Epidemiology

Cysticercosis is the most common parasitic infection of the CNS worldwide, particularly in Central and South America, India, Africa, East Asia, Eastern Europe, and other developing countries. However, neurocysticercosis involving the osseous spine is very rare, with the incidence ranging from 1% to 3% of total cases of neurocysticercosis. Approximately 50 cases of spinal involvement have been reported. The disease can occur at any age, and there is no gender predilection.

Clinical Presentation

Patients may present with spinal inflammation induced by metabolites of the parasite or degenerated larva. Diverse neurologic signs and symptoms may result from compression by parasitic cysts. Extraspinal cysticerci may also be seen.

Pathophysiology

Humans become infected with *Taenia solium* by consuming undercooked pork containing infective cysticercus

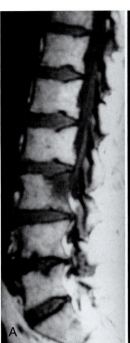
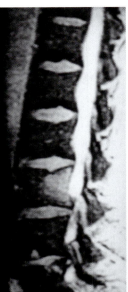
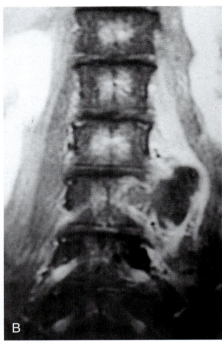

■ **FIGURE 18-22** *Cryptococcus* spondylitis. Sagittal T1W (**A**, *left*) and STIR (**A**, *right*) and coronal T1W (**B**) MR images demonstrate posterior half of L3 vertebral body signal alteration. Left paravertebral abscess formation is noticed with peripheral contrast enhancement. *(Courtesy of C. Andreula, Italy.)*

larvae. The larvae attach to the gastrointestinal mucosa, mature within the gut, and form adult tapeworms that produces infective eggs. Contamination of the pig's diet with human feces containing *T. solium* eggs results in infection of the intermediate host, completing the cycle. Infected patients who pass the eggs in their feces may reinfect themselves or infect others by a fecal-oral route of infection. The cysticercus larvae may breach the gut wall and spread hematogenously to the CNS and muscle.

Spinal cysticercosis can be classified as extraspinal (e.g., vertebral body) or intraspinal (including extradural, subarachnoid, and intramedullary sites). The most common forms of spinal cysticercosis are subarachnoid and intramedullary. These are known to be associated with cysticerci in the posterior fossa perhaps because of caudal migration of the parasites from the cerebral to the spinal subarachnoid space.[28] Spinal lesions are mostly racemose cysts, which are larger than the parenchymal lesions and lack scolices.

Pathology

The meningeal cysts are small and colorless. With time, the meninges become inflamed, thickened, and fibrotic. The spinal cord is less commonly involved.

Subarachnoid larvae can cause arachnoiditis. The cyst is usually 1 to 2 cm in diameter and contains a single invaginated scolex. After degeneration, the cysts become fibrotic and devolve into a firm white nodule that eventually calcifies. The cyst wall is sparsely cellular and consists of three histologic layers: an outer cuticular layer, a middle cellular layer, and an inner reticular or fibrillary layer. As long as the encysted larvae remain viable, the inflammatory fluid is contained within the cyst and the surrounding

parenchyma shows minimal reaction. After the cysticerci die, leakage of cyst contents leads to perifocal inflammation and infiltration by inflammatory cells and enclosure within a zone of granulation tissue.

Imaging

Spinal cysticercosis is commonly associated with intracranial cysticercosis, so the imaging evaluation of these patients should include both the head and the spine.

CT

CT identifies cysticerci as focal cystic lesions in the subarachnoid space. Calcifications are rarely seen with spinal cysticerci, because they are mostly the racemose-subarachnoid form of the parasite, which rarely dies.

MRI

MRI typically shows cystic areas with a signal intensity similar to CSF. Occasionally, a scolex may be identified as an isointense nodule within the cyst cavity. With progressive degeneration, cysts may show irregular peripheral contrast enhancement.[12] The appearance of the tissue surrounding the cyst varies with the immune status of the host. Minimal rim enhancement indicates no host response. Perilesional edema indicates a positive immunologic response. The intramedullary cystic forms may cause secondary syringomyelia. The subarachnoid forms may induce a homogeneous sheet-like arachnoiditis over the surface of the spinal cord. Use of the high spatial resolution sequences such as constructive interference in steady state (CISS) may detect many subarachnoid lesions not seen on conventional studies.

HYDATID DISEASE

This parasitic infection of the spine and adjacent soft tissue is caused by the cyst stage of infestation by a tapeworm of the genus *Echinococcus.* Alternative names include hydatic cyst disease, hydatidosis, and echinococcosis.

Epidemiology

Hydatid disease is most widespread in the Mediterranean basin, Central Europe, the Middle East, Australia, New Zealand, Latin America, and South Africa. The disease occurs more often in children and adolescents than in adults and is far more common in males than females, because these groups are more closely associated with animal care.[29] The parasites rarely invade the spine primarily, so spinal involvement is uncommon (0.5%-2% of cases).

Clinical Presentation

Spinal hydatidosis is usually diagnosed when the cysts compress the nerve roots or spinal cord. The specific neurologic deficits depend on the level of compression. Typically there is no fever. Otherwise, the clinical findings are similar to those of chronic pyogenic spondylodiscitis. Extravertebral lesions of the liver, abdomen, lungs, and so on, are frequently present in patients who present for spinal symptoms. Medical treatment is usually not sufficient to treat spinal cysts.

Pathophysiology

Echinococcosis is caused by the larval stage of the tapeworm *Echinococcus granulosus* (cystic hydatid disease), *E. multilocularis* (alveolar hydatid disease), *E. vogeli* (polycystic type), or *E. oligarthus.*

Humans are accidentally infected by consuming food contaminated with canine feces containing infective echinococcal eggs. *E. granulosus* and *E. multilocularis* are the most significant for human disease. *E. granulosus* normally has a domestic cycle in dogs and sheep. It produces unilocular hydatid cysts that then produce daughter cysts and scolices only by internal budding. *E. multilocularis* has a sylvatic cycle in wild carnivores and herbivores. It causes alveolar or multilocular hydatid disease, which results from invasive growth of cysts by external budding.

Echinococcus larvae (oncospheres) migrate from the gut into the body to infect the viscera, particularly liver and lung, and the spine. Some larvae are destroyed where they lodge. Others grow. By the end of the third week the host responds by forming a fibrous capsule (the pericyst) around the maturing parasitic cyst. Early mature cysts typically measure about 1 cm in diameter. If the cyst lodges in tissue that can accommodate its expansion without significant functional impairment, the cyst may continue to expand. The fully developed hydatid cyst is filled with fluid and typically unilocular and less frequently multilocular or "chambered." The wall of the hydatid cyst has three layers. The inner layer (endocyst) is a thick, nucleated germinative membrane and is the active layer of the parasite. The second layer (ectocyst) is an acellular, laminated, keratinous, mucopolysaccharide membrane of variable thickness, which is secreted by the nucleated germinal layer. It is strongly periodic acid–Schiff positive and shows acidophilic-staining with Gomori, methenamine silver, and Best's carmine stains. Microvillous extensions of the inner germinal layer cells protrude through the mucopolysaccharide membrane and provide nutrients. The third layer (pericyst) develops from the host response to the parasite and is composed of granulation tissue with fibroblasts, giant cells, and eosinophils.

Within the spine, echinococcosis has a predilection for the vertebral bodies of the thoracic (50%), lumbar (20%), sacral (20%) and cervical (10%) regions. There is special attraction to the center and pedicle of the thoracic vertebrae due to portovertebral shunts.[30,31] The cysts usually begin their growth in the vertebral bone marrow and may progress around the neural arch, through the anterior cortex into adjacent ribs, and through the posterior cortex into the canal. Within the spine, hydatid cysts do not form the typical spherical shape. Instead, vertebral cysts are microvesicular and invasive.[32] They permeate and slowly destroy cancellous bone, follow the path of least resistance to reach the cortex, and then penetrate the cortex to reach the paraspinal tissue. The disc is usually not involved, and the dura always remains intact.

Alveolar echinococcosis presents as a typical mass lesion with central necrosis, small cysts, calcifications, surrounding edema, and heterogeneous contrast enhancement.

Pathology

Vertebral involvement manifests as bone expansion with cysts that contain clear colorless fluid and granular deposits of protoscoleces, the so-called hydatid sand. The wall of a cyst is 2 to 3 mm thick. It consists of an inner germinal layer (endocyst) to which oval capsules are attached, an intermediate laminated cuticular layer (ectocyst), and an outer layer (pericyst) of fibrous tissue derived from the host. There may be lymphocytic cuffing of adjacent blood vessels.

Imaging

Because spinal echinococcosis is usually associated with more diffuse involvement of the body, imaging studies evaluate the head, thorax, and abdomen, as well as the spine.

Radiography

Plain radiographs demonstrate a nonspecific destructive lesion. Multilocular osteolysis with loss of cortical definition is the most common finding.

CT

CT is the preferred modality for displaying the extent of bony involvement. Cortical destruction with irregular margins, marrow erosion, and asymmetric involvement of the spinal canal suggest a multilocular, cystic lesion.

MRI

On MRI, echinococcal infection of the spine appears as well-defined or ill-defined lesions with CSF-like signal intensity and no or minimal contrast enhancement (Figs. 18-23 and 18-24). Typical spherical lesions are uncommon. Degenerated cysts may show signal alterations. Epidural or paraspiral soft tissue extensions generally show a "bunch of grapes" morphology. MRI is the preferred study for evaluating compression of the spinal cord and nerve roots.

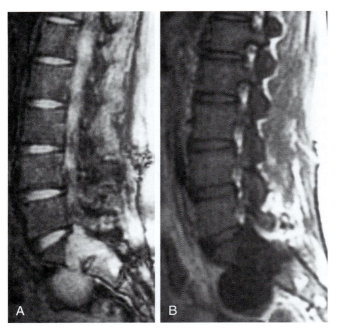

■ **FIGURE 18-23** Vertebral hydatid cyst. Sagittal T1W (**A**) and T2W (**B**) MR images demonstrate signal alteration of S1 and S2 in continuity with a well-defined paravertebral cystic lesion ventral to S1. The signal of the lesion is similar to that of cerebrospinal fluid. There is relative preservation of the S1-2 intervertebral disc.

KEY POINTS: HYDATID DISEASE

■ The extensive destruction and expansion of the bone in hydatid disease may mimic primary (e.g., osteosarcoma, chondrosarcoma, aneurysmal bone cysts) or metastatic bone neoplasms (e.g., renal cell, thyroid) and tuberculous or pyogenic spondylitis.
■ The pattern of contrast enhancement in imaging studies and the clinical and laboratory findings are helpful in the differential diagnosis.

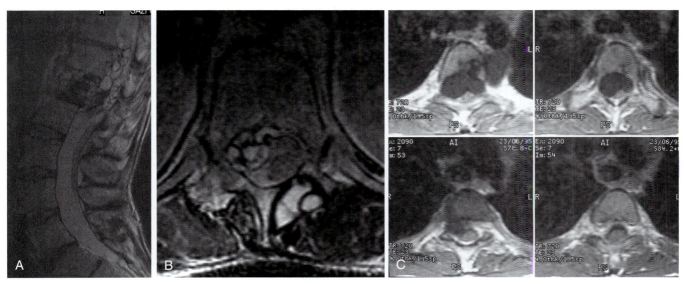

■ **FIGURE 18-24** Spinal epidural hydatid cysts. Sagittal (**A**) and axial (**B**) T2W MR images show multiple hydatid cysts in the epidural space of the T11 to L1 levels. Anterosuperiorly located hydatid cysts into the L1 vertebral body are also seen. Sclerotic changes are noticed at the posterior half of L1 due to prior curettage. The axial images demonstrate the epidural and also paraspinal multiple hydatid cysts at left posterior to spinous process and at right to lamina. The dural sac is displaced to posterior and left. Axial postcontrast T1W (**C**) MR image of a different patient demonstrates anterior epidural hydatid cyst with compression to spinal cord. Another paraspinal hydatid cyst is located posterior to the aorta. There is also an intravertebral hydatid cyst with ill-defined border. No enhancement is noted.

SCHISTOSOMIASIS

A parasitic infection of the spine and adjacent soft tissue can be caused by parasitic trematodes of the genus *Schistosoma*. It is also referred to as bilharziasis.

Epidemiology

This infection affects about 200 million individuals in 74 countries of Latin America, Africa, and Asia. Spinal cord schistosomiasis is one of the most frequent causes of non-traumatic myelopathies in endemic areas. The prevalence of CNS involvement varies from 1% to 30% of infected individuals. The infection can occur at any age, and males are affected more than females.

Clinical Presentation

Very few patients are symptomatic early in the disease. Later on, the patients may manifest signs of meningitis, myeloradiculitis, or transverse myelitis. However, there are no specific pathognomonic signs or symptoms. The response to the medical treatment is good, and, for this reason, early diagnosis is essential, but difficult.

Pathophysiology

There are three species of the trematode genus *Schistosoma*: *S. mansoni*, *S. japonicum*, and *S. hematobium*. Humans are infected when cercariae, released into the water from the snail intermediate host, directly penetrate the skin. Cercariae migrate through the skin to dermal veins and then to the pulmonary vasculature and liver. *Schistosoma* larvae mature in the liver and then migrate intravascularly to specific areas of the mesenteric or vesicular circulation.[33] The eggs release enzymes that allow them to dissolve their way from the small venules in which they are deposited into the lumen of bladder or bowel. These enzymes are allergenic and induce granulomatous inflammation and fibrosis where the eggs are deposited. *S. mansoni* passes preferentially to colonic mesenteric venules, so it produces egg granulomas in the CNS and spine more commonly than the other *Schistosoma* species. The ova usually reach the spine by the

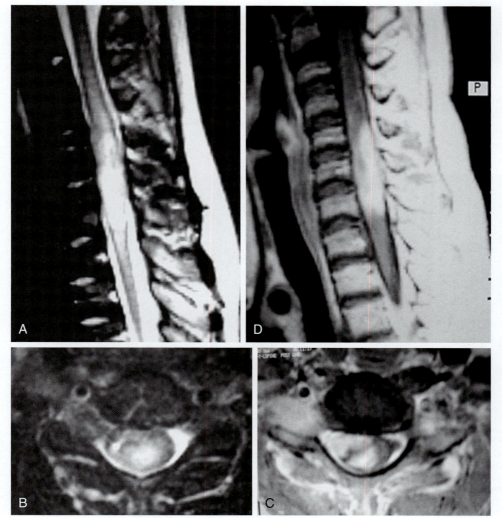

■ **FIGURE 18-25** Spinal schistosomiasis. Sagittal STIR (**A**), axial T2W (**B**), and sagittal (**C**) and axial (**D**) postcontrast T1W MR images demonstrate expansion of the cord at lower cervical and upper thoracic levels with edema, shown as high signal intensity on the T2W image. The lesion is seen as located centrally on the axial T2W image. Marked contrast enhancement at the affected area is evident. *(Courtesy of C. H. Zee, United States.)*

inferior vena cava, so schistosomiasis most commonly affects the thoracic and lumbar regions.[33]

Pathology

Granulomas may aggregate over the surface of the spinal cord and may occasionally invade the dura. There is marked swelling of affected spinal cord segments. Miliary granulomas may be scattered throughout the spinal cord. At times, the lesion may be solitary and mimic a tumor.

Histologically, the host response to the ova varies from none to a florid granulomatous inflammation with multinucleated giant cells, marked fibrosis, and adjacent gliosis. Eosinophils are usually present.

Imaging

Radiography

There is no prominent plain radiographic finding. Myelography may show an enlarged spinal cord mimicking an intramedullary mass.

CT

CT shows diffuse cord enlargement with patchy contrast enhancement.

MRI

MRI is the imaging modality of choice for evaluation of spinal schistosomiasis. T2W images show increased signal extending diffusely over several segments, enlargement of the cord at the level of the granuloma, and heterogeneous contrast enhancement (Fig. 18-25).

KEY POINTS: SCHISTOSOMIASIS

- The key differential diagnoses are those diseases that cause cord expansion, including multiple scleroses, acute disseminated encephalomyelitis (ADEM), transverse myelitis, intramedullary neoplasms, and abscesses.
- Immunologic tests and clinical findings are useful in the differential diagnosis.

SUGGESTED READINGS

Dagirmanjian A, Schils J, McHenry M. MR imaging of spinal infections. MRI Clin North Am 1999; 7:525-538.

Sharif HS. Role of MR imaging in the management of spinal infections. A JR Am J Roentgenol 1992; 158:1333-1345.

Sharif HS, Morgan JL, Al Shahed MS, Al Thagafi MYA. Role of CT and MRI in the management of tuberculous spondylitis. Radiol Clin North Am 1995; 33:787-804.

Stabler A, Reiser MF. Imaging of spinal infection. Radiol Clin North Am 2001; 39:115-135.

Tali ET. Spinal infections. Eur J Radiol 2004; 50:120-133.

Tyrrell PNM, Cassar-Pullucino VN, McCall IW. Spinal infection. Eur Radiol 1999; 9:1066-1077.

Van Tassel P. MRI of spinal infections. Topics Magn Reson Imaging 1994; 6:69-81.

REFERENCES

1. Heller RM, Szalay EA, Green NE. Disc space infection in children: MRI. Radiol Clin North Am 1988; 26:207-209.
2. Jinkins JR, Bazan III C, Xiong L. MR of disc protrusion engendered by infectious spondylitis. JCAT 1996; 20:715-718.
3. Ross JS. Discitis, osteomyelitis and epidural abscess. In Core Curriculum in Neuroradiology: Part II. Neoplasms and Infectious Diseases, 1996, pp 201-206.
4. Wolansky LJ., Heary RF, Patterson T, et al. Pseudosparing of end plate: A potential pitfall in using MRI to diagnose infectious spondylitis. AJR Am J Roentgenol 1999; 172:777-780.
5. Calli C, Yunten N, Kitis O, Zileli M. Diffusion weighted MRI in spondylodiscitis and vertebral malignancies. Neuroradiology 2001; 43:55.
6. Tali ET, Celik H, Ucar M, et al. Comparison of spinal DWI and ADC values to differentiate the spinal infections, tumors and degenerative changes. Presented before the Radiology Society of America annual meeting, Chicago, 2005.
7. Rothman SL. The diagnosis of infections of the spine by modern imaging techniques. Orthop Clin North Am 1996; 27:15-31.
8. Wetzel FT, La Rocca H. Griesel's syndrome: a review. Clin Orthop Relat Res 1989; 240:141.
9. Ledermann HP, Schweitzer ME, Morrison WB, Carrino JA. MRI findings in spinal infections: rules or myths? Radiology 2003; 228:506-514.
10. Bass SN, Ailani RK, Shekar R, Gerblich AA. Pyogenic vertebral osteomyelitis presenting as exudative pleural effusion. Chest 1998; 114:642-647.
11. Tang HJ, Lin HJ, Liu YC, Li CM. Spinal epidural abscess—experience with 46 patients and evaluation of prognostic factors. J Infect 2002; 45:76-81.
12. Lury K, Smith JK, Castillo M. Imaging of spinal infections. Semin Roentgenol 2006; 41:363-379.
13. Mitten RW. Vertebral osteomyelitis in the dog due to *Nocardia*-like organisms. J Small Anim Prac 1974; 15:563-570.
14. Atalay B, Azap O, Cekinmez M, et al. Nocardial epidural abscess of the thoracic spinal cord and review of the literature. J Infect Chemother 2005; 11:169-171.
15. Almeida A. Tuberculous of the spine and spinal cord. Eur J Radiol 2005; 55:193-201.
16. Shanley DJ. Tuberculous of the spine: imaging features. AJR Am J Roentgenol 1995; 164:659-664.
17. Gouliamos AD, Kehagias DT, Lahanis S, et al. MR imaging of tuberculous vertebral osteomyelitis: pictorial review. Eur Radiol 2001; 11:575-579.
18. Gillams AR, Chadda B, Carter AP. MR appearances of the temporal evaluation and resolution of infectious spondylitis. AJR Am J Roentgenol 1996; 166:903-907.
19. Chang MC, Wu HTH, Lee CH, et al. Tuberculous spondylitis and pyogenic spondylitis. Comparative magnetic resonance imaging features. Spine 2006; 31:782-788.
20. Tekkök IH, Berker M, Ozcan OE, et al. Brucellosis of the spine. Neurosurgery 1993; 33:838-844.
21. Görgülü A, Albayrak BS, Görgü üE, et al. Spinal epidural abscess due to *Brucella*. Surg Neurol 2006; 66:141-147.
22. Mousa AM, Bahar RH, Araj GF, Koshy TS. Neurological complications of *Brucella* spondylitis. Acta Neurol Scand 1990; 81:16-23.
23. Chemm RK, Wang S, Jaovisidha S, et al. Imaging of fungal, viral, and parasitic musculoskeletal and spinal diseases. Radiol Clin North Am 2001; 39:357-378.

24. Kim CW, Perry A, Currier B, et al. Fungal infections of the spine. Clin Orthop Relat Res 2006; 444:92-99.

25. Williams RL, Fukui M, Meltzer CC, et al. Fungal spinal osteomyelitis in the immuno-compromised patients: MR findings in three patients. AJNR Am J Neuroradiol 1999; 20:381-385.

26. Andemahr J, Isenberg J, Prokop A, Rehm KE. *Candida* spondylitis: a case report and review of the literature. Unfallchirurg 1998; 101:955-959.

27. Munk PL, Lee MJ, Poon PY, et al. *Candida* osteomyelitis and disc space infection of the lumbar spine. Skeletal Radiol 1997; 26:42-46.

28. Leite CC, Jinkins JR, Escobar BE, et al. MR imaging of intramedullary and intradural-extramedullary spinal cysticercosis. AJR Am J Roentgenol 1997; 169:1713-1717.

29. Turgut M. Hydatidosis of central nervous system and its coverings in the pediatric and adolescent age groups in Turkey during last century: a critical review of 137 cases. Child Nerv Syst 2002; 18:670-683.

30. Iplikcioglu C, Kokes F, Bayar A. Spinal invasion of pulmonary hydatidosis: computed tomographic demonstration. Neurosurgery 1991; 29:467-468.

31. Robinson RG. Hydatid disease of spine and its neurologic complications. Br J Surg 1959; 47:301-306.

32. Ozek MM. Complications of central nervous system hydatid disease. Pediatr Neurosurg 1994; 20:84-91.

33. Shail E, Siequeira B, Haider A, Halim M. Neuroschistosomiasis myelopathy: case report. Br J Neurosurg 1994; 8:239-242.

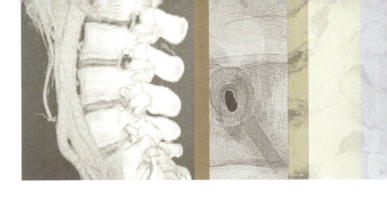

CHAPTER 19

Infections of the Spinal Cord

E. Turgut Tali and Serap Gultekin

SPINAL MENINGITIS

Spinal meningitis is infection of the spinal cord, leptomeninges, and subarachnoid space by various pathogens. It is also called infectious arachnoiditis.

Epidemiology

The incidence of bacterial meningitis is 2 to 3 per 100,000. It occurs most commonly in newborns, in infants aged 3 to 8 months, and in adults at the second and sixth decades. Spinal meningitis occurs less frequently than intracranial meningitis.

Clinical Presentation

The nature and the course of spinal meningitis vary with the virulence of the infective agent and the response of the host. It may present with flu-like symptoms. The neurologic manifestations are frequently limited to irritability, paresthesias, and sphincter dysfunction. Generally, the cranial meninges are also involved, leading to the typical signs and symptoms of nausea, vomiting, photophobia, inactivity, irritability, somnolence, and meningismus (stiff neck).

Pathophysiology

The infection is transmitted to the spine by hematogenous spread from extraspinal foci of infection, contiguous spread from adjacent spondylodiscitis or spinal epidural abscesses, direct inoculation, and an unexplained source of infection. The course depends on the virulence of the organism, the number of inoculating organisms, and the immunologic status of the patient.

Spinal meningitis is classified in accord with the specific class of infective agent.

Pyogenic leptomeningitis is the most common intradural infection of the spine. In adult patients, *Neisseria meningitidis, Staphylococcus aureus,* and *Streptococcus* species are the leading causes of infection. In the newborn,

group B *Streptococcus,* gram-negative bacilli, and *Listeria monocytogenes* are the main causes of infection.

Tuberculosis caused by *Mycobacterium tuberculosis* is the most common cause of granulomatous spinal meningitis. Tuberculous leptomeningitis commonly occurs together with tuberculous myelitis and tuberculous radiculitis. Frequently, intradural spinal tuberculosis presents with, or shortly after, intracranial tuberculosis. Less often, spinal tuberculous meningitis may be secondary to tuberculous spondylitis (uncommon) or may present as the sole primary infection (rare).[1] Tuberculomas may form on the inner aspect of the dura. Tuberculomas tend to excavate into the cord, so leptomeningeal tuberculosis may be difficult to distinguish from dural disease or intramedullary tuberculoma.

Pathologically, the meninges, cord, and nerve roots demonstrate congestion and exudates. As the exudate organizes, the coated nerve roots adhere to each other. The subarachnoid space narrows, becomes loculated, or is focally obliterated, leading to compartmentalization of the thecal sac, secondary syringomyelia, and/or hydrocephalus.

Brucellosis is another cause of granulomatous spinal infection, with 2% to 30% spinal involvement. Inflammatory vasculitis may develop during the course of the disease and permit the organism to pass into the cerebrospinal fluid (CSF). The spondylitis and meningitis may occur simultaneously during the acute stage, with the symptoms of one masking those of the other.[2]

Spinal cryptococcosis usually manifests as an infiltrating granulomatous mass that expands within the extradural or intradural extramedullary space to compress the spinal cord. Cryptococcal meningitis is frequently seen in AIDS patients, in whom the meningeal inflammatory reaction may be minimal and meningeal enhancement is uncommon.

Cysticercosis is the most common parasitic infection of the spinal leptomeninges. It is thought to result from direct CSF seeding of the larvae throughout the subarachnoid space from a source in the cerebrum. Intramedullary cysticercosis is much less common than subarachnoid infestation.

Viral spinal meningitis is extremely rare.

Pathology

Pyogenic and coccidioidal meningitides form a purulent exudate in the subarachnoid space. Fungal meningitides form small nodules (noncaseous granulomas) within thick, opacified meninges.

Pyogenic spinal meningitis induces an inflammatory infiltrate, first of polymorphonuclear leukocytes, then lymphocytes. These purulent exudates distend the subarachnoid space and penetrate into the perivascular spaces of the spinal cord. Bacteria then stimulate the production of cytokines and other inflammatory products.

Tuberculous meningitis causes an infiltration of lymphocytes and mononuclear cells and leads to formation of granulomas (tubercles). The tubercles show a central area of caseous necrosis, an intermediate layer of epithelioid cells, and a peripheral ring of lymphocytes. Perivascular inflammation may lead to vasculitis. The numbers of acid-fast bacilli vary, and the bacteria may become undetectable after treatment has begun.

Coccidioidal meningitis causes a meningeal reaction similar to tuberculosis, with organisms surrounded by epithelioid cells, giant cells, lymphocytes, and plasma cells. There may be small abscesses with noncaseous necrosis and vasculitis. In the tissues, the fungi form large spherules.

Imaging

Imaging studies may be positive or negative, so negative imaging does not exclude meningitis. The diagnosis of meningitis usually depends on CSF analysis and clinical symptoms. Unfortunately, MRI has low specificity for differentiating infectious meningitis from a leptomeningeal neoplastic process.

Radiography

Plain radiographs show no specific findings.

CT

CT has only a limited role in this disease. The density of the CSF may be increased by the infiltrate. The inflamed meninges may enhance. Calcifications may develop along the meninges, particularly in the healed stage of tuberculous meningitis.

MRI

Bacterial meningitis may extend to involve all segments of the spine. Precontrast T1-weighted (T1W) imaging may be normal or reveal nonspecific findings such as increased signal intensity of the CSF, irregular cord outline, and thickened dura. MRI commonly displays clumped nerve roots, an indistinct interface between the spinal cord and CSF, adhesions of the membranes, focal or diffuse obliteration of the subarachnoid space, and (multi)loculation of the subarachnoid space (Figs. 19-1 to 19-3). T2-weighted (T2W) imaging has limited use, since the high signal intensity of CSF may obscure the meningeal structures, but it may show focal or diffuse cord enlargement. Postcontrast T1W imaging typically shows an inflamed pia-arachnoid, may show inflamed dura and nerve sheaths, and may display abnormalities within the spinal cord. The enhancement pattern may be linear (most common), nodular, or diffuse. No significant correlation has been found between the pattern or severity of enhancement and either the severity of symptoms or the specific infective agent.[3] In acute meningitis, precontrast MRI may appear entirely normal whereas postcontrast MRI demonstrates the lesions in detail. In chronic healed meningitis, precontrast MRI usually shows the findings whereas postcontrast MRI detects no enhancement and adds no further information.

The MRI features of tuberculous leptomeningitis closely resemble those of pyogenic meningitis (see Fig. 19-2).[4]

Fungal spinal meningitis is very uncommon. Coccidioidal meningitis preferentially involves the basal cisterns and upper cervical subarachnoid space (see Fig. 19-3), leading to thickened, inflamed cervical meninges, possible cord infarction, and hydrocephalus. Candidiasis and histoplasmosis may also present as leptomeningitis.

Spinal cryptococcosis may manifest as a granulomatous mass that infiltrates the extradural or intradural extramedullary spaces and compresses the spinal cord. In AIDS patients and other immunocompromised hosts, cryptococcal meningitis may cause only minimal meningeal inflammation and minimal meningeal enhancement.

Viral meningitis shows no specific imaging findings. In AIDS patients, cytomegalovirus (CMV) may cause lumbosacral polyradiculopathy with meningeal enhancement on postcontrast MRI.

Cysticercosis of the leptomeninges and CSF exhibits discrete cystic lesions with signal very close to that of CSF. These cysts are particularly well shown by T2W MRI sequences with very high spatial resolution (e.g., constructive interference in steady-state sequences [CISS]). The rims of the cysts may show ring-like enhancement on contrast-enhanced MRI (Fig. 19-4). Racemose forms, with or without septal-capsular enhancement, are common in the CSF. Subarachnoid cysticercosis may cause homogeneous arachnoiditis that extends over the surfaces of the spinal cord in a sheet. Congenital lesions such as arachnoid and dermoid cysts should be considered in the differential diagnosis of the spinal cysticercosis.[5]

Hydatidosis of the CSF may also manifest as solitary or multiple cysts with signal similar to CSF. The cyst walls rarely enhance. Multiple daughter cysts and sterile cysts may be found together (Fig. 19-5).

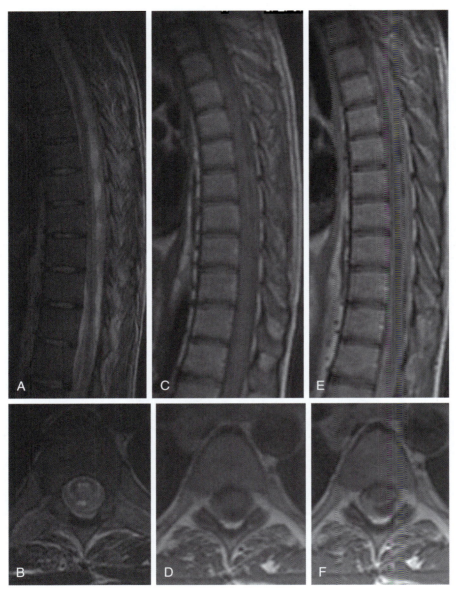

■ **FIGURE 19-1** Spinal bacterial meningitis. Sagittal (**A**) and axial (**B**) T2W and sagittal (**C**), axial (**D**), precontrast sagittal (**E**), and postcontrast axial T1W (**F**) images demonstrate thickened meninges with adhesion, loculations, obliteration of the subarachnoid space, absence of the spinal cord/CSF differentiation, and irregular cord outline. The thickened meninges show marked linear contrast enhancement.

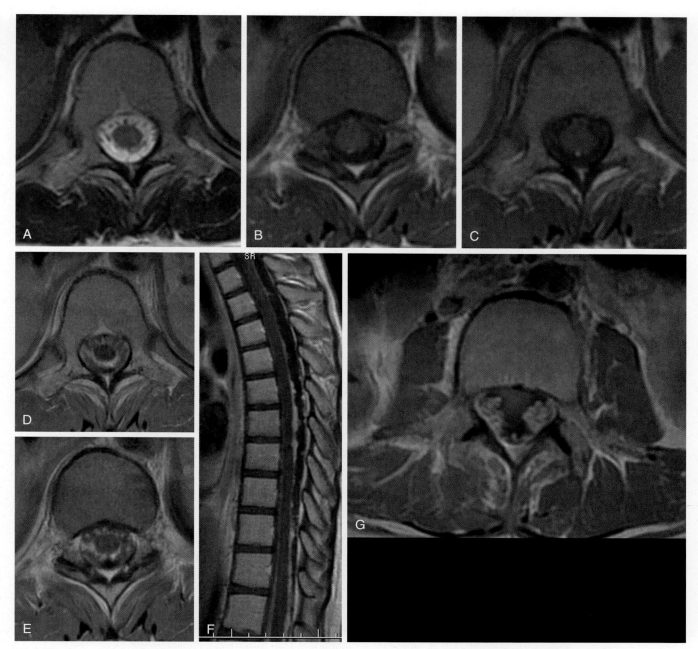

■ **FIGURE 19-2**   Spinal tuberculous meningitis. Axial T2W (**A**), precontrast axial T1W (**B, C**), postcontrast axial T1W (**D, E**), and postcontrast sagittal T1W (**F**) MR images show irregularly thickened meninges encasing the spinal cord with a marked irregular linear and nodular pattern of enhancement. The roots of the cauda equina are thickened and clumped and show marked contrast enhancement (**G**).

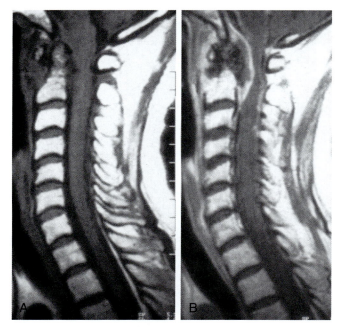

■ FIGURE 19-3 Coccidioidal spinal meningitis. Sagittal precontrast (**A**) and postcontrast (**B**) T1W MR images show obliteration of the subarachnoid space at the foramen magnum and upper cervical levels. Diffuse, marked linear pachymeningeal enhancement and mild leptomeningeal enhancement are observed. Inflammation surrounding the deformed odontoid process encroaches on and narrows the spinal canal. *(Courtesy of A. Hasso, USA.)*

KEY POINTS: SPINAL MENINGITIS

■ The MRI findings in patients with intradural extramedullary infections are quite similar to those of leptomeningeal tumor spread. Contrast agent administration increases the sensitivity but does not affect the specificity.

■ Fine linear enhancement of the cord surface also may be detected in sarcoidosis. Concurrent systemic manifestations and elevated angiotensin-converting enzyme level help in the diagnosis.

■ Arachnoiditis is another entity that must be taken into account in the differential diagnosis of enhancing nerve roots and meninges. Arachnoiditis is the inflammatory process of the spinal leptomeninges, seen as intradural clumping of the spinal nerve roots. Previous myelography, surgery, trauma, and subarachnoid hemorrhage may also be the predisposing factors of arachnoiditis. The exudative material around the nerve roots eventually causes adhesions, finally resulting in the obliteration of nerve root sheets and clumping of the roots. Early thickening of the nerve roots, later clumping, and dural adhesions appear with blunting of axillary root sleeves. Depending on the severity of the adhesions, stenosis or complete block of the spinal canal and also compartmentalization of the thecal sac with resultant mass effect on the cord may be seen. T2W imaging in the axial plane can display centrally clumped or peripheral adherent roots. Contrast enhancement of nerve roots is an infrequent finding that is often uncertain and useless for the correct diagnosis.

■ A rare chronic inflammatory hypertrophy of the dura, pachymeningitis hypertrophica of unknown origin, shows similar findings of meningitis.[6]

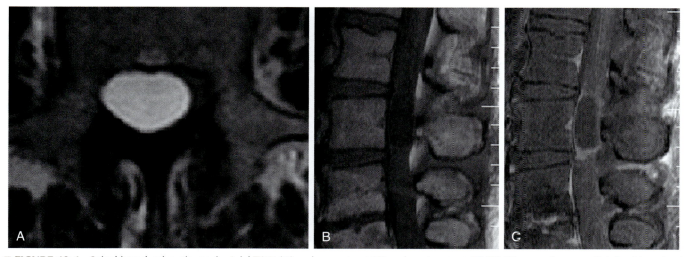

■ FIGURE 19-4 Spinal intradural cysticercosis. Axial T2W (**A**) and precontrast (**B**) and postcontrast (**C**) T1W images show a well-defined intradural extramedullary cystic lesion with the signal similar to that of cerebrospinal fluid. Mild ring-like peripheral contrast enhancement is also observed. *(Courtesy of C. H. Zee, USA.)*

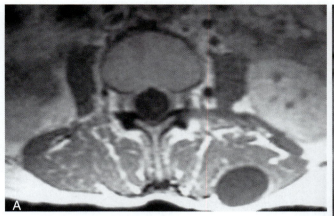

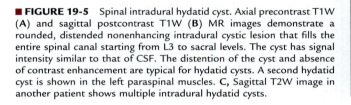

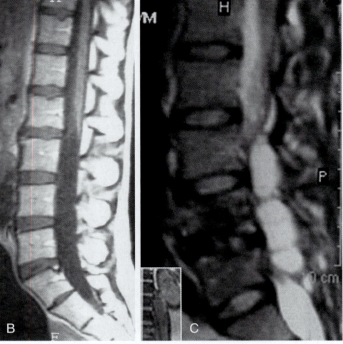

■ **FIGURE 19-5** Spinal intradural hydatid cyst. Axial precontrast T1W (**A**) and sagittal postcontrast T1W (**B**) MR images demonstrate a rounded, distended nonenhancing intradural cystic lesion that fills the entire spinal canal starting from L3 to sacral levels. The cyst has signal intensity similar to that of CSF. The distention of the cyst and absence of contrast enhancement are typical for hydatid cysts. A second hydatid cyst is shown in the left paraspinal muscles. **C,** Sagittal T2W image in another patient shows multiple intradural hydatid cysts.

MYELITIS/SPINAL ABSCESS

Infection of the spinal cord may be associated with necrosis. This can also be referred to as intradural intramedullary spinal cord abscess.

Epidemiology

Infection of the spinal cord is a rare clinical entity. The lesion can start as spinal venous thrombosis with resultant ischemic infarction that is later complicated by bacterial involvement. Postvaccinal occurrence or preceding infection is common in children whereas the acquired immunodeficiency syndrome (AIDS) is one of the major causes in adults. Often the exact etiology of myelitis is unknown and bacteria, fungi, viruses, and parasites may be the cause.

Pyogenic infection occurs most often. Similarly, the incidence of granulomatous infection of the cord is relatively low with tuberculosis as the most common cause. Children and adults (mean age: 34) and males are frequently affected. No specific ethnicity is defined.

Clinical Presentation

Spinal cord abscess is difficult to diagnose clinically, because the major symptoms have an insidious onset. Acute infection of the spinal cord may first present as mild back pain, then advance to paresthesias with a rising level of sensory impairment, and culminate in complete transverse myelitis. The most common neurologic deficits are sensory, motor, and sphincter dysfunction. Subacute or chronic myelitis tends to mimic a neoplasm. There may be recurrent bouts of radiculomyelitis with intervals of normal neurologic function. Rapid development of flaccid paraparesis may eventuate in permanent diminution or loss of tone with reduced deep tendon reflexes. Overall, sensory impairment is less prominent than motor impairment. Proprioception and vibratory sensation are usually preserved with no spasticity.

Ultimately, paralysis develops in 58% of cases, usually as a late finding after irreversible neurologic impairment has already occurred.[7]

Pathophysiology

In adults and children, bacterial myelitis and cord abscess usually reflect secondary hematogenous spread from a primary cardiopulmonary focus. Up to 40% of pediatric cases may be associated with spinal dysraphism or other congenital spinal malformations. *Staphylococcus aureus, S. epidermidis, Bacteroides, Haemophilus* species, and *Listeria monocytogenes* are the major organisms causing bacterial cord abscesses.

Tuberculous meningitis may lead to syringohydromyelia. This generally results from inflammatory edema and ischemia in the early period of the disease. Focal scarring in the subarachnoid space impedes free circulation of CSF, thus forcing CSF into the central canal of the spinal cord via Virchow-Robin spaces, finally giving rise to focal cystic dilatations that will eventually coalesce to form a syrinx. Later in the course of tuberculous meningitis, chronic arachnoiditis may loculate the subarachnoid space.

Pathology

The spinal cord is swollen and may discharge pus after myelotomy. The dura is tense owing to the underlying swollen cord.

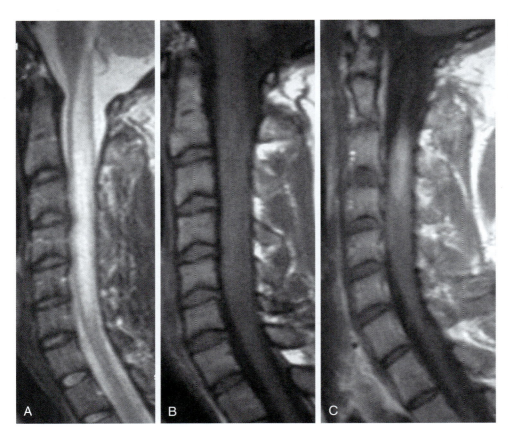

■ FIGURE 19-6 Pyogenic myelitis. Sagittal T2W (**A**), precontrast sagittal T1W (**B**), and postcontrast sagittal T1W (**C**) MR images demonstrate fusiform enlargement of the cord between C1 and C6. The T2W image shows increased signal, although the precontrast T1W image shows no signal abnormality. The postcontrast image demonstrates ring-like enhancement.

Irrespective of the agent, the infected cord demonstrates edema, perivascular inflammation, and variable degrees of vascular compromise, which may lead to vascular thrombosis, cord ischemia, and infarction. Histopathology shows inflammation with polymorphonuclear leukocytes, monocytes, squamous epithelial cells, and histiocytes.

Tuberculomas are composed of a caseous center and a surrounding granulomatous reaction that includes giant cells, lymphocytes, and fibrosis. They may spontaneously become cystic, fibrous, or calcified.

Imaging

Obtaining the correct diagnosis is extremely difficult on imaging criteria alone. History, laboratory findings, and histology are usually required for understanding the lesions shown by imaging. It is important to note that an infected syrinx may simulate an intramedullary abscess, particularly in children with congenital spinal malformations.

Radiography

Plain radiographs are not helpful in the diagnosis of myelitis.

CT

CT has limited use for this diagnosis. The cord contour may be normal or expanded, and the cord surface may be ill defined and irregular. The degree of contrast enhancement varies with the stage of infection.

MRI

MRI findings vary widely with the stage of the disease: from initial mild edema, to definite cord swelling with mild or no contrast enhancement, to prominent edema and abscess formation with diffuse, patchy, or ring enhancement (Fig. 19-6; see also Box 19-1). T2W imaging displays the cord expansion intramedullary signal abnormalities, and necrotic center of the lesion. Diffusion weighted imaging may show restricted diffusion, similar to cerebral abscesses. However, lack of diffusion restriction does not exclude abscess.[8]

MRI findings of tuberculous myelitis and abscesses are usually nonspecific. Tuberculous myelitis commonly displays focal spinal cord swelling, high signal edema, nodular lesions, and contrast enhancement (Fig. 19-7). The tuberculous exudate is usually isointense to hypointense on T1W imaging, isointense to hyperintense on T2W imaging, and hyperintense on fluid-attenuated inversion recovery (FLAIR) imaging, with marked enhancement. Noncaseating granulomas resemble bacterial abscesses and are hypointense on T1W imaging and hyperintense on T2W imaging with homogeneous nodular enhancement. Caseating granulomas with solid centers have isointense to hypointense signal on T1W and T2W images with heterogeneous/peripheral ring enhancement (see Fig. 19-7). Caseating granulomas with necrotic centers have

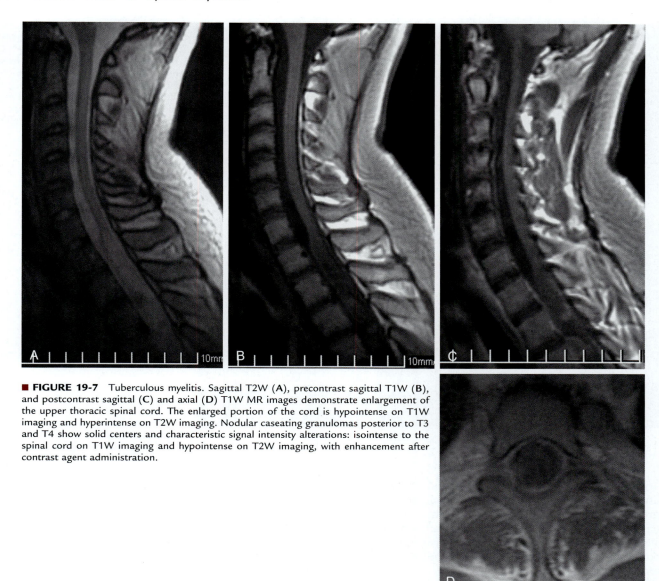

■ **FIGURE 19-7** Tuberculous myelitis. Sagittal T2W (**A**), precontrast sagittal T1W (**B**), and postcontrast sagittal (**C**) and axial (**D**) T1W MR images demonstrate enlargement of the upper thoracic spinal cord. The enlarged portion of the cord is hypointense on T1W imaging and hyperintense on T2W imaging. Nodular caseating granulomas posterior to T3 and T4 show solid centers and characteristic signal intensity alterations: isointense to the spinal cord on T1W imaging and hypointense on T2W imaging, with enhancement after contrast agent administration.

BOX 19-1   MRI for Evaluation of Myelitis

PATIENT HISTORY

A 35-year-old man with neck pain of 1 month's duration was admitted to hospital. He also had sensory disturbances and diminished motor functions in his arms. Elevated sedimentation rate and white blood cell count were remarkable laboratory findings. Neurologic examination showed paraparesis and diminished deep tendon reflexes.

TECHNIQUE

MRI examination of the cervical spine with contrast administration was performed. Pre- and postcontrast axial and sagittal T1W, axial and sagittal T2W, and STIR sagittal images were obtained.

FINDINGS

There is normal height and alignment of the vertebral bodies. The vertebral marrow signal is normal. The intervertebral discs are normal in height and hydration. There is no evidence of disc herniation, spinal stenosis, or nerve root compression.

There is expansion of the spinal cord with increased T2 signal extending caudad from C3 to C7. Two nodular hypointense lesions are noted posterior to C4 (5 mm) and C5 (3 mm). The lesion posterior to C4 shows ring-like enhancement, whereas the caudal lesion shows marked homogeneous enhancement after intravenous administration of gadolinium. The differential diagnosis includes granulomatous myelitis (tuberculous?, fungal?) or other infiltrating neoplasms.

Leptomeningeal enhancement suggests the presence of infection or infiltration of the leptomeninges.

IMPRESSION

This patient may have cervical myelitis.

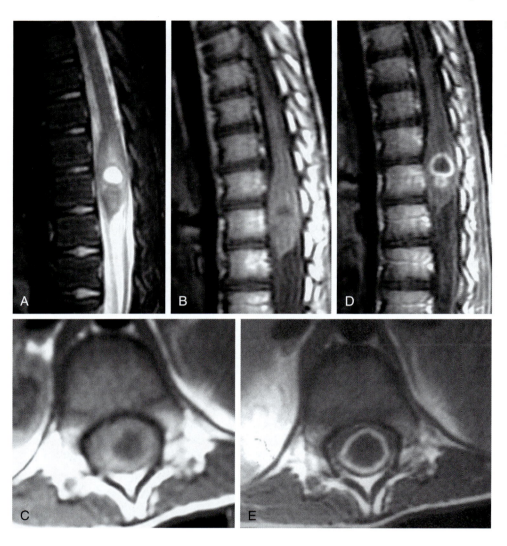

■ **FIGURE 19-8** Intramedullary cysticercosis. Sagittal T2W (**A**), precontrast sagittal T1W (**B**), precontrast axial T1W (**C**), and postcontrast sagittal (**D**) and axial (**E**) T1W MR images demonstrate a well-defined intramedullary cystic mass of the thoracic spinal cord. The cord shows typical fusiform expansion, peripheral edema, and ring-like enhancement. Almost homogeneous enhancement is seen in a smaller intramedullary advanced-stage cyst situated caudad to the first.

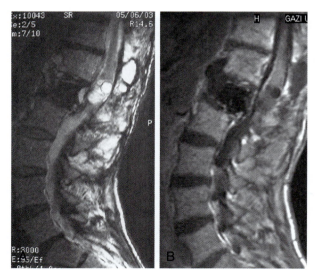

■ **FIGURE 19-9** Hydatid cysts of the conus and cauda equina. Sagittal T2W (**A**) and T1W (**B**) MR images show multiple well-defined hydatid cysts of the cauda equina and conus and expansion of the cord. The signal alterations of the L1 vertebral body are due to prior surgery. Multiple paraspinal hydatid cysts lie anterior to the L1 vertebra.

isointense to hypointense signal on T1W, hyperintense signal on T2W, ring enhancement, and, usually, peripheral edema. Healed tuberculous myelitis may cause calcifications within the spinal cord and neighboring meninx.

Syringohydromyelia, a well-known complication of tuberculous radiculomyelitis, may also be detected.

Intramedullary cysticercosis may cause syringomyelia together with typical cystic lesions (Fig. 19-8). MRI frequently shows an intramedullary cyst with an enhancing mural lesion or ring-like enhancement

Intramedullary hydatid cyst is very rare. MRI demonstrates a discrete cystic lesion with signal intensity very similar to CSF on T1W and T2W and no contrast enhancement (Fig. 19-9). Degenerated or infected cysts may have higher signal on T1W and T2W, may enhance, and may calcify.

VIRAL MYELITIS

Viral myelitis is an acute infection of the spinal cord caused by direct viral attack or postviral immunologic attack. It can be known as nongranulomatous infective viral myelitis or acute transverse myelitis.

KEY POINTS: MYELITIS/ SPINAL ABSCESS

- Intramedullary tumors may simulate spinal cord granulomas. Both show fusiform dilatation of the cord and similar patterns of enhancement. Tumors generally have an insidious clinical onset. The symptoms are nonspecific. Concurrent intracranial infection, meningitis, or spondylitis increase the likelihood of spinal infection over tumor.
- Nongranulomatous infective myelitis typically exhibits mild cord enlargement and patchy enhancement. This can often be distinguished from the more marked cord expansion and more marked enhancement seen with intramedullary neoplasms. Diffusion weighted imaging may show restricted diffusion in abscesses but no restricted diffusion in necrotic tumors.
- Noninfective inflammatory conditions such as multiple sclerosis, transverse myelitis, and sarcoidosis may sometimes be indistinguishable from infective myelitis. CSF antigen titers and viral cultures may be useful in the diagnosis.
- Cord infarction and cavernous malformations are the other diseases in the differential diagnosis.

Epidemiology

Viral myelitis is more common in immunocompromised and in younger individuals. Its overall incidence is 1 per 100,000 per year. No gender difference or ethnic predilection is known.

Clinical Presentation

The initial phase usually begins with flu-like symptoms: fever, malaise, anorexia, muscle aches, and back pain. Later symptoms and signs vary from mild sensory disturbance to paraplegia/quadriplegia, depending on the causative viral agent. Neurologic manifestations of advanced disease include weakness of the limbs, asymmetric reflexes, sensory disturbances, and sphincter dysfunction. Muscle tremors, rigidity, clonic spasms, and painful hypersensitivity may also be seen.

Pathophysiology

Viruses are the most common agents to infect the spinal cord: herpesvirus, poliovirus, cytomegalovirus, and human immunodeficiency virus (HIV) are the leading ones.

Herpesviruses are double-stranded DNA viruses. Most frequently they cause encephalitis, but some also cause myelitis and polyradiculitis (Fig. 19-10). Herpes zoster may cause neurologic symptoms after the dermatomal vesicular rash appears. Herpes zoster is caused by reactivation of herpesviruses latent in the dorsal root ganglia and typically affects posterior horns first. The virus is rarely isolated from the CSF, but antivirus antibody titers may be shown to be elevated. Herpes simplex virus-2 (HSV-2) can produce HSV myelitis with rapidly progressive neurologic dysfunction and extensive spinal cord necrosis. It also can produce a relapsing transverse myelitis.

CMV polyradiculomyelitis causes radicular pain, rapidly progressive paraparesis in the lower extremities, and urinary retention.

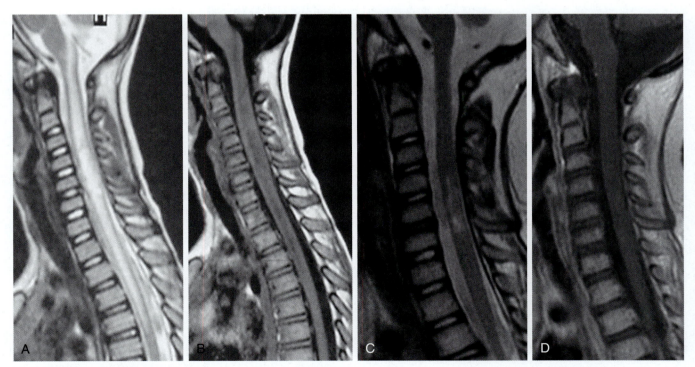

■ **FIGURE 19-10**   Spinal viral myelitis. Sagittal T2W (**A**) and T1W (**B**) MR images show fusiform enlargement and signal alteration of the entire cervical and upper thoracic cord. The cord signal is heterogeneously hypointense on T1W imaging but homogeneously hyperintense on T2W imaging. Post-treatment follow-up sagittal T2W (**C**) and T1W (**D**) images demonstrate gliosis posterior to C4 and C5.

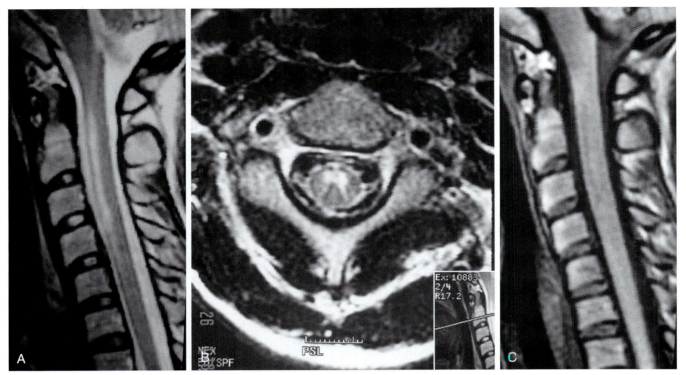

■ **FIGURE 19-11** Spinal poliomyelitis. Sagittal T2W (**A**), axial T2W (**B**), and sagittal T1W (**C**) MR images show moderate expansion of the cord and a vertically oriented band along the entire ventral surface of the cord. The band is hyperintense on T2W imaging, is hypointense on T1W imaging, and conforms to the ventral horns of the cord. This finding is typical for poliomyelitis.

There are three kinds of polioviruses (types 1, 2 and 3). Poliovirus infection is generally spread by the fecal-oral route, so it is more common in infants, in young children, and in regions with poor hygiene. The virus causes poliomyelitis by selectively invading the motor neurons of the spinal cord and brain stem, causing flaccid asymmetric muscle weakness (Fig. 19-11).

West Nile virus infection is associated with a myriad of clinical features ranging from a subclinical febrile illness to severe neurologic deficits. Common symptoms include fever, headache, nausea, meningismus, myalgia, rash, and tremors. In addition, a subset of patients exhibits features of an acute, usually asymmetric, flaccid paralysis.

Pathology

The leptomeninges may become infected and show clouding and congestion. Transmission of herpes zoster virus from the ganglion down the sensory nerve to the skin produces acute inflammation of the nerve, which may eventually result in demyelination, wallerian degeneration, and sclerosis. In the acute phase of poliovirus infection, the spinal cord is congested particularly on the anterior horns of the spinal cord.

The replication of herpes zoster in the sensory ganglion results in intense inflammation, neuronal destruction, focal hemorrhage, lymphocytic pleocytosis, and intranuclear inclusion bodies.

CMV radiculomyelitis causes inflammatory polymorphonuclear neutrophils to infiltrate the spinal cord, nerve roots, and dorsal root ganglia.

In poliovirus infection, motor neurons show swelling or necrosis. Continuing severe inflammation and microglial nodules are associated with severe loss of motor neurons at the affected segment of the cord. By 4 to 6 weeks after the onset of symptoms, many plasma cells can be seen in the same areas. Years after an attack of acute poliomyelitis, further muscle weakness may signify persistent perivascular inflammation from post-poliovirus syndrome.

Imaging

Radiography

Plain radiographs are not used in the diagnoses of viral myelitis.

CT

Contrast-enhanced CT examination may reveal mild contrast enhancement in the swollen cord.

MRI

Nongranulomatous infective viral myelitis causes edema and swelling of one or multiple segments of the spinal cord, particularly the cervical and thoracic cords (see Figs. 19-10 and 19-11). The MRI features of herpes zoster myelitis are nonspecific and indistinguishable from other forms of myelitis. Typically, MRI shows spinal cord lesions in a dermatomal distribution affecting the spinal segments that conform to the skin lesions. Slight enlargement of the cord with patchy contrast enhancement is often noted. On serial MR images the degree of enhancement ranges from marked to none and does correlate with the clinical status.[4,9,10] MRI of HSV-2 myelitis shows spinal cord enlargement, increased signal intensity on T1W imaging, and contrast enhancement. Necrotizing CMV myelitis is an opportunistic spinal infection seen in 3.4% of spinal autopsies. The cauda equina is thickened on noncontrast studies. There is diffuse enhancement of the cauda equina, the surface of the conus, and the meninges. Proton density and T2W images reveal a hyperintense band along the entire ventral surface of the cord in poliomyelitis (see Fig. 19-11). Enteroviral encephalomyelitis characteristically affects the brain stem and cervical spinal cord.[4,11] West Nile virus causes hyperintensity of the anterior horns of the cervical spinal cord resembling the features of poliomyelitis. Cauda equina enhancement and parenchymal spinal cord signal abnormalities are also seen.[4,12,13]

KEY POINTS: VIRAL MYELITIS

- Nongranulomatous infective myelitis may have mild cord enlargement with patchy enhancement. Such cases can be distinguished from the severe cord enlargement and marked enhancement typically found with intramedullary neoplasms.
- Inflammatory conditions such as multiple sclerosis, idiopathic transverse myelitis, and acute disseminated encephalomyelitis (ADEM) may sometimes be indistinguishable from infective myelitis. Clinical findings, CSF antigen titers, and viral cultures may be useful in the differential diagnosis. Idiopathic transverse myelitis typically affects long segments of the spinal cord, whereas multiple sclerosis causes focal lesions that extend over only one to two segments and often affects multiple discontinuous sites.

HIV MYELITIS

Myelopathy can result from primary HIV infection. It is sometimes referred to as AIDS or HIV myelopathy.

Epidemiology

HIV frequently affects the nervous system, producing neurologic symptoms, which can be severe. Although opportunistic infections (e.g., toxoplasmosis, cryptococcosis) and tumors (e.g., lymphoma) often produce CNS disease in patients with AIDS, many neurologic diseases are a direct result of HIV infection. HIV may affect the nervous system in two ways: (1) by direct HIV invasion producing myelitis, vacuolar myelopathy and tract pallor, and (2) by permitting opportunistic infections to flourish. Vacuolar myelopathy is the most common pathologic finding at postmortem examination of HIV patients.[5] For unknown reasons, however, it affects HIV-positive males far more often than HIV-positive females. HIV myelopathy has a prevalence of 20% to 55% but causes symptoms in only 10%, so it is usually not diagnosed clinically. HIV myelitis is found in 5% to 8% of AIDS patients and opportunistic infections in 9.5% of spinal AIDS autopsies.

Clinical Presentation

AIDS-related vacuolar myelopathy typically presents late in the disease with gradual onset of fatigue and slowly progressive spastic paraparesis. Less commonly, vacuolar myelopathy causes monoparesis or tetraparesis with impaired vibration and joint position sense. Ataxia, spastic bladder, sphincter abnormalities, and erectile dysfunction may also be seen. Vacuolar myelopathy is generally limited to the thoracic cord, so the arms are usually spared. With the progression, patients experience asymmetric lower extremity weakness, severe spastic paraparesis with painful spasms, and clonus. Sensory impairment varies from paresthesias to deficits.

Pathophysiology

HIV causes progressive depletion of the CD4 helper subset of lymphocytes, leaving the nervous system vulnerable to infection by CMV, HSV, or human T-cell lymphocytotrophic virus III. HIV may also infect the CNS directly.

The pathogenesis of vacuolar myelopathy is controversial. Many patients with HIV have increased numbers of macrophages within the spinal cord. Because CD+ helper cells produce cytokines and because cytokines inhibit macrophage activity, the large increase in macrophage activity may simply reflect the decreased numbers of CD+ helper T cells. Substances produced by the macrophages have toxic effects on oligodendrocytes and myelin, resulting in myelin damage and intramyelinic swelling, which then appears as vacuole formation. Clinically, this causes progressive myelopathy.

Tract pallor affects the distal axonal gracile tract and is believed to be caused by degeneration of dorsal root ganglion cells. It may result from direct infection of the dorsal root ganglion by HIV or from infection by human T-cell lymphotrophic virus type 1, CMV, or herpesvirus. Tract pallor correlates with sensory neuropathy.

HIV myelitis may involve both the gray matter and the white matter of the spinal cord. It is frequently related to severe HIV encephalitis.[5]

Pathology

Gross examination of spinal cord is normal. Vacuolar myelopathy affects the dorsal and lateral columns predominantly, causing spongy degeneration and loss of myelin with relative preservation of the axons. The vacuolization is usually symmetric. It can extend to the other portions of the cord and can progress to severe demyelination with axonal damage and reactive gliosis. In children, diffuse demyelination with axonal loss and inflammatory infiltrate are common features.

Imaging

MRI

MRI is essential for evaluating the AIDS myelopathy. MRI displays vacuolar myelopathy as cord atrophy with signal abnormalities that extend along the white matter tracts laterally and symmetrically over multiple contiguous segments. There is no mass effect.[5] Contrast enhancement is usually absent, but some lesions do enhance in a patchy pattern. Vacuolar myelopathy starts in the mid to lower thoracic cord and extends progressively rostrad as the disease becomes more severe. In contrast, HIV myelitis shows multifocal, asymmetric changes.

> ### KEY POINTS: HIV MYELITIS
>
> ■ The differential diagnosis of an enhancing lesion in the spinal cord in an AIDS patient includes CMV, HSV-2, fungal myelitis, lymphoma, and other neoplasms. The presence of hemorrhage in the lesion may suggest HSV-2. Meningeal enhancement may be found with CMV and herpesvirus infections and with tuberculosis, nocardiosis, toxoplasmosis, and lymphoma but is usually not seen with cryptococcal infection. Cord edema is not a prominent feature of HIV myelitis or vacuolar myelopathy. In contrast, toxoplasmosis and lymphoma cause extensive, multilevel cord swelling.

IDIOPATHIC TRANSVERSE MYELITIS

This clinical syndrome has many causes and is defined as an inflammatory disorder involving both halves of the spinal cord. It results in bilateral motor, sensory, and autonomic dysfunction. It is also called idiopathic acute transverse myelopathy (IATM). The terms *myelopathy* and *myelitis* are often used interchangeably because both refer to involvement of the spinal cord by some pathologic events. However, *myelopathy* is generic and implies no particular etiologic factor, whereas *myelitis* refers to inflammatory diseases of the spinal cord.[14]

Epidemiology

The incidence of IATM (i.e., the number of new cases per year) is estimated as approximately five new cases per million people per year.[15] There is no gender predilection or familial predisposition.[16] The majority of cases occur in the late winter. IATM shows one peak in the age group 10 to 19 years and another in the 30- to 39-year range. It is uncommon in children. Young adults may develop IATM as the first presentation of multiple sclerosis (MS). Older adults may develop IATM as a manifestation of spinal cord ischemia (spinal cord stroke). Children with IATM often report an antecedent illness, so the condition may result from direct infection of the spinal cord or CSF, or from an immune-mediated cross reaction between the infective agent and the host nervous tissue.

Clinical Presentation

Symptoms develop rapidly. In approximately half the patients signs and symptoms worsen within hours to weeks. A common presenting symptom is limb weakness of varying severity. Tingling, numbness, and diminished sensation below the level of involvement are other typical symptoms. Bowel and bladder dysfunction, back pain, and radicular pain may also be seen. Recovery varies from absent to complete. Even though IATM is a monophasic illness, recurrence may be seen in rare instances. MS may develop in patients with IATM. MS patients commonly show oligoclonal bands on CSF analysis.

Pathophysiology

The cause of IATM is unknown. It may be associated with prior viral infection or vaccination, autoimmune phenomena, or small vessel vasculopathy. At present, IATM is considered to be an autoimmune process with an indirect autoimmune attack on the spinal cord.

Imaging

MRI

MRI helps to identify IATM in almost 40% of cases but may be negative. Short tau inversion recovery (STIR) sequences appear to be the most sensitive for depicting the spinal cord lesions, even if they are sensitive to movement artifacts. If STIR is not available, conventional spin-echo sequences are useful and more sensitive than fast spin-echo sequences (Fig. 19-12).[15]

Characteristic imaging abnormalities include enlargement/swelling of the spinal cord extending over more than two vertebral segments. IATM typically affects the central portion of the thoracolumbar cord but affects the cervical cord in 10% of cases and may extend into the conus (see Fig. 19-12). The lesions are isointense to mildly hypointense on T1W imaging and hyperintense on T2W imaging (see Fig. 19-12). There is inconspicuous patchy/punctate contrast enhancement, which is not usually as extensive as the signal alteration. Meningeal and radicular enhancement may also be apparent, although usually mild. The zones of altered signal alteration may appear "geographic," that is, restricted to the anterior or posterior aspects of the cord or confined to either the gray matter or the white matter. The extent of involvement does not correlate with the severity of the clinical presentation or the outcome. Cerebral imaging can be useful for elucidating the cause of the myelitis, particularly in MS-associated forms of the disease.[17]

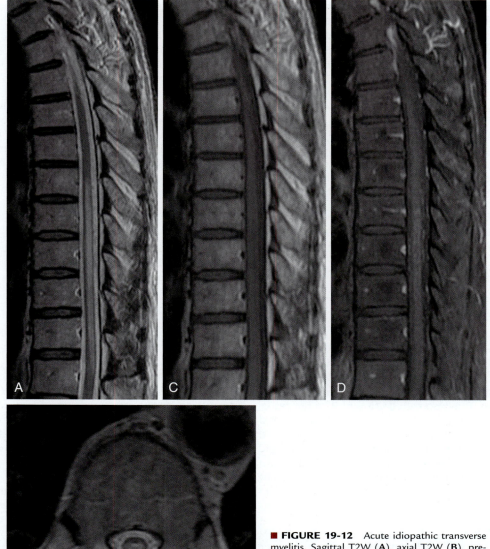

■ **FIGURE 19-12** Acute idiopathic transverse myelitis. Sagittal T2W (**A**), axial T2W (**B**), precontrast sagittal T1W (**C**), and postcontrast sagittal T1W (**D**) images show abnormal signal intensity extending over approximately five segments of the thoracolumbar spinal cord. The cord is hyperintense on T2W imaging, is isointense on T1W imaging, and shows no contrast enhancement. (*Case courtesy of S. Cheng-Yu Chen, Republic of China.*)

KEY POINTS: IDIOPATHIC TRANSVERSE MYELITIS

■ In the appropriate clinical setting, the pattern of abnormalities on MRI can suggest a strong presumptive diagnosis of IATM.

■ Differential diagnoses of intramedullary lesions may be based on the location of the lesion in the cross section of the cord.[18]

■ Cord swelling, with or without increased T2 signal, can be observed in a wide variety of conditions.

■ The principal specific and treatable causes of IATM include trauma, granulomatous meningomyelitis (especially tuberculosis), and vascular malformations that present as acute hemorrhage (or ischemia), particularly intramedullary cav-

ernous malformation in which siderotic signal shortening is distinctive.[17]

■ MRI can help to distinguish between IATM and the myelopathy associated with multiple sclerosis (MS). Findings that favor MS include (1) a short craniocaudal extent of the lesion (<two vertebral segments in 86%, with only 14% extending farther), (2) involvement of less than 50% of the diameter of the cord, (3) multifocal lesions (with greater than one 1 cord lesion seen in 50% of MS); (4) insignificant parenchymal swelling, (5) tendency to involve the dorsal columns, (6) homogeneous or ring-like contrast enhancement, and (7) concurrent brain lesions (~90%).[17]

KEY POINTS: IDIOPATHIC TRANSVERSE MYELITIS—cont'd

- Neuromyelitis optica (Devic's disease) is considered a variant of multiple sclerosis but is also associated with autoimmune diseases and differs from multiple sclerosis in its tendency to involve more than three vertebral segments of the cord. Even though it is considered rare in children, Devic's disease may be indistinguishable from IATM when MRI shows increased T2 signal in the spinal cord, optic neuritis has not developed, and no intracranial abnormality is seen on the MRI.[17]
- Rare, complex disorders of the spinal cord in childhood, such as systemic lupus erythematosus, mixed connective tissue diseases, idiopathic eosinophilic syndrome, and Hopkins syndrome are more difficult to exclude on neuroimaging studies alone. In all of these conditions, MRI findings may be normal or variable and nonspecific.[17]
- Symptoms, signs, and radiologic findings of intramedullary sarcoidosis are no different from those of other intramedullary pathologic processes. Multiple enhancing nodules and associated meningeal enhancement may aid in the differential diagnosis.

SUGGESTED READINGS

Bernaerts A, Vanhoenacker FM, Parizel PM, et al. Tuberculosis of the central nervous system: overview of the neuroradiological findings. Eur Radiol 2003; 13:1876-1890.

Gero B, Sze G, Sharif H. MR imaging of intradural inflammatory diseases of the spine. Am J Neuroradiol 1991; 12:1009-1019.

Provenzale JM, Jinkins JR. Brain and spine imaging findings in AIDS patients. Radiol Clin North Am 1997; 35:1127-1166.

Sharif HS. Role of MR imaging in the management of spinal infections. AJR Am J Roentgenol 1992; 158:1333-1345.

Tali ET, Gultekin S. Spinal infections. Eur Radiol 2005; 15 599-607.

Van Tassel P. Magnetic resonance imaging of spinal infections. Top Magn Reson Imaging 1994; 6:69-81.

REFERENCES

1. Chang KH, Han MH, Choi YW, et al. Tuberculous arachnoiditis of the spine: findings of the myelography, CT and MR imaging. Am J Neuroradiol 1989; 10:1255-1262.
2. Mousa AM, Bahar RH, Araj GF, et al. Radiological complications of brucella spondylitis. Acta Neurol Scand 1990; 81:16-23.
3. Rothman SL. The diagnosis of infections of the spine by modern imaging techniques. Orthop Clin North Am 1996; 27:15-23.
4. Lury K, Smith JK, Castillo M. Imaging of spinal infections. Semin Roentgenol 2006; 41:367-379.
5. Leite CC, Jinkins JR, Escobar BE, et al. MR imaging of intramedullary and intradural-extramedullary spinal cysticercosis. AJR Am J Roentgenol 1997; 169:1713-1717.
6. Smith AS, Blaser SI. Infectious and inflammatory processes of the spine. Radiol Clin North Am 1991; 29:809-827.
7. Simon JK, Lazareff JA, Diament MJ, Kennedy WA. Intramedullary abscess of the spinal cord in children: a case report and review of the literature. Pediatr Infect Dis J 2003; 22:186-192.
8. Thurnher MM, Bammer RB. Diffusion-weighted magnetic resonance imaging of the spine and spinal cord. Semin Roentgenol 2006; 48:795-801.
9. Quencer RM, Post MJ. Spinal cord lesions in patients with AIDS. Neuroimaging Clin North Am 1997; 7:359-373.
10. Hirai T, Korogoi Y, Hanatake S, et al. Case report: varicella-zoster virus myelitis—serial MR findings. Br J Radiol 1996; 69:1187-1190.
11. Cheng-Yu C, Changa Y-C, Huanga C-C, et al. Acute flaccid paralysis in infants and young children with enterovirus 71 infection: MR imaging findings and clinical correlates. AJNR Am J Neuroradiol 2001; 22:200-205.
12. Kraushaara G, Patela R, Storehama GW: West Nile Virus: a case report with flaccid paralysis and cervical spinal cord MR imaging findings. AJNR Am J Neuroradio 2005; 26:26-29.
13. Jeha LE, Sila CA, Lederman RJ, et al: West Nile virus infection: a new acute paralytic illness. Neurology 2003; 61:55-59.
14. Brinar VV, Habek M, Brinar M, et al. The differential diagnosis of acute transverse myelitis. Clin Neurol Neurosurg 2006; 108:278-283.
15. Jeffery DR, Mandler RN, Davis LE. Transverse myelitis: retrospective analysis of 33 cases, with differentiation of cases associated with multiple sclerosis and parainfectious events. Arch Neurol 1993; 50:532-535.
16. Scotti G, Gereveni S. Diagnosis and differential diagnosis of acute transverse myelopathy: the role of neuroradiological investigations and review of the literature. Neurol Sci 2001; 22:S69-S73
17. Andronikou S, Jonathan GA, Wilmshurst J, Hewlett R. MRI findings in acute idiopathic transverse myelopathy in children. Pediatr Radiol 2003; 33:624-629.
18. Thurnher M, Cartes-Zumelzu F, Mueller-Mang C. Demyelinating and infectious diseases of the spinal cord. Neuroimaging Clin North Am 2007; 17:37-55.

Spinal Inflammation

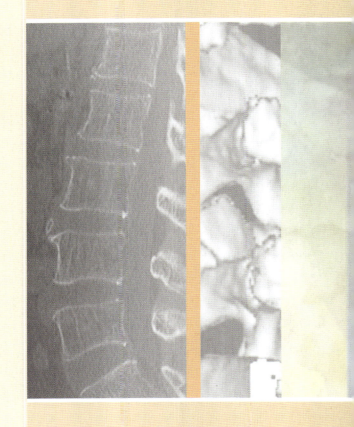

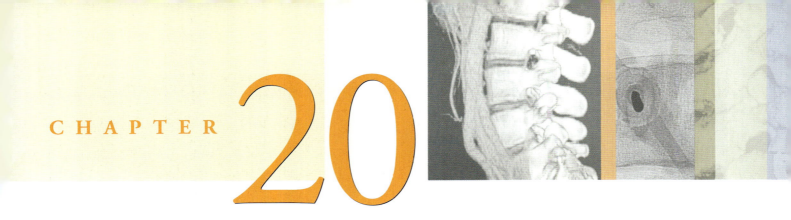

CHAPTER 20

Inflammation of the Spinal Column

Kenneth Michael Lury

Noninfective inflammations of the vertebral spine can be caused by seronegative spondyloarthropathies or by seropositive rheumatoid arthritis. The seronegative spondyloarthropathies include ankylosing spondylitis, psoriatic arthritis, reactive arthritis, arthritis associated with inflammatory bowel diseases, and undifferentiated arthritis.[1,2]

ANYLOSING SPONDYLITIS

Epidemiology

Ankylosing spondylitis is the most frequent seronegative inflammatory spinal disease in adults and the prototype for other members of the spondyloarthropathies.[2] The prevalence of this disorder is estimated at 0.1% to 0.2% in the general population. Ankylosing spondylitis primarily affects young males, with a male-to-female ratio of 4 to 10 : 1. The peak age at onset is 15 to 35 years, with a mean age of 26 years. In 15% to 20% of patients, the disease begins in the second decade of life. In 10%, onset occurs after age 39 years.

Ankylosing spondylitis classically begins in the sacroiliac joints and then affects the thoracolumbar and lumbosacral spinal junctions. The disease typically ascends as it progresses, involving the mid lumbar, the upper thoracic, and then the cervical vertebrae. However, the disease does not always conform to this ascending pattern. In general, atypical patterns occur more frequently in women, but spinal disease without sacroiliac joint involvement is unusual in either sex. The cervical spine becomes ankylosed late in the course of the disease, leading to restriction in neck movement and head rotation. Eventually, the spine becomes completely rigid, with loss of its normal curvatures and movement.

Patients with ankylosing spondylitis test negative for rheumatoid factors. HLA-B27 is present in 95% of patients, but only a small percentage of all individuals positive for HLA-B27 actually develop the disorder.[3] Therefore, this test cannot be used diagnostically.

Clinical Presentation

Inflammatory spinal disease typically presents in patients younger than age 40 years with back pain that is insidious in onset, persists for at least 3 months, is associated with morning stiffness, and improves with exercise.[4] Ankylosing spondylitis is the most common inflammatory spinal disease in adults and the prototype for all of the spondyloarthropathies. It usually starts in the sacroiliac joints early in the disease and progresses to involve other parts of the axial skeleton later. Inflammatory back pain is most frequently located at the lower part of the back, partly as alternating buttock pain. The pain may spread to multiple other locations in the spine, typically at night. The disorder tends to follow a more mild and benign course in females.[2]

Pathophysiology

Ankylosing spondylitis is a distinct disease entity characterized by inflammation of multiple articular and para-articular structures. The inflammation frequently results in bony ankylosis of the joints. The term *ankylosing* derives from the Greek word *ankylos*, meaning "stiffening of a joint." *Spondylos* means "vertebra"; *spondylitis* refers to inflammation of one or more vertebrae. Ankylosing spondylitis is usually classified as a chronic and progressive form of seronegative arthritis. It has a predilection for the axial skeleton (particularly the sacroiliac joints), the spinal facet joints, and the paravertebral soft tissues. Extraspinal manifestations of the disease include peripheral arthritis, iritis, pulmonary involvement, and systemic upset.[3]

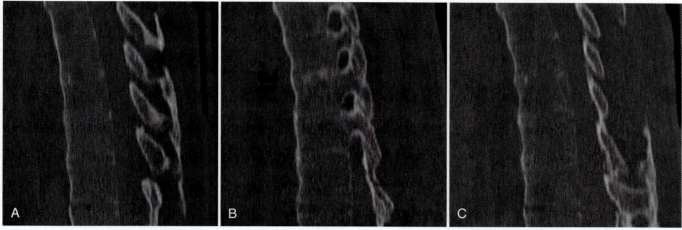

■ **FIGURE 20-1** Ankylosing spondylitis. **A to C,** Sagittal reformatted MDCT images of the thoracic spine demonstrate bony ankylosis of the ventral portion of multiple contiguous vertebral bodies. There is also confluent ankylosis of the spinous processes and facets.

The basic pathologic lesion of ankylosing spondylitis occurs at the entheses. These are the sites at which the ligaments, tendons, and joint capsules attach to the bone. Cellular infiltration by lymphocytes, plasma cells, and polymorphonuclear leukocytes is associated with erosion and eburnation of the subligamentous bone. The inflammation forms new bone within the outer layers of the annulus fibrosus of the intervertebral discs. The margins of the disc are invaded by hyperemic granulation tissue arising from the subchondral bone. This tissue replaces the disc fibers with new bone. Insufficiency fractures and traumatic fractures of the affected vertebrae also occur. Another important sign of spondyloarthritis is enthesitis. This affects the interspinal and supraspinal ligaments of the vertebral spine and the interosseous ligaments in the retroarticular space of the sacroiliac joints.[3]

Imaging

CT

CT is useful for documenting the presence of ankylosing spondylitis in patients whose initial sacroiliac joint radiographs are normal or equivocal. Features such as joint erosions, subchondral sclerosis, and bony ankylosis are visualized better on CT than on radiographs. However, normal variants of the sacroiliac joint may simulate the features of sacroiliitis. CT supplements bone scintigraphy in evaluating areas of increased radionuclide uptake, particularly in the spine. Bony lesions such as pseudarthroses, fractures, spinal canal stenosis, and facet inflammatory disease are well detected using CT, particularly with multiplanar reformatting into coronal, sagittal, or oblique images (Fig. 20-1). Other useful applications of CT include the assessment of costovertebral disease, manubriosternal disease, dural ectasia, and paraspinal muscle atrophy. Multidetector CT (MDCT) is superior to radiographs and to MRI for showing the number of lesions and demonstrating fracture morphology.[3] In patients with advanced disease, MDCT is the primary modality for evaluating cervical spine fractures (Fig. 20-2).[3] MDCT complements MRI,

which better shows spinal cord and soft tissue injuries. CT is accurate for diagnosing complications of ankylosing spondylitis, such as spinal pseudarthrosis, fractures, and vertebral scalloping from dural ectasia.[3]

MRI

MRI may contribute to the early diagnosis of sacroiliitis. MRI detection of synovial enhancement correlates with disease activity as measured by laboratory inflammatory markers.[3] MRI is superior to CT for detecting abnormal cartilage, bone erosions, and subchondral bone changes.[3] It is also sensitive for assessing disease activity early in the course of ankylosing spondylitis. Affected sites include the discovertebral junctions and peripheral joints. In general, areas of increased T2 signal intensity correlate with the presence of edema or vascularized fibrous tissue (Fig. 20-3).

In established disease, MRI can assess the integrity of the intervertebral discs and spinal ligaments and display spinal fractures. MRI detects pseudarthroses, diverticula associated with cauda equina syndrome, and spinal canal stenosis.[3] In patients with complications of fractures or pseudarthroses, MRI demonstrates any compromise of the spinal canal or spinal cord injury. MRI is very helpful in patients with neurologic symptoms, especially those with a symptom-free interval after initial diagnosis and those with neurologic deterioration after established spinal cord injury from trauma.[3] Advantages of MRI include direct visualization of cartilage abnormalities, detection of bone marrow edema, improved detection of bone erosions, and lack of ionizing radiation.[3]

Early in ankylosing spondylitis, the spinal lesions mainly involve the intervertebral discs, the adjacent edges of the vertebrae, and the rims. The cartilage and the subchondral bone are involved secondarily.[2] Neither MRI nor CT is diagnostic of spondylitis/spondylodiscitis specifically early in the disease.[3] However, it is possible to differentiate between the noninfective spinal inflammation of spondyloarthropathy and infectious spondylitis/spondylodiscitis *if* the bacterial infection has already spread to adjacent

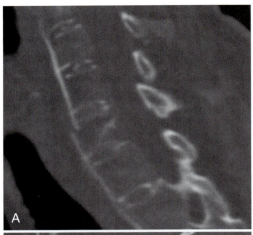

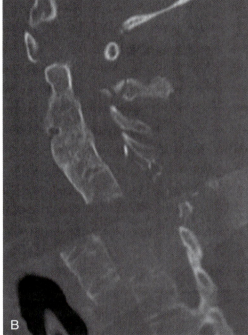

■ **FIGURE 20-2** Ankylosing spondylitis. Lateral radiographs of the cervical spine in two different patients with cervical fracture. **A,** Fracture through the calcified anterior longitudinal ligament is well seen. **B,** Because the discs, ligaments, and vertebral bodies are "ankylosed," they break off and are displaced as one solid structure.

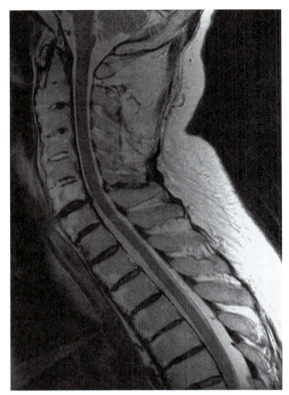

■ **FIGURE 20-3** Ankylosing spondylitis. Sagittal T2W MR image shows abnormal increased signal within multiple contiguous and noncontiguous vertebral bodies as well as abnormal signal in the intervening discs. Anterior syndesmophytes also demonstrate abnormal signal.

structures. Noninfectious spondyloarthropathy does not spread outside the bone and ligament, so evidence of such spread implicates infection. MRI is sensitive enough to detect early inflammation of the axial skeleton in both spondyloarthritis and rheumatoid arthritis.[2]

Radiography

Radiographs are the single most important imaging technique for detection, diagnosis, and follow-up of patients with ankylosing spondylitis.[3] Bony morphology, subtle calcifications, and ossifications are well demonstrated radiographically. Early spondylitis manifests as small erosions at the corners of the vertebral bodies with surrounding reactive sclerosis, findings designated the "shiny corner sign" or "Romanus lesion." Squaring of the verte-

bral bodies is another characteristic feature of ankylosing spondylitis and is caused by a combination of corner erosions and periosteal new bone formation along the anterior aspect of the vertebral body. Squaring is most easily appreciated in the lumbar spine, where the anterior border of the vertebral body is normally concave. Further inflammation is associated with formation of syndesmophytes: ossifications of the outer fibers of the annulus fibrosus that form bony bridges between the inflamed corners of adjacent vertebrae. Ossification also occurs within the fibers of the adjacent paravertebral connective tissue. Ossification of the posterior interspinous ligaments links sequential spinous processes into a solid vertical midline "bone," which causes a dense line on frontal radiographs. In similar fashion, the apophyseal and costovertebral joints are frequently affected by erosions and then ossification and eventually fuse. Complete fusion of the vertebral bodies by syndesmophytes and related ossifications produces the "bamboo spine" (Fig. 20-4). The intervertebral discs may calcify at single or multiple levels, usually in association with apophyseal joint ankylosis and adjacent syndesmophytes.

In established ankylosing spondylitis, fractures usually occur at the thoracolumbar and cervicothoracic junctions. Upper cervical spine fractures and atlantoaxial subluxations are rare. Spinal fractures are characteristically transverse (i.e., horizontal) rather than vertical or oblique and are called "chalk stick" fractures.[3] They extend from

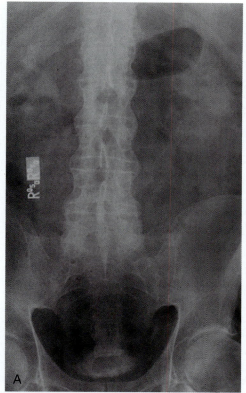

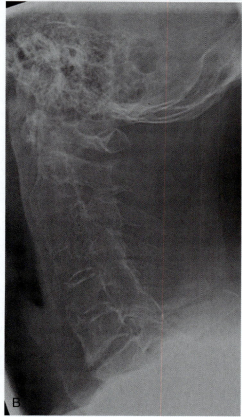

■ **FIGURE 20-4** Ankylosing spondylitis. Lateral radiograph of the cervical spine (**A**) and anteroposterior radiograph of the lumbar spine (**B**) demonstrate confluent ankylosis of the vertebral bodies and facets.

anterior to posterior and frequently pass through the unossified disc.

Pseudarthroses are seen radiographically as areas of discovertebral destruction and adjacent sclerosis. These changes are referred to as the Anderson lesion and may resemble disc infection. Pseudarthrosis usually develops secondary to a previously undetected fracture or at an unfused segment. Therefore, an important imaging feature of ankylosing spondylitis is the involvement of the facet joints, which is seen as a linear hypodense area with sclerotic borders.

The spinal abnormalities found in ankylosing spondylitis may also be encountered in other diseases, such as enteropathic arthropathy, psoriasis, and Reiter syndrome. Careful analysis and classification of bony outgrowths in the vertebrae help to differentiate among these conditions. Flowing anterior ossification is a feature of diffuse idiopathic skeletal hyperostosis. Paravertebral ossification is present in both psoriasis and Reiter syndrome. Syndesmophytes are found in alkaptonuria as well as ankylosing spondylitis.

Spinal pseudarthrosis in ankylosing spondylitis may produce marked discovertebral destructive changes that resemble infective spondylodiscitis. The detection of posterior element fractures or defects is an important distinguishing clue in diagnosing these patients with ankylosing spondylitis.[3] The spondyloarthritides often share common features of aggressive erosions, bone density preservation, and proliferative bony response to inflammation. These features along with asymmetric involvement of the appendicular skeleton, sacroiliitis, and spine abnormalities usually allow differentiation of ankylosing spondylitis from rheumatoid arthritis and other inflammatory arthritides based on imaging studies.[5]

PSORIATIC ARTHRITIS

Epidemiology

Psoriatic arthritis is a unique inflammatory arthritis associated with psoriasis. Its exact prevalence is unknown, but estimates vary from 0.3% to 1% of the population. The prevalence of psoriasis among patients with arthritis in the general population is 2% to 3%. Inflammatory arthritis occurs in 2% to 3% of the general population, but among patients with psoriasis the prevalence of inflammatory arthritis varies from 6% to 42%.[6]

Clinical Presentation

Typically, psoriatic arthritis initially presents as a mild oligoarticular disease. It becomes polyarticular and a severe disease in at least 20% of patients. Patients with psoriatic arthritis who present with polyarticular disease have an increased risk for disease progression. Health-related quality of life is reduced among patients with this disease.

Pathophysiology

The histopathologic correlate of MRI bone edema has not been defined in psoriatic arthritis.[7]

Imaging

MRI

Psoriatic arthritis shares MRI features with rheumatoid arthritis and spondyloarthropathy. On MRI, the synovitis of psoriatic arthritis appears indistinguishable from the synovitis of rheumatoid arthritis.[7] Although in some patients the synovitis observed conforms to a typical rheumatoid pattern, in others the inflamed tissue extends far beyond the joint capsule and involves adjacent structures, such as thickened collateral ligaments and periarticular soft tissue. The erosions themselves consist of a break in the cortical bone overlying a region of altered signal intensity with definite margins. Psoriatic arthritic erosions can be large, ill-defined areas in the subcortical bone with increased signal on short tau inversion recovery (STIR) and T2-weighted (T2W) imaging with fat saturation. They may enhance on postcontrast T1-weighted (T1W) fat saturation sequences.[7]

Radiography

Radiographically, the spondylitis and reactive arthritis of psoriatic arthritis are chunky and asymmetric, as compared with the smooth, fine, symmetric changes of ankylosing spondylitis.[7]

REACTIVE ARTHRITIS

Reactive arthritis (Reiter syndrome) is an acute nonpurulent seronegative arthritis that complicates an infection elsewhere in the body.

Epidemiology

Reactive arthritis is associated with HLA-B27, which is not always present in affected individuals, particularly in the presence of human immunodeficiency virus (HIV).[8] When reactive arthritis occurs in African Americans, it is frequently HLA-B27 negative.

In the United States, the frequency of reactive arthritis is estimated at 3.5 cases per 100,000 individuals.[8] It is reported most frequently in whites. The male-to-female ratio following venereal disease is 5 to 10:1. The peak onset is in persons aged 15 to 35 years. Reactive arthritis is rarely seen in children; if it does occur it almost always follows an enteric infection.[8]

Clinical Presentation

An estimated 1% to 3% of all patients with a nonspecific urethritis develop an episode of arthritis.[8] Most patients have severe symptoms lasting weeks to 6 months. Fifteen to 50 percent have recurrent bouts of arthritis. Chronic arthritis or sacroiliitis occurs in 15% to 30% of patients. Symptoms generally appear within 1 to 3 weeks but can range from 4 to 35 days from the onset of the urethritis/cervicitis or diarrhea. Symptoms include fever (usually low grade), malaise, myalgias (early), low back pain with radiation to the buttocks or thighs, and asymmetric joint stiffness primarily involving the knees, ankles, and feet. Symptoms become worse with rest or inactivity.[8]

Pathophysiology

Reactive arthritis is triggered by enteric or urogenital infections.

Imaging

CT

Paravertebral calcifications may be seen as the initial manifestation of reactive arthritis, in contrast to the syndesmophytes seen in early ankylosing spondylitis. Erosions of the anterior corners of the vertebral bodies are rare in reactive arthritis.[9]

MRI

There is no specific role for MRI in the diagnosis of reactive arthritis.

Radiography

In early reactive arthritis radiographs may show no abnormalities. Two typical findings are unilateral or bilateral sacroiliitis and asymmetric paravertebral comma-shaped ossification involving the lower thoracic and upper lumbar vertebrae.[8]

RHEUMATOID ARTHRITIS

Epidemiology

The prevalence of rheumatoid arthritis is approximately 1% of the adult population in Europe and North America (range: 0.3%-2.1%).[10] The prevalences are higher in some Native American groups and lower in the Caribbean. Worldwide, the incidence is about 3 cases per 10,000 population.

Severe rheumatoid arthritis occurs at approximately four times the expected rate in first-degree relatives of individuals with seropositive disease.[10] Approximately 10% of patients with rheumatoid arthritis have an affected first-degree relative. Women are affected approximately three times more often than men. Disease onset is most frequent during the fourth and fifth decades of life, with 80% of patients developing disease between the ages of 35 and 50 years. The incidence of rheumatoid arthritis is more than six times greater in 60- to 64-year-old women compared with 29-year-old women.[10] Older patients are more likely to have lesions in the lower spine.[10]

Clinical Presentation

Rheumatoid arthritis affects the cervical spine primarily.[10] Abnormalities in the thoracic and lumbar spine are relatively rare. The appendicular joints and the cervical spine are affected earlier and more often than the rest of the axial skeleton. In prospective studies, 83% of patients develop anterior atlantoaxial subluxation within 2 years of disease onset.[10] Features of spinal involvement in rheumatoid arthritis include erosive synovitis, ligamentous subluxation, osteopenia, and vertebral body fractures.[10]

Pathophysiology

Rheumatoid arthritis is a chronic multisystemic disease of unknown cause. Synovitis within the joints of the cervical spine causes destruction of the articular cartilage with direct extension of rheumatoid pannus into the spinal canal.[10] Simultaneous involvement of the ligaments causes laxity and rupture, promoting instability and subluxation. Together, these factors lead to compression of the spinal cord or nerve roots and may even compress the vertebral arteries. Progressive disease can also trigger a cascade of events causing destruction, osteoporosis, instability, and fractures of the vertebral bodies or the posterior neural arches. The entire cervical spine is involved in the rheumatoid process. Changes may extend superiorly to the occiput and inferiorly to the cervicothoracic junction. Specifically, synovial and cartilaginous articulations, the joints of Luschka, tendinous and ligamentous attachments, and soft tissues of the cervical region can all be damaged. Atlantoaxial subluxation is the result of erosive rheumatoid synovitis in the atlantoaxial, atlanto-odontoid, and atlanto-occipital joints and in the synovium-lined bursa between the anterior arch of C1, the odontoid process, and the transverse ligament. Normally, C1-C2 subluxation is prevented by the transverse ligament, which interconnects the lateral masses of the atlas behind the odontoid process and maintains the normal position of the dens. The alar ligaments and, to a lesser extent, the apical ligaments also play a role in stability of this region.[10]

A characteristic feature of rheumatoid arthritis is persistent inflammatory synovitis.[10]

Mediators of joint destruction include phospholipase A_2, prostaglandin E_2, and plasminogen activators. The proliferating fibroblasts and inflammatory cells form a granulation tissue—the rheumatoid pannus—within the joint. The synovial inflammation causes cartilage destruction and bone erosion, which usually involves the peripheral joints in a symmetric distribution.[10] Subsequently, joint deformity occurs.

Imaging

CT

CT is indicated for preoperative assessment of neurologic deficits and severe pain. Subluxations of a degree likely to cause paralysis need to be identified, because better outcomes are recorded with earlier intervention (Fig. 20-5).[10]

MRI

MRI is indicated for abnormal measurements on radiographs (see later), unremitting suboccipital/cervical pain,

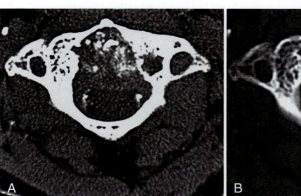
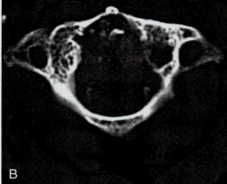
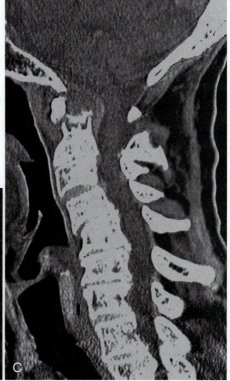

■ **FIGURE 20-5** Rheumatoid arthritis. Axial MDCT images. Bone (**A**) and soft tissue (**B**) windows and sagittal reformatted MDCT (**C**) images of the cervical spine demonstrate soft tissue mass surrounding the dens. There is severe erosion of the dens as well as erosion of the anterior arch of C1. The soft tissue mass is bulging posteriorly and impinging on the spinal canal at the level of the foramen magnum. At other levels note diffuse, severe disc space narrowing and erosions of vertebral end plates.

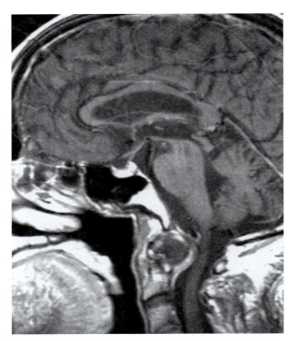

■ FIGURE 20-6 Rheumatoid arthritis. Sagittal T1W MR image enhanced with gadolinium. Peripherally enhancing soft tissue surrounds and is destroying the dens. This extends posteriorly to compress the spinal cord at the cervicomedullary junction.

progressive/severe subluxations, symptoms of cord/brain stem compression, and vertebral artery compression.[10] It demonstrates directly the relationship of the odontoid to the medulla and brain stem and any abnormal signal within the spinal cord. Edema of the cord is associated with a poor clinical status, poor prognosis, and poor postoperative outcome (Fig. 20-6).[10]

Radiography

Plain film radiography is the primary modality for imaging rheumatoid arthritis of the spine. Lateral radiographs in flexion and extension show the sagittal dimension of the spinal canal, any subluxations that narrow the canal, and, specifically, any atlantodental instability. The sagittal diameter of the spinal canal is a better predictor of the development of paralysis than the degree of subluxation of one vertebral body on another. The normal sagittal diameter of the spinal canal from C3 to C7 is 14 to 23 mm.[10] A sagittal diameter of at least 14 mm is critical at all levels in the cervical spine, because 14 mm is the minimum space required to house the normal, uncompromised spinal cord, cerebrospinal fluid, and dura.[10] Atlantoaxial subluxation manifests as abnormal separation between the anterior arch of the atlas and the odontoid process of the axis. Generally, the interosseous interval between the posterior surface of the anterior arch of the atlas and the anterior aspect of the odontoid process should not exceed 2.5 mm in adults.[10] Destruction of the atlantoaxial complex by rheumatoid pannus causes subsequent atlantoaxial subluxation, basilar impression, and erosion of the dens axis. Destruction of the apophyseal joints in the lower cervical segments causes multilevel subluxations and the charac-

teristic "stepladder configuration" in 10% to 20% of patients.[10] In most patients, the subluxations are not fixed in one abnormal position. Rather, changes in alignment can be demonstrated on lateral radiographs taken during flexion and extension of the neck.[11] Rarely, the spinal cord may be compressed by extradural rheumatoid nodules.[10]

SARCOIDOSIS

Pathophysiology

Sarcoidosis is a systemic granulomatous disease of unknown etiology that has been shown to affect nearly every organ system. Osseous involvement occurs in 1% to 13% of patients, typically in the small tubular bones of the hands and feet. Sarcoidosis is usually treated with corticosteroid.[12]

Imaging

CT

In patients with vertebral sarcoidosis, plain radiographs and CT show diverse lytic lesions with or without peripheral sclerosis, mixed lytic and sclerotic lesions, and purely sclerotic lesions. The lesions may be multiple, may extend into the pedicles, and often preserve the disc spaces.[13]

MRI

Sarcoidosis may affect both the vertebral column and the spinal cord. Within the vertebral column, sarcoid may cause lytic lesions with sclerotic borders that enhance on MRI (Fig. 20-7).[13] These findings can mimic widespread vertebral involvement with metastatic disease, infection, or lymphoma.[12] Multiple levels of involvement and sparing of intervertebral discs are suggestive of sarcoidosis; however, precise diagnosis is only possible with histopathologic verification.[13] At times, the intervertebral discs may enhance.[13]

Radiography

Radiographs may be normal or show lytic lesions at multiple levels.[14]

DIALYSIS-RELATED AMYLOIDOSIS

Pathophysiology

Dialysis-related amyloidosis is a recently recognized complication of long-term hemodialysis. Histologic examination of excised fibrous tissues shows that a unique form of amyloid derived from circulating β_2-microglobulin is deposited in the intervertebral discs, apophyseal joints, and ligaments.[15,16] Marked macrophage reaction is observed around the amyloid in severe cases. The amyloid deposition and reactive cytokine-mediated inflammation are closely related to the pathogenesis of destructive spondyloarthropathy.[17]

Dialysis-related amyloid disease most commonly affects the cervical spine.[15] However, amyloid deposition, destruc-

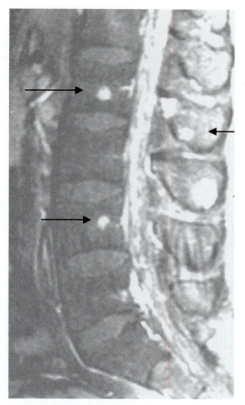

■ **FIGURE 20-7** Sarcoidosis. Sagittal T1W post-gadolinium fat-saturated MR image of the lumbar spine demonstrates enhancing nodules (*arrows*) within the posterior elements of L2 and L3 and within the L2 and L4 vertebral bodies.

tive spondyloarthropathy, and hypertrophy of extradural soft tissues may involve the lumbar spine and lead to compression of the thecal sac and cauda equina.

Imaging

CT

In destructive spondyloarthropathy, CT characteristically shows severe narrowing of the intervertebral spaces, erosions and geodes of adjacent vertebral end plates, and absence of significant osteophytosis (Fig. 20-8).[16]

MRI

MRI shows the extent and distribution of bony, articular, and soft tissue involvement in destructive spondyloarthropathy. MRI also helps to distinguish destructive spondyloarthropathy from infectious spondylitis. Amyloid deposits are not cellular and do not have large amounts of water. In destructive spondyloarthropathy, therefore, the abnormalities at the discovertebral junction have low to intermediate signal intensity, between that of fibrocartilage and that of muscle, on all pulse sequences.[15] Some heterogeneity in the signal intensity may be evident on T2W imaging. Some lesions have signal intensities similar to that of adjacent bone marrow. Inflammatory masses, acute or chronic synovitis, and brown tumors of hyper-

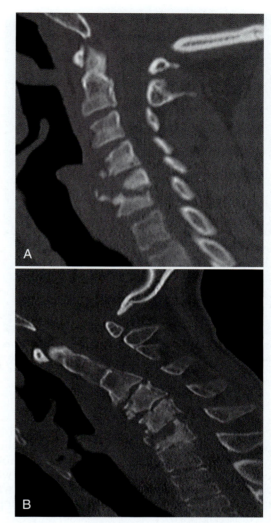

■ **FIGURE 20-8** Destructive spondyloarthropathy (amyloid deposition) in two different patients. **A** and **B**, Reformatted MCDT images of the cervical spine in the sagittal plane show, at multiple levels, severe narrowing of the intervertebral spaces, erosions and sclerosis of adjacent vertebral plates, malalignment, and exaggerated kyphosis.

parathyroidism, however, have long T2 relaxation times and high signal intensity on T2W imaging.[15]

Radiography

In destructive spondyloarthropathy, conventional radiography shows subarticular radiolucent lesions, usually with thin sclerotic margins. In the axial skeleton, a rapidly progressive destructive spondyloarthropathy, commonly involving the cervical spine, may simulate infectious discitis. Characteristic findings on radiographs include progressive narrowing of the disc space, extensive, poorly defined end plate erosions, and modest subchondral sclerosis that may progress substantially over a period of months. The facet joints also can be involved.[15]

ANALYSIS

Sample reports for the entities discussed here are presented in Boxes 20-1 to 20-4.

BOX 20-1 Evaluation of Ankylosing Spondylitis

PATIENT HISTORY

Back pain.

CT

Technique

Axial MDCT using soft tissue and high-definition bone algorithm was performed. Multiplanar reformatted images of the cervical spine were then obtained in the sagittal and coronal planes.

Findings

There is ankylosis of the dorsal and ventral aspects of the vertebral bodies, the uncovertebral joints, the facet joints, and the spinous processes. End plate erosion involves multiple cervical vertebral bodies. There are transverse fractures involving the C4-C5 disc, the inferior end plate of C4, and the superior portion of the C6 vertebral body. There is a fracture through the C2 spinous process and the posterior elements of C4 through C6. The fractured segment from C4-C6 is displaced completely ventral to the remaining cervical spinal column.

Impression

There is ankylosing spondylitis of the cervical spine complicated by post-traumatic fractures/displacements. MRI would be helpful to assess the spinal cord.

RADIOGRAPHY

Technique

Anteroposterior, lateral, and oblique views were obtained of the cervical and lumbar spine.

Findings

On the lateral film of the cervical spine there are bridging syndesmophytes ventrally. There is loss of definition of the facet joints, indicating ankylosis. On the anteroposterior view of the lumbar spine there are "flowing" syndesmophytes along the lateral aspects of the vertebral bodies bilaterally. The sacroiliac joints are sclerotic, and the joint space cannot be visualized.

Impression

Ankylosing spondylitis of the cervical and lumbar spine and the sacroiliac joints is evident.

MRI

Technique

Noncontrast multiplanar T1W and T2W and STIR images were obtained. After gadolinium administration, multiplanar T1W images were obtained with fat saturation technique.

Findings

There is abnormal high T2 signal in the discs from C2-C3 through C5-C6. There is abnormal high T2 signal in the end plates and vertebral bodies of C1 through C7 as well as in the ventral corners of T9-T12. Confluent anterior syndesmophytes extend from C2 to C6, and these have abnormal high T2 signal as well.

Impression

Ankylosing spondylitis of the cervical spine is evident.

BOX 20-2 Evaluation of Rheumatoid Arthritis

PATIENT HISTORY

Back pain; positive rheumatoid factor.

CT

Technique

Axial MDCT images of the cervical spine were obtained using soft tissue and high-definition bony algorithm. These were reformatted to display sagittal and coronal plane images.

Findings

Sagittal reformatted MDCT images of the cervical spine soft tissue windows demonstrate soft tissue mass surrounding the dens. There is severe erosion of the dens as well as erosion of the anterior arch of C1. The soft tissue mass bulges posteriorly and impinges on the spinal canal at the level of the foramen magnum. Other levels show diffuse severe disc space narrowing and erosions of the vertebral end plates.

Impression

Rheumatoid arthritis of the cervical spine with pannus surrounding the dens and impingement on the spinal canal.

MRI

Technique

Noncontrast multiplanar T1W and T2W and STIR images were obtained. After gadolinium administration, multiplanar T1W images were obtained with fat saturation technique.

Findings

There is peripherally enhancing soft tissue surrounding and destroying the dens. This extends posteriorly to compress the spinal cord at the cervicomedullary junction.

Impression

Pannus involving the dens extends posteriorly to compress the spinal cord at the cervicomedullary junction. This may be seen in rheumatoid arthritis or crystal arthropathy.

BOX 20-3 Evaluation of Sarcoidosis

PATIENT HISTORY

Back pain; hilar adenopathy.

TECHNIQUE

Noncontrast multiplanar T1W and T2W and STIR images were obtained. After gadolinium administration, multiplanar T1W images were obtained with fat saturation technique.

FINDINGS

Sagittal T1W post-gadolinium fat-saturated images of the lumbar spine demonstrate enhancing nodules within the posterior elements of L2 and L3 and within the L2 and L4 vertebral bodies.

IMPRESSION

The findings are not specific. In a patient with known systemic sarcoidosis, the findings strongly suggest spinal column involvement. Metastatic disease and lymphoma should also be considered.

BOX 20-4   Evaluation of Destructive Spondyloarthropathy

PATIENT HISTORY

Back pain; end-stage renal disease.

TECHNIQUE

After axial MDCT using soft tissue and high-definition bony algorithm, multiplanar reformatted images of the cervical spine were obtained in the sagittal and coronal planes.

FINDINGS

Reformatted MDCT images of the cervical spine in the sagittal plane show, at multiple levels, severe narrowing of the intervertebral space, erosions and sclerosis of adjacent vertebral end plates, malalignment, and exaggerated kyphosis.

IMPRESSION

In a patient with end-stage renal disease on long-term dialysis, the findings are very suggestive of amyloidosis (destructive spondyloarthropathy).

KEY POINTS: DIFFERENTIAL DIAGNOSIS

- In ankylosing spondylitis, complete fusion of the vertebral bodies, facets, and spinous processes by syndesmophytes produces bamboo spine.
- All the noninfectious spondyloarthropathies are typically confined by anatomic boundaries. They characteristically do not affect adjacent tissue. Therefore, it is often possible to differentiate between noninfectious spinal inflammation of spondyloarthropathy and infectious spondylitis/spondylodiscitis by identifying the extension of infection into adjacent structures.
- Radiographically, destructive spondyloarthropathy is characterized by severe narrowing of the intervertebral disc space, erosions and geodes of adjacent vertebral end plates, and absence of significant osteophytosis on CT.
- Typical changes in rheumatoid arthritis are the destruction of the atlantoaxial complex by rheumatoid pannus with subsequent atlantoaxial subluxation, basilar impression, and erosion of the dens axis. However, gout and pseudogout may appear similar.

SUGGESTED READINGS

El-Khoury GY, Kathol MH, Brandser EA. Seronegative spondyloarthropathies. Radiol Clin North Am 1996; 34:343–357.

Helliwell PS, Taylor WJ. Classification and diagnostic criteria for psoriatic arthritis. Ann Rheum Dis 2005; 64:3–8.

Olivier I, Salvaran C, Cantini F, et al. Ankylosing spondylitis and undifferentiated spondyloarthropathies: a clinical review and description of a disease subset with older age at onset. Curr Opin Rheumatol 2001; 13:280–284.

Rajesh K, Brent L. Spondyloarthopathies. Am Fam Physician 2004; 69:2853–2860.

REFERENCES

1. Peters KM. Non-infective inflammations of the vertebral spine. Z Orthop Ihre Grenzgeb 2007; 145:R1-R19.
2. Bollow M, Enzweiler C, Taupitz M, et al. Use of contrast enhanced magnetic resonance imaging to detect spinal inflammation in patients with spondyloarthritides. Clin Exp Rheumatol 2002; 20(Suppl 28):S167-S174.
3. Peh W. Ankylosing spondylitis. Available at http://www.emedicine.com/radio/topic41.htm. Last updated May 5, 2005; accessed 6/30/2007.
4. Grandbois L, Lomasney LM, Demos TC, Tehrani R. Radiologic case study: seronegative spondyloarthropathy associated with Crohn's disease. Orthopedics 2005; 28:1296, 1375-1379.
5. Calin J, Porta J, Fries F, Schurman DJ. Clinical history as a screening test for ankylosing spondylitis. JAMA 1977; 237:2613-2614.
6. Gladman DD, Antoni C, Mease P, et al. Psoriatic arthritis: epidemiology, clinical features, course, and outcome. Ann Rheum Dis 2005; 64:14-17. Accessed from ard.bmj.com on 6/21/2007.
7. McQueen F, Lassere M, Østergaard M. Magnetic resonance imaging in psoriatic arthritis: a review of the literature. Arthritis Res Ther 2006; 8:207.
8. Scoggins T, Boyarsky I. Reactive arthritis. Available at http://www.emedicine.com/emerg/topic498.htm. Last updated February 15, 2007. Accessed 6/30/2007.
9. Resnick D. Diagnosis of Bone and Joint Disorders, 3rd ed. Philadelphia, WB Saunders, 1995, p 1114.
10. Calleja M, Hide G. Rheumatoid arthritis, spine. Available at http://www.emedicine.com/radio/topic836.htm. Last updated March 28, 2006. Accessed 6/30/2007.
11. Hermann KG, Bollow M. Magnetic resonance imaging of the axial skeleton in rheumatoid disease. Best Pract Res Clin Rheumatol 2004; 18:881-907.
12. Campbell SE, Reed CM, Liem T, et al. Radiologic-pathologic conference of Brooke Army Medical Center: vertebral and spinal cord sarcoidosis. AJR Am J Roentgenol 2005; 184:1686-1687.
13. Poyanli A, Poyanli O, Sencer S, et al. Vertebral sarcoidosis: imaging findings. Eur Radiol 2000; 10:92-94.
14. Lisle D, Mitchell K, Crouch M, Windsor M. Case report: sarcoidosis of the thoracic and lumbar spine: imaging findings with an emphasis on magnetic resonance imaging. Australas Radiol 2004; 48:404-407.
15. Cobby MJ, Adler RS, Swartz R, Martel W. Dialysis-related amyloid arthropathy: MR findings in four patients. AJR Am J Roentgenol 1991; 157:1023-1027.
16. Marcelli C, Pérennou D, Cyteval C, et al. Amyloidosis-related cauda equina compression in long-term hemodialysis patients: three case reports. Spine 1996; 21:381-385.
17. Ohashi K, Hara M, Kawai R, et al. Cervical discs are most susceptible to beta 2-microglobulin amyloid deposition in the vertebral column. Kidney Int 1992; 41:1646-1652.

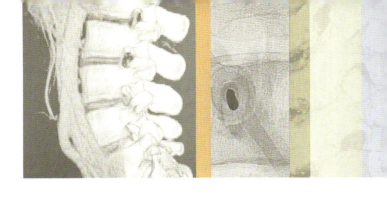

21

Inflammation of the Spinal Cord

J. Keith Smith

Noninfectious inflammatory spinal cord lesions include multiple sclerosis (MS), acute transverse myelitis (ATM), neuromyelitis optica (NMO), neurosarcoidosis, and Guillain-Barré syndrome (GBS). Except for MS, these entities are rare. The disease etiologies are incompletely understood but seem to involve immune system activation as a significant event. Recent discoveries, such as the recognition of a serum autoantibody to the membrane protein aquaporin-4 in patients with NMO, have led to better understanding of these diseases and changes in their classification. It is likely that further changes will occur as these entities are better understood.

The imaging features of these inflammatory lesions of the spinal cord are typically nonspecific and overlap with other conditions such as spinal cord neoplasm, spinal cord infarction, and dural arteriovenous fistulas. The key to differential diagnosis is the extent or pattern of lesion(s) and associated clinical and imaging findings. For this reason MRI of the brain may be very useful in narrowing or supporting the differential diagnosis.

SPINAL CORD MULTIPLE SCLEROSIS

Multiple sclerosis is an inflammatory demyelinating disease of the central nervous system (CNS) with multiple lesions disseminated in time and space.

Epidemiology

MS most commonly presents between ages 30 and 40 years but can occur at almost any age. Females are affected twice as often as males. The incidence of disease varies from 1 per 100,000 in equatorial regions to 30 to 80 per 100,000 in northern Europe and the United States.

Clinical Presentation

The clinical presentation of spinal MS depends on lesion location. The most common symptoms are paresthesia, weakness, gait disturbance, and bowel and bladder dysfunction. Among patients who present with spinal cord lesions, 90% will have brain lesions visible on MRI. The natural history and prognosis of the various clinical forms of MS are presented elsewhere.

Pathophysiology

MS is a chronic, inflammatory demyelinating disease of the CNS. The pathogenesis is incompletely understood. The traditional understanding of the disease process has been that T cells autoreactive to myelin cause an inflammatory reaction, which is followed by recruitment of macrophages and microglia and myelin destruction. More recent studies have highlighted the heterogeneity of MS lesions and the heterogeneity of immunologic mechanisms, which vary with the stage of disease and from lesion to lesion at each stage. Alternative immunologic mechanisms of injury, including antibody and complement activation, hypoxic injury, and oligodendroglial metabolic defects, seem to play a role in many lesions.[1,2] The apparent climatic variation in incidence has stimulated the hypothesis that pathogenesis may be, at least in part, related to infectious agents.

Genetic factors in MS are not well understood. There is a weak familial tendency, and those of western European ethnicity are at increased risk.

Pathology

MS lesions (plaques) show inflammation composed of T cells and macrophages. There is focal demyelination. Axons are usually at least partly preserved.[1,2]

Imaging

MRI is the imaging modality of choice. All patients with suspected spinal cord MS should have an MRI unless it is contraindicated. If the patient with spinal cord symptoms has a contraindication to MRI, myelography with post-myelogram CT should be performed to exclude a cord-compressing lesion as the cause of the symptoms. If patients present with spinal cord symptoms, and a lesion which may be MS is seen on spinal MRI, brain MRI should be performed, because 90% of patients will have concomitant brain lesions.

MRI

The typical spinal cord lesions of MS show high signal intensity on T2-weighted (T2W) images. They are peripherally located within the cord on axial images and occupy less than half of the cross-sectional area of the spinal cord (Fig. 21-1). Typically, the lesions are less than two

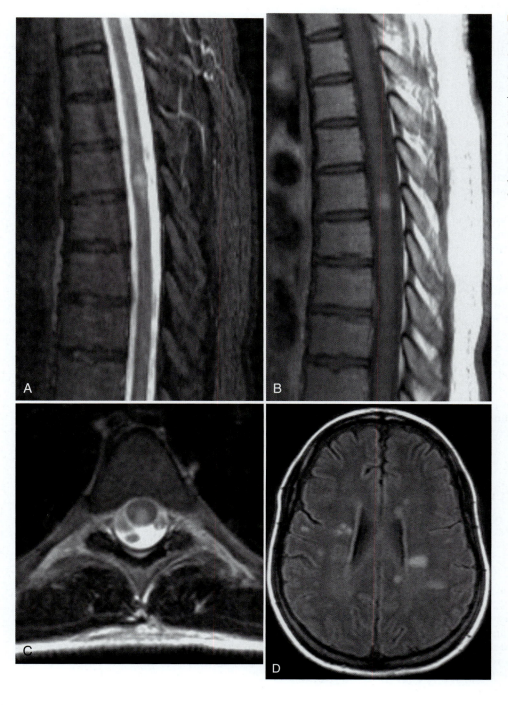

■ **FIGURE 21-1** Spinal cord multiple sclerosis. T2W (**A**) and T1W postcontrast (**B**) sagittal and T2W axial (**C**) MR images of the thoracic spine show a small lesion (less than one vertebral body in craniocaudal dimension) with high signal on T2W image and some central enhancement. There is slight cord expansion, with little surrounding edema. On the axial image, the lesion occupies less than half of the cross-sectional cord area. **D,** FLAIR axial MR image of the brain at the level of the lateral ventricles reveals multiple white matter lesions in the subcortical and periventricular white matter, supporting the diagnosis of multiple sclerosis.

vertebral bodies in vertical length.[3] The extent of T2 signal correlates with the degree of demyelination.[4] On T1-weighted (T1W) images, lesions are isointense to hypointense. There is variable enhancement after intravenous contrast agent administration, especially in acute and subacute (1-2 months) lesions. Enhancement may be nodular, ring-like, or homogeneous. Unlike in the brain, fluid-attenuated inversion recovery (FLAIR) images are insensitive to lesions in the spinal cord. Cord edema and swelling are not prominent. Cord atrophy may be seen in the late stages.

Occasionally, MRI findings are indistinguishable from those of spinal cord tumor, with avid enhancement, edema, and mass effect.[5]

It is challenging to try to apply advanced MRI techniques to lesions of the spinal cord, owing to the small size of the cord and artifacts from respiratory motion, cardiac motion, cerebrospinal fluid pulsations, and motion of the spinal cord itself. In patients with MS, diffusion tensor imaging of the spinal cord shows decreased fractional anisotropy and increased mean diffusivity in lesions and in normal-appearing white matter.[6,7] Several authors report decreased magnetization transfer ratios in MS lesions and in the normal-appearing white matter of the spine.[8,9]

ACUTE TRANSVERSE MYELITIS

Acute transverse myelitis (ATM) is a focal inflammatory disorder of the spinal cord that results in motor, sensory, and autonomic dysfunction. Symptoms should be bilateral, with a clearly defined sensory level. Symptoms should progress, with a nadir between 4 hours and 21 days from onset of symptoms. Spinal cord compression should be excluded as a cause of the symptoms. Inflammation of the spinal cord should be documented by cerebrospinal fluid pleocytosis or elevated IgG levels, or by spinal cord enhancement on MRI.[10] Alternate names for this disorder include acute myelitis, idiopathic acute transverse myelitis, and idiopathic transverse myelopathy.

Epidemiology

ATM has an incidence of about 4 new cases per million people per year in the United States. All ages are affected, but there is a bimodal age distribution with one peak between 10 and 19 years of age and a second peak between 30 and 39 years of age. There is no sex predilection.

Clinical Presentation

Affected patients present with acute or subacute signs and symptoms of motor, sensory, and autonomic dysfunction localizable to the spinal cord. There is usually a clearly defined rostral level of the sensory deficit. The symptoms progress to a maximum between 4 hours and 21 days, with bladder dysfunction, inability to move the legs, and paresthesia and numbness. Autonomic dysfunction is manifest as urinary urgency, inability to void, or bowel or bladder incontinence. Evidence of inflammation within the spinal cord can be provided by detecting pleocytosis or elevated IgG level within the cerebrospinal fluid, or by

MRI that displays spinal cord enhancement after intravenous administration of a contrast agent. Patients with a spinal cord infarction or spinal vascular malformations may have similar clinical presentations and imaging appearances.

Pathophysiology

ATM may occur as an isolated "idiopathic" entity or in association with prior radiation, direct cord infection, systemic diseases (e.g., lupus, Behçet's disease, sarcoid), or nonspinal neoplasms (i.e., paraneoplastic syndrome). When the transverse myelitis is associated with a systemic disease, the pathogenesis varies with the systemic disease. For example, patients with lupus-associated transverse myelitis have CNS vasculitis. Neurosarcoid lesions are often associated with noncaseating granulomas (see later).[11]

Paraneoplastic cases of transverse myelitis may be caused by autoantibodies formed against tumor antigens that are shared with or are similar to antigens found on neuronal cells. Such a pathogenesis can be found in some patients with small cell lung cancer who form an autoantibody called collapsin response mediator protein-5 (CRMP-5-IgG). Females with breast cancer may form an anti-amphiphysin IgG.[1]

A variety of humoral and cellular immune derangements have been proposed as possible mechanisms for the tissue injury seen in idiopathic ATM.[1] In about half the cases of idiopathic ATM there is an antecedent respiratory, gastrointestinal, or systemic illness. These cases are referred to as parainfectious to indicate that the cord injury may have been caused by direct infection of the spinal tissue by the organism, direct cord infection with cord injury caused by immune-mediated damage against the agent, or remote infection followed by a systemic immune response leading to an immune-mediated injury to the noninfected spinal cord.[11] The list of infectious agents associated with idiopathic ATM is long and includes several herpesviruses, *Listeria monocytogenes*, *Staphylococcus* species, and *Streptococcus*. Idiopathic ATM has been associated with antigens against pinworms and even dust mites. ATM has also been reported after various vaccinations. In most of these reported associations, a direct causative effect has not been proven.

Optic neuritis associated with longitudinally extensive transverse myelitis (LETM) (covering more than three vertebral levels) may be designated as LETM or neuromyelitis optica (NMO). This entity is associated with the autoantibody NMO-IgG, which is directed against the cell membrane water channel protein aquaporin-4. This entity is discussed in more detail in the next section.

Some patients who present with idiopathic ATM have MS or will later meet the criteria for MS. In most cases, the spinal cord lesions of MS involve short segments (two or fewer vertebral body levels) and do not involve the cord bilaterally at the same level. Spinal cord involvement with MS was discussed earlier.

Many patients with idiopathic transverse myelitis have elevated levels of non–organ-specific serum autoantibodies such as antinuclear antibody (ANA), extractable nuclear antibody (ENA), or Sjögren's syndrome A antibodies (SSA).

Whether these patients should be considered to have idiopathic transverse myelitis, and how they should be classified, is controversial.

There is no clear genetic defect or inheritance of ATM, although some of the diseases associated with myelitis have an increased incidence in association with certain HLA subtypes.

Pathology

Biopsy is not recommended in suspected cases of transverse myelitis. The histologic description of lesions is mostly anecdotal, with biopsies performed on tumor-like lesions or at autopsy. Principal findings include inflammation and variable demyelination. The inflammation may involve the gray and/or white matter. There is focal infiltration by monocytes and lymphocytes and astroglial and microglial activation. Later in the course of disease, macrophages are more prominent and there may be cystic areas.[12]

Imaging

MRI is the imaging modality of choice for all patients with suspected ATM unless specifically contraindicated. If the patient with possible ATM has a contraindication to MRI, myelography with postmyelographic CT should be performed to exclude a cord-compressing lesion as the etiology of the patient's symptoms.[10,12]

MRI

The MRI findings of ATM are nonspecific. MRI may even be normal during the first 24 to 48 hours of symptoms. Common findings include high T2 signal occupying more than two thirds of the cross-sectional area of the cord (88%) and extending over a length of three to four or more vertebral segments (53%) (Fig. 21-2). Some cases (47%) showed a small area of signal isointense to cord in the center of the hyperintensity on axial T2W images. Spinal cord expansion (47%) and focal, peripheral cord enhancement (53%) after intravenous contrast agent administration may be seen.[13] The thoracic cord is the most commonly affected region.

It is not always possible to distinguish between the imaging appearance of ATM and intramedullary spinal cord tumors. Generally, tumors enhance more strongly, may have a central cavity, and are less homogeneous on T2W images. Tumors more commonly expand the cord and/or deform the exterior contour of the cord. ATM is not usually associated with spinal cord cavity or syrinx, whereas tumors frequently are.[13]

When trying to distinguish between ATM and the spinal cord lesions of MS, the longitudinal and cross-sectional extent of the lesion is important. In most cases, the spinal cord lesions of MS are smaller and peripherally located in the cord. They do not involve the cord bilaterally and involve only short segments of the cord (two or fewer vertebral body levels). Lesions of ATM occupy more than two thirds of the cross-sectional cord area and extend three or more vertebral segments in length.[3,13,14]

Evaluation of the spinal cord using diffusion tensor imaging (DTI) has been reported in patients with ATM.[15] Renoux and associates found decreased fractional anisotropy in areas of T2 signal abnormality in patients with ATM, compared with the spinal cords of normal subjects. Interestingly, they also found areas of decreased fractional anisotropy in normal-appearing areas of the ATM patients' spinal cords, away from the lesions of signal abnormality evident on T2W imaging. In some cases, these fractional anisotropy lesions not visible on T2W images corresponded to the patient's symptoms. This implies that there are significant areas of spinal cord injury that may only be detectable when studied with DTI.

NEUROMYELITIS OPTICA

Neuromyelitis optica is a severe CNS demyelinating syndrome characterized by optic neuritis and myelitis. This disorder is also known as Devic's syndrome, Devic's disease, longitudinally extensive transverse myelitis (LETM), and Japanese opticospinal MS.

Epidemiology

The epidemiology of NMO is similar to that of MS. NMO can occur at any age, but mean age of onset is 38 years. The female-to-male ratio is 2 or 3:1. Compared with MS, NMO makes up a relatively greater proportion of CNS demyelinating disease in people of nonwhite backgrounds. The true incidence of NMO is in question, because the diagnostic criteria are being revised.

Clinical Presentation

The clinical presentation depends on the site of the lesions. Optic neuritis leads to visual disturbance and blindness. Myelitis causes weakness and bowel and bladder dysfunction. For some time after it was described, NMO was considered a monophasic disease, with spinal cord and bilateral optic nerve inflammation, sparing the rest of the nervous system. Many considered it a variant of MS. More recently, the requirement for bilateral optic nerve involvement of NMO has been relaxed. In fact, it is now recognized that many patients with LETM have NMO. Patients with NMO may have demyelinating lesions elsewhere in the brain and still be considered as having NMO. It has also been recognized that most patients with NMO have a relapsing clinical course.[16]

Pathophysiology

Recently, a serum biomarker has been described that is greater than 90% specific for NMO. It is called NMO-IgG. This biomarker is an autoantibody that binds to the membrane protein aquaporin-4. This protein forms the principal water channel involved in cellular membrane water homeostasis in the CNS and is localized to the astrocytic foot processes and abluminal side of blood vessels in the spinal cord.[17,18] Similar to patients with MS, about a third of NMO patients have a personal history of some other autoimmune disease and about half have seropositivity for non–organ-specific autoantibodies. The genetics of NMO

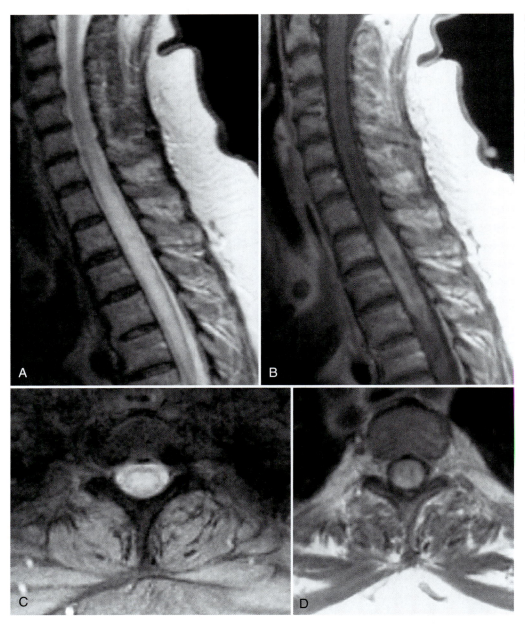

■ **FIGURE 21-2** Transverse myelitis. T2W (**A**) and T1W postcontrast (**B**) sagittal and T2W (**C**) and T1W postcontrast (**D**) axial MR images of the cervical spine show a large lesion (greater than three vertebral bodies in craniocaudal dimension) with high signal on T2W image and central enhancement. There is extensive cord expansion, with significant edema. On the axial image, the lesion occupies the entire cross-sectional cord area.

are poorly understood, but there is a weak familial tendency and about two thirds of NMO patients have a familial history of some autoimmune disease.

Pathology

NMO lesions are characterized histologically by deposits of IgG and IgM along with products of complement activation in a vasculocentric pattern. Affected blood vessels have thickened, hyalinized walls. This vasculocentric pattern of immune complex deposition in NMO patients mimics the distribution of aquaporin-4 membrane protein found in the CNS of normal controls.[19] This immune complex deposition leads to inflammatory cellular infiltrate, demyelination, and, in severe cases, areas of necrosis.

Imaging

MRI is the imaging modality of choice. All patients with suspected NMO should have an MRI unless MRI is contraindicated. If the patient with spinal cord symptoms has a contraindication to MRI, myelography with post-myelographic CT should be performed to exclude a cord-compressing lesion as the etiology of the patient's symptoms.

MRI

MRI of NMO reveals spinal cord and optic nerve lesions (Fig. 21-3). The areas of involvement show swelling and edema with high T2 signal intensity. There may be contrast enhancement.[16,20] The spinal cord lesion is

■ **FIGURE 21-3** Neuromyelitis optica. T2W sagittal (**A**) and T1W postcontrast axial (**B**) MR images of the cervical spine show a large lesion (greater than three vertebral bodies in craniocaudal dimension) with high signal on T2W image and patchy enhancement. There is cord expansion, with edema. On the axial image, the lesion occupies the entire cross-sectional cord area. These findings are compatible with transverse myelitis. T2W (**C**) and T1W postcontrast fat-suppressed (**D**) axial MR images through the orbits show heterogeneously elevated T2 signal and diffuse enhancement of the entire length of both optic nerves, from optic neuritis.

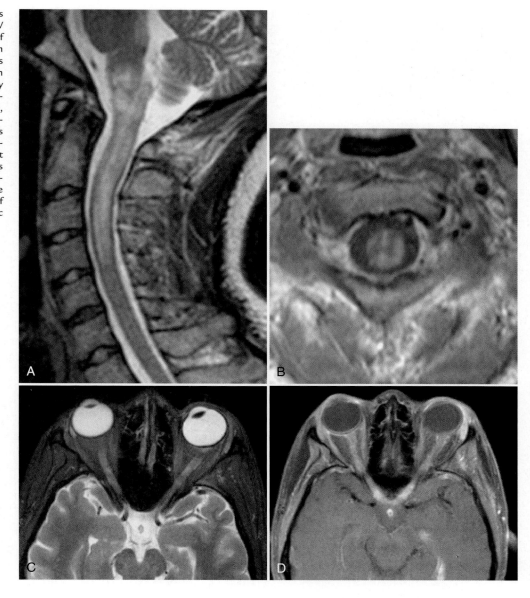

indistinguishable from other transverse myelitides, with high T2 signal occupying more than two thirds of the cross-sectional area of the cord and extending over a length of three or more vertebral segments. Enhancement is variable. Optic nerve lesions may be unilateral or bilateral, with or without enhancement.

The MRI appearance of spinal cord lesions changes through the course of disease. Initially, there is cord swelling and gadolinium enhancement, which resolve over weeks to months. Importantly for the purposes of using formal NMO diagnostic criteria, a longitudinally extensive lesion may later appear to break up into several shorter fragments or shrink to a length of less than three vertebral segments. Therefore, when interpreting cord MRI studies it is important to know the temporal relationship between the scan and the onset of symptoms. If there is a very long cord lesion, this is diagnostically useful regardless of the time since clinical symptom onset. If, however, a spinal

cord lesion fails to meet the three-segment criterion, the neuroradiologist must determine whether MRI was performed during an acute myelitis attack or during a remission period to properly interpret the results.

Brain lesions are relatively common in patients with otherwise typical NMO. Up to 60% of patients studied with serial brain MRI scans over several years after NMO onset developed nonspecific subcortical white matter lesions. Therefore, the presence of MRI-demonstrable brain lesions does not exclude the diagnosis of NMO, even if the lesions meet the radiologic criteria for MS. However, when recurrent optic neuritis, myelitis, or a combination occurs and the presenting brain MRI is normal or shows lesions that fail to meet MS criteria, the likelihood of NMO rises markedly. In many patients, the MRI brain lesions localize to the sites of high aquaporin protein concentration: the spinal cord, optic nerves, hypothalamus, and periventricular region.[16,21]

Using DTI, Yu and associates found that NMO patients had a higher average mean diffusivity and a lower average fractional anisotropy in areas of white matter connected with the spinal white matter tracts or optic nerve and normal mean diffusivity and fractional anisotropy in areas such as the corpus callosum without direct connection to spine or optic nerves. They concluded that secondary degeneration caused by lesions in the spinal cord and optic nerve might be responsible for this abnormality.[22,23]

SARCOIDOSIS

Sarcoidosis is an idiopathic systemic disease characterized histologically by the formation of noncaseating granulomas. The disease affects all parts of the body, especially the lungs and lymph nodes.

Epidemiology

Sarcoidosis can affect patients of all ages and races but is most common in the third and fourth decades. The incidence is estimated at approximately 20 per 100,000 among whites. African Americans and North European whites have the highest disease incidence. Women are more frequently affected than men.

CNS involvement is common in autopsy series of sarcoidosis, with about one fourth of patients with systemic disease showing histologic evidence of CNS involvement. Symptomatic premortem CNS involvement is not common (about 5% of cases). Imaging evidence of CNS disease, however, is seen in about 10% of patients with systemic disease. It is estimated that fewer than 1% of patients have isolated CNS involvement, without systemic evidence of disease. In cases with symptomatic CNS involvement the CNS symptoms are frequently the presenting features. For that reason, it is important for the radiologist to recognize the imaging manifestations of neurosarcoidosis. Unfortunately, the imaging manifestations of CNS sarcoidosis are protean.[24,25]

Clinical Presentation

Clinical symptoms of neurosarcoidosis depend on the site of granulomatous involvement and are nonspecific. Facial nerve paralysis (central or peripheral type) and vision loss are common symptoms, as are signs of meningeal irritation, headache, and seizure. The signs and symptoms of sarcoidosis can easily be confused with MS, including weakness, paresis, paresthesia, diplopia, and dysarthria. Less common are symptoms of diabetes insipidus such as intense thirst and polyuria, stemming from involvement of the hypothalamus or pituitary gland. Hydrocephalus is another uncommon clinical feature. Spinal cord involvement may present clinically with lower extremity weakness and other nonspecific signs of myelopathy.

Pathophysiology

The exact cause of sarcoidosis is unknown. Genetic factors that may confer increased susceptibility to sarcoidosis include the major histocompatibility complex and com-plement receptor gene. The granuloma formation is initiated by T lymphocytes responding to a specific, but unknown antigen. RNA and DNA from mycobacteria and propionibacteria have been detected in sarcoidosis lesions, suggesting a possible etiologic link.[24]

Pathology

The diagnosis of definite neurosarcoidosis is confirmed by biopsy showing noncaseating granulomas, with an absence of organisms or other etiologic agents. In many cases, biopsy is not possible or not desirable, owing to the site of involvement. The granulomatous involvement usually involves primarily the leptomeninges, with intramedullary spread via the perivascular spaces.

Imaging

MRI is the imaging modality of choice, so patients with suspected spinal sarcoidosis should have an MRI unless the MRI is contraindicated. If MRI is contraindicated, myelography with post-myelogram CT can be performed to exclude a cord-compressing lesion as the cause of the patient's symptoms.

MRI

The spinal lesions of sarcoidosis usually appear as fusiform enlargement of the spinal cord in the cervical or upper thoracic level (Fig. 21-4). On MRI, the spinal cord is enlarged with high signal intensity on T2W images, low signal intensity on T1W images, and patchy enhancement after contrast agent administration. Sarcoidosis may frequently involve the leptomeninges or dura, in isolation or in combination with intramedullary (parenchymal) lesions.

Junger and coworkers[26] proposed an MRI classification of intraspinal sarcoidosis in four stages, correlated with possible histologic stages of the disease:

Phase 1: early inflammation shows linear leptomeningeal enhancement along the spinal surface after gadolinium administration.
Phase 2: secondary centripetal spread of the leptomeningeal inflammatory process through the Virchow-Robin spaces shows parenchymal involvement with faint postcontrast enhancement and diffuse swelling.
Phase 3: less prominent swelling associated with less prominent focal or diffuse enhancement. The size of the cord can be normal.
Phase 4: resolution of the inflammatory process with normal size or atrophy of the spinal cord and no enhancement.

Phases 2 and 3 are the most frequent at clinical presentation. This classification scheme is rarely used clinically but is conceptually useful for understanding the different patterns seen on imaging studies. Other findings, such as calcifications, cyst formation, and extradural involvement are rarely found. Preoperative suggestion of intraspinal sarcoidosis may alert the pathologist to look carefully for granulomas and giant cells because sarcoidosis can mimic

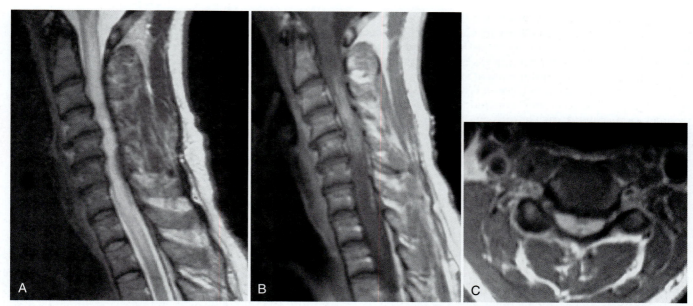

■ **FIGURE 21-4** Neurosarcoidosis myelitis. T2W (**A**) and T1W postcontrast sagittal (**B**) and T1W postcontrast axial (**C**) MR images of the cervical spine show a lesion measuring three vertebral bodies in craniocaudal dimension, with high signal on T2W image and central enhancement. On the axial image, the lesion occupies the entire cross-sectional cord area. The presence of systemic sarcoidosis suggested the diagnosis of neurosarcoidosis myelitis, which was confirmed at biopsy.

neoplasm and lead to misinterpretation of a frozen pathologic section.

Correct diagnosis and early treatment with corticosteroids can minimize the neurologic complications of sarcoidosis and decrease disease morbidity in 42% of cases. MRI shows post-treatment changes or recurrence on follow-up after corticosteroids. Koike and colleagues[27] showed the imaging improvement of intraspinal lesions does not correlate well with clinical improvement.

GUILLAIN-BARRÉ SYNDROME

Guillain-Barré syndrome (GBS) is a clinical syndrome with acute demyelinating polyneuropathy. It is also know as ascending paralysis, acute inflammatory demyelinating polyradiculoneuropathy (AIDP), acute motor axonal neuropathy (AMAN), and acute motor and sensory axonal neuropathy.

Epidemiology

GBS is the most common cause of acute flaccid paralysis in humans. The incidence is 1 to 2 cases per 100,000 population per year, with all ages and races affected.[28,29]

Clinical Presentation

The clinical presentation of GBS is symmetric, progressive motor weakness of more than one limb, with hyporeflexia or areflexia and little or no sensory changes (flaccid paralysis). Paralysis is frequently bilateral and symmetric. Cranial nerve and autonomic dysfunction are common. Respiratory paralysis may occur and require ventilatory support.

Pathophysiology

GBS is an immune-mediated attack on the myelin sheath of Schwann cells of motor (and less commonly, sensory) peripheral nerves. Genetics has not been firmly established, but there is probably an association between GBS and certain HLA subtypes. Frequently, there is a recognized antecedent illness. A number of viral and bacterial infections and vaccinations have been reported to precede development of GBS. The most commonly identified organism is *Campylobacter jejuni*. It is thought that certain lipopolysaccharides found on the outer surface of *C. jejuni* are similar in molecular structure to gangliosides on human nerve cell surfaces. After infection with *C. jejuni,* this "molecular mimicry" causes some subjects to develop antibodies against the lipopolysaccharides that cross-react with nerve cell gangliosides, leading to the immune-mediated attack against nerves.[28-31]

Pathology

Biopsy is rarely performed in GBS. Histologically, GBS is characterized by thickened nerve roots with focal, segmental demyelination. Axonal degeneration may also occur. There are perivascular and endoneural inflammatory infiltrates with lymphocytes and macrophages.

Imaging

MRI is the imaging modality of choice, and patients with suspected GBS should have an MRI unless MRI is contraindicated. If MRI is contraindicated, myelography with post-myelographic CT can be performed to exclude a

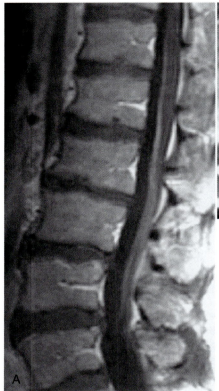
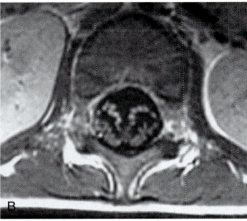

■ **FIGURE 21-5** Guillain-Barré syndrome. T1W postcontrast sagittal (**A**) and T1W postcontrast axial (**B**) MR images of the cauda equina show smooth, diffuse enhancement of the lumbar nerve roots. There is preferential involvement of the ventral roots, which is very suggestive of Guillain-Barré syndrome.

cord-compressing lesion as the cause of the patient's symptoms.

MRI

In patients with GBS, MRI may show slight, smooth enlargement and contrast enhancement of the spinal nerve roots of the cauda equina (Fig. 21-5). There is preferential enhancement of the ventral (motor) nerve roots in most patients, so this pattern is strongly suggestive of GBS.[32] The spinal cord is usually normal. There may be variable pial enhancement on the distal cord surface.

ANALYSIS

Imaging findings of the spinal cord inflammatory lesions are mostly nonspecific and in some cases may overlap those of spinal cord neoplasm or vascular lesions (spinal cord infarct or dural arteriovenous fistula). The key to differential diagnosis is the extent or pattern of lesion(s) and associated clinical and imaging findings. For this reason, MRI of the brain may be very useful in narrowing or supporting the differential diagnosis.

MS spinal cord lesions are commonly multiple, usually do not involve the entire cross-sectional area of the cord, and are usually less than three vertebral body segments in craniocaudal extent. Brain white matter lesions are frequently present at the time of presentation.

ATM is more commonly a single lesion that involves a longer segment of spinal cord (more than three vertebral segments) and occupies most of the cross-sectional area of the cord. Idiopathic ATM is a diagnosis of exclusion,

with other causes of spinal cord inflammation excluded by history, physical, and laboratory findings. Common nonidiopathic causes of ATM include radiation therapy, systemic diseases such as lupus or Behçet's disease, or an association with nonspinal neoplasms (i.e., paraneoplastic).

NMO is a clinical syndrome with ATM and optic neuritis. Diagnosis is supported by presence of serum NMO-IgG, an autoantibody that binds to the membrane protein aquaporin-4. Usually, brain MRI at presentation does not meet imaging criteria for MS. NMO frequently follows a relapsing clinical course.

Neurosarcoidosis may be suspected if there is a history of systemic sarcoidosis or if leptomeningeal or dural involvement is prominent.

Guillain-Barré syndrome may show slight, smooth enlargement and contrast enhancement of the spinal nerve roots of the cauda equina, with preferential enhancement of the ventral nerve roots in most patients. The spinal cord is normal.

KEY POINTS: DIFFERENTIAL DIAGNOSIS

■ All entities discussed may show nonspecific T2 signal abnormality and enhancement.
■ The pattern and distribution of lesions or associated findings may point to the diagnosis.
■ MRI is the imaging modality of choice for spinal cord lesions.

BOX 21-1   MRI for Suggested Neuromyelitis Optica

PATIENT HISTORY

A 34-year-old male patient presented with a history of loss of vision and lower extremity weakness.

COMPARISON STUDIES

There were no relevant comparison studies available at the time of interpretation.

TECHNIQUE

Multiplanar and multisequence MRI images of the brain, cervical, thoracic, and lumbar spine with and without intravenous contrast agent administration were obtained using our cranial nerve II imaging protocol.

FINDINGS
Brain

Both optic nerves are enlarged and demonstrate marked heterogeneous enhancement, involving the intraorbital, intracanalicular, and prechiasmatic portions. No mass lesion or intracranial hemorrhage is present. There is abnormal FLAIR signal noted in the superior cerebellar peduncles, right greater than left, both mammillary bodies, the periventricular white matter in the region of the atria of the lateral ventricles, and the walls of the third ventricle. These areas of abnormal FLAIR signal demonstrate enhancement.

Cervical

Abnormal T2 signal extends from the pontomedullary junction inferiorly to the C4-5 level. The cord is expanded and demonstrates patchy enhancement. This abnormal signal and enhancement involves the entire cross section of the cord from the C1 to C3 level.

Thoracic

The intervertebral discs are normal. No central canal or neural foraminal stenosis is seen. The vertebral bodies demonstrate normal height, signal, and alignment. The thoracic cord is normal in appearance.

Lumbar

The intervertebral discs are normal. No central canal or neural foraminal stenosis is seen. The vertebral bodies demonstrate normal height, signal, and alignment. The conus medullaris ends at a normal level.

IMPRESSION

Abnormal signal intensity is evident with enhancement in the optic nerves and multiple locations of the brain parenchyma, including the medulla and upper cervical cord. These findings are nonspecific, but the pattern and distribution of findings are highly suggestive of neuromyelitis optica.

SUGGESTED READINGS

Byun WM, Park WK, Park BH, et al. Guillain-Barré syndrome: MR imaging findings of the spine in eight patients. Radiology 1998; 208:137-141.

Hickman SJ, Miller DH. Imaging of the spine in multiple sclerosis. Neuroimaging Clin North Am 2000; 10:689, 704, viii.

Kaplin AI, Krishnan C, Deshpande DM, et al. Diagnosis and management of acute myelopathies. Neurologist 2005; 11:2-18.

Smith JK, Matheus MG, Castillo M. Imaging manifestations of neurosarcoidosis. AJR Am J Roentgenol 2004; 182:289-295.

Wingerchuk DM, Lennon VA, Pittock SJ, et al. Revised diagnostic criteria for neuromyelitis optica. Neurology 2006; 66:1485-1489.

REFERENCES

1. Pittock SJ, Lucchinetti CF. The pathology of MS: new insights and potential clinical applications. Neurologist 2007; 13:45-56.
2. Lassmann H, Bruck W, Lucchinetti CF. The immunopathology of multiple sclerosis: an overview. Brain Pathol 2007; 17:210-218.
3. Tartaglino LM, Friedman DP, Flanders AE, et al. Multiple sclerosis in the spinal cord: MR appearance and correlation with clinical parameters. Radiology 1995; 195:725-732.
4. Bot JC, Blezer EL, Kamphorst W, et al. The spinal cord in multiple sclerosis: relationship of high-spatial-resolution quantitative MR imaging findings to histopathologic results. Radiology 2004; 233:531-540.
5. Braverman DL, Lachmann EA, Tunkel R, et al. Multiple sclerosis presenting as a spinal cord tumor. Arch Phys Med Rehabil 1997; 78:1274-1276.
6. Agosta F, Benedetti B, Rocca MA, et al. Quantification of cervical cord pathology in primary progressive MS using diffusion tensor MRI. Neurology 2005; 64:631-635.
7. Hesseltine SM, Law M, Babb J, et al. Diffusion tensor imaging in multiple sclerosis: assessment of regional differences in the axial plane within normal-appearing cervical spinal cord. AJNR Am J Neuroradiol 2006; 27:1189-1193.
8. Filippi M, Bozzali M, Horsfield MA, et al. A conventional and magnetization transfer MRI study of the cervical cord in patients with MS. Neurology 2000; 54:207-213.
9. Hickman SJ, Hadjiprocopis A, Coulon O, et al. Cervical spinal cord MTR histogram analysis in multiple sclerosis using a 3D acquisition and a B-spline active surface segmentation technique. Magn Reson Imaging 2004; 22:891-895.
10. Transverse Myelitis Consortium Working Group. Proposed diagnostic criteria and nosology of acute transverse myelitis. Neurology 2002; 59:499-505.
11. Kerr DA, Ayetey H. Immunopathogenesis of acute transverse myelitis. Curr Opin Neurol 2002; 15:339-347.
12. Kaplin AI, Krishnan C, Deshpande DM, et al. Diagnosis and management of acute myelopathies. Neurologist 2005; 11:2-18.
13. Choi KH, Lee KS, Chung SO, et al. Idiopathic transverse myelitis: MR characteristics. AJNR Am J Neuroradiol 1996; 17:1151-1160.
14. Tartaglino LM, Croul SE, Flanders AE, et al. Idiopathic acute transverse myelitis: MR imaging findings. Radiology 1996; 201:661-669.
15. Renoux J, Facon D, Fillard P, et al. MR diffusion tensor imaging and fiber tracking in inflammatory diseases of the spinal cord. AJNR Am J Neuroradiol 2006; 27:1947-1951.

16. Wingerchuk DM. Diagnosis and treatment of neuromyelitis optica. Neurologist 2007; 13:2-11.
17. Pittock SJ, Lucchinetti CF. Inflammatory transverse myelitis: evolving concepts. Curr Opin Neurol 2006; 19:362-368.
18. Wingerchuk DM, Lennon VA, Pittock SJ, et al. Revised diagnostic criteria for neuromyelitis optica. Neurology 2006; 66:1485-1489.
19. Roemer SF, Parisi JE, Lennon VA, et al. Pattern-specific loss of aquaporin-4 immunoreactivity distinguishes neuromyelitis optica from multiple sclerosis. Brain 2007; 130:1194-1205.
20. de Seze J, Lebrun C, Stojkovic T, et al. Is Devic's neuromyelitis optica a separate disease? A comparative study with multiple sclerosis. Mult Scler 2003; 9:521-525.
21. Wingerchuk DM. Neuromyelitis optica. Int MS J 2006; 13:42-50.
22. Yu CS, Lin FC, Li KC, et al. Diffusion tensor imaging in the assessment of normal-appearing brain tissue damage in relapsing neuromyelitis optica. AJNR Am J Neuroradiol 2006; 27:1009-1015.
23. Yu CS, Zhu CZ, Li KC, et al. Relapsing neuromyelitis optica and relapsing-remitting multiple sclerosis: differentiation at diffusion-tensor MR imaging of corpus callosum. Radiology 2007; 244:249-256.
24. Schlegel U. Neurosarcoidosis: diagnosis and therapy. Fortschr Neurol Psychiatr 1987; 55:1-15.
25. Lury KM, Smith JK, Matheus MG, et al. Neurosarcoidosis—review of imaging findings. Semin Roentgenol 2004; 39:495-504.
26. Junger SS, Stern BJ, Levine SR, et al. Intramedullary spinal sarcoidosis: clinical and magnetic resonance imaging characteristics. Neurology 1993; 43:333-337.
27. Koike H, Misu K, Yasui K, et al. Differential response to corticosteroid therapy of MRI findings and clinical manifestations in spinal cord sarcoidosis. J Neurol 2000; 247:544-549.
28. Yu RK, Usuki S, Ariga T. Ganglioside molecular mimicry and its pathological roles in Guillain-Barré syndrome and related diseases. Infect Immun 2006; 74:6517-6527.
29. Yuki N, Odaka M. Ganglioside mimicry as a cause of Guillain-Barré syndrome. Curr Opin Neurol 2005; 18:557-561.
30. Koga M, Gilbert M, Takahashi M, et al. Comprehensive analysis of bacterial risk factors for the development of Guillain-Barré syndrome after *Campylobacter jejuni* enteritis. J Infect Dis 2006; 193:547-555.
31. Kuwabara S. Guillain-Barré syndrome. Curr Neurol Neurosci Rep 2007; 7:57-62.
32. Byun WM, Park WK, Park BH, et al. Guillain-Barré syndrome: MR imaging findings of the spine in eight patients. Radiology 1998; 208:137-141.

PART TWELVE

Operative Considerations

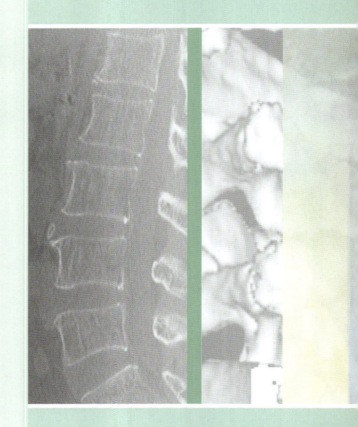

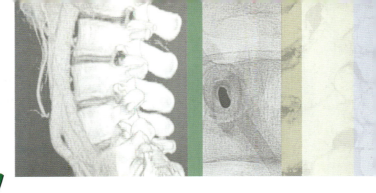

CHAPTER 22

Imaging Preparation for Surgery

Cynthia T. Chin

The spine and the peripheral nervous system remain diagnostically challenging to image owing to the extensive bony canal, relatively small size of the neural elements, and multiplicity of clinical symptoms.

A wide variety of techniques are available for imaging the spine. MRI is the procedure of choice for evaluation of many of the musculoskeletal and neurologic diseases of the spine. The musculoskeletal system includes the vertebral bodies, intervertebral discs, intervertebral foramina, ligaments, and facet joints. The portions of the nervous system evaluated include the spinal cord, spinal roots, and caudal portion of the brain stem and cerebellum. Conventional radiographs, bone radionuclide scans, positron emission tomography (PET), CT, CT myelography, and CT angiography are additional modalities that provide complementary information with indications depending on the disease entity being evaluated—degenerative disease, infection, tumor, and trauma—all of these modalities are instrumental when evaluating the spine in a surgical patient.

DEGENERATIVE DISEASE

Imaging and Pain

Radiographic correlation of symptoms in patients with back pain is a difficult task. A number of findings are not significantly more frequent in patients with back pain compared with controls. Incidental findings may include transitional vertebrae, spina bifida occulta, asymmetric facet joint orientation, facet joint osteophytes, Schmorl's nodes, and increased lordosis.

Demonstrating inflammatory changes and the relationship of pain to disc protrusions on MRI is controversial. No correlation has been demonstrated between the size,

side, or level of herniation and the degree of disability, pain, or frequency of neurologic symptoms, even in patients with concomitant central or foraminal stenosis.[1]

The use of a contrast agent has not clarified the relationship between disc herniation, inflammation, and symptoms. Nerve root enhancement may be seen in symptomatic and asymptomatic patients with and without disc herniations. In one study of asymptomatic volunteers, 53% demonstrated nerve root enhancement that was found likely to be related to caudally draining veins accompanying the nerve root.[2]

A high prevalence of disc bulges and protrusions has been demonstrated on lumbar spine MRI in asymptomatic patients. In addition, Schmorl's nodes, annular defects, and facet arthropathy were also found to be present in patients without back pain. These findings therefore may frequently be coincidental, and a patient's clinical situation must be evaluated in conjunction with the findings on MRI.[3]

Development of functional spine imaging may greatly facilitate the evaluation of spondylostenosis, radiculopathy, and myelopathy and aid the surgeon in the diagnosis and treatment of the patient with spine pain.

Spinal Stenosis

Central Stenosis

Routine Imaging

Central canal stenosis is characterized by distortion or compression of the thecal sac or obliteration of the adjacent epidural fat. This is predominantly due to impingement by osteophytes, facet joints, thickening of the ligaments, and bulging of the intervertebral discs. Although

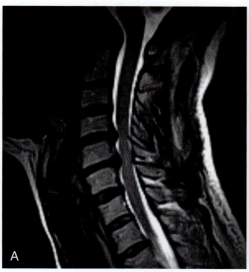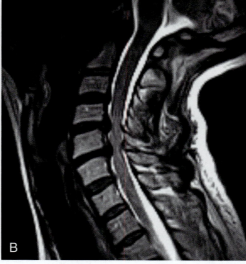

■ **FIGURE 22-1** Cervical upright MRI. Upright sagittal T2W sequences of the cervical spine in neutral (**A**) and extension (**B**) positions demonstrate increase in the degree of canal stenoses and cord compression at C4-5 and C5-6 with the neck in extension. *(Courtesy of Sean Bryant, MD.)*

the size of the central canal has a wide range of normal values and MRI can overestimate the degree of stenosis, specific quantitative data have been published.

Within the cervical spine, the most accurate assessment of spinal canal size can be obtained from sagittal T2-weighted (T2W) fast spin-echo sequences. CT has been considered the study of choice for assessing cervical foraminal stenosis because the margins of the normal foramen, central canal, and osteophytes are so well demonstrated. On MRI, gradient-echo sequences can be used, although there is some degree of motion and magnetic susceptibility artifact. In the cervical spine, the normal diameter of the canal is greater than 13 mm in the sagittal plane.[4] A sagittal measurement of 10 to 13 mm is considered borderline spinal stenosis.[5]

Central stenosis in the lumbar spine has been characterized numerically as an area less than 1.5 cm^2 or an anteroposterior diameter of less than 11.5 mm.[6] In clinical practice, the degree of stenosis is usually described qualitatively as mild, moderate, or severe rather than quantitatively. The thecal sac is distorted from a typically round morphology to a horizontally flattened, oblong shape. In severe cases, a trilobed configuration may result.

Functional Imaging

A limitation in evaluation of spinal stenosis is due to the fact that patients are routinely imaged in the supine position. Routine spine imaging in the static-recumbent position precludes evaluation of the effects of gravity and associated increased mass effect on the spine and discs. Patients experience signs and symptoms during dynamic-kinetic maneuvers. This is not possible to assess with standard conventional imaging of the spine with the patient in static recumbency.

Upright MRI

Open MRI scanners with upright and recumbent imaging capabilities facilitate partial or full weight bearing and simultaneous kinetic maneuvers that can reveal radio-logically occult but clinically relevant weight bearing–dependent disease not visible on a static-recumbent examination and unmasked by positional imaging technique with relative potential decreased sensitivity in demonstrating relevant pathology of central and lateral stenoses (Figs. 22-1 and 22-2).[7,8]

Because upright MRI scanners are not widely available, axial loading devices may be another approach for functional imaging of the spine patient. Axial loading devices apply forces that are a percentage of a patient's weight on the patient's spine. This is done with a harness compression device that the patient wears. The increased axial load simulates the patient in an upright position and may reveal central and lateral stenoses not evident on conventional supine spine imaging.[9]

Central Stenosis and Myelopathy

Cervical spondylotic myelopathy is the most common cause of spinal cord dysfunction in older individuals. Controversy remains in terms of the optimal timing and indications for surgical intervention. It would be of benefit to define clinical and MRI predictors of outcome. A crucial question regarding when to perform spinal decompression relies on the evaluation for myelopathy. When clinical examination and electrodiagnostic studies are equivocal and there is radiographic evidence of significant stenosis, an important question is whether surgical decompression should be performed to prevent irreversible damage to the spinal cord. Conventional radiographic MRI evaluation of spinal cord compromise due to spondylotic changes may be insensitive and relatively delayed. When increased T2 signal is evident within the spinal cord, the patient's symptoms may be irreversible. Intramedullary spinal cord changes in signal intensity in patients with cervical spondylotic myelopathy can be reversible (hyperintensity on T2W imaging) or nonreversible (hypointensity on T1-weighted [T1W] imaging). The regression of areas of hyperintensity on T2W imaging is associated with a better prognosis, whereas the T1W hypointensity is an expression of irreversible damage and, therefore, the

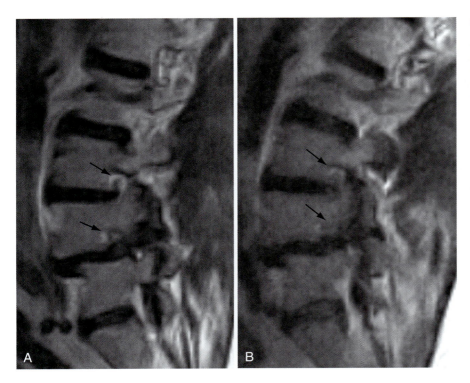

■ **FIGURE 22-2** Lumbar upright MRI. Upright sagittal T2W sequences of the lumbar spine in neutral (**A**) and extension (**B**) positions demonstrate L4-5 spondylolisthesis with increase in the degree of L3-4 and L4-5 foraminal narrowing (*arrows*) with the spine in extension. (*Courtesy of Sean Bryant, MD.*)

worst prognosis. Patients with high intramedullary signal change on T2W imaging who do not have clonus or spasticity may experience a good surgical outcome and may have reversal of the MRI abnormality. A less favorable surgical outcome is predicted by the presence of low intramedullary signal on T1W imaging, clonus, or spasticity. These data suggest that there may be a window of opportunity to obtain optimal surgical outcomes in patients with cervical spondylotic myelopathy.[10-13]

Diffusion-Weighted Imaging

Diffusion-weighted imaging (DWI) is more sensitive and has a higher negative predictive value than T2W imaging for the early detection of cervical spondylotic myelopathy. Because the results of surgical treatment are better in mildly affected patients than in severely affected patients, the diagnosis of cervical spondylotic myelopathy must be made as early as possible and with highly sensitive tools.

DWI has been extremely helpful in evaluating lesions in the brain such as acute infarction, abscess, and neoplasm. The image contrast it provides is dependent on detecting random microscopic molecular water motion, which can be significantly altered in various disease states.[14] Its use in spine imaging is being developed for evaluation of the spinal cord and potential causes of myelopathy.[15]

The lesion formation in the spinal cord is not precisely understood. Increase in pressure from cord compression may induce chronic hypoperfusion, with ischemic or hypoxic injury leading to subsequent vacuolization of gray and white matter. DWI of the spinal cord may be more sensitive than conventional T2W imaging for evaluation of patients with cervical myelopathy and demonstrating

spinal cord changes compatible with an increase in water diffusion and changes in diffusion direction. The underlying pathologic process may represent water increase in myelomalacia, chronic ischemia, inflammation, and cavitation. Changes may be located primarily in the interstitial space where molecules may flow from the subarachnoid space into the central spinal cord or destruction of cell membranes may result in increased water diffusion. Demyelination may also result in increased water diffusion.

Given the high sensitivity and high negative predictive value of DWI, this technique may facilitate decision making and make adequate treatment possible, especially for patients in whom clinical examination reveals discrete symptoms.[15]

Cerebrospinal Fluid Flow

Various hydrodynamic changes occur in cerebrospinal fluid (CSF) flow in cervical spinal stenosis. Dynamics of CSF flow are altered in areas of canal stenosis. Spinal stenosis does not alter the cord or CSF velocities at the C2 level but increases the velocity of CSF in the anterior CSF space below the stenotic segment when the stenosis is assessed by cord and dural sac area measurements. When the stenosis is assessed by relating the cord area to the dural sac area, a statistical correlation between narrow spinal canal and high velocities in the anterior CSF space below the stenotic segment is found.[16,17] Phase-contrast CSF flow imaging and the sensitivity to demonstrate abnormal CSF dynamics in patients with stenoses may therefore be a helpful imaging tool in evaluating patients with stenosis and equivocal clinical examination findings of myelopathy (Fig. 22-3).

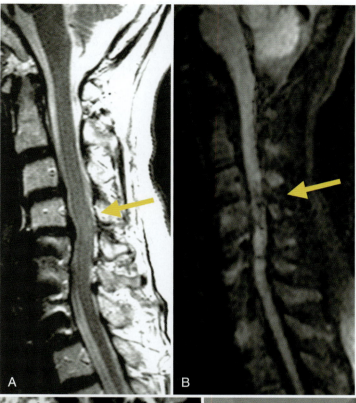

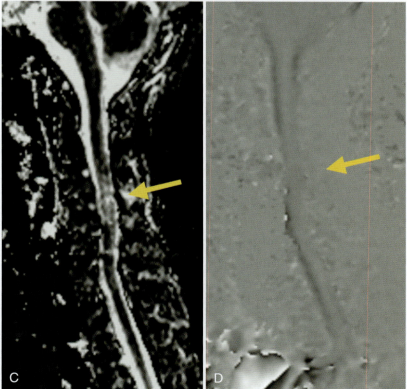

■ **FIGURE 22-3** Cervical spondylotic myelopathy. A 67-year-old woman with myelopathy underwent surgical decompression with clinical improvement. **A,** Sagittal T2W MR sequence of the cervical spine demonstrates C5-7 anterior fusion with adjacent segment stenosis at C4-5 and subtle abnormal increased cord signal. Diffusion-weighted MR image (**B**) and associated apparent diffusion coefficient map (**C**) demonstrate increased diffusion within the cord at C4-5. Corresponding obstruction to CSF flow is identified at C4-5 (**D**) (*arrows*).

Peripheral Stenosis

Routine Imaging

Peripheral stenosis involves the lateral recess and foramen and can occur alone or in combination with central stenosis. The measurement of the lateral recess is the distance between the anterior portion of the superior articular facet and the posterior portion of the vertebral body. A measurement of 4 mm or less is usually associated with symptoms. Foraminal stenosis may be the result of disc bulge, facet hypertrophy, or vertebral body osteophyte encroachment on the neural foramen. Foraminal size is best assessed on sagittal unenhanced T1W images as epidural fat outlines the nerve roots and dorsal root ganglion within the foramen.

In the cervical spine where there is relative paucity of epidural fat, axial gradient-echo sequences are obtained because they demonstrate good contrast between CSF and the neural elements. CT myelography may occasionally show foraminal disc displacement or foraminal spurs that MRI may not demonstrate.[18] The concordance between CT myelography and MRI is high (86%), and MRI is considered to be nearly equivalent to that of CT myelography for evaluation of degenerative disease in the cervical spine.[4,19] In addition, CT myelography provides limited information on the status of the spinal cord and is associated with the numerous risks and potential complications of the invasive procedure. CT myelography therefore is generally used as a supplemental test in patients who are going to have surgery or who have indeterminate MRI findings.[20]

Foraminal Stenoses and Radiculopathy

MRI has been used extensively in evaluation of cervical and lumbar radiculopathy because of its sensitivity in visualizing degenerative changes. However, its specificity is limited because changes may be found in a large percentage of asymptomatic patients.

Preoperative clinical evaluation of the levels to include for surgical decompression may sometimes be equivocal in patients with multilevel disease. Correlation with electrodiagnostic studies is often helpful. Corroborative evidence with imaging of the peripheral nerves and potential detection of intraneural edema may provide important information corresponding to clinically relevant levels of nerve compromise and aid in surgical planning.

Magnetic Resonance Neurography

MR neurography (MRN) is tissue-selective imaging directed at identifying and evaluating characteristics of nerve morphology. Visualization of the fascicular structure of the nerves is made possible by exploiting differences in the water content and connective tissue structure of the fascicles and perineurium compared with the surrounding epineurium.

Standard MRI techniques allow the detection of nerves. However, there is low conspicuity of these structures from the surrounding tissues. The inherent problems of low signal intensity and low conspicuity are addressed by suppressing signal from the adjacent non-neural structures such as blood vessels and fat in muscle and marrow. The use of T2 fat-saturated and inversion recovery sequences allows for optimal conspicuity of peripheral nerves. Standard T1W and T2W sequences can display the anatomy of the adjacent muscle, bone, vessels, and nerves as they are outlined by fat planes. Because of its small size, abnormal signal on T2W sequences within a nerve is often obscured by signal in adjacent fat. Fat suppression techniques are crucial to identifying normal and abnormal nerve tissue. Frequency-selective fat resonance saturation and short tau inversion recovery (STIR) are two common techniques used for fat saturation. The STIR method provides a uniform and consistent fat saturation and maintains high T2 contrast and is therefore more reliable compared with the frequency-selective fat saturation method. The disadvantages of the STIR sequences include a relatively lower signal-to-noise ratio and sensitivity to blood-flow artifacts. Flow saturation bands may be utilized to attenuate the accompanying blood-flow phase shift artifacts.[21]

On MRN, abnormal increased signal on T2W and STIR sequences is observed in symptomatic spinal nerves. This increased signal in symptomatic patients may be seen associated with or without electrodiagnostic abnormalities and may therefore be a highly sensitive technique in increasing the specificity of selecting patients who might benefit most from surgical decompression.

MRN is a sensitive technique for detecting signal change in proximal lumbar and cervical nerve roots compared with standard spine MRI. Among patients with clinical evidence of cervical radiculopathy, significant signal change was observed 2 to 3 cm distal to the site of nerve root compression on STIR sequences in the affected nerve roots.[22]

MRN may be particularly helpful in assessing the structural integrity of specific nerve roots in patients with diffuse anatomic change in the spine (i.e., multilevel degenerative disc or spondylotic changes). Abnormal nerve root signal in this setting draws further diagnostic attention to a specific segment of the spine (i.e., lateral recess syndrome detected by CT myelography) (Fig. 22-4).

Extraspinal Radiculopathy

Conventional MRI techniques may provide excellent visualization of the spinal cord, the central canal, and the neuroforamina in patients with back and leg pain. However, these techniques do not evaluate the extraforaminal lumbosacral plexus and sciatic nerves. In some patients with leg pain resembling lumbosacral radicular sciatica who have normal routine lumbar MRI evaluations, symptoms may be attributable to extraforaminal sciatic nerve injury or compression. MRN may identify causative anatomic abnormalities and direct clinical treatment. In patients with normal routine imaging of the spine and radicular symptoms, MRN may reveal nerve signal abnormality indicating an extraspinal cause for the patient's symptoms, such as sciatica related to compression at the sciatic notch or brachial plexus impingement at the thoracic outlet (Fig. 22-5).[23-25]

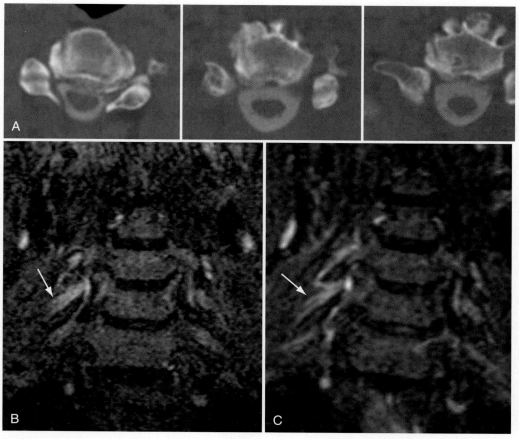

■ **FIGURE 22-4**   Multilevel stenoses. Multilevel severe bilateral foraminal stenoses are demonstrated on axial CT myelography (**A**) in a patient with right upper extremity pain. Preoperative MR neurogram (**B**) demonstrates abnormal increased signal (*arrow*) on the coronal STIR sequence of the cervical plexus within the right C6 root. Postoperative MR neurogram (**C**) status post right C6 foraminotomy demonstrates interval decrease in size and abnormal signal of the right C6 root (*arrows*).

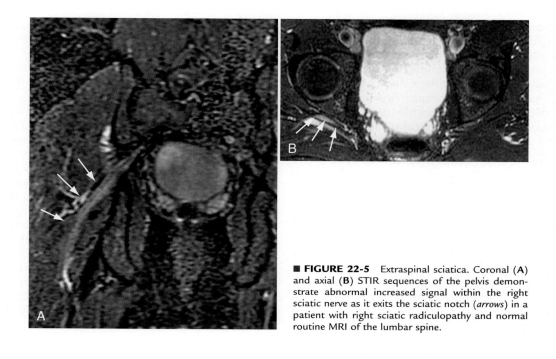

■ **FIGURE 22-5**   Extraspinal sciatica. Coronal (**A**) and axial (**B**) STIR sequences of the pelvis demonstrate abnormal increased signal within the right sciatic nerve as it exits the sciatic notch (*arrows*) in a patient with right sciatic radiculopathy and normal routine MRI of the lumbar spine.

DISC DISEASE

Disc herniation is best depicted by MRI compared with the other modalities. MRI not only provides morphologic information but also improves disc herniation visualization due to better soft tissue contrast of MRI relative to CT. Midline, posterolateral, and lateral herniations are well seen on T1W images owing to displacement of high signal intensity fat in the epidural space and foramen. Plain radiographs and CT are best used to show bony abnormalities.

A normal intranuclear cleft may be seen in the lumbar intervertebral discs beginning in adolescents as a dark, uniformly thin band of low signal intensity within the midportion of normal discs. By age 30, intranuclear clefts are commonly seen in the majority of lumbar intervertebral discs.[26]

With disc degeneration there is disc dehydration and compromise of the annular integrity. These changes manifest as decrease in disc height and decreased signal on T2W images. In severe disc degeneration, the disc may be collapsed and often will contain gas (nitrogen).[27] CT may be more sensitive than MRI in detection of gas in degenerating discs.

Radial annular tears may be seen as small focal areas of increased signal intensity on T2W sequences. Annular tears may enhance after intravenous administration of gadolinium.[28]

On T1W images, the disc herniation appears isointense and slightly hyperintense relative to the intervertebral portion of the disc. On T2W images, the herniated portion is typically more intense than the degenerating intervertebral disc. This may be due to increased water content or granulation tissue infiltrating the disc. With intravenous administration of gadolinium, enhancement is commonly seen peripherally involving the disc margins. This may represent the presence of displaced epidural veins or inflamed epidural tissue. Use of gadolinium does not significantly increase the diagnosis of posterior or posterolateral disc herniations but is helpful in demonstrating lateral and intraforaminal disc herniations.

Free disc fragment or *sequestered disc* refers to a disc fragment no longer in continuity with the parent disc material. These fragments can migrate inferiorly or, less commonly, superiorly relative to the parent disc level and rarely into the thecal sac to become an intradural disc fragment.

Nerve root and thecal sac compression is well shown on T1W images, particularly in the axial plane. The involved nerve root sleeve may have slightly higher signal than normal, and the nerve root itself may enhance with gadolinium, possibly indicating an inflammatory response to disc material. MRI is very sensitive in detecting sequestered disc fragments. Free fragments more commonly migrate inferiorly than superiorly and can be found anterior or posterior to the posterior longitudinal ligament, which is best seen on sagittal MR sequences.

In myelography, disc herniations are demonstrated only indirectly due to thecal sac deformity and individual nerve root sleeve filling defects. Myelography allows upright projections with full weight bearing, which can demonstrate small posterior central or posterolateral herniations that may not be seen on CT. Far lateral foraminal, extraforaminal, and anterior herniations will not be detected on myelography. The sensitivity for detecting posterior central L5-S1 herniations is also relatively poor because of the greater distance between the thecal sac and the posterior aspect of the disc.

Use of Gadolinium

Conditions in suspected degenerative disease in which the use of gadolinium preoperatively may be helpful include differentiating a lateral disc herniation from a nerve sheath tumor in the neural foramen. The disc will not enhance or may demonstrate subtle peripheral enhancement due to an associated inflammatory response.

Postoperatively, contrast-enhanced MRI is valuable in differentiating scar and residual or recurrent herniated disc. Contrast-enhanced CT has not been proven to be as effective as MRI.[29] Epidural scar is isointense with respect to disc on T1W images and relatively hypointense on T2W images.[30] Most discs detected postoperatively at the surgical site do not enhance.[31] Scar tissue within the epidural space enhances homogeneously. Scanning should be performed immediately after the contrast agent is administered. If scanning is delayed, the disc fragment may enhance, which would make it difficult to differentiate scar from disc material. Herniated discs can enhance, although the pattern is one of peripheral marginal enhancement.

The role for contrast-enhanced MRI in evaluation of postoperative arachnoiditis is more controversial. The most common finding is clumping of nerve rootlets in the thecal sac centrally or peripherally. The pattern of enhancement is variable, ranging from no enhancement to intense enhancement of the nerve roots.

Mimics of Disc Herniation

Epidural metastasis may on axial images resemble a disc herniation. The center of the epidural tumor tends to be located away from the disc level. Conjoined roots may sometimes be difficult to distinguish from disc herniations on plain CT but are easily see on MRI. Synovial cysts usually can be distinguished from herniated discs in the axial plane because typically they are located adjacent to the facet and have a peripheral rim of low signal intensity on T2W images.

INFECTION

Intervertebral discitis is an inflammatory condition that can result in disc and vertebral endplate destruction and subsequent osteomyelitis. Associated paraspinal masses can also be present, and 25% may also have involvement of additional disc levels.

Analysis of endplates is important in the diagnosis, differential diagnosis, and follow-up of inflammatory spine diseases. As early as 2 to 3 weeks, an ill-defined vertebral endplate may be seen and is one of the earliest radiographic signs of infectious spondylitis. However, plain films are frequently negative, and at the time of symptom onset only 25% of patients show unambiguous endplate destruction. Reduction of disc height is a relatively early sign that sometimes may precede endplate erosion. Two to 3 months after symptom onset, bony sclerosis can be identified radiographically. Sclerosis, severe disc space narrowing, bony ankylosis, and osteophytosis can be found in healed spondylitis. The radiographic findings, however, are often ambiguous; and complete healing often is confirmed only with stability on long-term follow-up. Both infectious spondylitis and tumors frequently are associated with osteolysis and vertebral body destruction. Tumors almost never enter the disc space, whereas infectious spondylitis results in disc destruction.

The sensitivity of bone scan for the detection of osteomyelitis is high (>90%). The specificity however is poor. The specificity is improved with the use of indium 111–labeled white blood cell scan, but the sensitivity is low (17%).[32] Precise assessment of extent and localization of inflammatory spine processes is not possible, and infection of bony elements and soft tissues cannot be differentiated on these radionuclide studies.

CT is less useful than MRI for the diagnosis of spondylitis. However, it is very helpful for guidance for percutaneous biopsy and drainage of intradiscal, paraspinal fluid collections and abscesses.

MRI is the imaging modality of choice for detecting spinal infection. Infectious spondylitis is characterized by bone marrow edema within two vertebrae adjacent to the involved disc. Although bone marrow edema is the earliest sign of infection, it is nonspecific. The earliest specific sign is evidence of destruction of the vertebral end plate. Disc space narrowing is common, and the signal of the disc is high on T2W sequences. The intranuclear cleft that is present in approximately 94% of normal discs is lost.[26] Osteomyelitis is seen as high signal intensity on T2W images involving the vertebral body. The affected disc and vertebral body typically enhance. The disc space can be totally obliterated in chronic osteomyelitis and discitis.

Healing of spondylitis is often associated with chronic signal alterations on MRI even when there is no clinical evidence of persistent infection. A reduction in the thickness of inflammatory soft tissue may be the earliest sign of healing. A high signal intensity rim on T1W images at the edge of the lesion represents healing; however, this is a relatively late sign, seen at a mean of 15 weeks. After several months, bone marrow in healed pyogenic spondylitis may show a higher signal on T1W images than noninvolved marrow. Degeneration of hematopoietic marrow is likely caused by obliteration of intramedullary vessels, preventing repopulation with red marrow cells. High signal within the disc on T2W images may decrease. Progression of bone or disc changes with increasing destruction does not necessarily indicate failed treatment. Progressive reduction in gadolinium enhancement may be a useful sign of healing.[33]

Infectious spondylitis must be differentiated from acute, inflammatory disc degeneration, which is also known as erosive intervertebral osteochondrosis. The clinical presentation may be similar with severe back pain and progressive symptoms. In erosive degenerative disease, there is bone marrow edema adjacent to the end plates and vascularization of the disc, which can simulate the appearance of infection. Erosive intervertebral osteochondrosis

is likely caused by a rapid disc degeneration without production of the typical osteophytes. Bone marrow edema in erosive osteochondrosis is identified within the two end plates adjacent to the involved disc and is band-like in shape and does not usually extend past the middle of the vertebral body to the opposite end plate. In addition, preservation of the low signal intensity end plate on T1W images can be observed. Within the disc, increased signal on T2W sequences may be seen, representing highly vascularized degenerative disc tissue. With administration of gadolinium, a pattern of band-like enhancement adjacent to the vertebral end plates can be seen as well as focal areas of enhancement within the annulus.[34]

Spinal infections such as discitis and osteomyelitis are commonly seen in clinical practice. Spinal abscesses in the epidural space, paraspinal space, and bone are important complications of spinal infection. Abscesses in the epidural space frequently are surgical emergencies, because the mass effect from the abscesses and adjacent phlegmonous tissues can result in spinal cord compression and permanent neurologic deficit if it is not treated rapidly. Abscesses in the bony structures of the spine can result in bone weakening and spinal instability. Thus, techniques that could help in the accurate and early detection of spinal abscesses are valuable. Diffusion-weighted images could help to increase the conspicuity of spinal abscesses.

Osseous abscess and epidural abscess are hyperintense relative to the surrounding tissues on diffusion-weighted images and hypointense on apparent diffusion coefficient (ADC) maps, correlating with reduced diffusion and findings of previously published reports that describe a similar appearance in abscess cavities in the brain and liver (Fig. 22-6).[35]

EXTRADURAL LESIONS

The most frequent cause of extradural vertebral malignancy is metastasis. Conventional radiographs and bone scintiscans demonstrate marrow abnormalities indirectly. The standard radiograph is not as sensitive to most active bone processes as is the bone scintiscan. As much as 50% of cortical bone must be destroyed before becoming visible on radiographs, and radiographic abnormalities often lag scan findings by weeks to months. The degree of uptake on the bone scintiscan does not correlate with the benign or malignant nature of the tumor being imaged. Most bone metastases show markedly increased production of immature, reactive bone, accounting for the prominent uptake on the bone scintiscan. Bone scintigraphy has excellent sensitivity for detecting metastases from prostate, breast, lung, and head/neck primary tumors. However, metastases that are less likely to induce an osteoblastic response will be less easily visible. These include round cell tumors such as lymphomas, leukemias, and myelomas, which may produce osteoclast-activating and osteoblast-inhibiting factors. In addition, highly vascular or anaplastic tumors (including some tumors of renal, lung, and thyroid origin) may produce little reactive bone and not be apparent on the scan. Slowly growing tumors that elicit little osteoblastic response may also be difficult to detect.

MRI is more sensitive than conventional radiography, bone scintigraphy, or CT in detection of both metastatic

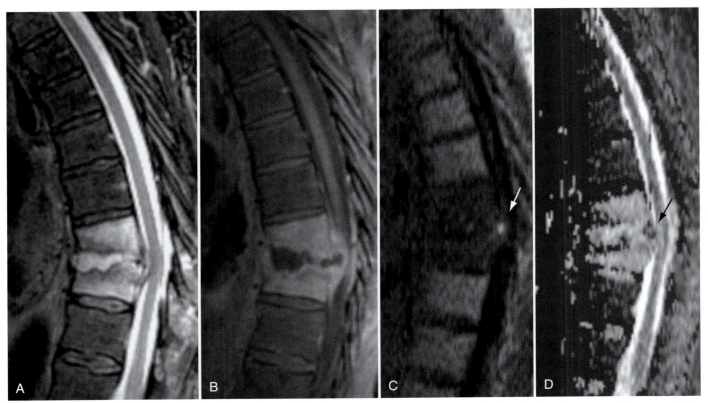

■ **FIGURE 22-6** Epidural abscess. Sagittal T2W (**A**) and postcontrast T1W (**B**) MR sequences through the thoracic spine demonstrate disc osteomyelitis and epidural abscess. There is reduced diffusion within the epidural abscess on the diffusion-weighted image (**C**) and associated apparent diffusion coefficient map (**D**) (*arrows*).

disease and primary malignant bone tumors.[36,37] The T1W sequence is the most valuable sequence in evaluation of vertebral metastases because the high fat content of marrow allows for excellent tissue contrast between normal and abnormal areas. Normal fatty marrow is relatively high in signal on T1W sequences, whereas pathologic processes including metastatic disease will manifest as low signal on T1W sequences. On T2W sequences, lesions may appear hyperintense, isointense, or hypointense; therefore, these sequences play a secondary role to T1W images. Myeloma, lymphoma, and leukemia may manifest as diffuse low signal on T1W images owing to diffuse marrow infiltration.

The use of a contrast agent may not be helpful in vertebral lesion detection. By enhancing the lesion to the intensity of the surrounding marrow, administration of a contrast agent may actually mask vertebral lesions.[38] Contrast enhancement is beneficial in the detection and characterization of epidural, intradural, and intramedullary processes. It should be administered to all patients with a known primary malignancy to exclude leptomeningeal disease and subarachnoid spread, which can occur in isolation of osseous or marrow abnormalities.

Differentiation of benign osteoporotic compression fractures from pathologic vertebral collapse is a dilemma often encountered in elderly patients. In the first 3 to 6 months after fracture, increased water content can be identified in both benign and malignant fractures and is therefore dark on T1W sequences and bright on fat-saturated T2W sequences. Both benign and pathologic fractures enhance and both will take up radiotracer on nuclear bone scans.

In general, a pathologic cause is suggested when there is evidence of adjacent osseous metastatic disease, when there is involvement of the posterior elements, and when there is cortical destruction and associated abnormal soft tissue.

Diffusion imaging in the spine may be helpful in differentiating benign and pathologic fractures with evidence for reduced diffusion manifested as high signal intensity in pathologic fractures and facilitated diffusion manifested as low signal in benign osteoporotic fractures (Fig. 22-7).[39]

INTRADURAL EXTRAMEDULLARY TUMORS

For the differentiation of the various nerve sheath tumors, no consistent radiographic features may be relied on for definitive distinction of schwannoma from neurofibroma on MRI. The importance of the distinction for surgical planning involves the anticipation of gross resection of the peripherally originating, eccentric focal schwannoma around which the nerve fascicles are splayed compared with the relatively more infiltrative neurofibroma through which the fascicles are intimately incorporated and therefore unlikely to be resected without nerve deficit.

The "target sign" on T2W MR sequences has been described predominantly with neurofibromas but can be

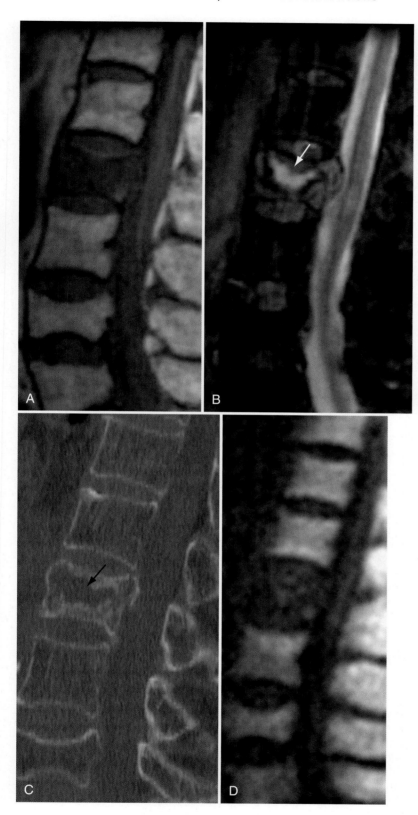

■ **FIGURE 22-7** Benign compression fracture. Sagittal T1W (**A**) and T2W (**B**) MR sequences through the lumbar spine demonstrate an L1 benign osteoporotic compression fracture with associated fluid cleft on MRI and CT scan (**C**) (*arrows*). **D,** There is increased diffusion compatible with benign fracture.

seen with both schwannomas and neurofibromas, demonstrating relative central low T2 signal on the background of higher T2 signal. Pathologically, the correlate may represent central fibrocollagenous tissue and predominant myxoid tissue. In schwannomas, the cellular components are usually distributed more randomly. The majority of peripheral nerve sheath tumors that demonstrate the target sign are benign neurofibromas. When the target sign is seen in schwannomas, it is generally attributed to a central distribution of the more cellular Antoni type A cells surrounded by the relative hypocellular Antoni type B cells.[40,41]

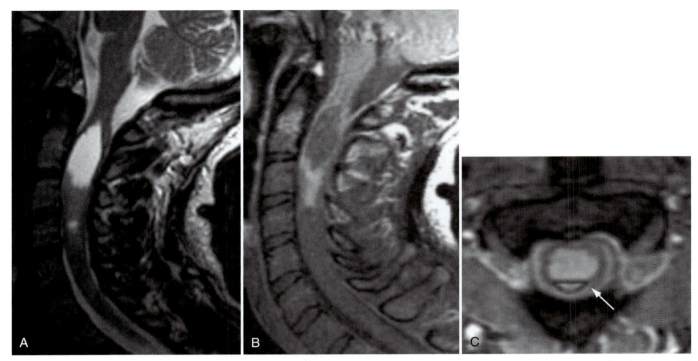

■ **FIGURE 22-8** Ependymoma. Sagittal T2W (**A**) and postcontrast T1W MR (**B**) sequences of the cervical cord demonstrate an enhancing mass with associated hemorrhage and hematocrit level (*arrow*) on the axial gradient-echo sequence (**C**).

Malignant peripheral nerve sheath tumors are difficult to distinguish radiographically from benign nerve sheath tumors. When noted, rapid growth and associated bony destruction may be of concern.[42] CT and MRI are an effective means of delineating lesions and their relationship to surrounding structures, but they are not considered sufficiently accurate to distinguish benign from malignant nerve sheath tumors. Fluorodeoxyglucose (FDG)-labeled PET has limited value in distinguishing schwannomas from malignant peripheral nerve sheath tumors or other malignant soft tissue tumors. Schwannomas generally have a high tumor-to-background ratio with elevated standardized uptake values. The wide range of standardized uptake values for FDG uptake in benign schwannomas appears to be explained by different degrees of cellularity. However, the reason high FDG accumulation is found in benign tumors such as schwannoma remains unclear. Needle biopsy from various portions of the tumor may be necessary to exclude malignancy.[43]

INTRAMEDULLARY LESIONS

MRI is the modality of choice for visualization of the spinal cord. Notwithstanding its unsurpassed sensitivity, MRI has limited specificity and cannot differentiate the wide variety of possible causes of intramedullary lesions.

Neoplasm

The differentiation of neoplastic from non-neoplastic entities is crucial to the surgeon. Three important MRI features in evaluation of intramedullary tumors include the presence of cord expansion, enhancement, and associated cysts. MRI findings may correctly suggest the histologic diagnosis in 70% of cases. However, the differentiation of

ependymoma from astrocytoma is difficult with MRI alone. Spinal cord ependymomas are the most common type in adults, and cord astrocytomas are most common in children. Both entities constitute up to 70% of all intramedullary neoplasms. A central location within the spinal cord, presence of a cleavage plane, intense homogeneous enhancement, and presence of hemosiderin are imaging features that favor an ependymoma. Intramedullary astrocytomas are usually eccentrically located within the cord, are ill defined, and have patchy enhancement after intravenous contrast material administration. Even with these characteristics, it may not be possible to differentiate these two entities on the basis of imaging features alone (Fig. 22-8).[44]

Multiple Sclerosis

Most focal plaques are less than two vertebral body lengths in size, occupy less than half the cross-sectional diameter of the cord, and are characteristically located peripherally.[45] Lesions within the cord are twice as likely to involve the cervical cord compared with the lower levels.[46] When an isolated cord lesion is demonstrated, obtaining a head MRI is helpful for detecting additional lesions and supporting a diagnosis of primary demyelinating disease. However, 10% to 15% of patients with spinal cord lesions have no intracranial disease (Fig. 22-9).[47]

The lesions appear as foci of increased signal on T2W images and possible low signal intensity on T1W sequences. There may be associated cord expansion during the acute phase of the disease and cord atrophy in the late stages. In one series, more than half of cord plaques longer than two vertebral segments were accompanied by cord atrophy or swelling. Cord swelling occurred only in patients with relapsing-remitting multiple sclerosis and in

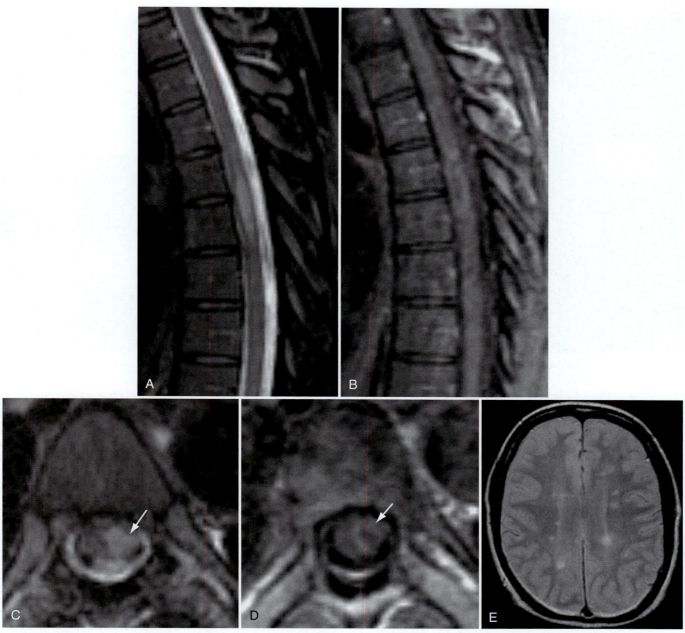

■ **FIGURE 22-9** Multiple sclerosis. Sagittal T2W (**A**) and postcontrast T1W (**B**) MR sequences through the thoracic cord demonstrate a focal intramedullary lesion without significant expansion. Axial T2W sequence (**C**) demonstrates the peripheral location of the lesion within the left hemicord. There is incomplete marginal enhancement of the lesion evident on the axial postcontrast image (**D**) compatible with a primary demyelinating process (*arrows*). Axial T2W sequence through the brain (**E**) reveals multiple deep periventricular and callosal white matter foci compatible with multiple sclerosis.

patients with Devic's syndrome.[48] Diffuse cord abnormalities have been shown to correlate with primary or secondary progressive clinical multiple sclerosis subtypes.[49]

The presence of enhancement appears to correlate with active disease.[50] In very old plaques, there is evidence of wallerian degeneration and iron deposition has been demonstrated at the edge of plaques that may account for some foci of low signal intensity seen on the T2W sequences. There is lack of precise correlation between clinical and MR spinal cord activity because newly detected plaques are not necessarily associated with new clinical signs.[47,48,51]

Acute Transverse Myelopathy

The MR appearance of this acute inflammatory monophasic process is quite variable. Although the regions of abnormal cord T2 hyperintensity can range in size, they tend to extend for three or more spinal segments and, unlike multiple sclerosis plaques, generally involve more than two thirds the cross-sectional area of the cord on transverse images.[52-55]

MRI of the head is useful because approximately one third of these patients will demonstrate intracranial lesions typical of multiple sclerosis. These patients have a high probability of developing clinical multiple sclerosis. It has been shown that in those patients with small, ovoid, enhancing cord lesions without cord swelling there was a high likelihood of developing clinically definitive multiple sclerosis. Those patients who demonstrated long segments of cord swelling with inhomogeneous gadolinium enhancement did not develop multiple sclerosis.[52,54,55]

Subacute Necrotizing Myelopathy

Most cases of this rare progressive myelopathy that occurs frequently in elderly patients are thought to be related to spinal dural arteriovenous fistula (AVF). In an analysis of patients with suspected spinal dural AVFs who underwent spinal angiography, myelography, and MRI, all of the patients who were diagnosed with spinal dural AVFs by spinal angiography demonstrated vessels on supine myelography and abnormal T2 hyperintense signal within the cord on MRI. Gadolinium enhancement was seen in 88%. Mass effect and flow voids were seen in fewer than half the patients. In patients with negative spinal angiograms, vessels were demonstrated on supine myelography in 92%. However, very few patients (17%) demonstrated abnormal cord signal on T2W images (Fig. 22-10).[56]

AIDS

Vacuolar myelopathy is a spongy degeneration in the spinal cord predominantly involving the posterior and lateral columns and is the most common spinal cord disease in patients with AIDS. On MRI, there may be atrophy and symmetric abnormal hyperintense signal on T2W sequences within the dorsal columns over several spinal segments. There is no cord swelling, and characteristically there is no enhancement.[57,58]

Subacute Combined Degeneration

Subacute combined degeneration (SCD) is a complication of vitamin B_{12} deficiency. MRI demonstrates abnormal increased signal within the dorsal columns on T2W sequences. There is corresponding improvement of these radiologic findings along with improvement in clinical function after vitamin B_{12} supplementation.

Nitrous oxide toxicity can also result in a pathophysiologic process and radiologic picture identical to SCD due to inactivation of cobalamin.

Radiation Myelopathy

The incidence of radiation myelopathy correlates with total radiation dose, dose per fraction, and length of spinal cord irradiated. A 50% incidence of radiation myelopathy can be expected if the cord has received between 68 and 73 Gy and only 5% when the cord receives between 57 and 61 Gy.[59] The time course for development of radiation myelopathy demonstrates two peaks: one at 12 to 14 months and the second at 24 to 28 months

MRI findings are variable with no correlation between the MR appearance and the latency period.[59] Less than 8

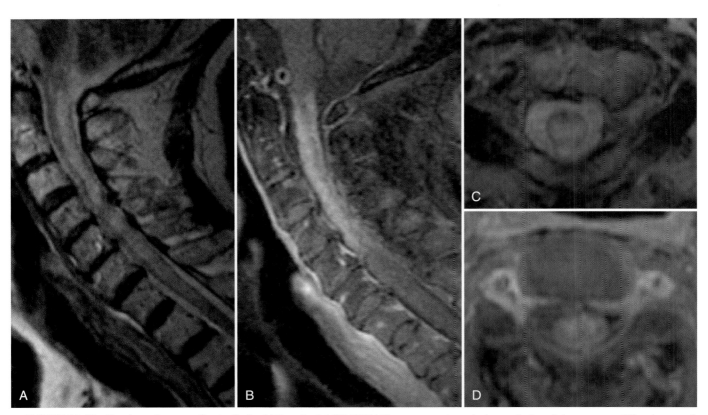

■ **FIGURE 22-10** Dural arteriovenous fistula. Sagittal (**A**) and axial (**C**) T2W MR sequences through the cervical cord demonstrate diffuse increased signal without expansion. There is diffuse enhancement of the lesion on postcontrast sagittal (**B**) and axial (**D**) T1W MR sequences. There was occlusion of the left transverse sinus with associated dural arteriovenous fistula to the left occipital artery.

months after symptom onset, low T1 signal and high T2 signal may be seen within a long segment of the spinal cord, possibly with cord swelling and focal enhancement. Imaging after 3 years following symptom onset usually reveals cord atrophy (Fig. 22-11).

TRAUMA

Plain film radiographs have a high spatial resolution and may be the initial screening imaging tests ordered by many physicians, serving as a guide for further imaging techniques. Plain films are particularly useful in cases of trauma for detection of fractures and alignment of vertebral bodies. In the cervical spine, oblique radiographs may be helpful in demonstrating spurs not seen on MRI. There is a good correlation between uncovertebral spurs and myelographic impingement associated with cervical radiculopathy. In the lumbar spine, oblique radiographs provide an excellent view of the pars interarticularis and detection of spondylolysis. Lateral radiographs in flexion and extension may provide information on spine stability.

CT is the best method for detecting bone fragments and canal compromise in acute spinal injury. Some limitations with CT include the potential to miss fractures in the axial plane and partial volume averaging masking or mimicking fractures.

CT aids in visualizing the C1, C2, C6, and C7 vertebrae, which may be difficult to visualize on plain films. CT is helpful in assessing the degree of cervical subluxation, fractures of the lateral masses, articular processes, and dens.

MRI reliably reveals intrinsic cord injury. Abnormalities in acute cord injury include intramedullary hemorrhage and swelling. In severe trauma, lacerations and cord transections are present. MRI can also demonstrate subluxations, fractures, ligamentous tears, and traumatic disc herniations.

Those patients with acute spinal cord injury and normal MRI findings have the best prognosis. Those patients with cord hemorrhage tend to have the poorest prognosis. Patients with isointensity on T1W images and high signal intensity on T2W images have some potential for reversible change and improved outcome.[60-62] The sequelae of significant cord trauma may be atrophy, myelomalacia, post-traumatic syrinx, arachnoid cyst, and arachnoiditis.

Good quality three-view radiographs (anteroposterior, lateral, and open-mouth/odontoid) of the cervical spine exclude most unstable injuries, with sensitivity as high as 92% in adults and 94% in children. The diagnostic performance of helical CT scanners may be even greater, with reported sensitivity as high as 99% and specificity of 93%. Missed injuries are usually ligamentous and may only be detected with MRI or dynamic plain radiographs.[63]

Common methods for cervical spine evaluation in injured patients are plain radiographs, cervical CT, and functional flexion/extension views. Cervical CT is the most efficient imaging tool in detecting skeletal injuries, showing a sensitivity of 100% compared with a single cross-table lateral view with a sensitivity of only 63%. Functional radiography or MRI is also necessary, because plain radiographs and CT may fail to detect significant ligamentous injuries in 6% of the patients.[64,65]

CONGENITAL CONDITIONS AND MYELOGRAPHY

MRI will demonstrate the abnormalities in patients with scoliosis, congenital cysts, spinal cord herniation through a congenital dural defect, or spinal cord adhesion. However, myelography is a valuable imaging tool in these cases and can more clearly identify the pertinent anatomy and should therefore be considered an important imaging step for surgical planning.

Meningeal Cysts

Meningeal cysts are fluid collections lined with arachnoid that herniate through the dura (diverticula) or within the dura. Most of these are diverticula with communication to the subarachnoid space rather than true cysts and can result in cord compression and myelopathy as well as radiculopathy.

Treatment options include aspiration, fibrin glue injection, and surgical ligation and packing with a myofascial flap. Documenting the presence or absence of communication with the subarachnoid space is important to determine if the patient would be a candidate for nonoperative management as well as the potential for operative care. In the absence of communication with the subarachnoid space, or communication via a narrow neck, aspiration with fibrin glue injection may be an option in addition to surgery. Delayed imaging up to 60 minutes after injection to detect slow filling is an important component to the myelographic evaluation.

Spinal Cord Herniation

The thoracic spinal cord can become anteriorly displaced, or herniated, through a congenital ventral dural defect and result in muscle atrophy, weakness, or Brown-Séquard syndrome. The MRI appearance of an abrupt curvature of the spinal cord associated with absence of the ventral subarachnoid space and an "empty canal" dorsal to the cord is highly suggestive of idiopathic spinal cord herniation. The differential diagnosis includes cord compression by an arachnoid cyst. Myelography is diagnostic in excluding the presence of a cyst and demonstrating the site of the cord herniation. Intraspinal CSF flow studies in which phase-contrast pulse sequence cine MRI is used are also helpful and can display a normal pattern dorsal to the spinal cord (Fig. 22-12).[66]

Scoliosis

In patients with congenital scoliosis, it is important to evaluate for additional associated anomalies. When the scoliosis is significant, MRI is often limited in demonstrating the pertinent anatomy of the cord and filum. Surgical planning involves identifying the termination of the conus and presence of associated tethered cord, diastematomyelia, and fatty filum. CT myelography can be superior to MRI in patients with severe scoliosis in demonstrating the level of the conus, presence of a split cord, and associated bony bar (Fig. 22-13).

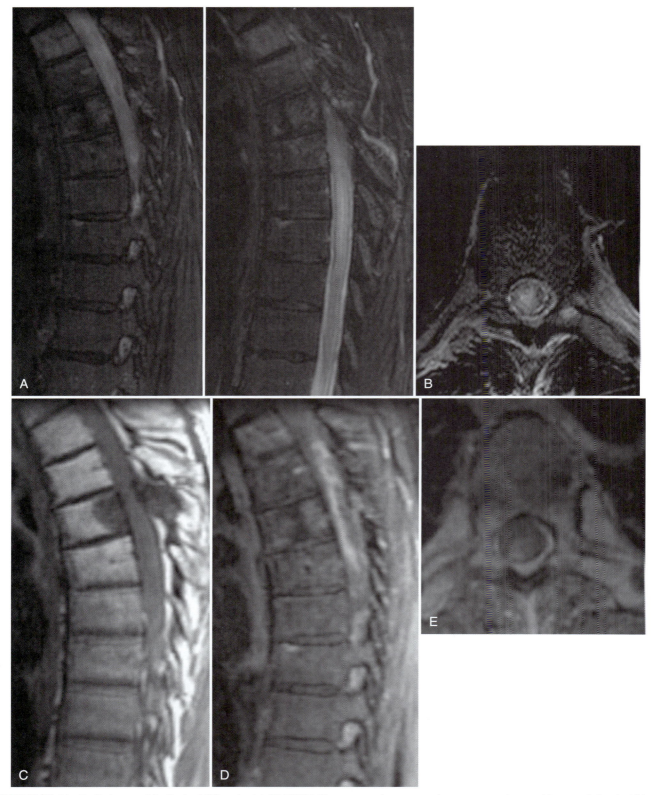

■ **FIGURE 22-11**   Radiation myelitis. Sagittal (**A**) and axial (**B**) T2W MR sequences demonstrate long segment abnormal increased signal within the thoracic spinal cord involving the entire transverse dimension compatible with edema. The precontrast sagittal T1W (**C**) MR sequence demonstrates the osseous metastatic lesion, which was previously irradiated. Sagittal (**D**) and axial (**E**) postcontrast T1W sequences demonstrate enhancement within the cord at the irradiated level.

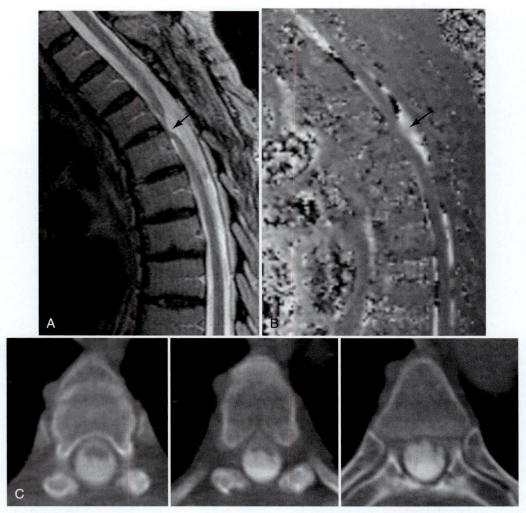

■ **FIGURE 22-12**   Idiopathic spinal cord herniation. Sagittal T2W (**A**) sequence demonstrates herniation of the thoracic spinal cord through a ventral dural defect (*arrow*). Phase-contrast CSF flow study (**B**) shows patent flow dorsal to the herniated spinal cord, confirming the absence of a cyst (*arrow*). Axial CT myelogram (**C**) demonstrates the characteristic morphology of the ventral herniated spinal cord with the "empty canal" appearance.

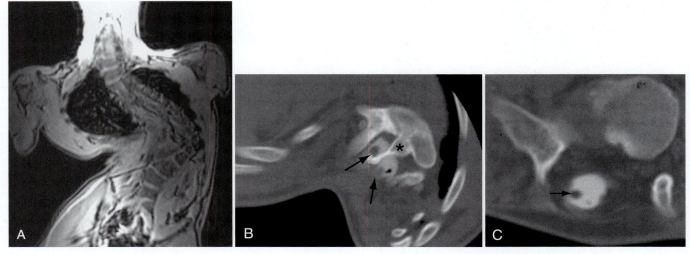

■ **FIGURE 22-13**   Scoliosis. Coronal scout spine MRI view (**A**) shows a severe thoracolumbar levoscoliosis. Axial CT myelogram images show a diastematomyelia (**B**) with a bony bar (*asterisk*) and two spinal cords (*arrows*), as well as the presence of a fatty filum (**C**) (*arrow*).

CT ANGIOGRAPHY

Whereas diagnostic conventional angiography remains the mainstay for evaluation of vascular malformations, recent advances in MR angiography and CT angiography have allowed reliable identification of the artery of Adamkiewicz and are very helpful for preoperative imaging of vascular compromise and compression and displacement by tumor or trauma. Preoperative imaging for identifying the artery of Adamkiewicz may result in significantly lower rates of spinal cord ischemia in patients undergoing thoracoabdominal aortic or descending thoracic aortic repair (Fig. 22-14).[67]

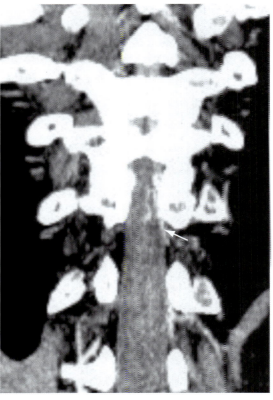

■ **FIGURE 22-14** Coronal CTA demonstrates the artery of Adamkiewicz originating at the left T10 level (*arrow*).

KEY POINTS

■ Dynamic functional spine imaging may unmask degenerative spine pathologic processes not demonstrated on routine spine imaging in the static-recumbent position.

■ Diffusion-weighted imaging may be helpful in evaluation of patients with cervical spondylotic myelopathy.

■ Magnetic resonance neurography allows demonstration of nerve pathology and is useful in evaluation of patients with multilevel and extraspinal radiculopathy.

■ CT myelography is useful for evaluation of congenital spinal conditions.

REFERENCES

1. Jinkins JR. MR of enhancing nerve roots in the unoperated lumbosacral spine. AJNR Am J Neuroradiol 1993; 14:193-202.
2. Jinkins JR, Whittemore AR, Bradley WG. The anatomic basis of vertebrogenic pain and the autonomic syndrome associated with lumbar disk extrusion. AJR Am J Roentgenol 1989; 152:1277-1289.
3. Jensen MC, Brant-Zawadzki MN, Obuchowski N, et al. Magnetic resonance imaging of the lumbar spine in people without back pain. N Engl J Med 1994; 331:69-73.
4. Jahnke RW, Hart BL. Cervical stenosis, spondylosis, and herniated disc disease. Radiol Clin North Am 1991; 29:777-791.
5. Sherman JL, Nassaux PY, Citrin CM. Measurements of the normal cervical spinal cord on MR imaging. AJNR Am J Neuroradiol 1990; 11:369-372.
6. Ullrich CG, Binet EF, Sanecki MG, Kieffer SA. Quantitative assessment of the lumbar spinal canal by computed tomography. Radiology 1980; 134:137-143.
7. Ferreiro Perez A, Garcia Isidro M, Ayerbe E, et al. Evaluation of intervertebral disc herniation and hypermobile intersegmental instability in symptomatic adult patients undergoing recumbent and upright MRI of the cervical or lumbosacral spine. Eur J Radiol 2007; 62:444-448.
8. Wessberg P, Danielson BI, Willen J. Comparison of Cobb angles in idiopathic scoliosis on standing radiographs and supine axially loaded MRI. Spine 2006; 31:3039-3044.
9. Danielson B, Willen J. Axially loaded magnetic resonance image of the lumbar spine in asymptomatic individuals. Spine 2001; 26:2601-2606.
10. Alafifi T, Kern R, Fehlings M. Clinical and MRI predictors of outcome after surgical intervention for cervical spondylotic myelopathy. J Neuroimaging 2007; 17:315-322.
11. Shimomura T, Sumi M, Nishida K, et al. Prognostic factors for deterioration of patients with cervical spondylotic myelopathy after nonsurgical treatment. Spine 2007; 32:2474-2479.
12. Mastronardi L, Elsawaf A, Roperto R, et al. Prognostic relevance of the postoperative evolution of intramedullary spinal cord changes in signal intensity on magnetic resonance imaging after anterior decompression for cervical spondylotic myelopathy. J Neurosurg Spine 2007; 7:615-622.
13. Yukawa Y, Kato F, Yoshihara H, et al. MR T2 image classification in cervical compression myelopathy: predictor of surgical outcomes. Spine 2007; 32:1675-1678; discussion 1679.
14. Schaefer PW, Grant PE, Gonzalez RG. Diffusion-weighted MR imaging of the brain. Radiology 2000; 217:331-345.
15. Demir A, Ries M, Moonen CT, et al. Diffusion-weighted MR imaging with apparent diffusion coefficient and apparent diffusion tensor maps in cervical spondylotic myelopathy. Radiology 2003; 229:37-43.
16. Lee KH, Chung TS, Jeon TJ, et al. Application of spatial modulation of magnetization to cervical spinal stenosis for evaluation of the hydrodynamic changes occurring in cerebrospinal fluid. Korean J Radiol 2000; 1:11-18.
17. Parkkola RK, Rytokoski UM, Komu MES, Thomsen C. Cerebrospinal fluid flow in the cervical spinal canal in patients with chronic neck pain. Acta Radiol 2000; 41:578-583.
18. Van de Kelft E, van Vyve M. Diagnostic imaging algorithm for cervical soft disc herniation. J Neurol Neurosurg Psychiatry 1994; 57:724-728.
19. Frocrain L, Duvauferrier R, de Korvin B, et al. [Comparison of MRI and scanning coupled with myelography in the diagnosis of cervicobrachial neuralgia]. J Radiol 1988; 69:99-102.
20. Zanetti M, Hodler J. [Vertebra pain in advanced age: radiological diagnosis]. Schweiz Rundsch Med Prax 1996; 85:1360-1372.
21. Maravilla KR, Bowen BC. Imaging of the peripheral nervous system: evaluation of peripheral neuropathy and plexopathy. AJNR Am J Neuroradiol 1998; 19:1011-1023.

22. Dailey AT, Tsuruda JS, Goodkin R, et al. Magnetic resonance neurography for cervical radiculopathy: a preliminary report. Neurosurgery. 1996; 38:488-492; discussion 492.

23. Filler AG, Haynes J, Jordan SE, et al. Sciatica of nondisc origin and piriformis syndrome: diagnosis by magnetic resonance neurography and interventional magnetic resonance imaging with outcome study of resulting treatment. J Neurosurg Spine 2005; 2:99-115.

24. Lewis AM, Layzer R, Engstrom JW, et al. Magnetic resonance neurography in extraspinal sciatica. Arch Neurol 2006; 63:1469-1472.

25. Dailey AT, Tsuruda JS, Filler AG, et al. Magnetic resonance neurography of peripheral nerve degeneration and regeneration. Lancet 1997; 350:1221-1222.

26. Aguila LA, Piraino DW, Modic MT, et al. The intranuclear cleft of the intervertebral disk: magnetic resonance imaging. Radiology 1985; 155:155-158.

27. Grenier N, Grossman RI, Schiebler ML, et al. Degenerative lumbar disk disease: pitfalls and usefulness of MR imaging in detection of vacuum phenomenon. Radiology 1987; 164:861-865.

28. Ross JS, Modic MT, Masaryk TJ. Tears of the anulus fibrosus: assessment with Gd-DTPA-enhanced MR imaging. AJR Am J Roentgenol 1990; 154:159-162.

29. Yang PJ, Seeger JF, Dzioba RB, et al. High-dose I.V. contrast in CT scanning of the postoperative lumbar spine. AJNR Am J Neuroradiol 1986; 7:703-707.

30. Bundschuh CV, Modic MT, Ross JS, et al. Epidural fibrosis and recurrent disk herniation in the lumbar spine: MR imaging assessment. AJR Am J Roentgenol 1988; 150:923-932.

31. Hueftle MG, Modic MT, Ross JS, et al. Lumbar spine: postoperative MR imaging with Gd-DTPA. Radiology 1988; 167:817-824.

32. Whalen JL, Brown ML, McLeod R, Fitzgerald RH Jr. Limitations of indium leukocyte imaging for the diagnosis of spine infections. Spine 1991; 16:193-197.

33. Gillams AR, Chaddha B, Carter AP. MR appearances of the temporal evolution and resolution of infectious spondylitis. AJR Am J Roentgenol 1996; 166:903-907.

34. Stabler A, Baur A, Kruger A, et al. [Differential diagnosis of erosive osteochondrosis and bacterial spondylitis: magnetic resonance tomography (MRT)]. Rofo 1998; 168:421-428.

35. Eastwood JD, Vollmer RT, Provenzale JM. Diffusion-weighted imaging in a patient with vertebral and epidural abscesses. AJNR Am J Neuroradiol 2002; 23:496-498.

36. Algra PR, Bloem JL, Tissing H, et al. Detection of vertebral metastases: comparison between MR imaging and bone scintigraphy. RadioGraphics. 1991; 11:219-232.

37. Avrahami E, Tadmor R, Dally O, Hadar H. Early MR demonstration of spinal metastases in patients with normal radiographs and CT and radionuclide bone scans. J Comput Assist Tomogr 1989; 13:598-602.

38. Smoker WR, Godersky JC, Knutzon RK, et al. The role of MR imaging in evaluating metastatic spinal disease. AJR Am J Roentgenol 1987; 149:1241-1248.

39. Baur A, Stabler A, Bruning R, et al. Diffusion-weighted MR imaging of bone marrow: differentiation of benign versus pathologic compression fractures. Radiology 1998; 207:349-356.

40. Jee WH, Oh SN, McCauley T, et al. Extraaxial neurofibromas versus neurilemmomas: discrimination with MRI. AJR Am J Roentgenol 2004; 183:629-633.

41. Banks KP. The target sign: extremity. Radiology 2005; 234:899-900.

42. Pilavaki M, Chourmouzi D, Kiziridou A, et al. Imaging of peripheral nerve sheath tumors with pathologic correlation: pictorial review. Eur J Radiol 2004; 52:229-239.

43. Beaulieu S, Rubin B, Djang D, et al. Positron emission tomography of schwannomas: emphasizing its potential in preoperative planning. AJR Am J Roentgenol 2004; 182:971-974.

44. Koeller KK, Rosenblum RS, Morrison AL. Neoplasms of the spinal cord and filum terminale: radiologic-pathologic correlation. RadioGraphics 2000; 20:1721-1749.

45. Tartaglino LM, Friedman DP, Flanders AE, et al. Multiple sclerosis in the spinal cord: MR appearance and correlation with clinical parameters. Radiology 1995; 195:725-732.

46. Larsson EM, Holtas S, Nilsson O. Gd-DTPA-enhanced MR of suspected spinal multiple sclerosis. AJNR Am J Neuroradiol 1989; 10:1071-1076.

47. Kidd D, Thorpe JW, Kendall BE, et al. MRI dynamics of brain and spinal cord in progressive multiple sclerosis. J Neurol Neurosurg Psychiatry 1996; 60:15-19.

48. Wiebe S, Lee DH, Karlik SJ, et al. Serial cranial and spinal cord magnetic resonance imaging in multiple sclerosis. Ann Neurol 1992; 32:643-650.

49. Lycklama à Nijeholt GJ, Barkhof F, Scheltens P, et al. MR of the spinal cord in multiple sclerosis: relation to clinical subtype and disability. AJNR Am J Neuroradiol 1997; 18:1041-1048.

50. Poser CM, Paty DW, Scheinberg L, et al. New diagnostic criteria for multiple sclerosis: guidelines for research protocols. Ann Neurol 1983; 13:227-231.

51. Trop I, Bourgouin PM, Lapierre Y, et al. Multiple sclerosis of the spinal cord: diagnosis and follow-up with contrast-enhanced MR and correlation with clinical activity. AJNR Am J Neuroradiol 1998; 19:1025-1033.

52. Campi A, Filippi M, Comi G, et al. Acute transverse myelopathy: spinal and cranial MR study with clinical follow-up. AJNR Am J Neuroradiol 1995; 16:115-123.

53. Choi KH, Lee KS, Chung SO, et al. Idiopathic transverse myelitis: MR characteristics. AJNR Am J Neuroradiol 1996; 17:1151-1160.

54. Holtas S, Basibuyuk N, Fredriksson K. MRI in acute transverse myelopathy. Neuroradiology 1993; 35:221-226.

55. Tartaglino LM, Flanders AE, Rapoport RJ. Intramedullary causes of myelopathy. Semin Ultrasound CT MR 1994; 15:158-188.

56. Gilbertson JR, Miller GM, Goldman MS, Marsh WR. Spinal dural arteriovenous fistulas: MR and myelographic findings. AJNR Am J Neuroradiol 1995; 16:2049-2057.

57. Chong J, Di Rocco A, Tagliati M, et al. MR findings in AIDS-associated myelopathy. AJNR Am J Neuroradiol 1999; 20:1412-1416.

58. Sartoretti-Schefer S, Blattler T, Wichmann W. Spinal MRI in vacuolar myelopathy, and correlation with histopathological findings. Neuroradiology 1997; 39:865-869.

59. Marcus RB Jr, Million RR. The incidence of myelitis after irradiation of the cervical spinal cord. Int J Radiat Oncol Biol Phys 1990; 19:3-8.

60. Schaefer DM, Flanders A, Northrup BE, et al. Magnetic resonance imaging of acute cervical spine trauma: correlation with severity of neurologic injury. Spine 1989; 14:1090-1095.

61. Flanders AE, Schaefer DM, Doan HT, et al. Acute cervical spine trauma: correlation of MR imaging findings with degree of neurologic deficit. Radiology 1990; 177:25-33.

62. Silberstein M, Tress BM, Hennessy O. Prediction of neurologic outcome in acute spinal cord injury: the role of CT and MR. AJNR Am J Neuroradiol 1992; 13:1597-1608.

63. Sciubba DM, McLoughlin GS, Gokaslan ZL, et al. Are computed tomography scans adequate in assessing cervical spine pain following blunt trauma? Emerg Med J 2007; 24:803-804.

64. Platzer P, Jaindl M, Thalhammer G, et al. Clearing the cervical spine in critically injured patients: a comprehensive C-spine protocol to avoid unnecessary delays in diagnosis. Eur Spine J 2006; 15: 1801-1810.

65. Goradia D, Linnau KF, Cohen WA, et al. Correlation of MR imaging findings with intraoperative findings after cervical spine trauma. AJNR Am J Neuroradiol 2007; 28:209-215.

66. Miyake S, Tamaki N, Nagashima T, et al. Idiopathic spinal cord herniation: report of two cases and review of the literature. J Neurosurg 1998; 88:331-335.

67. Yoshioka K, Niinuma H, Ehara S, et al. MR angiography and CT angiography of the artery of Adamkiewicz: state of the art. RadioGraphics 2006; 26(Suppl 1):S63-S73.

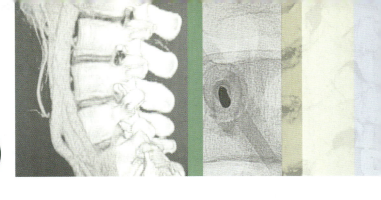

CHAPTER 23

Intraoperative Neurophysiologic Monitoring

Donald Jacob Weisz

First described more than 40 years ago,[1,2] intraoperative neurophysiologic monitoring (IONM) is now used routinely in many surgical procedures that carry risk to the brain, spinal cord, and peripheral nervous system. These include closure of intracranial aneurysms and arteriovenous malformations; resections of intracranial tumors; repair of carotid artery disease; relief of spinal compressions caused by degenerative spondylosis, tumor, or trauma; and treatment of spinal vascular malformations. IONM is particularly useful (1) to detect potential problems that may be addressed intraoperatively before irreversible complications occur; (2) to differentiate neural tissue from non-neural tissue before the tissue is cut (e.g., a nerve hidden by or within tumor); (3) to determine whether a planned maneuver or procedure can be accomplished safely (e.g., balloon test occlusion before embolization); and (4) to identify a maneuver or event that may have led to an intraoperative complication (i.e., as a tool for retrospective analysis).

IONM is also used in radiology suites to detect reversible events during endovascular procedures.[3] This chapter provides a general overview of IONM by identifying the types of neurophysiologic signals that can be recorded intraoperatively, including the pathways that generate the signals, by identifying the procedures that now use IONM routinely and how IONM is used in those procedures, and by addressing the increasing use of IONM in endovascular procedures.

MONITORED NEUROPHYSIOLOGIC ACTIVITIES

The neurophysiologic activities used for IONM can be considered in three major categories:

1. *Monitoring sensory systems:* assessing neurophysiologic activity elicited by stimulation of one of the sensory systems
2. *Monitoring motor systems:* assessing electromyographic (EMG) and neurophysiologic activity elicited by activation of descending and segmental motor pathways
3. *Monitoring locally generated activity:* assessing electroencephalograms (EEGs) and extracellular neuronal spikes

Monitoring Sensory Systems

Somatosensory Evoked Potentials (SSEPs)

SSEPs are elicited by the averaging of neural responses to electrical stimuli that are applied to peripheral nerves.[4] Averaging is necessary for sensory evoked potentials because the response to each stimulus is small relative to background electrical activity. Typical stimulation sites for intraoperative SSEPs are the median or ulnar nerve at the wrist and the posterior tibial nerve at the ankle or knee. Recordings are typically made at both peripheral sites (to verify that the stimulation is constant) and central sites in the spinal cord and brain.

The pathway for upper limb SSEPs includes the ulnar (or median) nerve, the brachial plexus, the tractus cuneatus in the posterior column of the cervical cord, the nucleus cuneatus, the medial lemniscus, the ventral posterior nucleus of the thalamus, the thalamocortical radiations, and the primary somatosensory cortex along the lateral convexity of the anterior parietal lobe. Recordings are typically made at Erb's point (located on the side of the neck, 2 to 3 cm above the clavicle, at the lateral root of the brachial plexus), the cervical spine, and the scalp overlying the somatosensory cortex.

The pathway for lower limb SSEPs includes the posterior tibial nerve (usually stimulated at the ankle), the tractus gracilis in the posterior column of the thoracic and cervical spinal cord, the nucleus gracilis, the medial lemniscus, the ventral posterior nucleus of the thalamus, the thalamocortical radiations, and the primary somatosensory cortex along the midline. Potentials are typically recorded at many locations, including the popliteal fossa, lumbar spine, and scalp overlying the leg region of the somatosensory cortex.

SSEP monitoring is widely used, because it is sensitive to ischemia; responsive to physical manipulation of peripheral nerves, spinal cord, and parietal cortex; and can be elicited easily. SSEPs and EEGs are the two neurophysiologic recordings used most widely during surgery.

Auditory Brain Stem–Evoked Responses (BAERs)

BAERs are elicited by the presentation of brief auditory clicks to the ear. The auditory pathway includes the cochlea, the cochlear nerve, and multiple pathways through the lower pons, the lateral lemniscus, and the inferior colliculus of the midbrain. Auditory potentials above the midbrain cannot be recorded in the operating room because these potentials are suppressed by general anesthesia. BAERs are very sensitive to both stretch and compression of the cochlear nerve. Mild to moderate stretch results in increased latency with smaller effects on amplitude. Compression typically reduces the amplitude of the BAERs in a graded manner.

Visual Evoked Responses (VEPs)

VEPs are elicited by either flashes of a strobe light positioned 20 to 30 cm in front of a patient's eyes or by flashes from light-emitting diodes (LEDs) embedded in eye goggles. The flashes activate, sequentially, the layers of the retina (yielding an electroretinogram), the fibers in the optic nerve and tract, the lateral geniculate nucleus in the thalamus, and the visual cortex in the occipital lobe. Although VEPs are a staple of diagnostic neurophysiology laboratories, they are infrequently used in the operating room. Reasons for this include the low number of cases in which the visual system is at risk, the high sensitivity of VEPs to changing levels of anesthesia, and the substantial variability of their amplitudes intraoperatively. Nevertheless, VEPs can be useful in cases of tumor resection in or near visual structures and in cases involving the posterior circulation of the brain.

Monitoring the Motor System

Motor Evoked Potentials (MEPs)

MEPs are elicited by transcranial electrical stimulators that deliver trains of high energy, which are closely spaced electrical pulses. In *normal* patients, such multi-pulse transcranial electrical stimulation can evoke muscle contractions (despite the general anesthesia) by facilitating the motor neurons in the spinal cord. In *patients with*

significant paresis, however, monitoring of the motor system may require more invasive epidural recording, if it can be accomplished at all.

MEPs are typically recorded bilaterally from muscles in both hands and both legs during spine surgery even if the surgical site is below the cervical spine. The MEPs from the hand muscles serve as controls for systemic factors during thoracic or lumbar surgery. MEPs do not require signal averaging, because MEPs are large relative to ongoing background muscle activity. Direct spinal cord recordings are used much less frequently than are MEPs from muscle, but direct recordings are extremely helpful during invasive spinal cord surgeries (e.g., resection of intramedullary spinal cord tumors[5]).

Free-Run and Electrically Triggered EMG

Transcranial electrical stimulation activates only a small fraction (<5%) of the motor fibers in any muscle. That is, the vast majority of motor neurons in the cord are not monitored by transcranial MEPs. Many additional techniques have been employed to improve monitoring of motor function in the spinal cord and motor nerve roots.[6] Each of these involves the recording of either free-run or electrically triggered EMG.

Free-run EMG can be monitored continuously during surgeries or procedures that place cranial or peripheral motor nerves at risk. Transient discharges of EMG may signal that a motor nerve has been mechanically manipulated or has experienced trauma, particularly when specific patterns of EMG activity are seen in the records (e.g., neurotonic discharges). EMG that is elicited by electrical stimulation of nerves, nerve roots, or descending fiber tracts can be monitored to (1) discriminate nervous system from non–nervous system tissue (e.g., during tumor resection); (2) monitor the integrity of a pathway at risk by repeatedly measuring the threshold stimulation necessary to elicit a motor response (e.g., the facial nerve during resection of acoustic neuroma); (3) determine if an implanted device impinges dangerously close to a motor nerve or root (e.g., during pedicle screw placement), and (4) test the integrity of reflex arcs by stimulating sensory input and recording reflexive motor responses (e.g., Hoffmann reflex). The Hoffmann reflex is elicited by electrically stimulating the sensory nerve at the knee that contains 1a afferents from muscle spindles in the muscles that then are activated via a reflex arc.

Monitoring Local Cortical Activity (EEG)

Spontaneous EEG

The EEG is the summed electrical activity that is recorded at the scalp. Its primary generators are postsynaptic potentials from large cortical neurons that lie in close physical proximity to the recording site. The frequencies and amplitudes of EEG activity reflect the functional state of the brain and correlate well with levels of alertness and stages of sleep. Certain patterns of EEG may predict underlying brain pathology (e.g., seizures due to a brain lesion). The EEG is sensitive to levels of local or global ischemia,[7] so it is useful for monitoring endovascular procedures.

Electrocorticography (ECoG)

Recordings in the operating room can also be made from electrodes placed directly on the surface of the brain. These electrodes can be used for identification of the locus for seizure generation and for neurophysiologic mapping of cortical areas (e.g., motor and somatosensory cortex).[8]

Extracellular Spikes Using Microelectrode Recordings

The monitoring of extracellular spikes by high-impedance microelectrodes is commonly used for localization of targets during the placement of electrodes for deep brain stimulation (DBS).[9] At present, DBS electrodes are implanted primarily for movement disorders (e.g., Parkinson's disease and dystonia), but clinical trials are now planned or under way for the use of DBS technology in the treatment of psychiatric disorders, including obsessive-compulsive disorder and major depression.[10] The techniques for monitoring extracellular spikes are quite different from those used to monitor sensory and motor function. Microelectrodes are placed stereotactically deep within the brain. They have much higher impedance than the electrodes used for sensory and motor monitoring, and the analysis and interpretation of microelectrode recordings focuses on the rates and patterns of neuronal firing rather than on the latencies and amplitudes used for somatosensory and motor evoked potentials. After recording, the microelectrode is withdrawn and the DBS electrode is then chronically implanted at the target, defined both by radiographic images and neuronal recordings.

PROCEDURES

Spinal Surgeries

IONM was developed in large part to monitor neural function during procedures to correct spinal deformities. In the early 1970s, for example, scoliosis surgery carried a neurologic morbidity of approximately 0.7%.[11] In a large multicenter study involving more than 51,000 cases, patients undergoing scoliosis surgery who were monitored by experienced neurophysiologists had significantly lower levels of postoperative morbidity than those whose surgeries were not monitored or were monitored by inexperienced teams.[12] The effectiveness of IONM in reducing intraoperative morbidity in patients with scoliosis has led surgeons to use IONM in a wide range of spine surgeries that involve more localized levels of the spine (e.g., posterior cervical decompression and instrumentation).[13,14]

A combination of SSEPs, MEPs, spontaneous EMG, and triggered EMG can be used to monitor patients undergoing spine surgery. These recordings are sensitive to many intraoperative events, such as traumatic manipulation of the cord or peripheral nerve, ischemia, cord compression, and excessive traction (e.g., while correcting a scoliosis). SSEPs represent the first and still primary method for monitoring spinal cord function during invasive spine surgery.

Lower limb SSEPs are used to monitor the entire length of the cord. Upper limb SSEPs are useful for surgeries at the upper levels of the cervical cord and as systemic controls (e.g., for blood pressure and anesthesia) during thoracic and lumbar surgeries. SSEPs, however, are sensitive only to disruptions of the ascending somatosensory system, so there is always the potential for loss of motor function despite preservation of the SSEPs.[15] Therefore, MEPs have rapidly been included for spinal monitoring. It is expected that MEPs will be used nearly as often as SSEPs for intraoperative monitoring of spinal surgeries in the future.

Continuous monitoring of spontaneous EMG is not used widely at this time but may be employed during spinal surgeries to give warning of excess stretching of a motor nerve or root (e.g., by a retractor). Triggered EMG can be used to discriminate nerve roots from tumor or other tissue and to determine the integrity of a nerve or nerve root.

Placement of Pedicle Screws

Fixation of the spine using pedicle screws has grown in popularity over the past 2 decades. Experienced surgeons place the screws properly within the pedicle and vertebral body in a high percentage of cases. Misplacement of screws too close to a nerve, however, can produce neurologic consequences (primarily root irritation) in up to 1.0% of screw placements.[16]

In the 1990s, a monitoring technique was developed for identifying misplaced screws that could cause root irritation. The method involves delivering electrical stimuli to either the walls of the hole during drilling and/or the screw after it is placed into the pedicle and then recording from muscles that are innervated by the root at the level of the screw.[17] Electrical stimulation of a screw that is too close to a root will trigger a muscle response at a lower level of current (e.g., <7 mA) than will one placed properly in the middle of the pedicle and vertebral body (e.g., >15 mA). The greater the distance between the screw and the root, the higher the current level needed to trigger a muscle response. Screws determined to be placed incorrectly can then be reoriented in the same hole or, if that is not possible, moved to a different pedicle.

Pedicle screw monitoring would appear to be especially important for minimally invasive surgeries that permit only limited visualization of the operative field versus open surgeries that provide a wide surgical exposure. Whereas the minimally invasive approach has many benefits (e.g., pain reduction, reduced length of stay), there is a higher potential for misplaced screws because of the reduced exposure and consequent restricted view.

Surgeries with Risk of Global or Hemispheric Ischemia

Global or hemispheric ischemia is always a concern in surgical cases involving the larger vessels in the body (e.g., carotid artery, descending aorta, ascending aorta) especially in patients with a history of diabetes, hypertension, and cardiovascular problems. Because recordings from the cerebral cortex are more sensitive to ischemic

Left parietal cortex

C3/F Average
3.00 uV/div

Right parietal cortex

C4/F Average
3.00 uV/div

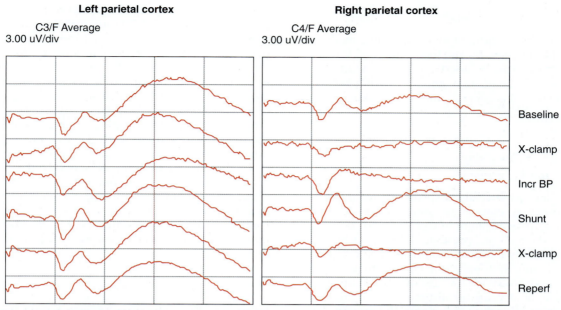

Baseline

X-clamp

Incr BP

Shunt

X-clamp

Reperf

■ **FIGURE 23-1** Neurophysiologic monitoring for hemispheric ischemia using upper limb SSEPs. SSEPs elicited by bilateral median nerve stimulation were recorded throughout the case. Representative SSEPs from the left and right parietal cortices are shown (x-axis = 100 ms). The first set of traces represents the baseline SSEPs, which were recorded just prior to cross-clamping of the right carotid artery (Baseline). Immediately after cross-clamping, the SSEP from the right parietal cortex became very small while the left SSEP was unchanged (X-clamp). Increasing the blood pressure led to an improvement in amplitude, but the SSEP still did not return to baseline (Incr BP). A shunt was established around the clamped portion of the carotid to increase the blood supply to the right hemisphere. After shunting, the BP was lowered to pre-clamp values. With shunting, the right parietal SSEP returned to baseline (Shunt). Near the end of the repair of the right carotid, the artery had to be cross-clamped to complete the repair. For a brief period the SSEP was reduced in amplitude (X-clamp) but quickly returned to baseline when carotid repair was complete and the artery was reperfused (Reperf).

insults than are recordings from the spinal cord or from subcortical structures, cortical EEG, cortical evoked potentials (either somatosensory or visual), and MEPs are candidates for this application of IONM. In general, reductions in cortical blood flow below approximately 15 mL/100 g/min result in the total loss of cortical evoked potentials (either SSEPs or VEPs). Historically, EEG and/or SSEPs have been used to monitor surgical procedures that carry risk of global ischemia.[18] However, MEP monitoring is increasingly used for this purpose. VEPs can also be used for to monitor cortical ischemia, but they are seldom employed, because the amplitudes of cortical VEPs are more variable intraoperatively than are SSEPs.

Figure 23-1 illustrates the use of upper limb SSEPs to monitor a patient for hemispheric ischemia. The patient was a 67-year-old hypertensive man undergoing a right-sided carotid endarterectomy. The standard practice of the surgical team is selective use of bypass shunting because of the risk, although very small, that the placement of the bypass could cause an embolus to be released into the arterial system. At this hospital, therefore, shunting around the cross-clamped segment of the carotid artery is performed only if neurophysiologic recordings indicate that shunting is needed. In this patient the surgeon was notified immediately after cross-clamping that bypass shunting would be needed to maintain normal SSEPs. The patient awakened postoperatively with no change in his neurologic status compared with preoperative function.

Surgeries of Brain with Risk of Focal Ischemia or Local Insult

The usefulness of IONM in detecting focal ischemia or a local insult depends primarily on the structures that are at risk. The diverse modalities for monitoring evoked potentials reflect the need to activate different neural circuits.

Upper limb SSEPs are used extensively in cases that affect the middle cerebral artery, because it is this artery that supplies blood to the arm and hand region of the primary somatosensory cortex. Upper limb SSEPs are also sensitive to infarcts in the thalamocortical radiation. Lower limb SSEPs are monitored in cases involving the anterior cerebral artery, because this artery supplies blood to the leg region of the primary somatosensory cortex.

MEPs achieved by *direct cortical stimulation* are widely used to guide a surgeon who is removing diseased tissue near to the motor cortex.

MEPs achieved by *transcranial* stimulation are used by some centers to monitor procedures that place the blood supply to the cortex and/or brain stem at risk, because such MEPs are sensitive to ischemia in the corticospinal tracts. Transcranial MEP monitoring is not used for brain surgery in other centers, however, because (1) the transcranial electrical stimulation inevitably produces contractions of the head and neck muscles, (2) the surgeons fear that the motor stimulation could cause the patient to move at an inopportune time, and (3) the use of muscle relaxants precludes MEP monitoring. Even though the patients' heads are secured during cranial procedures, many surgeons do not believe that the risk of monitoring via MEPs is worth the additional information the MEPs provide.

ECoG can be used for intraoperative identification of the central sulcus.[8] When recorded from the surfaces of brain, deep to the dura, potentials evoked by median nerve stimulation show opposite polarity in the motor cortex and the somatosensory cortex. In almost all cases, therefore, the central sulcus lies between the two sites with reverse polarity. This technique is especially useful for differentiating the motor cortex from the somatosensory cortex when tumors alter the morphology to such an extent that simple identification is difficult or when a minicraniotomy affords only limited surgical exposure.

As yet, if one excludes EEG and cerebral oximetry, IONM cannot provide specific functional information noninvasively for large areas of the cerebral cortex. These include the vast span of the frontal cortex anterior to the motor cortex, the noneloquent areas of the temporal and parietal lobes excluding the primary somatosensory cortex, and the occipital lobe excluding visual cortex. The sensory areas of the thalamus, of course, can be monitored by recording the appropriate sensory evoked potential.

Posterior Fossa Surgeries

IONM is frequently used during surgery to resect a cerebellopontine angle tumor (e.g., acoustic neuroma), for vestibular nerve section, for microvascular decompression of cranial nerves V, VII, and VIII, for clipping of aneurysms along the basilar artery, and for posterior fossa AVMs. Auditory BAERs are recorded whenever the cochlear nerve is involved directly in the surgery or when the cochlear nerve may be stretched by retraction (e.g., during surgery for microvascular decompression of a cranial nerve). Spontaneous and triggered EMG can be recorded for any cranial nerves that have motor function.

Surgeries for the resection of tumors in the brain stem or cervicomedullary junction pose great risk to any motor nuclei that lie in the vicinity of the tumor or in the path of the surgical approach. In addition, tumors frequently distort the anatomy, making it much more difficult to identify critical brain stem structures. A variant of triggered EMG monitoring was developed specifically to minimize morbidity during the resection of intramedullary tumors.[19,20] Essentially, electrical stimulation is applied directly to the surface of the brain stem or spinal cord while recording from the muscles innervated by cranial nerves VII, IX, X, and XII. In a similar manner, the corticospinal tract at the level of the cerebral peduncle can also be mapped by recording from appropriate muscles in the face, neck, and upper and lower limbs while stimulating descending motor tracts.[21]

Many other structures in the posterior fossa cannot be monitored without resorting to invasive procedures. The cerebellum cannot be monitored using sensory or motor evoked potentials, and monitoring provides little or no specific information for areas rostral to the inferior colliculus. The white matter tracts in the brain stem are composed primarily of ascending sensory and descending motor fibers. These tracts, however, are more resistant to ischemia than are cortical structures. Therefore, although SSEPs and MEPs are frequently monitored during posterior fossa surgery, they are not nearly as valuable as when the surgeries involve areas that are more sensitive to the effects of local or global ischemia. The exception, of course, is when direct stimulation of motor tracts is possible.

MONITORING ENDOVASCULAR PROCEDURES

Neurophysiologic monitoring during endovascular procedures was first reported more than 20 years ago.[22,23] Since that time, however, only a few case reports have addressed the monitoring of endovascular procedures on spinal AVMs[24] and the coiling of an intracranial aneurysm.[25] In each of these case reports, a change in neurophysiologic recordings led to an alteration of the surgical plan.

Retrospective reviews of neurophysiologic monitoring for endovascular procedures of the spine are also sparse.[3,27] One study reviewed the impact of neurophysiologic monitoring on 110 embolizations of spinal AVMs under general anesthesia in 85 consecutive patients.[3] In almost 30% of these, the safety of the surgical plan was tested provocatively by injections of both a short-acting barbiturate (to block neuronal activity in the gray matter) and lidocaine (to block axonal conduction in the white matter). SSEPs and MEPs were monitored throughout all procedures. In 30% of tested patients, embolization was not performed, because the provocative tests revealed loss of MEPs or decrease in SSEP amplitude greater than or equal to 50% of baseline. There were no false-negative results. False-positive results could not be assessed, because the procedures were abandoned after a positive provocative test.

The same authors subsequently studied a separate set of 60 provocative tests performed during 84 planned spinal embolizations in 52 patients.[26] The provocative test was positive in 19 of the 52 patients (either MEP loss or SSEP decline). In 6 of the 19 patients, embolization was aborted. These 6 were treated by alternate means. The other 13 patients were safely embolized by a modified procedure, including advancing the catheter to a place that yielded a negative test result, using coils or dilute particles instead of N-butyl-cyanoacrylate (NBCA), or embolizing with NBCA but with reduced force. One false-negative test occurred in this series, when embolization of the anterior spinal artery led to a transient increase in spasticity, despite the prior negative provocative test.

The value of neurophysiologic monitoring for intracranial procedures was assessed in 35 consecutive patients undergoing a total of 50 endovascular procedures,[27] including balloon test occlusions, embolization using Guglielmi detachable coils, and permanent vessel occlusions. Patients who failed the provocative test were not treated by embolization or were treated only after a bypass graft was placed to protect the circulation distal to the vessel to be occluded. The neurophysiologic monitoring changed therapeutic management in 5 of 35 patients. The authors concluded that neurophysiologic monitoring was a valuable guide to therapeutic decision making.

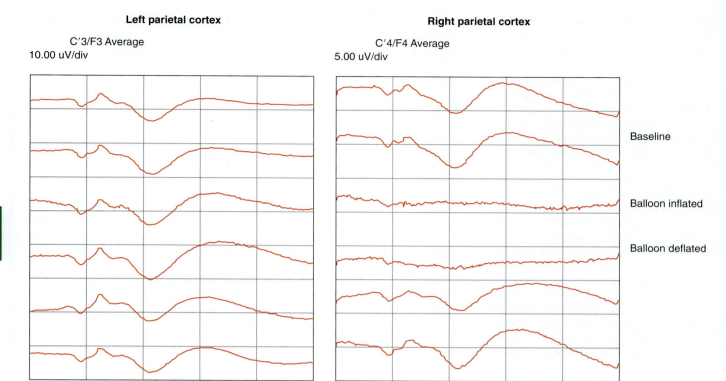

Left parietal cortex

C'3/F3 Average
10.00 uV/div

Right parietal cortex

C'4/F4 Average
5.00 uV/div

Baseline

Balloon inflated

Balloon deflated

■ **FIGURE 23-2**   Representative SSEPs recorded from the left and right parietal cortices are shown (x-axis = 100 ms) before, during, and immediately after a balloon test occlusion. Note that the baseline responses from the right parietal cortex are approximately 50% of the size of those from the left cortex (y-axis scaling is different in the figure). The balloon was deflated immediately after the test because of the loss of the SSEP from the right parietal cortex. See text for additional explanation.

Figure 23-2 illustrates neurophysiologic monitoring during a balloon test occlusion in the radiology suite. This 61-year-old woman presented with a tumor that encased the right carotid artery. The endovascular procedure was performed to determine whether the carotid artery could be cross-clamped or sacrificed during surgery. The figure shows SSEPs elicited by stimulation of the right and left median nerves. The first two sets of baseline SSEPs were recorded immediately before a balloon was inflated in the right carotid artery at the level of the tumor. The next two sets of SSEPs were recorded immediately after the balloon was inflated. Within seconds of the inflation, the SSEP from the right parietal cortex flattened. The balloon was immediately deflated and the SSEPs recovered within 2 minutes. The patient awoke at her neurologic baseline.

SUMMARY

Intraoperative neurophysiologic monitoring is now an established part of many surgical procedures. Neurophysiologic techniques are being used increasingly to monitor endovascular procedures performed in radiology suites. The data published thus far indicate a real role for such monitoring, especially in patients at risk for ischemic insult to the brain or spinal cord during embolizations or arterial procedures.

KEY POINTS

- Intraoperative neurophysiologic monitoring (IONM) is widely used to detect an intraoperative problem while intervention is still possible, to detect and identify neural tissue, and to determine the safety of a planned procedure (e.g., balloon test occlusion).
- Over the past 10 years, the types of neurophysiologic recordings available to the monitoring specialist are more numerous and are more refined than those that existed during the first 30 years of IONM. The types of cases for which IONM is commonly used are much more numerous as well.
- In spite of this growth and development, IONM is not frequently used for procedures performed by interventional neuroradiologists or endovascular neurosurgeons in radiology suites. This is the case even when IONM is commonly requested by surgeons when treating the same disease or condition in the operating room.
- There appears to be a just cause for an expansion of IONM in the radiology setting, particularly in patients for whom there is potential risk of ischemic insult to the brain or spinal cord (e.g., embolization, tumor resection, or artery repair).

SUGGESTED READINGS

Boyd SG, Rothwell JC, Cowan JM, et al. A method of monitoring function in corticospinal pathways during scoliosis surgery with a note on motor conduction velocities. J Neurol Neurosurg Psychiatry 1986; 49:251-257.

Kothbauer KF. Neurosurgical management of intramedullary spinal cord tumors in children. Pediatr Neurosurg 2007; 43:222-235.

Macdonald DB. Intraoperative motor evoked potential monitoring: overview and update. J Clin Monit Comput 2006; 20:347-377.

Nash CL Jr, Lorig RA, Schatzinger LA, Brown RH. Spinal cord monitoring during operative treatment of the spine. Clin Orthop Relat Res 1977; (126):100-105.

Sala F, Bricolo A, Faccioli F, et al. Surgery for intramedullary spinal cord tumors: the role of intraoperative (neurophysiological) monitoring. Eur Spine J 2007; July 26 (Epub ahead of print).

Schneider JR, Novak KE. Carotid endarterectomy with routine electroencephalography and selective shunting. Semin Vasc Surg 2004; 17:230-235.

Sutter M, Deletis V, Dvorak J, et al. Current opinions and recommendations on multimodal intraoperative monitoring during spine surgeries. Eur Spine J 2007; Aug 15 (Epub ahead of print).

REFERENCES

1. Larson SJ, Sances A Jr. Evoked potentials in man: neurosurgical applications. Am J Surg 1966; 111:857-861.

2. Perez-Borja C, Meyer JS. Electroencephalographic monitoring during reconstructive surgery of the neck vessels. Electroencephalogr Clin Neurophysiol 1965; 18:162-169.

3. Sala F, Niimi Y, Berenstein A, Deletis V. Neuroprotective role of neurophysiological monitoring during endovascular procedures in the spinal cord. Ann N Y Acad Sci 2001; 939:126-136.

4. Toleikis JR. American Society of Neurophysiological Monitoring. Intraoperative monitoring using somatosensory evoked potentials. A position statement by the American Society of Neurophysiological Monitoring. J Clin Monit Comput 2005; 19:241-258.

5. Kothbauer KF, Deletis V, Epstein FJ. Motor-evoked potential monitoring for intramedullary spinal cord tumor surgery: correlation of clinical and neurophysiological data in a series of 100 consecutive procedures. Neurosurg Focus 1998; 4(5):e1.

6. Leppanen RE, Abnm D, American Society of Neurophysiological Monitoring. Intraoperative monitoring of segmental spinal nerve root function with free-run and electrically-triggered electromyography and spinal cord function with reflexes and F-responses. A position statement by the American Society of Neurophysiological Monitoring. J Clin Monit Comput 2005; 19:437-461 (Epub 2006; Jan 25).

7. Torres F, Frank GS, Cohen MM, et al. Neurologic and electroencephalographic studies in open heart surgery; a preliminary report. Neurology 1959; 9:174-183.

8. Nuwer MR, Banoczi WR, Cloughesy TF, et al. Topographic mapping of somatosensory evoked potentials helps identify motor cortex more quickly in the operating room. Brain Topogr 1992; 5:53-58.

9. Gross RE, Krack P, Rodriguez-Oroz MC, et al. Electrophysiological mapping for the implantation of deep brain stimulators for Parkinson's disease and tremor. Mov Disord 2006; 21(Suppl 14): S259-S283.

10. Hardesty DE, Sackeim HA. Deep brain stimulation in movement and psychiatric disorders. Biol Psychiatry 2007; 61:831-835.

11. MacEwen GD, Bunnell WP, Sriram K. Acute neurological complications in the treatment of in the treatment of scoliosis. A report of the Scoliosis Research Society. J Bone Joint Surg Am 1975; 57:404-408.

12. Nuwer MR, Dawson EG, Carlson LG, et al. Somatosensory evoked potential spinal cord monitoring reduces neurologic deficits after scoliosis surgery: results of a large multicenter survey. Electroencephalogr Clin Neurophysiol 1995; 96:6-11.

13. Eggspuehler A, Sutter MA, Grob D, et al. Multimodal intraoperative monitoring (MIOM) during cervical spine surgical procedures in 246 patients. Eur Spine J 2007; July 4 (Epub ahead of print).

14. Sutter M, Eggspuehler A, Grob D, et al. The diagnostic value of multimodal intraoperative monitoring (MIOM) during spine surgery: a prospective study of 1,017 patients. Eur Spine J 2007 (Epub ahead of print).

15. Krieger D, Adams HP, Albert F, et al. Pure motor hemiparesis with stable somatosensory evoked potential monitoring during aneurysm surgery: case report. Neurosurgery 1992; 31:145-150.

16. Lonstein JE, Denis F, Perra JH, et al. Complications associated with pedicle screws. J Bone Joint Surg Am 1999; 81:1519-1528.

17. Calancie B, Madsen P, Lebwohl N. Stimulus-evoked EMG monitoring during transpedicular lumbosacral spine instrumentation: initial clinical results. Spine 1994; 19:2780-2786.

18. Cloughesy TF, Nuwer MR, Hoch D, et al. Monitoring carotid test occlusions with continuous EEG and clinical examination. J Clin Neurophysiol 1993; 10:363-369.

19. Morota N, Deletis V, Constantini S, et al. The role of motor evoked potentials during surgery for intramedullary spinal cord tumors. Neurosurgery 1997; 41:1327-1336.

20. Strauss C, Romstock J, Nimsky C, Fahlbusch R. Intraoperative identification of motor areas of the rhomboid fossa using direct stimulation. J Neurosurg 1993; 79:393-399.

21. Yingling CD, Ojemann S, Dodson B, et al. Identification of motor pathways during tumor surgery facilitated by multichannel electromyographic recording. J Neurosurg 1999; 91:922-927.

22. Berenstein A, Young W, Ransohoff J, et al. Somatosensory evoked potentials during spinal angiography and therapeutic transvascular embolization. J Neurosurg 1984; 60:777-785.

23. Hacke W, Zeumer H, Berg-Dammer E. Monitoring of hemispheric or brainstem functions with neurophysiologic methods during interventional neuroradiology. AJNR Am J Neuroradiol 1983; 4:382-384.

24. Sala F, Niimi Y, Krzan MJ, et al. Embolization of a spinal arteriovenous malformation: correlation between motor evoked potentials and angiographic findings: technical case report. Neurosurgery 1999; 45:932-937; discussion 937-938.

25. Horowitz MB, Crammond D, Balzer J, et al. Aneurysm rupture during endovascular coiling: effects on cerebral transit time and neurophysiologic monitoring and the benefits of early ventriculostomy: case report. Minim Invasive Neurosurg 2003; 46:300-305.

26. Niimi Y, Sala F, Deletis V, et al. Neurophysiologic monitoring and pharmacologic provocative testing for embolization of spinal cord arteriovenous malformations. AJNR Am J Neuroradiol 2004; 25:1131-1138.

27. Liu AY, Lopez JR, Do HM, et al. Neurophysiological monitoring in the endovascular therapy of aneurysms. AJNR Am J Neuroradiol 2003; 24:1520-1527.

CHAPTER 24

Vertebral Body Augmentation Procedures: Vertebroplasty and Kyphoplasty

Ronit Gilad, David M. Johnson, and Aman B. Patel

Compression fractures of vertebral bodies affect approximately 750,000 people each year in the United States and up to 25% of postmenopausal women.[1,2] The leading cause of vertebral compression fractures is osteoporosis, a disease that affects 44 million Americans.[2] Younger patients taking corticosteroids for medical problems such as lupus, asthma, and rheumatoid arthritis may also suffer from osteoporotic compression fractures.[3] Other, less common causes of vertebral body compression fractures or deformities are severe trauma to healthy bone, metastatic or other neoplastic lesions, and prior, healed infections such as osteomyelitis or tuberculosis.[2,3]

Patients with vertebral compression fractures often present with acute or chronic back pain. As a result of the pain, these patients often experience limited mobility that leads to osteoporosis and progressive vertebral body collapse.[3] In the thoracic spine, significant sagittal kyphosis may lead to decreased vital capacity of the lungs, with increased respiratory difficulties.[2] The first line of treatment for vertebral compression fractures is conservative therapy. This may include pain medication, calcium and vitamin D supplements, short-term bed rest (because prolonged inactivity can lead to further bone loss), external bracing, and physical therapy. Pain from the spinal fracture can last for several months, but if the fracture heals well with conservative treatment the pain will usually improve significantly within a few days or weeks.[4]

Patients are typically evaluated with imaging studies that may include plain radiographs, CT, MRI, or radionuclide bone scintiscans.[2] Lateral radiographs demonstrate the loss of vertebral body height resulting from the fracture and the sagittal alignment of the spine. Axial and sagittal reformatted CT images (Fig. 24-1) demonstrate any retropulsed bone fragments in addition to the loss of vertebral height. Preoperatively, CT is helpful for assess-ing the integrity of the posterior cortex and for planning the needle trajectory. MRI provides excellent anatomic detail. T1-weighted and short tau inversion recovery (STIR) sequences show edema of acute fractures (Fig. 24-2). MRI also reveals any other lesions or injuries that may contribute to the patient's back pain. In patients with no evidence of osteoporosis and otherwise unexplained compression of the vertebra, it is important to obtain both a noncontrast and a contrast-enhanced MRI to exclude malignancy. Radionuclide bone scans are useful for patients who are unable to have an MRI. A bone scan (Fig. 24-3) will demonstrate activity in an acute fracture and in a chronic, nonhealed fracture. However, bone scans will not demonstrate activity in chronic, healed fractures. Bone scans are also useful for detecting the presence of occult metastases.[2,5]

Vertebroplasty is an image-guided, minimally invasive, nonsurgical therapy used to strengthen a vertebral body that has been weakened by osteoporosis, malignant lesion, or treated infection.[1] This procedure was initially developed in France in 1984 and was first introduced in the United States in 1994.[2] The purpose of strengthening a compression deformity is to decrease pain, increase the patient's functional abilities, permit the patient to return to the previous level of activity, and prevent further vertebral collapse.[3] Vertebroplasty is accomplished by injecting a cement mixture through a needle into the fractured bone under fluoroscopic or CT guidance.[2,3] Kyphoplasty is a variant form of vertebroplasty that was introduced in 1998 to address several concerns posed by those performing simple vertebroplasty, specifically, the potential for cement to extravasate into the spinal canal, neural foramen, or venous plexus and the failure of vertebroplasty to restore the vertebra to normal height.[2] In kyphoplasty, a balloon catheter is introduced into the fracture

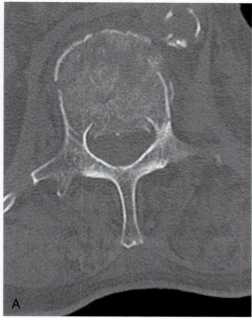

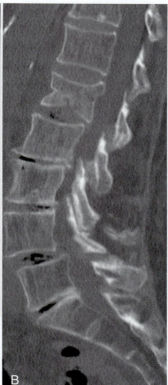

■ FIGURE 24-1   Axial (**A**) and sagittal (**B**) CT scans show an L1 compression fracture. Note the bony retropulsion with narrowing of the spinal canal on the axial view.

■ FIGURE 24-2   Sagittal STIR MR sequence shows characteristics suggestive of an acute compression fracture of T8. There does not appear to be an underlying neoplastic lesion. Note the retropulsed fragments and cord signal changes.

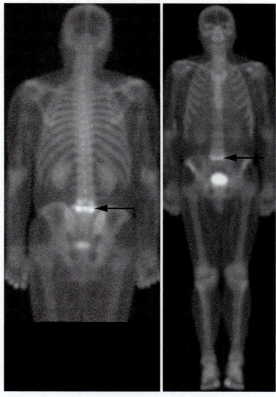

■ FIGURE 24-3   Bone scintigraphy demonstrates increased uptake of the L5 vertebral body (*arrows*), suggestive of an acute or unhealed fracture.

site and, under fluoroscopic guidance, is inflated until the fracture is reduced or until it is unsafe to continue. The cavity created by the inflated balloon is then filled with cement.[2,3]

INDICATIONS

Indications for treating patients with spinal augmentation procedures, vertebroplasty, or kyphoplasty include failure of conservative therapy, prolonged immobility, and progressive kyphotic deformity on serial imaging studies.[1] Specific types of fractures respond poorly to conservative therapy and may be better treated with augmentation early on. These include thoracolumbar junction fractures, burst fractures, and significant anterior wedge compression fractures.[2] Such fractures can heal in compressed or flattened wedge shape, precluding later treatment by minimally invasive spinal augmentation procedures.[2,3] Thus, they should be treated early, before the spinal deformity becomes irreparable.

Vertebral augmentation may also be an alternative to more extensive surgery. Spinal instrumentation/fusion surgery requires prolonged general anesthesia and may be accompanied by substantial blood loss. Postoperative complications include infection, instrumentation failure, prolonged pain from the surgery itself and consequently prolonged immobility, and the attendant complications of deep vein thrombosis, pulmonary embolus, and pneumonia. A patient with multiple comorbidities and/or advanced age may not be able to tolerate such prolonged surgery and should be considered for minimally invasive vertebral body augmentation instead.[1,3] Similarly, in patients with severe diffuse osteoporosis or destructive metastases the residual weakened vertebrae may not be able to support the mechanical constructs used for spinal instrumentation, so these patients should also be considered for minimally invasive vertebral augmentation to prevent further collapse of their vertebral bodies.[1,2]

Patients with metastatic lesions may also be treated with vertebroplasty or kyphoplasty for palliative pain control.[6] Vertebral augmentation is now being performed before chemotherapy or radiation therapy. It has the advantage of relieving pain rapidly and adding structural support to the weakened bone. Additionally, the cement does not interfere with subsequent chemotherapy or radiation therapy. As with osteoporotic fractures, identifying and treating the symptomatic lesion is paramount. Lesions confined to the vertebral body often result in localized back pain at that level. Radicular symptoms, myelopathy, or focal weakness should raise suspicion of epidural or foraminal extension of the lesion and necessitate neurosurgical consultation.[5] Any mass lesion, unusual-appearing compression fracture, or fracture in a patient with a history of cancer should be sampled during the procedure. In addition to their role in treating metastatic lesions, vertebroplasty and kyphoplasty have been shown to be effective in treating painful hemangiomas and fractures from multiple myeloma.[3,5]

A patient with a history of treated infection, osteomyelitis, or tuberculosis may develop progressive kyphosis leading to increased back pain.[7] In such patients, active infection should first be ruled out by CT, MRI, or radionu-

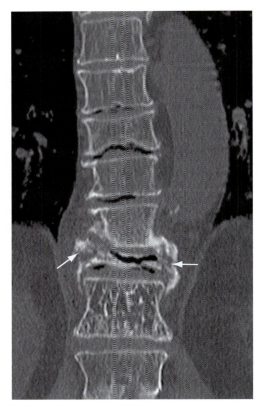

■ FIGURE 24-4 CT scan, coronal view, demonstrates avascular necrosis with collapse of the vertebral body and an associated intervertebral vacuum cleft (*arrows*).

clide bone scan. However, a biopsy and culture should still be performed at the time of the procedure. In osteomyelitis, the disc space is often involved and there may be subsequent anterior subluxation of one vertebral body over another. This situation may necessitate surgical correction of sagittal alignment and internal stabilization.[2,7]

Avascular necrosis is another cause of painful fracture deformity. This unstable lesion most commonly results from prior infection, chronic corticosteroid use, alcoholism, and radiation therapy. Imaging studies typically demonstrate a collapsed vertebral body with an intravertebral vacuum cleft or fluid collection (Fig. 24-4).[8] Such a cleft is a good prognostic sign, indicating that vertebroplasty is highly likely to relieve the patient's pain.[9]

CONTRAINDICATIONS

Contraindications to these procedures include an uncorrectable coagulation disorder, active infection in the area (including the overlying skin, prevertebral soft tissues, and vertebral body or disc), spinal cord compression, and posterior vertebral body fracture with cortical disruption (which allows the cement to leak into the spinal canal). The relative weight of these contraindications is under debate.[1] Other relative contraindications include vertebral body collapse greater than 75%, epidural extension of disease with more than 20% involvement of the spinal canal diameter, and preoperative radiculopathy.[2] Recent literature does not substantiate the fear that cement may

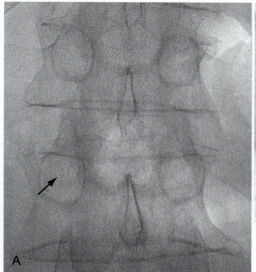

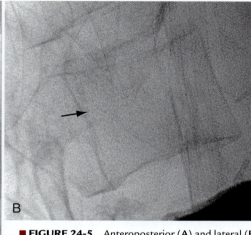

■ **FIGURE 24-5**   Anteroposterior (A) and lateral (B) fluoroscopy images showing the desired entry point and trajectory (*arrows*) for a transpedicular approach.

leak into the spinal canal from a compression or burst fracture with posterior vertebral cortical disruption.[10]

EQUIPMENT

Vertebroplasty and kyphoplasty should be performed in an interventional radiology suite or in an operating room. The room should contain fluoroscopy equipment (biplane preferable), an adjustable table, and viewing monitors. Typically, vertebroplasty or kyphoplasty kits with all the necessary equipment are used for the procedure. They include 11-gauge bone needles, cement (polymethyl methacrylate [PMMA]), and the cement delivery device. PMMA comes as separate liquid and powder components that must be mixed before use. In vertebroplasty kits, the cement delivery device consists of a rotating syringe-like apparatus that allows for controlled delivery of the cement into the vertebral body. Kyphoplasty kits also contain balloon catheters that are inflated with an insufflator to create the cavity within the vertebral body. Thereafter, the cement is usually delivered through a hand plunger system, which is also provided in the kit.

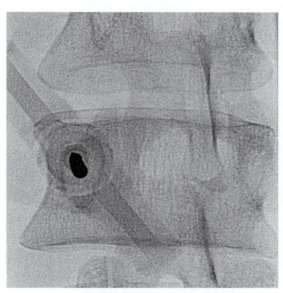

■ **FIGURE 24-6**   Anteroposterior tube angled toward the point of entry such that the interventionalist is looking directly down the pedicle.

TECHNIQUE

Anatomy and Approaches

The precise vertebral body level being treated must first be confirmed on real-time fluoroscopy before beginning the procedure. It is important to center on the vertebral body in question and to align the vertebral end plates in both the anteroposterior and lateral views. Transpedicular and parapedicular approaches are typically used for this procedure. In the transpedicular approach (Fig. 24-5), the anterior aspect of the needle remains on the ipsilateral side of the vertebral body. Therefore, a bilateral approach is often necessary to deliver cement to both sides of the vertebral body.[11] To perform the transpedicular approach, the anteroposterior tube should be angled toward the side of the pedicle being entered such that the operator is looking directly down the pedicle as if it were down a

barrel (Fig. 24-6). The needle enters the pedicle at the upper, outer quadrant and is advanced to the anterior third of the vertebral body. This procedure is then repeated on the contralateral side to place cement into both halves of the vertebral body.

Alternatively, a unipedicular transpedicular approach may be used. For the unipedicular approach, the anteroposterior tube is angled to obtain an oblique "Scotty dog" view of the affected vertebra. The needle is then passed into the pedicle at the eye of the dog and advanced to the anterior third of the vertebral body (Fig. 24-7). This positions the needle tip close to midline from which cement passes to both sides simultaneously.[11] Care must be used when delivering cement because it may travel into the venous plexus.

The parapedicular approach is useful for treating vertebrae with small pedicles and for performing vertebral augmentation when the pedicle is destroyed by tumor.

For thoracic vertebrae, the needle is inserted superolateral to the pedicle, through the costovertebral joint. Using a steeper cranial-caudad projection, the operator can advance the needle into the anterior half of the vertebral body, where it is well positioned for either vertebroplasty or kyphoplasty.

Technical Aspects

The procedure is performed in a step-wise manner:

1. Place the patient prone on the table of the interventional suite or operating room and administer anesthesia and prophylactic antibiotics.
2. Confirm the location of the vertebral body being treated by placing a radiopaque instrument on the patient's back. Then, position the anteroposterior and lateral tubes even with the superior and inferior end plates of the vertebra. Align the pedicle to be accessed between the end plates to ensure that the needle stays within the vertebral body.
3. After preparing and draping the patient's back in the standard surgical fashion, anesthetize the entry point with lidocaine.

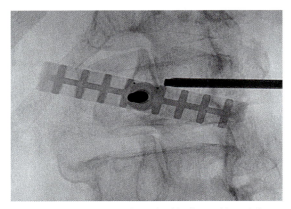

■ **FIGURE 24-7** Anteroposterior tube ideally positioned for a unipedicular approach, such that the "Scotty dog" is visible and the trocar/bone needle is "in the eye."

4. Use a 20-gauge spinal needle to anesthetize the periosteum with lidocaine. Confirm the trajectory with both anteroposterior and lateral tubes.
5. Use a No. 11 blade to make the skin incision and then advance an 11-gauge bone needle with trocar under fluoroscopic guidance into the anterior one third of the vertebral body.
6. If the approach is to be bilateral, consider placing both bone needles in proper position before delivering the cement. If multiple levels are to be treated, consider placing all of the bone needles in the desired locations before delivering the cement. The cement components (liquid and powder) are mixed off to the side of the field and must be allowed to set for several minutes. The consistency must be somewhat viscous to allow control of delivery.
7. After removing the inner trocar, inject the cement slowly through the needle in a controlled fashion under fluoroscopic guidance. If leakage is detected, stop the cement administration to allow the cement to set before continuing with the injection.
8. Once the desired cement fill is obtained and confirmed on fluoroscopy, remove the needle. There are situations in which reinforcement of the pedicles is also desired. In such cases a "tail" of cement may be left along the pedicular tract. Otherwise, the remaining cement in the needle may be pushed into the vertebral body with a plunger before the needle is removed.
9. After the bone needle is removed, apply pressure over the wound for 5 to 10 minutes before placing a sterile dressing.

In vertebroplasty, the cement is injected into the vertebral body immediately after the bone needles are in place. The idea is to provide structural support via extension of the cement throughout the bony trabeculae of the cancellous vertebral body. The goal is to fill much of the anterior portion, or the anterior wedged portion, of the vertebral body (Fig. 24-8). Extravasation of cement into the disc space, spinal canal, or venous structures is undesirable and should alert the operator to halt the injection. Vertebroplasty does not restore vertebral body

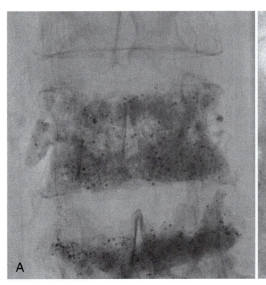

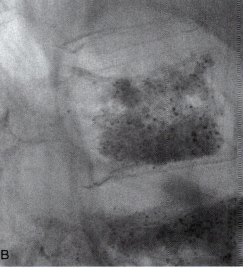

■ **FIGURE 24-8** Anteroposterior (**A**) and lateral (**B**) views of a vertebroplasty after cement injection.

height, except in certain cases where intravertebral clefts are present.

In kyphoplasty, a balloon catheter is inserted into the vertebral body through the cannula after removing the inner trocar. The balloon is then inflated with a mixture of contrast agent and saline while monitoring fluoroscopically. Pressures of 100 to 300 psi are generally utilized to distend the balloon and create the cavity within the vertebra (Fig. 24-9). The balloon is subsequently deflated, and the cement is delivered into the void created in the cancellous bone (Fig. 24-10). In addition to creating a cavity, the balloon may reduce the fracture and provide some restoration of vertebral height. Occasionally, the balloon may protrude through an end plate. When this happens, an eggshell technique may be used to limit cement leakage. A small amount of cement is placed in the cavity. The balloon is reinserted and inflated slightly to displace the cement into the defect and seal the leak. Once the cement hardens, the balloon is removed and cement deposition is continued.[12]

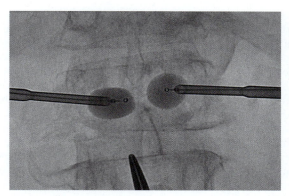

■ **FIGURE 24-9** Anteroposterior view of a kyphoplasty after balloon inflation.

CONTROVERSIES

Percutaneous vertebroplasty and kyphoplasty are minimally invasive procedures used to treat vertebral compression deformities, especially those associated with osteoporotic fractures. Although both procedures have been shown to be highly effective, with low complication rates, there have been no prospective clinical trials directly comparing the two procedures. The decision as to which procedure to use is largely based on individual experiences and retrospective series published in the literature.[13]

Many explanations have been offered for the pain relief associated with delivery of polymethyl methacrylate into a compression fracture site. In addition to improving mechanical stability, bone cement may also cause pain relief through thermal necrosis and chemotoxicity to the intraosseous pain receptors.[1,2] Some authors suggest a slightly greater improvement in pain scores with vertebroplasty compared with kyphoplasty, although this is not statistically significant.[3] With vertebroplasty, cement is allowed to infiltrate the bony trabeculae, so the cement may affect more pain receptors. In contrast, with kyphoplasty the cement is preferentially confined to the cavity created by the balloon, so less cement travels through the bony trabeculae.[2,14] The outcomes reported for pain relief with each procedure are discussed in detail in the next section.

Recently, kyphoplasty has been criticized for incurring a greater economic cost than vertebroplasty with little difference in clinical outcome. Vertebroplasty is usually performed with conscious sedation and local anesthesia in an outpatient setting. Kyphoplasty utilizes general anesthesia or a greater level of sedation because of the greater severity of pain endured by the patient when the balloon is inflated. This may necessitate an admission and incur additional hospital costs. In addition, the balloons themselves add to the cost of the procedure. It is estimated that

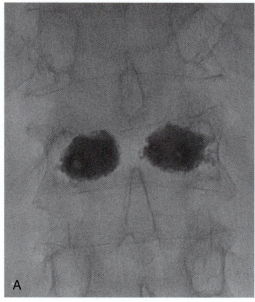

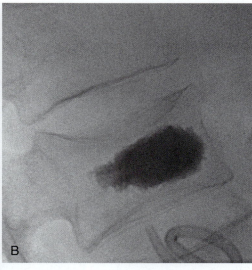

■ **FIGURE 24-10** Anteroposterior (**A**) and lateral (**B**) views of a kyphoplasty after cement injection.

kyphoplasty costs 2 to 2.5 times more than vertebroplasty owing to additional equipment, anesthesia, and hospital expenses.[13]

OUTCOMES

Much of the literature on vertebroplasty and kyphoplasty comes from retrospective studies and case series. There are few prospective, randomized controlled trials comparing vertebroplasty with kyphoplasty or either procedure with conservative therapy.[3] The studies done include a small number of patients, so the statistical power of these studies is low. In addition, most studies report follow-ups of only 12 to 36 months. No studies describe the long-term outcomes of these procedures.[2] Both procedures are very effective in reducing pain, and multiple studies have shown statistically significant reduction in pain scores regardless of the pain scales used. For osteoporotic compression fractures, pain relief has been reported in 70% to 100% of patients.[14] Regardless of the etiology of the compression deformity, patients experience a pain reduction of 60% to 70% with vertebroplasty and 55% to 60% with kyphoplasty.[1,3] Although the difference between the procedures is statistically significant in some studies, the clinical significance of this difference may not be substantial, because pain reduction of 33% or greater can be meaningful to a patient.[1,15] Furthermore, patients experience significant improvement in mobility, physical function, mental function, and decreased use of analgesics after both procedures.[2,13]

One of the theoretical advantages of kyphoplasty is fracture reduction and vertebral height restoration, although results vary significantly among case series.[2] Greater fracture reduction and vertebral height restoration are achieved in acute fractures compared with chronic fractures.[4] Although height restoration has been associated with reduced kyphosis, no significant correlation has been found between height restoration and pain relief.[13] A relative correction of kyphosis may improve sagittal alignment, and overall stability may lead to long-term pain reduction. Interestingly, with multiple-level kyphoplasty, the kyphotic angle and sagittal balance are not significantly improved over that achieved by a single-level kyphoplasty.[16] Consideration may therefore be given to using a combined vertebroplasty/kyphoplasty approach in multiple-level fracture situations. Some improvement in kyphosis has also been reported in vertebroplasty, suggesting the reduced kyphosis may also result from improved posture from pain relief.[13] Fracture reduction may also occur with vertebroplasty. Exaggerating patient extension during positioning can facilitate this.[14]

Most of the studies evaluating vertebroplasty and kyphoplasty have included patients with *osteoporotic* compression fractures. More recent literature has addressed the treatment and results in patients with *pathologic* fractures. The mechanism of pain relief with cement injection into neoplastic tissue is even less well characterized than that of cement injection into osteopenic fractured bone. However, in patients with *osteolytic* metastatic lesions, vertebroplasty provides an analgesic effect in 68% to 73% at 6 months.[17] In patients with *osteoblastic* metastases, analgesic effects of 64% to 86% are seen within 1 month

TABLE 24-1. Complication Rates of Vertebroplasty and Kyphoplasty

Complication	Vertebroplasty	Kyphoplasty
Cement leak	5%-20%	0%-7%
Symptomatic cement leak	<1%	<1%
New compression fracture	15%-19%	11%-14%
Infection	<0.1%	<0.5%
Hematoma	<0.5%	<0.5%
Medical complications	<0.1%	0.5%-1%

of the procedure and in up to 92% within 6 months. The degree of analgesia appears to correlate with the degree of cement filling within the lesion.[18] In the few studies of kyphoplasty in malignant lesions, pain reduction of 73% to 80% was observed at 1 year, with 56% height restoration and 0% clinically significant complication rate.[19,20] Thus far, both vertebroplasty and kyphoplasty have been demonstrated to be effective and safe in such lesions. More studies are necessary to characterize the outcomes and complications of minimally invasive vertebral augmentation in malignant lesions.

COMPLICATIONS

Minimally invasive vertebral body augmentation procedures have an exceedingly low risk of clinically significant complications, with an overall incidence in the range of 1% to 3%.[2,3] Table 24-1 lists the common complications of vertebroplasty and kyphoplasty reported in the literature and their respective rates. Cement leak is the most common complication encountered with both procedures, but it may not be clinically significant. Each study in the literature reports that the risk of cement leak is higher in vertebroplasty than kyphoplasty, presumably because, with vertebroplasty, the cement is injected directly into the bone under higher pressure.[3] In contrast, in kyphoplasty, cement is injected under low pressure into the hollow cavity created by the balloon, limiting inadvertent cement deposition.[14] Nevertheless, the rate of symptomatic cement leak, which includes radiculopathy, myelopathy, or any neurologic deficit, is low and there is no significant difference between vertebroplasty and kyphoplasty.[2,3]

In malignant lesions, the reported rate of asymptomatic cement leak has been as high as 86% in older series but is up to 20% in recent studies.[20] This is still higher than the leakage rate for benign fractures and may reflect the presence of defects in the posterior wall of the vertebra due to the malignancy.[13,18] In malignant lesions, cement leaks have been associated with epidural extension of the tumor and osteoblastic lesions. The leaks tend to happen suddenly and in an unpredictable manner because of the presence and heterogeneity of the soft tissue mass.[18] Fortunately, most of these cement leaks are asymptomatic. To combat some of the difficulties with leaks and soft tissue masses encountered in treating malignant lesions, tumor ablation is now being investigated. Laser-induced thermotherapy, coblation, or radiofrequency ablation is being used to create cavities before cement injection with promising preliminary results.[21]

The risk of developing a new postprocedural compression fracture is poorly understood. A patient with one osteoporotic compression fracture has increased risk of another compression fracture in the subsequent year. Either vertebroplasty or kyphoplasty may lead to new compression fractures, and the risk of fracture may be increased in the levels adjacent to the level treated.[3] The incidence of adjacent level fracture may be similar in treated and untreated patients. Identifying factors that predispose to adjacent level fracture may minimize this complication.[2] Several case reports indicate that leakage of cement into the intervertebral disc space during vertebroplasty may increase the risk of a new fracture in the adjacent vertebrae.[22,23] Since vertebroplasty usually has more cement leakage than kyphoplasty, this could explain the greater incidence of postprocedural adjacent level fractures that occur after vertebroplasty.

In osteoporosis, the spine is characterized by diffuse osteopenia. After an osteoporotic, fractured vertebral body is stabilized with cement, the biomechanics at adjacent levels are changed and there is increased motion and subsequent microinstability, predisposing the adjacent levels to compression fractures.[23,24] This instability is likely magnified by a kyphotic fulcrum, suggesting why kyphotic deformities may be progressive.[25] The fracture reduction and the restoration of vertebral height gained by kyphoplasty may provide the extra sagittal alignment needed to prevent adjacent level instability and compression fracture formation. A recent review of the literature suggests that the incidence of adjacent level fracture is indeed lower with kyphoplasty versus vertebroplasty.[25] However, other studies have shown that height restoration is, instead, a risk factor for developing adjacent level compression fractures.[22,24] Infection of the vertebral body and cement complex is rare, with only five cases of infected vertebroplasty described as individual case reports. To date, there have been no reports of infected kyphoplasty. Of the five infected vertebroplasties, three yielded grampositive cocci and two showed no organisms. All five patients had significant comorbidities as well as systemic infections within a month before the procedure, suggesting that the infection may result from hematogenous spread of distant infection in these cases.[26] Although there is no definitive evidence for the use of routine perioperative antibiotics in preventing infection, one dose of antibiotics with gram-positive coverage is typically administered before the procedure.[14]

The imaging appearance of an infected vertebroplasty has not been fully characterized. Imaging studies may show lucency around the cement and evidence of bone destruction on CT, increased T2 signal on MRI, and increased uptake of tracer on radionuclide bone scan.[26] With or without these imaging findings, a strong clinical suspicion should lead to biopsy of the vertebroplasty site.

The medical complication rates of minimally invasive spinal augmentation procedures are exceedingly low—less than 1% regardless of procedure type and etiology of the compression deformity.[3] These medical complications include myocardial infarction, pulmonary embolism, and pneumonia. Risk factors associated with these medical complications include advanced age, multiple comorbidities, and the use of general anesthesia.[1,14] Although not statistically significant, the overall medical complication rate is slightly higher with kyphoplasty than with vertebroplasty, likely because general anesthesia is more frequently used in kyphoplasty.[13] Therefore, thorough preprocedural assessment by an anesthesiologist and/or a medical physician is important in minimizing the risk of medical complications. Individual case reports have documented rare and unusual complications such as cement embolus into the pulmonary and renal arteries, cardiac perforation, retroperitoneal hematoma, and rib fracture.[2,3]

POSTPROCEDURAL AND FOLLOW-UP CARE

Patients may typically sit up and walk once they have recovered from anesthesia. Vertebroplasty patients should be observed for 1 to 3 hours after the procedure and then be released. If general anesthesia was administered, as for kyphoplasty, the patient should be observed in the recovery room for several more hours or admitted overnight. Pain relief frequently occurs within several hours to 3 days after the procedure. Clinical follow-up involves assessing for pain and routine neurologic examination. Imaging is indicated if the patient fails to respond to the intervention, if a new fracture is suspected, or if there is a change in neurologic examination.[2]

KEY POINTS

- Osteoporotic compression fractures have become increasingly prevalent in the aging population.
- Indications for minimally invasive vertebral body augmentation include compression fracture or deformity secondary to osteoporosis, chronic corticosteroid use, neoplastic lesion, or treated infection.
- Proper imaging and thorough neurologic examination are critical in evaluating patients for vertebral body augmentation.
- Both vertebroplasty and kyphoplasty are minimally invasive procedures. Vertebroplasy is usually performed with local anesthesia and conscious sedation. Kyphoplasty usually requires general anesthesia.
- The controversy over which of these is preferable has not been resolved. Multiple published studies demonstrate that both vertebroplasty and kyphoplasty have favorable outcomes, with significant pain relief and low complication rates.

SUGGESTED READINGS

Binning MJ, Gottfried ON, Klimo P Jr, Schmidt MH. Minimally invasive treatments for metastatic tumors of the spine. Neurosurg Clin North Am 2004; 15:459-465.

Lewis G. Percutaneous vertebroplasty and kyphoplasty for the standalone augmentation of osteoporosis-induced vertebral compression fractures: present status and future directions. J Biomed Mater Res B Appl Biomater 2007; 81:371-386.

McKiernan FE. Kyphoplasty and vertebroplasty: how good is the evidence? Curr Rheumatol Rep 2007; 9:57-65.

Satre TJ, Mackler L, Birch JT Jr. Clinical inquiries: who should receive vertebroplasty? J Fam Pract 2006; 55:637-638.

Sequeiros RB, Binkert CA, Carrino JA. Bone augmentation past, present, and future. Semin Musculoskelet Radiol 2006; 10:111-123.

REFERENCES

1. De Negri P, Tirri T, Paternoster G, Modano P. Treatment of painful osteoporotic or traumatic vertebral compression fractures by percutaneous vertebral augmentation procedures: a nonrandomized comparison between vertebroplasty and kyphoplasty. Clin J Pain 2007; 23:425-430.

2. Lavelle W, Carl A, Lavelle ED, Khaleel MA. Vertebroplasty and kyphoplasty. Med Clin North Am 2007; 91:299-314.

3. Eck JC, Nachtigall D, Humphreys SC, Hodges SD. Comparison of vertebroplasty and balloon kyphoplasty for treatment of vertebral compression fractures: a meta-analysis of the literature. Spine J 2007; May 29 [Epub ahead of print].

4. Crandall D, Slaughter D, Hankins PJ. Acute versus chronic vertebral compression fractures treated with kyphoplasty: early results. Spine J 2004; 18:294-299.

5. Masala S, Fiori R, Massari F, Simonetti G. Vertebroplasty and kyphoplasty: new equipment for malignant vertebral fractures treatment. J Exp Clin Cancer Res 2003; 22(4 Suppl):75-79.

6. Brodano GB, Cappuccio M, Gasbarrini A, et al. Vertebroplasty in the treatment of vertebral metastases: clinical cases and review of the literature. Eur Rev Med Pharmacol Sci 2007; 11:91-100.

7. Mannes AJ, Grippo RJ, Anderson VL, et al. Percutaneous vertebroplasty as a palliative measure in the setting of chronic infection. J Pain Symptom Manage 2006; 31:382-384.

8. Mirovsky Y, Anekstein Y, Shalmon E, Peer A. Vacuum clefts of the vertebral bodies. AJNR Am J Neuroradiol 2005; 26:1634-1640.

9. Jang JS, Kim DY, Lee SH. Efficacy of percutaneous vertebroplasty in the treatment of intravertebral pseudarthrosis associated with noninfected avascular necrosis of the vertebral body. Spine 2003; 28:1588-1592.

10. Stoffel M, Wolf I, Ringel F, et al. Treatment of painful osteoporotic compression and burst fractures using kyphoplasty: a prospective observational design. J Neurosurg Spine 2007; 6:313-319.

11. Kim AK, Jensen ME, Dion JE, et al. Unilateral transpedicular percutaneous vertebroplasty: initial experience. Radiology 2002; 222:737-741.

12. Greene DL, Isaac R, Neuwirth M, Bitan FD. The eggshell technique for prevention of cement leakage during kyphoplasty. J Spinal Disord Tech 2007; 20:229-232.

13. Cloft HJ, Jensen ME. Kyphoplasty: an assessment of a new technology. AJNR Am J Neuroradiol 2007; 28:200-203.

14. Shen MS, Yong HK. Vertebroplasty and kyphoplasty: treatment techniques for managing osteoporotic vertebral compression fractures. Bull NYU Hosp Joint Dis 2006; 64:106-113.

15. Hanley MA, Jensen MP, Ehde DM, et al. Clinically significant change in pain intensity ratings in persons with spinal cord injury or amputation. Clin J Pain 2006; 22:25-31.

16. Pradhan BB, Bae HW, Kropf MA, et al. Kyphoplasty reduction of osteoporotic vertebral compression fractures: correction of local kyphosis versus overall sagittal alignment. Spine 2006; 31:435-441.

17. Weill A, Chiras J, Simon JM. Spinal metastases: indication for and results of percutaneous injection of acrylic chirurgical cement. Radiology 1996; 199:241-247.

18. Calmels V, Vallee JN, Rose M, Chiras J. Osteoblastic and mixed spinal metastases: evaluation of the analgesic efficacy of percutaneous vertebroplasty. AJNR Am J Neuroradiol 2007; 28:570-574.

19. Köse KC, Oguz C, Burak A, et al. Functional results of vertebral augmentation techniques in pathological vertebral fractures of myelomatous patients. J Natl Med Assoc 2006; 98:1654.

20. Fourney DR, Schomer DF, Nader R, et al. Percutaneous vertebroplasty and kyphoplasty for painful vertebral body fractures in cancer patients. J Neurosurg (Spine 1) 2003; 98:21-30.

21. Ahn H, Mousavi P, Chin I, et al. The effect of pre-vertebroplasty tumor ablation using laser-induced thermotherapy on biomechanical stability and cement fill in the metastatic spine. Eur Spine J 2007; 16:1171-1178.

22. Komemushi A, Tanigawa N, Kariya S, et al. Percutaneous vertebroplasty for osteoporotic compression fracture: multivariate study of predictors of new vertebral bode fracture. Cardiovasc Intervent Radiol 2006; 239:195-200.

23. Lin EP, Ekholm S, Hiwatashi A, Westesson PL. Vertebroplasty: cement leakage into the disc increases the risk of new fracture of adjacent vertebral body. AJNR Am J Neuroradiol 2004; 25:175-180.

24. Kim SH, Kang HS, Choi JA, Ahn JM. Risk factors of new compression fractures in adjacent vertebrae after percutaneous vertebroplasty. Acta Radiol 2004; 45:440-445.

25. Taylor RS, Fritzell P, Taylor RJ. Balloon kyphoplasty in the management of vertebral compression fractures: an updated systematic review and meta-analysis. Eur Spine J 2007; Feb 3 [Epub ahead of print].

26. Vats HS, McKiernan FE. Infected vertebroplasty: case report and review of literature. Spine 2006; 31:E859-E862.

CHAPTER 25

Complications of Surgery for Decompression of Spinal Stenosis and Disc Disease

Thomas Paul Naidich, Yakov Gologorsky, Girish M. Fatterpekar, and Tanvir F. Choudhri

Successful surgery for spondylosis and disc disease relieves the initial symptoms and, for cases in which stabilization is performed, provides solid fusion at the operative site. Complications of surgery can include failure to relieve the symptoms, failure of fusion, and any new problem resulting from the surgery itself. General complications of surgery include thrombophlebitis (2%-3%), pulmonary embolism (1%), and death (0.1%-0.3%). Risks of spinal surgery include incomplete fusions, graft/implant extrusion, infection, and injury to the spinal cord and nerve roots. Ischemic optic neuropathy causes vision loss in 0.03% to 0.2% of spinal surgeries.[1]

The specific risks of cervical surgery are transient and permanent vocal cord dysfunction, airway dysfunction, esophageal fistula, vertebral and carotid artery injury, and injury to the sympathetic trunk. In thoracolumbar surgery there is the risk of injury to the reproductive system and to the iliac vessels, aorta, and vena cava. Imaging studies must address the level of surgery, nature of surgery, success of the procedure, and the presence/absence of specific complications known to be associated with the surgery.

COMPLICATIONS OF CERVICAL SPINE SURGERY

Degenerative cervical spondylosis is common. The past decades have seen improvements in the recognition and diagnosis of the clinical features of spondylosis, increases in the number of treatment options, and improvements in surgical technique, instrumentation, perioperative anesthesia, and critical care management. Over the period 1993 to 2001, the number of cervical spinal fusions performed in the United States increased 433%, from 15 to 87/100,000 population for patients aged 40 to 59 years

and from 9 to 44/100,000 population for patients aged 60 years or older.[2] The primary indication for cervical fusion was degenerative disc disease (33/100,000 in 2001).[2]

At present, compressive cervical radiculopathy and/or myelopathy may be treated by several types of procedures:

1. *Anterior cervical discectomy for one disc level only (ACD).* This procedure utilizes an anterior approach to the cervical spine to decompress the spinal canal or neural foramen by removal of compressive disc herniations and/or disc/osteophyte complex *without* placement of any interbody bone graft or instrumentation. It has a limited role in modern spine surgery but may still be considered for patients with normal cervical lordosis, a single level of pathology, and minimal axial pain.
2. *Anterior cervical discectomy and fusion for one or multiple disc levels (ACDF).* In this procedure, an interbody arthrodesis (fusion) is added to the ACD. The fusion is typically performed with a structural graft construct involving autograft or allograft bone (Fig. 25-1A, B). A plate/screw construct (P) is frequently applied to provide additional structural support (ACDFP) (Figs. 25-1C and 25-2).
3. *Anterior cervical corpectomy for two or more disc levels (ACC).* This procedure utilizes a similar approach to the anterior spinal column. Thereafter, most of the center of one or more vertebral bodies is removed between the discectomy levels to provide additional decompression of the spinal canal. The bone defect is then reconstructed with a structural support such as a fibular strut graft or a titanium mesh cage (filled with autograft and/or allograft bone). A plate/screw construct is typically affixed to provide additional support for the construct (Fig. 25-3).

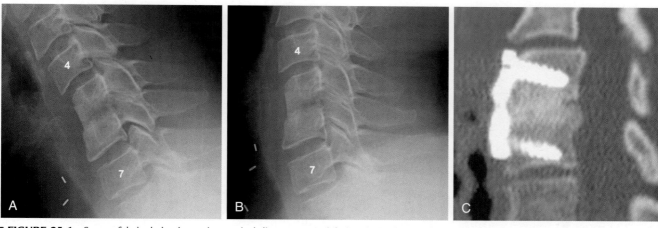

■ FIGURE 25-1   Successful single-level anterior cervical discectomy and fusion (ACDF). **A** and **B,** ACDF without instrumentation. Plain spine radiographs in flexion (**A**) and extension (**B**) demonstrate continuity of bony trabeculae across the C5-C6 fusion zone and absence of any motion at the level in flexion versus extension, signifying complete fusion. The C4-C7 vertebral bodies are well aligned and maintain normal curvature in both positions. **C,** ACDF with instrumentation. There is complete bony union with preserved density of the bone plug, continuity of bony trabeculae from C3 across the bone plug to C4, excellent bone surrounding and extending between the threads of the screws, proper seating of the fixation plate flush with the anterior surfaces of the vertebrae, proper placement of the plug at the anterior aspect of the interspace, consequent maintenance of the cervical lordosis, and absence of any prevertebral swelling.

4. *Posterior cervical decompression for one or more levels (PCD).* This procedure typically utilizes a laminectomy and/or foraminotomy to decompress the canal/foramen. Typically, posterior fusion is then achieved by lateral mass and/or pedicle screw instrumentation to provide spinal stability. Some surgeons prefer to decompress the spinal canal by laminoplasty rather than laminectomy. Laminoplasty *expands* the spinal canal by elevating the laminae and spinous processes dorsally and securing them in the new, expanded position with instrumentation.

5. *Combined anterior and posterior procedures for multilevel surgery (360-degree, circumferential surgery).* The anterior and posterior procedures can be performed as part of the same surgical procedure or on separate dates.

Zeidman and colleagues found an overall complication rate of 5.3% among 4,589 patients undergoing cervical spine surgery for diverse diseases.[3] A decade later, Fountas and coworkers found a mortality of approximately 0.1% (one esophageal perforation) and a morbidity of 19% in more than 1000 patients undergoing first ACDF for degenerative disc disease/spondylosis.[4] The true prevalence of postoperative complications is likely higher, because patient surveys uncover far more problems than are indicated in the surgical reports.[5] Complications specific to cervical spine surgery include incomplete cervical fusions (variably 7%-40%), graft extrusions and pseudarthroses (up to 10%), infection (0.4%-2%), nerve root injury (0.14%), spinal cord injury (~0.2%), transient vocal cord dysfunction (~3%), permanent voice changes (1%), esophageal perforation (0.4%), and vertebral artery injury (0.14%).[6,7] The anterior cervical approach may lead to additional surgery for complications of the bone graft (13%) and for accelerated adjacent level degeneration (7%). The posterior cervical approach may lead to C5 nerve palsy (6%, usually transient) and intractable axial pain postoperatively (28%).[8]

Both anterior and posterior cervical decompressions achieve better results when (1) the specific indications for surgery involve neurologic symptoms (radiculopathy and/or myelopathy), (2) the preoperative neurologic status is excellent, (3) only a single-level anterior cervical fusion is required, (4) the transverse area of the cord remains greater than or equal to 60% of normal, and (5) epidural spinal cord–evoked potentials are normal. Factors favorable for successful fusion with good short-term and long-term outcome include youth, male gender, short duration of symptoms, low intensity of pain, mild disability, good hand strength, an active range of neck motion, compression by soft disc (vs. osseous ridge), and single level of surgery.[9]

The clinical outcome after cervical decompression may be graded by Odom's criteria (Table 25-1).[10]

The role of smoking in spine surgery has been studied. Smoking reduces the rate of spinal fusion twofold to fourfold.[11] Chronic cigarette smoking impairs capillary ingrowth from viable adjacent recipient site bone, inhibits vascular growth into the graft, and results in fewer healthy pluripotent and osteoblastic bone-forming cells being available for recruitment. Nicotine decreases osteoblast cellular proliferation, interrupts collagen synthesis, and inhibits osteoblastic cellular metabolism. Free radicals from burning cigarettes destabilize membranes by lipid peroxidation and, thus, damage osteoblasts, endothelial cells, and leukocytes and impair osteoblastic mitochondrial oxidative function. Cigarette smoke products release endothelin by damaging endothelial cells and inhibit prostaglandin production, a powerful vasodilator and inhibitor of platelet aggregation. This leads to impaired bone blood flow and increased bone blood viscosity and microcirculatory occlusion. There is accelerated osteoporosis.[11] Overall, many studies have shown that smoking interferes with fusion success rates. However, other studies have not shown a detrimental effect on clinical outcome.[12]

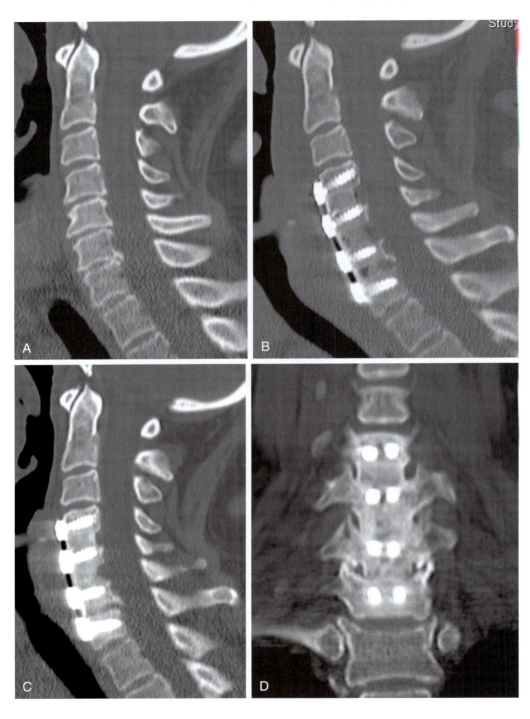

■ **FIGURE 25-2** Multi-level anterior cervical discectomy and fusion (ACDF). **A** to **C,** Serial sagittal reformatted CT images. **D,** Coronal reformatted CT image. **A,** Preoperative CT image shows degenerative disc disease with posterior spurs most marked at C4-C5-C6-C7. The prevertebral soft tissue is normal. **B,** Repeat CT 2 days after surgery shows three-level discectomy with decortication of the apposing end plates, placement of allograft interbody fusion plugs at the anterior aspects of the interspaces, and internal fixation with anterior cervical plate and screws. The cervical lordosis is maintained. The prevertebral soft tissue is now swollen. The cervical plate sits flush with the anterior border of the vertebral bodies. Nearly all screws are well placed, although the C5 screw rises up to the superior surface of the vertebra posterior to the plug. Small posterior spurs remain at C6-7. **C,** Six months later the prevertebral soft tissue has returned to normal. The bony trabeculae are continuous across the interspaces at C4-C5-C6, indicating fusion. Lucency persisting at C6-C7 raises the question of possible nonfusion at this level. **D,** Simultaneous coned-down coronal reformatted CT image confirms the fusion at C4-C5-C6 and the persistent lucency at C6-C7.

Complications of Anterior Cervical Approaches

Nonunions and Extrusions of Interbody Grafts and Strut Grafts

Successful fusion (arthrodesis) of the operated levels means complete bony union of the adjacent bones that is sufficiently strong to support the spine and avoid abnormal motion at the operated level. Nonfusion (failed fusion) signifies incomplete bony union and can potentially lead to abnormal motion at the segment, migration/angulation of the interposed bone grafts or strut grafts, and impingement upon sensitive nerves (Fig. 25-2).

Epidemiology

Single-Level Procedures

In 14 studies of a total of 939 patients with cervical disc degeneration treated by single-level and dual-level anterior interbody fusions, meta-analysis shows that discectomy

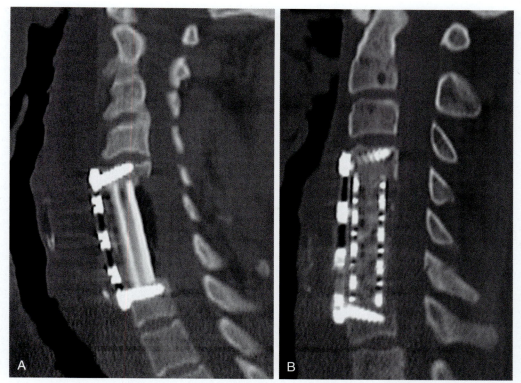

■ **FIGURE 25-3**   Successful anterior cervical corpectomies and fusion with decompression of the cervical spinal canal. Two patients. **A,** Strut graft. Sagittal reformatted cervical spine CT demonstrates anterior cervical corpectomy at C6 and C7 for a three-level discectomy and strut graft fusion from C5-T1. The canal is well decompressed. The superior screw is well angled but slightly high in position. The lower screw is well placed. The anterior cervical plate is flush with the vertebral bodies. The height and placement of the plate will not interfere with motion at adjoining levels. The strut graft is well positioned and well seated with maintenance of cervical lordosis. **B,** Cervical cage. Sagittal reformatted CT shows corpectomy at C5 and C6, decortication of the apposing surfaces of C4 and C7, placement of a bone-filled cage that has fused into a dense strut with direct continuity of bony trabeculae from C4 to C7, excellent bone about the anterior cervical screws, flush position of the plate against the vertebrae, and maintenance of normal cervical lordosis. (*A, from Naidich TP. Cervical spine decompression for spinal stenosis and disk disease: Complications of surgery. In Castillo M, Koeller KK, Mukherji SK. Neuroradiology Categorical Course Syllabus, pp 289-296. American Roentgen Ray Society, 107th Annual Meeting, Orlando, FL, 2007.*)

TABLE 25-1.   Odom's Clinical Outcome Ratings

Excellent	No complaint referable to cervical disease
	Able to perform daily occupation without impairment
Good	Intermittent discomfort referable to cervical disease
	No significant interference with work
Fair	Subjective improvement in symptoms
	Physical activity substantially impaired
Poor	Worsening or no improvement

From Wang JC, et al. Graft migration or displacement after multilevel cervical corpectomy and strut grafting. Spine 2003; 28:1016-1021; discussion 1021-1022.

alone has a shorter operation time, shorter hospital stay, and shorter absence from work than discectomy plus fusion and is equally effective for relieving pain and achieving good fusion (Table 25-2).[13-17] Single-level interbody fusions achieve successful arthrodesis in more than 90% of cases.[14] Use of rigid anterior instrumentation with plating does not increase the fusion rate and may add complications unique to the instrumentation.[15] For single levels there is no significant difference in the fusion rate for allografts versus autografts,[12] but autografts give better fusion rates than do cages.[13]

Multilevel Procedures

Multilevel procedures achieve complete fusion less often than single-level procedures.[14] For anterior cervical discectomy or corpectomy with instrumentation and plating, Bose reported fusion rates of 100% for two-level surgery; 98.3% for three-level surgery; and 77.8% for three-level surgery.[11] In a single series of 1015 patients with one-, two-, and three-level ACDF, the overall fusion rate was 94.5% at 12 months (one-level, 95.6%; two-level, 93.9%; and three-level, 90.5%).[4] Multilevel procedures performed by corpectomy and strut graft fuse successfully more often (93%) than do multiple sequential discectomies with multilevel interbody grafts (66%).[14] The bone grafts and strut grafts may settle, angulate, or migrate. In Hilibrand and colleagues' series, none of the interbody bone grafts became displaced or extruded, but 10.2% of the strut grafts became displaced or dislodged.[14] In Hughes and associates' series, fibular strut grafts settled an average of 6.7 mm (±5.7 mm) over 2 years and angulated about 2.5 degrees when no instrumentation was performed.[16]

Clinical Presentation

Nonfusion of the operated level can present as chronic pain. In the series of Bolesta and coworkers, the 8 patients

TABLE 25-2. Anterior Approaches to Fusion of the Cervical Spine: A Meta-analysis of Fusion Rates

	Outcome		
Type of Surgery	Total No. of Procedures	Fusion Rates (%)	Pseudarthrosis Rates (%)
One Disc Level			
ACD	73	84.9	15.1
1-level ACDF	1231	92.1	7.9
1-level ACDFP	339	97.1	2.9
Two Disc Levels			
2-level ACDF	422	79.9	20.1
2-level ACDFP	184	94.6	5.4
1-level corpectomy	73	95.9	4.1
1-level corpectomy with plating	56	92.9	7.1
Three Disc Levels			
3-level ACDF	123	65.0	35.0
3-level ACDFP	40	82.5	17.4
2-level corpectomy	88	89.8	10.2
2-level corpectomy with plating	53	96.2	3.8
Total	2,682	89.5	10.5

ACD, Anterior cervical discectomy; ACDF, ACD with fusion; ACDFP, ACDF with plating.
From Fraser JF, Härtl R. Anterior approaches to fusion of the cervical spine: A meta-analysis of fusion rates. J Neurosurg Spine 2007; 6:298-303.

who did not have complete fusion manifested no pain (4 patients), pain without need for further surgery (1 patient), and pain severe enough to require additional surgery (3 patients, with pain relief in 2 of the 3).[18]

Pathophysiology

Arthrodesis may require months to years to achieve the maximum degree of bone fusion. Multiple factors contribute to the rapidity and success of complete bone fusion, including adequate bone graft substrate, immobilization of the region being fused, and many host-related factors. Factors that predispose to nonunion include excessive motion/trauma at the operated level, smoking, diabetes, malnutrition, corticosteroid usage, and osteoporosis.

Imaging

Radiographic signs of successful fusion include (1) continuity of bone density and bony trabeculae across the interspace; (2) minimal loss of height at the operated disc space; (3) less than 3 degrees of movement at the operative site on flexion-extension series; (4) presence of a sclerotic line between the graft and the vertebral bone indicating bone remodeling with new bone formation at the junction; (5) absence of any lucent "halo" or periprosthetic lucency around the implant(s); and (6) integrity of the construct with no screw fracture, pullout, or plate buckling.[19] At times, there may also be resorption of anterior osteophytes (see Figs. 25-1 and 25-2).[20]

Postoperative Cervical Kyphosis

Over the length from C2 to C7, the normal lordotic curve is about 24 degrees (range: 10-34 degrees).[21] An angle of less than 10 degrees is hypolordotic. An angle of less than 0 degrees is kyphotic.[21]

Epidemiology

In 42 patients with single-level ACD, ACDF, or ACDFP, the extent of cervical lordosis from C2 to C7 did not change after ACD, ACDF, or ACDFP.[22] Kyphosis was seen at the operative level at 2 years in 75% of patients treated by simple ACD but in none of those treated by ACDF or ACDF with instrumentation.[22] In 25 patients with three-level and four-level ACDF and complete fusion, a lordotic curvature was achieved in 84%.[23] In 26 patients with four- and five-level surgeries, follow-up showed successful reconstruction of a lordotic curve in 20 (76.9%), a hypolordotic curve in 4 (15.4%), and a kyphotic curve in 2 (7.7%).[21]

Patient Presentation

Postoperative cervical kyphosis typically presents as axial or radicular pain but sometimes as head drop.

Pathophysiology

Initial resection of bone plus later resorption of the host bone and the interbody graft may lead to settling and angulation of the construct, with kyphosis.

Imaging

Plain radiographs, reformatted sagittal CT scans, and MR images display the overall curvature of the spine and enable precise measurements of the angle across the operative level (Fig. 25-4).

Adjacent Level Degenerative Disc Disease

The term *adjacent level degenerative disc disease* signifies new or accelerated degeneration of the disc and development or exaggeration of spondylosis at the levels adjacent to the operated level. This may be associated with new or worsened symptoms.

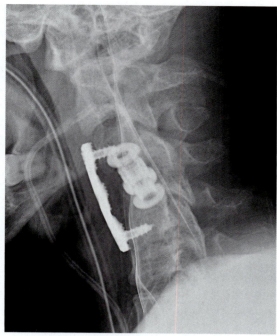

■ **FIGURE 25-4** Cervical kyphosis. Lateral spine radiograph shows abnormal cervical kyphosis after C4 corpectomy with placement of an expandable cage, anterior cervical plating, and screw fixation. The plate lies well anterior to the operated level, is slightly separated from the anterior surface of C3, and contacts only the most inferior portion of C5. There is no evidence of bony fusion.

Epidemiology

Among 42 consecutive patients treated by single-level ACD, ACDF, or ACDFP, radicular symptoms developed at a level adjacent to the site of surgery in 17% of all cases, specifically ACD, 17%; ACDF, 20%; and ACDFP, 20%.[22] Among 26 patients with long (four- or five-level) anterior cervical constructs, adjacent level disc degeneration developed in 19 (73%).[21]

Patient Presentation

Adjacent level disease may become symptomatic in as many as 15% of patients undergoing multilevel surgeries and may progress in 12%.[14,21,24] Ultimately, 2 (7.7%) of 26 patients undergoing four- and five-level procedures required surgery at levels adjacent to the index construct.[21]

Pathophysiology

Successful fusion of one or more spinal levels increases the biomechanical load on the adjoining levels. The increased load may lead to excessive motion at the adjoining levels, accelerated degeneration of the discs, stretching or damage to the ligaments, and new or more severe compression of emerging or traversing nerve roots.

Imaging

Serial imaging studies can assess the extent to which surgical hardware impinges on and distorts adjacent bony elements (Fig. 25-5). Serial studies document whether the levels adjoining the surgical site develop narrowing of the interspaces, spondylotic spurs, and subluxations of the vertebral bodies and posterior elements with flexion and extension. They also display any impingement of the surgical hardware on bone.

Hardware and Graft Failure

Hardware failure is a breakdown in the instrumentation used to stabilize the spine. Examples include broken or

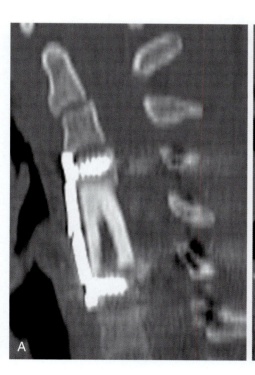

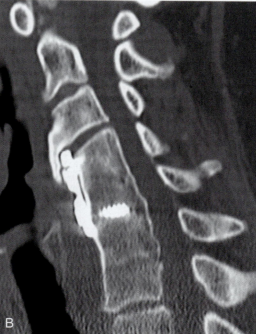

■ **FIGURE 25-5** High position of anterior cervical plates and adjacent level disease. Sagittal reformatted CT images. Two patients. **A,** C5 corpectomy with strut graft at C4-C6. The superior margin of the plate impinges on the anterior inferior margin of C3, limiting patient motion at C3-C4. **B,** Sagittal reformatted CT shows anterior C6-C7 fusion without instrumentation and anterior C3-C4 fusion with instrumentation. The C4-C7 surgical levels are well fused but exhibit cervical kyphosis. High position of the cervical plate and progressive degenerative change at C3-C4 led to growth of a robust anterior osteophyte that incorporates the upper margin of the anterior cervical plate.

TABLE 25-3. Graft Migration

Corpectomy Levels	No. of Patients Operated Upon	No. of Patients with Graft Migration	Incidence of Graft Displacement (%)
One	95	4	4.2
Two	76	4	5.3
Three	71	7	9.9
Four	6	1	16.7
Five	1	0	0
Total	249	16	6.4

loosened screws, screw extrusion, and/or anterior migration of the fixation plate. Graft failure is graft resorption, displacement, or migration precluding complete bony fusion, maintenance of normal disc height, and preservation of normal spinal curvature.

Epidemiology

Lowery and associates found hardware failure in 35% of anterior cervical plate fixations.[25] Fountas and coworkers reported a 0.1% rate of instrumentation failure for first ACDF.[4] With long-segment (four- or five-level) anterior cervical constructs, the fixation plate may impinge on adjacent levels either primarily (11.5%) or secondarily (owing to settling of the construct with telescoping at the end of a long construct) (15.4%) (total: 27%).[21] The geometry of long-segment constructs often changes over time but typically does not undergo catastrophic failure.[21] In patients treated with corpectomy and strut grafting, the incidence of graft migration increases with the number of levels treated, that is, with the length of the strut graft (Table 25-3).

Clinical Presentation

In Lowery and coworkers' series, the hardware failure did not endanger the patient.[25] However, mechanical failure has led to significant injury to the prevertebral tissue in other series.

Pathophysiology

Hardware failure may cause, or result from, failed fusion, destabilization of the construct, and erosion of prevertebral soft tissue structures. (See Esophageal Perforation, later.)

Imaging

Plain radiographs and CT scans with reformatted 2D and 3D images depict the integrity or disruption of the hardware, misplacement or loosening of the fixation screws, and collapse/angulation of the construct (Figs. 25-6 to 25-8).

Spinal Cord Injury

Spinal cord injury is damage to the spinal cord beyond that present before surgery.

Epidemiology

Fountas and coworkers reported cord contusions in 2 patients (0.2% of >1000 cases).[4]

Clinical Presentation

Both of the reported patients in Fountas and coworkers' series presented with postoperative worsening of preexisting myelopathy. In both patients there was gradual improvement over the next 6 weeks after intensive physical therapy and they returned to their preoperative functional level 12 weeks after the procedure. Neither showed neurologic deficits or myelopathic signs at the 12-month follow-up evaluation.[4]

Imaging

In Fountas and coworkers patients there was evidence on MR images of cord contusion.[4] Seichi and associates studied the incidence and significance of postoperative "expansion" of preexisting areas of T2 prolongation (high T2 signal intensity) in 114 patients with stenotic cervical myelopathy (Fig. 25-9).[26] They found abnormal postoperative expansion of the high intensity zone in 7/114 (6.1%) patients. Four of these 7 patients were symptomatic; 3 were not. After surgery, 9 patients (7.9%) suffered unilateral upper motor paresis with sparing of the lower extremity. Five of these 9 (56%) exhibited expansion of the high signal zone, correlating with distal paresis arising immediately after surgery (3 patients) or diffuse paresis (2 patients).[26] Four of the 9 (44%) showed no expansion of the zone. These 4 had solely unilateral proximal deltoid, biceps, and brachialis palsy first arising 4 to 6 days postoperatively.[26]

Pathophysiology

After reviewing 10 cases, Kraus and Stauffer suggested that the risk of spinal cord injury is increased by advancing instruments, such as nerve hooks, into the spinal canal to remove posterior osteophytes.[27]

Dysphagia (Pharyngeal-Esophageal Dysfunction)

Dysphagia is difficulty in swallowing and moving ingested material smoothly from the oropharynx into the stomach.

Epidemiology

Temporary dysphagia is found in up to 60% of patients after anterior cervical discectomy. It persists for more than 12 months in up to 12% of patients.[28] Fountas and coworkers found mild to moderate postoperative dysphagia in 9.5% of 1015 first ACDFs.[4] Ninety-five percent of these cases cleared completely within 2 to 7 days postoperatively. The rest improved slowly over 2 to 4 weeks after surgery.[4] In 310 patients undergoing ACD, Lee and coworkers found dysphagia in 54.0% at 1 month, 33.6% at 2 months, 18.6% at 6 months, 15.2% at 12 months, and 13.6% at 24 months after surgery.[29] Risk factors for

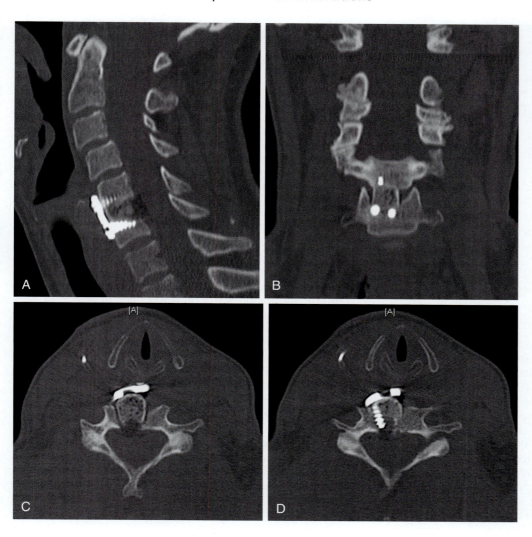

■ **FIGURE 25-6**   Recent anterior cervical discectomy and fusion (ADCF) with misplaced anterior cervical screw. Sagittal reformatted (**A**), coronal reformatted (**B**), and sequential direct axial bone algorithm CT images (**C, D**). The single C5 screw has complete bony purchase. The right C6 screw grooves the upper surface of C6 at the interface with the bone plug, achieving no real bony purchase.

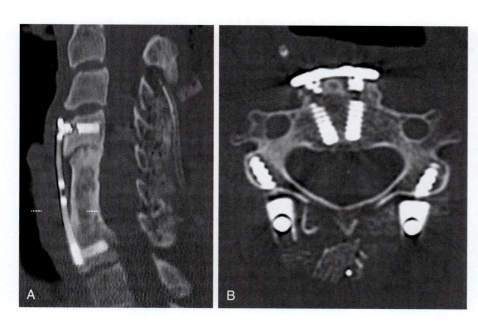

■ **FIGURE 25-7**   Broken cervical screws. Sagittal reformatted cervical spine CT (**A**) and axial bone algorithm CT (**B**) show breaks in the anterior ends of both C4 screws, slight anterior "springing" of the upper end of the anterior cervical plate away from the vertebra, and nonfusion between the upper end of the strut graft and C4, leading to the subsequent posterior cervical fusion. Note the posterior bone laid down for fusion, and the drain. In **B**, the lateral mass screws are well angled and well seated bilaterally. The "gaps" in these two screws are artifacts of the plane of section passing obliquely through the angled connection between the screws and the connectors to the vertical members. *(From Naidich TP. Cervical spine decompression for spinal stenosis and disk disease: Complications of surgery. In Castillo M, Koeller KK, Mukherji SK. Neuroradiology Categorical Course Syllabus, pp 289-296. American Roentgen Ray Society, 107th Annual Meeting, Orlando, FL, 2007.)*

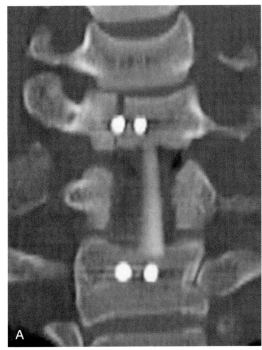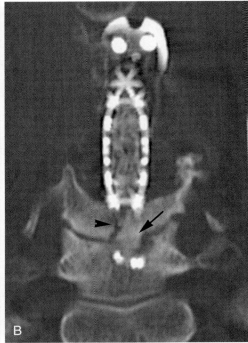

■ **FIGURE 25-8** Fractured vertebrae. Coronal reformatted CT scans. Two patients. **A,** C7 corpectomy with strut graft. The right C6 screw is intimately associated with the vertical C6 fracture. **B** The vertebral body interposed between the lower end of the interbody cage and the interbody bone plug (*arrow*) has fractured vertically (*arrowhead*) at the point of maximum vertical stress. (*B, from Naidich TP. Cervical spine decompression for spinal stenosis and disk disease: Complications of surgery. In Castillo M, Koeller KK, Mukherji SK. Neuroradiology Categorical Course Syllabus, pp 289-296. American Roentgen Ray Society, 107th Annual Meeting, Orlando, FL, 2007.*)

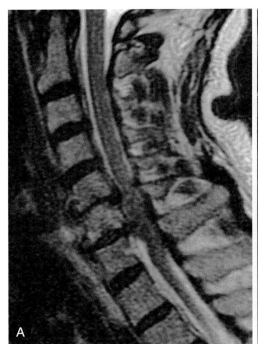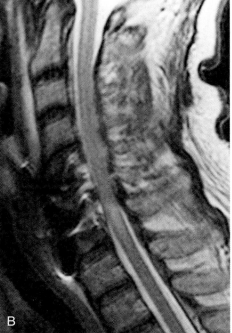

■ **FIGURE 25-9** Postoperative spinal cord edema. **A,** Preoperative T2-weighted sagittal cervical MR image shows marked stenosis of the spinal canal at C5-C7 with compression of the subarachnoid space and spinal cord. **B,** After multilevel anterior cervical discectomy and fusion with instrumentation, T2-weighted sagittal MRI shows decompression of the spinal canal and cord, with interval appearance of high signal edema within the decompressed spinal cord. (*From Naidich TP. Cervical spine decompression for spinal stenosis and disk disease: Complications of surgery. In Castillo M, Koeller KK, Mukherji SK. Neuroradiology Categorical Course Syllabus, pp 289-296. American Roentgen Ray Society, 107th Annual Meeting, Orlando, FL, 2007.*)

postoperative dysphagia that persists for at least 24 months include female gender (18.3% vs. 9.9% for males), revision surgery (27.7% vs. 11.3% primary surgery), and multilevel surgery (three or more levels) (19.3% vs. 9.7% for one- or two-level surgery). Dysphagia is also more common in elderly patients versus young patients.[4,29] In Lee and colleagues' series, the prevalence of dysphagia did *not* increase with use of instrumentation or with corpectomy versus discectomy.[29]

Clinical Presentation

Postoperative dysphagia manifests as pain with swallowing, difficulty in swallowing, coughing or choking with

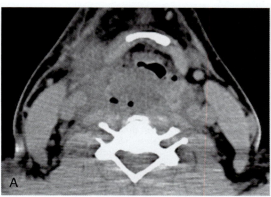
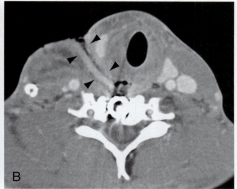

■ **FIGURE 25-10** Esophageal perforation. Two patients. **A,** Axial CT image shows a large retropharyngeal collection with air bubbles, representing phlegmon and abscess from esophageal perforation during the approach to the anterior cervical spine. **B,** Contrast-enhanced axial CT scan shows a squamous-lined esophagocutaneous fistula (*arrowheads*) created to divert secretions away from the esophageal perforation.

swallowing, new onset of heartburn, regurgitation of old food, feeling of throat blockage, and/or frequent throat clearing.[4] Typically, the dysphagia is more severe with solid food than with liquids.

Pathophysiology

Postoperative dysphagia may result from pressure by the retractor blades against the gut wall.[30,31] In 31 patients undergoing ACDF, Heese and associates showed that the mean pressure of the open retractor blades against the pharynx exceeded both the mean arterial pressure and the mean mucosal perfusion pressure of the pharynx.[30,31] In open position, therefore, retractors may reduce mucosal perfusion and cause local ischemia.[30,31]

Imaging

Barium swallow studies may show luminal narrowing, delayed transit, and/or laryngeal penetration/aspiration.

Esophageal Perforation

Esophageal perforation is the creation or later development of a full-thickness defect in the esophageal wall. The defect may be the result of (1) an immediate direct full-thickness injury, (2) a lesser injury that weakens the wall leading to later perforation, or (3) a peri-esophageal complication such as breakdown of the construct with instrument migration that erodes into the esophagus secondarily.

Epidemiology

Esophageal perforation is a rare complication of ACDF, with a reported incidence between 0%[32] and 1.62%.[33] Several recent large series (>1000 patients each) have found an incidence between 0.1% and 0.4%.[4,34,35]

Clinical Presentation

The perforation may present acutely in the intraoperative period (27%), shortly postoperatively (27%), or weeks to months (even years) later (45%).[34,36] Patients may present with progressive dysphagia, fever/sepsis, mediastinitis,

and/or wound drainage, swelling, crepitus, or abscess. The diagnosis may be confirmed with a Gastrografin swallowing study. Although nonoperative management has been used selectively with success, the treatment generally involves surgical repair. When all causes of esophageal perforation were analyzed, there is some evidence suggesting that earlier treatment may lead to a better outcome. The mortality rate was 20% when treatment was instituted less than 24 hours from diagnosis and 50% when it occurred in a more delayed fashion, but this was not a randomized study.[37]

Pathophysiology

Inadvertent perforation during surgery typically leads to immediate leak. Recognition of the perforation allows primary repair and, if needed, interposition of vital tissue. Such immediate repair may permit complete healing.[4] Unrecognized perforations can lead to esophagocutaneous fistula and/or potentially fatal mediastinitis. Alternatively, a leak can present in a delayed fashion, sometimes from erosion of instrumentation into the esophagus. Loosening of cervical fixation screws and/or plates, for example, may allow the displaced hardware to erode into the cervical esophagus (0.8%).[38] Extruded hardware that erodes into the esophagus has been reported to traverse the gastrointestinal tract and to exit orally or rectally, so the imager must be alert to the *absence* of any screws and should search for any "missing screw" whenever esophageal perforation occurs in the postsurgical patient.[39,40] Treatment of chronic esophageal perforation is difficult, may necessitate multiple surgical procedures over years, and may require sternocleidomastoid myoplasty and deliberate creation of an external fistula (Fig. 25-10B).

Imaging

CT and MRI with contrast enhancement may demonstrate paraesophageal abscess or air in the surgical bed (Figs. 25-10 to 25-12). However, air in the surgical field is normal in the early postoperative field. Increasing air on interval imaging should raise the suspicion for esophageal perforation. Both CT and MRI may be hard to interpret owing to postsurgical changes and instrumentation artifact (when present).

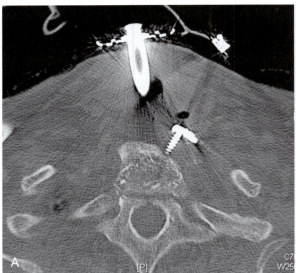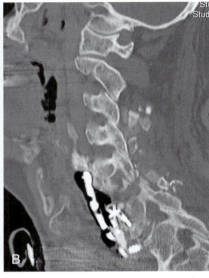

■ **FIGURE 25-11** Migration of instrumentation with esophageal perforation. **A,** Axial bone algorithm CT shows a tracheostomy, extrusion of the lower left fixation screw, anterior migration of the cervical plate, and prevertebral soft tissue swelling. **B,** Sagittal reformatted CT scan shows anterior migration of the lowest screw and plate. Air from an infected esophageal fistula surrounds the instrumentation. *(From Naidich TP. Cervical spine decompression for spinal stenosis and disk disease: Complications of surgery. In Castillo M, Koeller KK, Mukherji SK. Neuroradiology Categorical Course Syllabus, pp 289-296. American Roentgen Ray Society, 107th Annual Meeting, Orlando, FL, 2007.)*

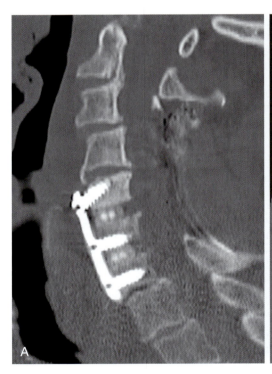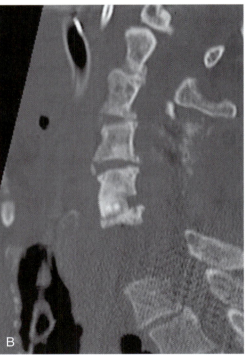

■ **FIGURE 25-12** Esophageal perforation and infection requiring corpectomy and removal of instrumentation. Serial sagittal reformatted CT images. **A,** Postoperative CT image shows anterior cervical discectomy and fusion at C5-C7 with interbody bone plugs at C5-C6 and C6-C7, plus later posterior laminectomy and fusion (posterior instrumentation not visible in the midline). The superior C5 screw has loosened, allowing the upper end of the cervical plate to separate from the anterior surface of C5. The prevertebral soft tissue is swollen. **B,** Three months later, repeat study shows interval removal of the instrumentation, the C7 vertebral body, and the C6-C7 bone plug. The remaining upper plug has fused to the undersurface of C5 but not to the superior surface of C6.

Airway Dysfunction

The term *airway complication* signifies any postoperative compromise of the airway, especially those that lead to prophylactic delay of extubation for more than 24 hours after surgery or to urgent/emergent re-intubation.

Epidemiology

Sagi and associates reported airway complications in 6% of more than 300 anterior cervical procedures. These required emergency re-intubation of the just-operated neck (with all attendant risks) in one third of cases (2%) and led to death in 0.3%.[28] Terao and coworkers encountered airway complications in 1.8% of anterior surgeries, 1.1% of posterior surgeries, and 70% of combined anteroposterior (360-degree procedures).[41] Risk factors for cervical edema include prolonged/difficult surgery involving high cervical exposures (C2, C3, or C4), exposure of more than three vertebral levels, combined anteroposterior surgery at the same time, operative time more than 5 hours, blood loss greater than 300 mL, and increased volume of crystalloid replacement. Histories of myelopathy, spinal cord injury, pulmonary problems, smoking, and anesthetic risk factors do not correlate with airway complications.[28]

TABLE 25-4. Prevertebral Soft Tissue Swelling after Anterior Cervical Discectomy and Fusion (ACDF) with Plate Fixation: Measurements in Neutral Position in 193 One- and Two-level ACDF*

Level	Preop Prox	Preop Dist	Postop Prox	Postop Dist	Day 1 Prox	Day 1 Dist	Day 2 Prox	Day 2 Dist	Day 3 Prox	Day 3 Dist	Day 4 Prox	Day 4 Dist	Day 5 Prox	Day 5 Dist
C2	3.6	3.5	6.4	4.5	8.4	5.0	13.1	8.5	11.2	8.7	9.2	6.1	8.1	4.9
C3	3.9	3.6	7.3	5.6	11.7	6.8	15.5	11.0	14.1	12.0	10.8	10.1	11.1	7.9
C4	5.9	6.2	9.8	9.7	13.0	11.1	16.6	13.2	15.1	14.5	13.5	12.6	13.9	11.1
C5	13.7	14.8	15.6	16.4	17.6	16.9	17.9	17.4	17.7	18.2	16.4	16.8	17.8	16.3
C6	15.6	15.3	17.2	17.1	18.5	17.6	17.7	17.0	18.0	18.1	17.8	18.1	18.9	17.6

*Comparison of prevertebral soft tissue between the proximal to C5 surgery group (*Prox*) and distal to C5 surgery group (*Dist*) in mm.
From Suk KS, Kim KT, Lee SH, Park SW. Prevertebral soft tissue swelling after anterior cervical discectomy and fusion with plate fixation. Int Orthop 2006; 30:290-294.

TABLE 25-5. "Normal" Prevertbral Soft Tissue Swelling after Elective Anterior Cervical Decompression and Fusion*

	Preoperative	2 Weeks	6 Weeks
C2	4.34 (3-8)	5.53 (3-17)	4.58 (3-11)
C3	5.04 (3-10)	7.35 (3-17)	5.4 (3-11)
C4	6.58 (3-18)	10.57 (3-22)	7.5 (3-18)
C5	12.06 (5-25)	17.81 (5-32)	13.06 (5-25)
C6	16.23 (7-25)	21.65 (15-35)	18.05 (10-27)
C7	15.31 (8-25)	21.03 (10-33)	17.94 (9-29)

Significant: *P* < 0.001 for all levels from preoperative to 2 weeks. *P* < 0.001 for all levels from 2 weeks to 6 weeks. *P* < 0.01 for C4, C6, C7 from preoperative to 6 weeks.
Not Significant: *P* > 0.05 for C2, C3 C5 from preoperative to 6 weeks.
*Mean soft tissue measurements (mm) for all levels and all time periods, with ranges.
From Sanfilippo JA Jr, et al. "Normal" prevertebral soft tissue swelling following elective anterior cervical decompression and fusion. J Spinal Disord Tech 2006; 19:399-401.

Clinical Presentation

Airway dysfunction typically presents as shortness of breath, decreased oxygen saturation, hypercapnia, and/or stridor. Acute airway obstruction nearly always results from pharyngeal edema, but hematoma, laryngeal obstruction (see later), and hardware slippage must be excluded. Normal postoperative soft tissue swelling increases markedly on the second day, is maximal at days 2 to 3, and gradually reduces from day 4 onward (Tables 25-4 and 25-5).[42-44] Therefore, extubation on postoperative day 1 and discharge to home may occur before maximal swelling. Epstein and associates recommended keeping patients intubated overnight and having the anesthesiologist remove the endotracheal tube to reduce the risk of such airway complications.[42]

Pathogenesis

For procedures cephalic to C5 the swelling is most marked at C2-C3. There is no difference in the degree of soft tissue swelling between one-level and two-level surgeries.

Imaging

Plain lateral cervical radiographs are often obtained postoperatively to assess vertebral alignment, instrument position, and airway patency. Tables 25-4 and 25-5 give the expected thickness of the prevertebral soft tissue in the postoperative period.

Transient and Permanent Vocal Cord Dysfunction

Vocal cord dysfunction represents unilateral (typical) or bilateral (potentially life-threatening) impaired function of the vocal cord (e.g., from impaired neurologic input), causing adduction of the affected vocal cord(s) with resultant airway compromise. Mechanical causes (e.g., hematoma from pressure/trauma) may also contribute. Laryngospasm is another cause of vocal cord dysfunction.

Epidemiology

The recurrent laryngeal nerve is injured in 0.07% to 11% of ACDs,[45] leading to transient (80%-90%) or permanent (10%-20%) dysfunction.[46,47] In two series totaling more than 1300 patients, symptomatic dysfunction of the recurrent laryngeal nerve was seen in 3%.[4,45] It develops equally frequently with left-sided versus right-sided surgical approaches.[4,45] Actual paralysis of the recurrent laryngeal nerve is reported in 0.6% of patients.

Clinical Presentation

Postoperative unilateral recurrent laryngeal nerve dysfunction manifests clinically as a wet quality of the voice and/or new postoperative hoarseness.[4] In Fountas and coworkers' series, all patients were treated conservatively and all showed spontaneous resolution of their symptomatology within a 12-week period.[4] Other series, however, show that the dysfunction may be permanent.

Pathogenesis

Review of recurrent laryngeal nerve dysfunction in 900 consecutive patients coming to anterior cervical spine surgery over 12 years disclosed that vocal cord dysfunction results in part from pressure on the nerve by the endotracheal tube and the retractors.[46] The retractors displace the larynx against the shaft of the endotracheal tube, leading to compression of the nerve.[46] Monitoring of cuff pressure in the endotracheal tube and periodic relaxation of the retractors to permit re-perfusion of the nerve have been reported to decrease the rate of transient vocal cord paralysis from 6.4% to 1.7%.[46] A more recent randomized study, however, found that cuff deflation did not affect the rate of transient laryngeal nerve dysfunction seen on laryngoscopy (about 15% in each group).[48]

The course of the recurrent laryngeal nerve is different on the two sides.[45] On the right side, the recurrent laryngeal nerve separates from the main trunk of the vagus nerve, passes anterior to and then beneath the subclavian artery, and then ascends in the tracheoesophageal groove. It frequently bifurcates before entering the larynx. On the left side, the recurrent laryngeal nerve descends parallel to the carotid artery, passes anterior to, under, and then posterior to the aortic arch at the ligamentum arteriosum, and then ascends within the tracheoesophageal groove (where it lies a little more medial than on the right side).

In a small minority of patients, the laryngeal nerve follows a variant course and is designated the "nonrecurrent" or "direct" laryngeal nerve. On the right, a direct inferior laryngeal nerve is reported in about 1% of patients and is often associated with aberrant subclavian artery.[45] On the left, a direct left inferior laryngeal nerve is rare and is mostly associated with right aortic arch.[45] These variants present unexpected risks to the operating surgeon.

Imaging

In addition to the usual information as to level, extent, and so on of cervical spondylosis and stenosis, *preoperative* assessment of patients for anterior cervical surgery should include review and specific reporting of (1) any preexisting laryngeal paralysis and (2) any anomalies of the aortic arch and great vessels that might raise concern about anomalous "direct" laryngeal arteries.

Postoperatively, three simple signs reliably identify vocal cord paralysis: (1) dilatation of the ipsilateral pyriform sinus, (2) thickening and medialization of the ipsilateral aryepiglottic fold, and (3) dilatation of the ipsilateral laryngeal ventricle (Fig. 25-13).[49] These findings should be sought and specifically commented on in each report on the postoperative patient. In rare patients with preexisting unilateral vocal cord paralysis, anterior cervical spine surgery may lead to bilateral vocal cord paralysis and require permanent tracheostomy.[50] Manski and colleagues advocate *preoperative* assessment of the vocal cords to avoid inducing bilateral paralysis.[50]

Vertebral and Internal Carotid Artery Injury

Arterial injury is any alteration in the lumen or wall of the vessel leading to narrowing, occlusion, intravascular clot with embolization, dissection, pseudoaneurysm, and/or rupture of the vessel.

Epidemiology

The vertebral artery is injured in 0.2% to 0.5% of ACDs, with an estimated incidence of 0.25% among 12,205 cervical spine procedures (0.25%).[51-53] Lacerations may occur at any spinal level.[52] Vertebral artery injury occurs more frequently with ACC (81% of vertebral artery lacerations) than with ACDF (19%).[52]

Pathogenesis

Causes of vertebral artery injury include excessive lateral drilling (which can occur from intraoperative loss of midline landmarks, especially with pathologic anatomy), excessive removal of lateral bone and disc, excessive lateral placement of hardware, and/or pathologic softening of bone by tumor or infection.[52] It is generally considered safe to resect bone laterally up to the medial margin of the uncinate process (uncovertebral joint of Luschka).[54] However, there is a less than 6-mm distance between the medial border of the uncinate process and the medial margin of the foramen transversarium. When the vertebral bodies are distracted, a "window" of approximately 6 mm opens between the uncinate process and the next-superior vertebra, exposing the vertebral artery to potential injury by drill, Kerrison punch, or curet.[54,55]

In addition, the course of the vertebral artery alters subtly as it ascends in the neck. From C6 to C3 the vertebral artery (1) courses medially at an angle of approximately 4 degrees to the midline and (2) passes progressively farther posteriorly. Therefore, the extent of lateral resection must be adjusted level by level during surgery. At C6-C7, the vertebral artery typically runs between the transverse process of C7 and the longus colli before entering the foramen transversarium at C6. Therefore, the longus coli should be retracted at the level of C6 and care taken to avoid extensive lateral dissection at C6-C7.[54,55]

The vertebral artery shows variable entry into the foramina transversaria (Table 25-6).[56-59] Imaging studies of 500 vertebral arteries showed that atypical entries are mostly unilateral (12.4% of patients) and rarely bilateral (0.8% of patients); are more common in women (66.7%) than in men (33.3%); and are nearly as frequent on the right (48.6%) as on the left (51.4%) sides.[56] In case of high

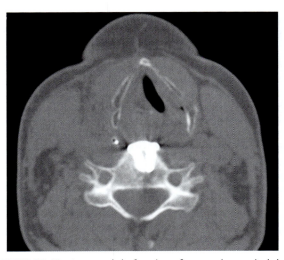

■ **FIGURE 25-13** Laryngeal dysfunction after anterior cervical decompression. Axial CT scan shows medialization of the right arytenoid and vocal cord due to dysfunction of the right recurrent laryngeal nerve. *(From Naidich TP. Cervical spine decompression for spinal stenosis and disk disease: Complications of surgery. In Castillo M, Koeller KK, Mukherji SK. Neuroradiology Categorical Course Syllabus, pp 289-296. American Roentgen Ray Society, 107th Annual Meeting, Orlando, FL, 2007.)*

TABLE 25-6.   Anomalous Entry of the Vertebral Artery into the Foramen Transversarium

References	Side(s)	C7	C6	C5	C4	C3
Bruneau et al.[56] 400 imaging studies	Both	0.8%	93.0%	5.0%	1.0%	0.2%
Daseler & Anson[59]	Right	4.2%	88.9%	6.1%		
	Left	6.6%	86.0%	7.1%		
379 cadavers 758 sides	Both	5.4%	87.5%	6.6%		

entry, the vertebral artery ascends anterior to the transverse processes, just posterior to the longus colli, unprotected by bone. Separate origin of the left vertebral artery from the aortic arch between the left common carotid artery and the left subclavian artery is found in 2.4% to 5.8% of cases. In such cases, the vertebral artery nearly always enters the foramen transversarium at C5.[57,58]

A major cause of vascular injury is the anomalous course of the vertebral artery. The vertebral artery makes a prominent medial loop in 2.0% to 2.7% of cases.[59,60] In Curylo and coworkers' series of seven medial loops, the loops were unilateral and were at C3 (three of seven), at C4 (three of seven), and at two levels (both C3 and C7).[60] The medial deviation of the arterial loop may take two forms. The vertebral artery may loop into a medially enlarged foramen transversarium (1.2% of patients).[60] In such a case the greatest medial deviation of the loop is at the level of the midbody of the vertebra, with normal position of the artery at the disc levels above and below. Alternatively, the artery may loop into the proximal portion of the intervertebral foramen close to the point of emergence of the nerve roots (0.8% of patients).[60] For these reasons, the vertebral artery may course medial to the uncovertebral joint, usually at C3, C4, or C5.[56] These anomalies may thin the pedicle and bring the vertebral artery medial to, or less than 1.5 mm from, the uncovertebral joint. In such cases, the "5.5-mm distance rule" from the uncinate process may not be applicable, leading to potential for injury. Such medially placed vertebral arteries are at risk of injury during surgery. In rare cases, the vertebral artery itself may be the cause of the radiculopathy.[60] Anterior cervical surgery with prolonged retraction of the carotid sheath may lead to internal carotid artery thrombosis with hemispheric infarction.[52]

Clinical Presentation

Injury to the vertebral artery may lead to massive hemorrhaging, pseudoaneurysm, vertebral artery thrombosis, arteriovenous fistula, embolization of the distal vertebral territory, brain stem infarction, and death. Arterial control/repair may be attempted by direct tamponade, coiling and/or stenting of the damaged segment, and occlusion of the vessel.[51]

Imaging

Foramina transversaria that *do not* contain a vertebral artery are substantially smaller than those that do.[56] Foramina transversaria in which the vertebral artery makes an

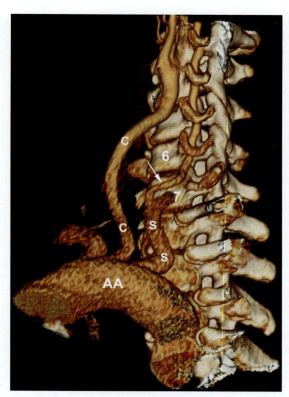

■ **FIGURE 25-14**   Entry of the vertebral artery into the foramen transversarium at C6. 3D-color reformatted CT scan. The left common carotid artery (C) and subclavian artery (S) arise from the aortic arch (AA). The left vertebral artery (*arrow*) arises from the subclavian artery, passes anterior to the transverse process of C7 (7), enters the foramen transversarium at C6 (6), and ascends within the foramina transversaria of the more cephalic vertebrae.

unusual medial loop are typically larger and more medially situated than usual. *Preoperatively*, therefore, the presence, sites, and sizes of the foramina transversaria should be noted and any anomalies of size or position reported to alert the surgeon to a potentially anomalous course, tortuosity, or redundancy of the vertebral artery, especially at any known surgical levels. By evaluation of the sites and sizes of the foramina transversaria, the imager can suggest which vertebral artery is dominant, suggest any anomalously high or low entry of the vertebral artery into the foramina transversaria, and suggest any medial looping of the artery that presents additional risk for surgery at that level. Unusual degenerative, traumatic, or neoplastic erosions of the spine that might alter surgical landmarks should also be noted and reported. 3D CT reformatted images display the spinal-arterial relationships especially well (Fig. 25-14).

Postoperatively, the relationship of spinal instrumentation to the expected (or known) course of the vertebral artery should be noted and any difficulties reported (Fig. 25-15). For specific imaging of potential injury of the vertebral artery, the caliber of the artery, compression or stenosis of the artery, smoothness or irregularity of the wall, filling defect potentially representing intraluminal platelet or red cell clot, leakage from the vessel, pseudoaneurysm, or perivascular hematoma should be reported and communicated rapidly. In the appropriate setting, endovascular therapy of vascular injury should be considered.

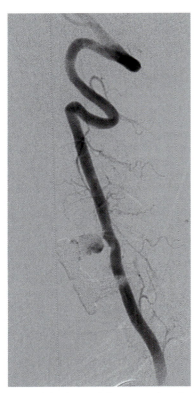

■ FIGURE 25-15 Vertebral artery injury. Lateral projection subtraction vertebral arteriogram demonstrates extravasation and pseudoaneurysm formation in relation to the upper vertebra of a single-level anterior cervical discectomy and interbody fusion (ACDF). Note the subtraction artifact from the instrumentation. *(From Naidich TP. Cervical spine decompression for spinal stenosis and disk disease: Complications of surgery. In Castillo M, Koeller KK, Mukherji SK. Neuroradiology Categorical Course Syllabus, pp 289-296. American Roentgen Ray Society, 107th Annual Meeting, Orlando, FL, 2007.)*

Sympathetic Nerve Injury with Horner's Syndrome

Second-order preganglionic pupillomotor sympathetic fibers exit the spinal cord approximately at the T1 level and then enter the cervical sympathetic chain where they ascend through the sympathetic chain to synapse in the superior cervical ganglion at the level of the bifurcation of the common carotid artery (C3-C4). Horner's syndrome is defined as a clinical triad of ptosis, miosis, and anhidrosis due to injury of this pathway.

Epidemiology

The sympathetic trunk is damaged in 0.1% to 4% of anterior cervical spine surgeries.[4]

Clinical Presentation

Damage to the sympathetic trunk may lead to Horner's syndrome with the triad of ptosis, miosis, and anhidrosis. In one case, temporary unilateral Horner's syndrome developed after surgery, ipsilateral to the surgical site, and resolved spontaneously within 6 weeks.[4]

Pathophysiology

Second-order preganglionic pupillomotor sympathetic fibers exit the spinal cord approximately at the T1 level

and then enter the cervical sympathetic chain where they ascend (near the longus coli muscles) until they synapse in the superior cervical ganglion at the level of the bifurcation of the common carotid artery (C3-C4). Because the trunk lies closer to the medial border of the longus colli at C6 than at C3 the risk of injury to the sympathetic trunk is greater with surgery for lower cervical spine disease.[61]

Imaging

There are no standard studies that depict the sympathetic nerves.

Postoperative Infection

Postoperative spinal infection is any infection of the operative or adjacent site that arises within the immediate postoperative period or later, even after a long delay.

Epidemiology

In large series, postoperative wound infections are reported in 1.2% to 8.5% of cases.[62] Pooled data from 843 patients show an overall infection rate of 3.9%: 2.2% in those receiving prophylactic antibiotics and 5.9% in those not receiving prophylactic antibiotics.[62] Infection rates as high as 10% are reported with instrumented spinal surgery.[63] Infections are very uncommon after purely anterior approaches to the spine (~1.5%).[4,12] They are significantly more frequent in posterior approaches. Combined anteroposterior approaches have the same infection rate as posterior approaches alone.[63] Risk factors for infection include smoking, diabetes, obesity, malnutrition, long-term alcohol abuse, prior infection, and prior spinal surgery. The risk of infection also increases with preoperative hospitalization greater than 1 week, surgery lasting more than 3 hours, and blood loss more than 1 liter.

Clinical Presentation

Spinal infections may present as persistent or increasing pain, sometimes associated with fullness, erythema, and/or drainage of serosanguineous/purulent material from the wound. Elevated patient temperature and inflammatory markers (e.g., erythrocyte sedimentation rate and C-reactive protein) are frequently seen, although the peripheral white blood cell count may not necessarily rise.

Spinal infections may be understood and classified into three groups in terms of two major factors: severity of infection and host resistance characteristics (Table 25-7).

Most patients in the first group can be successfully treated with a single irrigation and débridement and with closure over suction drainage tubes without use of an inflow irrigation system. Patients in the second group require an average of three irrigation-débridements. Patients in the third group are difficult to manage and have poor outcomes. Patients without normal host defense have higher rates of postoperative infection.

TABLE 25-7. Clinical Staging for Spinal Wound Infections (Modified Cierny Classification)

Severity of Infection		Host Characteristics	
Group	Anatomic Type	Physiologic Classification	Response
1	Single organism (superficial or deep)	A	Normal
2	Multiple organisms, deep	B	Local or multiple systemic disease (e.g., smoking)
3	Multiple organisms with myonecrosis	C	Immunocompromised (Injury Severity Score > 18)

From Sasso RC, Garrido BJ. Postoperative spinal wound infections. J Am Acad Orthop Surg 2008; 16:330-337.

Imaging

Contrast-enhanced studies (CT or MRI) can demonstrate enhancing collections in the surgical wound as well as other findings suggestive of potential infection, such as subcutaneous air, fascial dehiscence, and/or fat stranding. However, the imaging findings may be difficult to interpret in the postoperative setting, particularly in the case of instrument artifacts and early or smaller infections.

Postoperative Neck Hematoma

Postoperative hematoma is a new collection of blood in or near to the operative bed.

Epidemiology

Postoperative hemorrhage has been reported variably in 0.2% to 5.6% of cases.[4] In 1,015 first ACDF procedures, postoperative hemorrhage occurred in 5.6% of cases and required emergent surgical intervention in 2.4% of cases.[4] The incidence of hemorrhage was equal for one-level, two-level, and three-level ACDF.[4]

Clinical Presentation

Postoperative hemorrhage often presents as a neck mass. The mass may displace the trachea and esophagus, leading to dysphagia and even respiratory distress. Alternatively, hematoma deep within the operative bed may lead to spinal cord compression, with neurologic deficit appropriate to the level and extent of hemorrhage.

Pathogenesis

Postoperative bleeding leads to a cervical hematoma that may compress the spinal cord within the canal and/or displace the trachea. Risks factors for hemorrhage include coagulation abnormalities and excessive hypertension in the postoperative period. Coughing/straining in the postoperative period may also contribute to hematoma development, presumably from increased venous pressure.

Imaging

Imaging should display the full extent of the operative bed, the relationship of the aerodigestive tract to the operative site, the integrity of the surgical construct (if any), the integrity of the adjacent blood vessels, and the size and position of the spinal cord within the canal. Any contained hemorrhage or displacement/compression of the trachea, esophagus, or spinal cord by hemorrhage and any vascular abnormality that could be the source of hemorrhage should be delineated completely and rapidly to provide the data needed to determine and effect operative control of hemorrhage.

Inadvertent Durotomy

Unintentional opening into the dura mater by a slight "nick" or tear is designated an inadvertent durotomy. The underlying arachnoid may or may not be injured.

Epidemiology

Inadvertent durotomy is reported in 0.5% of first ACDF procedures.[4] Hannallah and colleagues reported cerebrospinal fluid leaks in 1% of both anterior and posterior cervical spine surgery. The incidence was greater (1) in men (1.56%) than in women (0.4%), (2) when surgery was performed to correct compression by ossified posterior longitudinal ligaments (12.5%), (3) for anterior revision surgery (1.92 %), and (4) for anterior corpectomy and arthrodesis (1.77 %).[64]

Clinical Presentation

Patients may demonstrate low-pressure positional headaches and other symptoms of cerebrospinal fluid (CSF) leak. When present, pseudomeningoceles typically manifest as fluctuant soft tissue masses within and adjacent to the operative bed. Complicating infection usually presents as fever with elevation of the white blood cell count and acute inflammatory markers (e.g., erythrocyte sedimentation rate, C-reactive protein). In Hannallah and coworkers' series of 20 patients with CSF leak, symptoms resolved by 3 days in 60%, by 1 week in 85%, by 4 weeks in 95%, and within 4 months in 100% of cases.[64] No patient suffered long-term sequelae. None had external CSF fistula, wound infection, or meningitis.[64] One (5%) developed a pseudomeningocele that closed after lumbar CSF drainage.

Pathogenesis

In Fountas and coworkers' series, dural perforation led to CSF leakage in five cases (0.5%).[4] In four of these cases the dural opening was accidental, whereas in one case the dura was intentionally opened for removing a large intradural disc fragment. In Hannallah and coworkers' study of 20 durotomies with CSF leak, 15 anterior dural tears resulted from use of a Kerrison rongeur for resection of the ossified posterior longitudinal ligament (14 durotomies) and use of a pituitary rongeur for anterior discectomy (1 durotomy). The five posterior dural tears resulted from use of electrocautery for posterior exposure

(2 durotomies), during posterior foraminotomy (1 durotomy), and during elevation of the lamina for posterior laminoplasty (2 durotomies).[64] Dural incision carries the potential for concurrent injury to the arachnoid mater or later bulging and weakening of the arachnoid mater by protrusion through the dural defect, leading to CSF leakage, pseudomeningocele, and potential infection.

Imaging

CSF leak may present as "edema" within the soft tissue at the operative site. The leakage may be documented and localized by intrathecal placement of positive contrast or radionuclide with subsequent imaging to depict the presence and site of leak. Pseudomeningoceles appear as small or large, deep or superficial, fluid-filled "pockets" within and enlarging the surgical bed. The collection may be confined to the level of surgery or may dissect craniad or caudad for multiple additional segments. The wall of the pseudomeningocele is typically thickened and shows contrast enhancement due to inflammatory reaction and granulation tissue, either sterile or infected. The paraspinal muscles and adjoining tissue may show simple postoperative edema or acute inflammation. In patients with severe concurrent infection, there may be discitis, osteomyelitis, paraspinal phlegmon or abscess, and draining sinuses.

Complications of the Posterior Cervical Approach

The major complications of posterior spinal surgery include spinal instability with (variably) progressive spinal deformity, postoperative radiculopathy, CSF leak with pseudomeningocele, infection, and adjacent segment degeneration (Fig. 25-16).

Spinal Instability (Postoperative Cervical Kyphosis)

Spinal instability is the inability of the spine to withstand normal movements without development of abnormal subluxation, neurologic dysfunction, and/or pain. Postoperative cervical kyphosis represents a type of instability that can complicate posterior cervical spine surgery.

Epidemiology

After posterior cervical spine surgery, the rate of postoperative cervical kyphosis varies widely from 0% to 33%.[65] The rate is higher for patients who do not have fusion performed and for patients with spinal cord dysfunction.

Clinical Presentation

As for anterior cervical procedures, the postoperative cervical kyphosis that complicates posterior cervical surgery typically presents as axial or radicular pain, sometimes with head drop.

Pathophysiology

The posterior cervical approach itself can predispose the patient to kyphosis, especially if there is injury or denervation of the posterior paraspinal muscles. Removal of the posterior elements (e.g., laminae, spinous processes, ligaments) can contribute to postoperative kyphosis due to loss of the posterior tension band. Because of their intrinsic denervation, patients with myelopathy/spinal cord injury are more likely to experience postoperative kyphosis, particularly without fusion/instrumentation.

Imaging

Postoperative kyphosis is readily apparent on standard radiographs. Dynamic flexion-extension views may help to determine the extent of deformity, whenever obtaining these views is judged safe. CT and MRI may provide additional details on the osseous and soft tissue anatomy and thus help to define the mechanism leading to kyphosis and guide decisions on surgical/medical management (e.g., the degree of neurologic compression).

Radiculopathy after Posterior Cervical Decompression

After posterior cervical decompression surgery, the patient may experience new radicular nerve symptoms and dysfunction in the postoperative period from a number of potential causes.

Epidemiology

Postoperative radiculopathy has been reported in 9% of 287 consecutive patients undergoing multilevel posterior cervical laminectomy for decompression of cervical spondylosis and ossification of the posterior longitudinal ligament.[66] Placement of pedicle screws carries a 0.4% incidence of radiculopathy.[6]

Clinical Presentation

Postoperative radiculopathy typically occurs 4 hours to 6 days after surgery, affects the C5 and C6 motor roots predominantly, and typically returns to baseline 2 weeks to 3 years (mean, 5.3 months) after surgery.[66] Patients treated for cervical spondylotic myelopathy generally recover better than those treated for ossification of the posterior longitudinal ligament.

Pathophysiology

Although a number of studies have described this condition, there is no definite known cause.

Imaging

CT and MRI display any direct impingement of spinal elements or surgical construct on the nerve roots and any enhancement signifying inflammation of the roots.

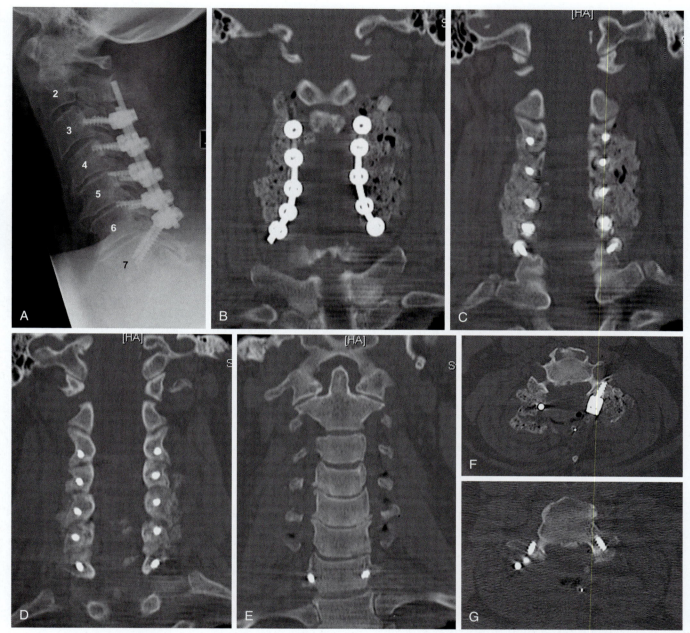

■ FIGURE 25-16 Multilevel posterior cervical laminectomy with internal fixation and bony fusion mass. **A,** Lateral spine radiograph. **B to E,** Coronal reformatted CT images displayed from posterior to anterior. **F and G,** Axial CT images. This patient underwent long segment posterior cervical decompression with bilateral laminectomies and internal fixation by lateral mass screws (C3-C6), pedicle screws (C7), and placement of bone fragments for fusion. The lateral radiograph (**A**) and coronal CT images (**B-E**) show expected normal alignment and trajectories of the screws, except for slight lateral position of the right C7 pedicle screw. **F,** Axial image shows good placement of the right lateral mass screw. **G,** Axial image shows good placement of the left C7 pedicle screw but lateral position of the right pedicle screw.

Vertebral Artery Injury

Vertebral artery injury is any alteration in the lumen or wall of the vessel leading to narrowing, occlusion, intravascular clot with progressive thrombosis or embolization, dissection, pseudoaneurysm, and/or rupture.

Epidemiology

Simple posterior cervical laminectomy and laminoplasty carry no significant risk of major arterial injury.[52] Cervical pedicle screw fixation carries a 0.3% to 0.6% risk of vertebral artery injury.[52,53] Lateral mass screws placed at C2 injure the vertebral artery in 4.1% to 8.2% of cases,[54] but lateral mass screws placed below C2 are not associated with arterial injury.[54] Vertebrojugular arteriovenous fistula has been reported after posterior cervical foraminotomy.[52]

Clinical Presentation

Vertebral artery injuries may present immediately or years later as hemorrhage at the operative site, arteriovenous fistula, pseudoaneurysm, thrombosis with emboli, cerebral ischemia, stroke, and death. Brain stem infarction is expected in 3.1% of patients when the left vertebral artery is occluded and in 1.8% when the right vertebral artery is ligated.[53] Acute ligation of the vertebral artery carries a 12% mortality.[53] Injury is best addressed either by direct repair or by endovascular control.

Pathophysiology

Arterial injury may result from primary trauma to the vessel or from secondary trauma consequent to manipulation and (dis)traction of adjacent bone elements.[54]

C1-C2

Most arterial injury occurs during placement of transarticular screws at C1-C2 (4.1% per patient, 2.2% per screw). In about 80% of the population, the vertebral artery makes an acute lateral bend in the lateral mass of C2, just under the superior articular facet. Up to 20% of the population has anomalous positioning of the vertebral artery and 18% has a high-riding C2 transverse foramen on at least one side, placing the vertebral artery at significant risk. Other anomalies include bending of the artery under the superior articular facet of the axis, which can then be too medial, posterior, or high, leading to a very narrow C2 isthmus. In 20% the inferior surface of the lateral mass of C2 is grooved by the vertebral artery to the extent that the pedicle is eroded and the lateral mass thinned. Typically, the C1-C2 transarticular screw is inserted 2 to 3 mm superomedial to the C2-C3 facet joint and is directed superomedially through the C2 pars and toward the anterior tubercle of C1. If the trajectory is too low or too lateral, the screws may intersect the vertebral artery.[54]

C3-C6

Lateral mass screws at C3-C6 may risk injury to the vertebral artery, especially if started too medial and/or not directed sufficiently lateral. Because of the anatomy, pedicle screws placed at C3-C6 carry the risk of arterial injury. The cortex of the pedicle is thinnest laterally, with consequent risk to the vertebral artery. C4 has the thinnest pedicle, so C4 pedicle screws carry the greatest risk of vertebral artery injury.[54]

Imaging

Preoperatively, CT and MRI can display the course of the arteries and their relationship to the pedicles, lateral masses, and expected trajectories of the fixation screws. Postoperatively, imaging can demonstrate any fracture, bone fragments, or instrumentation that may impinge on the vertebral artery, as well as any secondary hemorrhage.

Complications after Use of Lateral Mass Screws with Plating

In 1995, Heller and associates reported the complications observed in 78 consecutive patients treated with 654 screws (average, 8.4 screws per patient).[67] Calculated per screw insertion, the complications were nerve root injury (0.6%), facet violations (0.2%), vertebral artery injury (0%), broken screw (0.3%), screw avulsion (0.2%), and screw loosening (1.1%).[67] Calculated per patient, the complications were spinal cord injury (2.6%), iatrogenic foraminal stenosis (2.6%), broken plate (1.3%), lost reduction (2.6%), adjacent segment degeneration (3.8%), infection (1.3%), and pseudarthrosis (1.4%).[67]

Patients with symptomatic cervical myelopathy from circumferential cervical stenosis can be managed by single-stage, multilevel wide posterior laminectomy with lateral mass instrumented fusion.[68] In Sekhon's series of 50 consecutive patients, there was no mortality, no instrument-related neural or vascular injuries, and no need for subsequent ventral decompression.[68] Three patients (6%) had simple screw pullouts that did not affect their neurologic status. Kyphosis worsened slightly in 8 patients (4%). One patient (2%) required foraminotomy/posterior discectomy 1 year later at an adjacent level.[68] Other complications reported with laminoplasty include canal restenosis, decreased cervical motion, and loss of normal cervical lordosis.[69]

Complications of Cervical Transpedicular Screw Fixation

Because the pedicles of the cervical vertebrae are small from C3-C6 and larger at C2 and C7, traditional posterior cervical instrumentation achieves internal fixation by using lateral mass screws for cervical levels C3-C6 and pedicle screws only at the C2 and/or C7 levels. More recently, pedicle screws have also been used in the smaller pedicles at C3-C6.[53,70,71] Review of 94 pedicle screws implanted in 26 patients, mostly at C3 and C4, reveals that 20/94 screws (21%) were misplaced with reduction of mechanical strength, narrowing of the foramen transversarium less than 25%, and narrowing of the lateral recess, all with no clinical sequelae.[57] Another 8/94 screws (9%) caused a critical breech of the cortex, with 4 screws narrowing the foramen transversarium more than 25% without vascular injury and 3 screws traversing the intervertebral foramen, leading to transient paresis in 1 patient and new sensory loss requiring revision surgery in a second.[53] Yoshimoto and associates inserted 134 screws in 26 patients and experienced complete perforation of the pedicles in 5/134 screws (3.7%) (all in the first 10 patients) and partial perforation of the pedicle in another 10/134 patients (7.4%).[72] Bony union was achieved in all patients except 2 with cancer. No patient suffered neurologic complications from the pedicle screws.[72] In the series of Neo and colleagues, 18 consecutive patients underwent posterior cervical decompression for degenerative disease with placement of 86 pedicle screws at C2 to C6.[55] The screws breeched the pedicle cortex in 25/86 screws (29%).[53] Most screws deviated laterally (84%), violating the transverse foramen, but none injured the vertebral artery.[53]

Combined Anteroposterior "Circumferential" Cervical Spinal Decompression and Fusion

For selected complex cervical problems, especially those with instability, surgeons may undertake combined anterior and posterior cervical spinal decompression and fusion at the same session. Such "360-degree" surgery provides immediate stabilization, decreases anterior graft and instrument failure, and obviates use of postoperative halo fixation.[71] However, the surgery is longer and far more invasive, leading to increased risk of airway compromise (70%), among other problems. Kwon and colleagues routinely maintained patients treated by single-stage multilevel anterior cervical discectomy and posterior fusion in the intensive care unit overnight and then determined by cuff-leak test whether they could safely be extubated the next day. Half were not and had delayed extubation beyond day 1.[73]

COMPLICATIONS OF LUMBAR SPINE SURGERY

Spinal stenosis signifies constriction of the cross-sectional area of the spinal canal and/or neural foramina, typically leading to pain and neurologic deficit.[74] Spinal stenosis may arise anteriorly, posteriorly, or circumferentially, at one or multiple levels. Common causes of stenosis are degenerative osteophytes of the vertebral bodies, disc bulges or herniations, osteophytes from the facet joints, infolding-hypertrophy of the ligamenta flava, and excess deposition of epidural fat (epidural lipomatosis). Secondary degenerative spondylolisthesis and degenerative scoliosis may aggravate the primary stenosis.

Overview

Over the period 1993 to 2001 the number of lumbar spinal fusions performed in the United States increased 356%, from 13 to 63/100,000 population for patients aged 40 to 59 years and from 13 to 68/100,000 population for patients aged 60 years or older.[2] The primary indication for lumbar fusion was degenerative disc disease in 21/100,000 in 2001.[2]

Compressive lumbar myelopathy and radiculopathy may be treated in many ways (Figs. 25-17 to 25-21):

1. *Anterior lumbar discectomy and interbody fusion (ALIF).* In this procedure, an anterior/anterolateral incision is used to enter the extraperitoneal space, enabling *retro*peritoneal dissection to the ventral spine and associated vascular structures. After exposing the disc space (sometimes requiring mobilization and careful retraction of the vascular structures), the discectomy is performed. A structural graft, typically a bone plug or titanium cage filled with bone graft, is then placed

into the interspace. Instrumentation is sometimes used to stabilize the construct.
2. *Posterior lumbar laminectomy (or laminoplasty) and fusion (PLIF).* In this procedure, a midline skin incision is carried to the spinous processes and then deflected toward the side of surgery. The paraspinal muscle is stripped from the bone from medial to lateral to the level of the facets. A wide laminectomy is performed with resection of the ligamentum flavum (yellow ligament) and partial or complete removal of the cranial lamina. The lower one third of the inferior facet and the medial two thirds of the superior facet are resected to expose the pedicle of the vertebra as far laterally as possible. Such wide opening into the canal minimizes the neural retraction needed to reach the disc. The traversing nerve root and the dural sac are retracted medially to expose the disc. The disc and any osteophytes are then resected as far anteriorly and laterally as possible. The cartilaginous end plates are removed. The bony end plates are preserved to help support the interbody spacer, spread the load, and prevent subsidence.
3. *Transforaminal lumbar discectomy and interbody fusion (TLIF).* In this procedure the surgical approach is from the side. The pars interarticularis is resected, and the inferior facet is removed. Next the superior articular facet is reduced progressively until it is flush with the pedicle. The traversing nerve root is then mobilized and retracted medially, affording access to the disc via the foramen. Discectomy may then be performed across the disc to the opposite side.
4. *Circumferential (360-degree) decompression.* This procedure is performed in one or sequential sessions.

Successful Surgery

Seventy to 80% of patients operated on for lumbar spinal stenosis have a satisfactory outcome in the short term.[74] However, outcomes tend to deteriorate in the long term.[74] Jansson and colleagues analyzed the health-related quality of life in 263 Swedish patients before and after surgery for a lumbar herniated disc.[75] The quality of life improved in 74% of the patients but did not reach levels normal for the population as a whole. Predictors for poor outcome included a history of smoking, short preoperative walking distance, and a long history of back pain.[75]

Specific study of anterior lumbar interbody fusion with cages suggests that the most reliable sign of fusion is the presence of bridging bone anterior to the fusion cage ("sentinel sign").[76] Specific study of posterior lumbar interbody fusion using carbon fiber cages shows that the most useful plane for imaging is the coronal plane and the most reliable imaging sign of fusion is the presence of bony bridging through the hollows of the cages without signal alteration adjacent to the surface of the implant.[77] The bridging bone may display some inhomogeneity within the cage. MRI is able to show successful fusion by 12 months after surgery in many cases, but the imaging features become more evident after 24 months.[77] New bone may still form within and outside the cages between 12 and 24 months, indicating that the healing process is not complete by 12 months.[77]

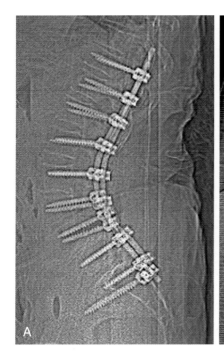

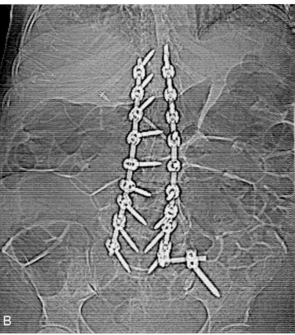

■ **FIGURE 25-17** Long segment posterior thoracolumbosacral fixation. Lateral (**A**) and frontal (**B**) scout views from a CT scan show the multilevel placement of pedicle screws, the left sacroiliac screw, and the paired connecting vertical elements (rods).

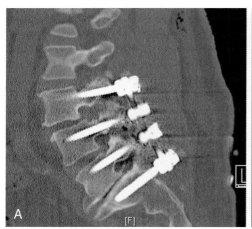

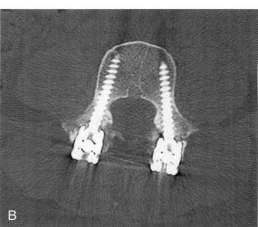

■ **FIGURE 25-18** Posterior lumbar laminectomy and L3-S1 fusion (PLIF). **A,** Sagittal reformatted CT scan. **B,** Axial CT scan. The pedicle screws align with, traverse, and are well seated within the pedicles, with no violation of the cortex. The lumbar lordosis is maintained.

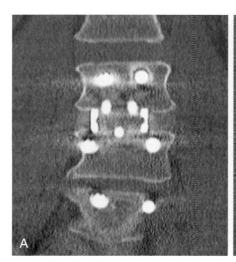

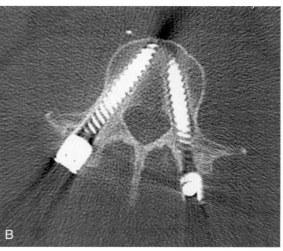

■ **FIGURE 25-19** Loosening of pedicle screw. **A,** Coronal reformatted bone algorithm CT scan. **B,** Axial bone algorithm CT image through the L3 pedicles. These images show a L3-L4 posterior lumbar interbody fusion with internal fixation by rods and pedicle screws at L3, L4, and L5. The bone plug is well seated against the apposing end plates of L3 and L4. The right L3 and both L4 and L5 pedicle screws show excellent bone density immediately adjacent to the screws with no "lucent halo" or sclerotic rim about the screw. The left L3 pedicle screw shows loss of bony trabeculae about the screw, creating a lucent halo with a thick sclerotic bone rim peripheral to the halo. This indicates loosening of the screw within the bone, creating a cylindrical cavity or "hollow sleeve" about the screw.

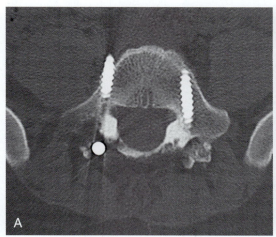

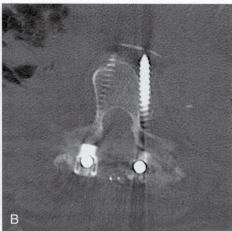

■ **FIGURE 25-20** Malposition of the pedicle screws. Axial CT scans. Two patients. **A,** The right pedicle screw protrudes beyond the margin of the vertebral body into the para-spinal soft tissue. **B,** The left pedicle screw passes lateral to the pedicle and the vertebral body.

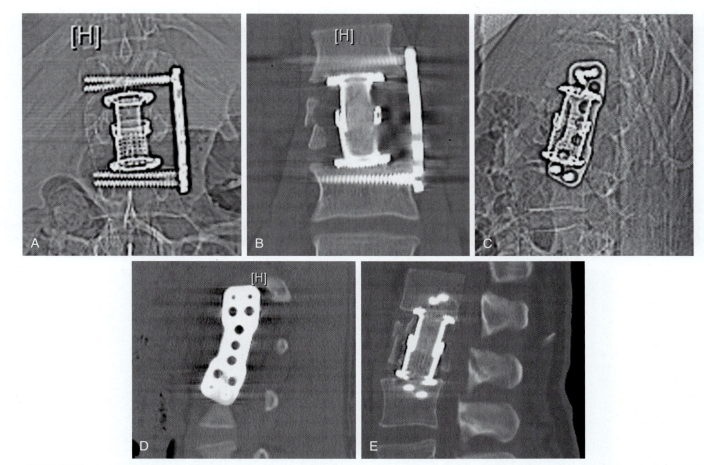

■ **FIGURE 25-21** Translumbar partial corpectomy with interbody fusion T12-L2 for spinal trauma. **A,** Frontal CT scout view. **B,** Coronal reformatted CT scan. **C,** Lateral CT scout view. **D** and **E,** Sagittal reformatted CT scans. These images show translumbar partial L1 corpectomy with placement of an expandable cage and lateral lumbar plate at T12-L2. The plate and cage align with the spine in two planes with no alteration in normal curvature. The screws fixing the plate to the vertebrae lie in separate planes to reduce risk of fracture. The cage seats well against the T12 and L2 vertebrae. There is continuity of bony trabeculae from lower T12 through the cage into upper L2, indicating solid bony fusion. Fracture lines are seen in the residual portion of L1.

General Complications of Thoracolumbar Surgery

Review of 1,223 anterior and posterior thoracic and lumbar surgeries performed for diverse diseases disclosed many general complications.[78] Serious nonspinal complications included death (0.33%), cardiac arrest (0.33%), pulmonary embolism (0.82%), acute respiratory distress syndrome (0.33%), respiratory arrest (0.08%), and cerebrovascular accident (0.25%).[78] Retrograde ejaculation is reported in up to 45% of men who have undergone ALIF.[79] Relatively minor, nonspinal complications included urinary tract infection (9.74%), urinary retention (0.9%), pneumonia (3.36%), and thrombophlebitis (0.9%).[78] Review of 27,576 lumbar disc operations in Sweden disclosed a 30-day death rate of 0.5 per 1000 surgeries.[80] A large prospective study by the Swedish Lumbar Spine Study Group[81] found the overall complication rate was 12% with PLIF alone, 22% with PLIF plus instrumentation (PLIFI), and 40% with 360-degree circumferential fusion.

Failed Back Syndrome

Failed back syndrome is persistent or recurrent pain after at least one previous lumbar surgery.[82]

Epidemiology

This syndrome occurs in 10% to 60% of patients after lumbar discectomy.[82]

Clinical Presentation

The typical presentation is persistent (or new) pain syndrome involving the back (and/or nerve roots).

Pathophysiology

Failed back syndrome may result from wrong diagnosis, insufficient surgery, insufficient rehabilitation, recurrent disc herniation, arachnoiditis, epidural fibrosis, infection, or mechanical instability.[82] Gejo and associates showed that surgical disruption of the paraspinal muscles caused by stripping the muscle from the laminae resulted in loss of muscular support and contributed to development of the failed back syndrome.[83] Gambardella and colleagues studied 74 patients and found significantly better clinical and MRI results in those patients in whom autologous fat grafts were placed around the exposed nerve roots to reduce epidural fibrosis.[84] However, a prospective controlled study of 186 discectomies showed that placement of autologous free-fat grafts does not reduce the incidence of failed back syndrome.[82] Paresthesias of the thigh or lower leg occurred as often in the treated as the control group.[82]

Imaging

Imaging studies for this entity focus on finding potentially treatable causes for the persistent pain (e.g., nonunion, instability, infection).

Surgical Site Infection

Surgical site infection is infection of a previously clean surgical site. Definitive diagnosis depends on culture of the organism from the surgical site. *Superficial surgical site infection* is infection isolated superficial to the dorsal fascia and is characterized by purulent discharge or cutaneous dehiscence with positive microbiologic testing. *Deep surgical site infection* is defined by imaging evidence of infection deep to the dorsal fascia, with or without positive microbial testing. *Acute infection* is an infection manifesting within 30 days of the surgical procedure.[85] *Delayed (late) infection* is infection presenting at the operative site more than 10 to 12 *months* after surgery (average, 27 months after surgery).[86]

Epidemiology

Superficial wound infections occur in 2.9% to 9.7% of posterior spinal instrumentations and often present early.[87,88] Deep wound infections occur in about 2.4% (range: 1% to 9.7%) of instrumented lumbar surgeries and may present early or late.[87] However, there is substantial variation in the infection rate associated with spinal surgery and fusion.[89] Multiple series show that the infection rate decreases with use of short-term prophylactic antibiotics and with increasing surgical experience.[63,86,88,90-92] Specific risk factors for infection include patient obesity, malnourishment, diabetes, corticosteroid therapy or other immunocompromise, nonelective (trauma) surgery, posterior versus anterior spinal surgery, prior spinal surgery, prior infection, length of procedure more than 3 hours, loss of blood more than 1 L, and greater length of stay in the hospital.[20,93] Lumbar discectomy with prophylactic antibiotics carries a 0.7% infection rate, which doubles to 1.4% with use of the operating microscope.[63] Percutaneous intradiscal procedures carry a 2.75% infection rate.[63] Overall, the incidence of infection is reported as 2.8% to 6%.[63] Interestingly, in one large series of 1,747 patients, the rate of surgical site infections was lower (0.62%) for those having just one procedure and higher (2.3%) for the first procedure of those undergoing multiple surgeries.[85]

Clinical Presentation

Acute infection typically presents as a pain that persists longer than the usual incisional pain, and pain that increases with time. Local physical signs include erythema and bulging at the closure, tenderness to palpation, copious drainage of increasingly turbid fluid or pus, and wound breakdown.[63] Constitutional signs of infection include patient temperature greater than 39°C (102.2°F), chills, sweats, and, in severe cases, hypotension, lethargy, confusion, and other signs of acute sepsis.[63] Delayed infection is often occult. It may present as increasing pain and tenderness at the incision site but constitutional signs are often the key indicators of infection. With deep infection, imaging evidence of failed fusion and inflammation may be crucial to diagnosis.[86] Superficial infections typically present early as erythema, swelling, and discharge. Deep infections may present late as subfascial seromas and paraspinal abscesses, possibly with concurrent osteomyelitis.[63]

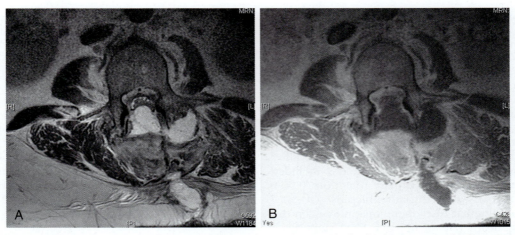

■ **FIGURE 25-22**   Axial lumbar MR images. **A,** Axial T2-weighted image shows prior posterior lumbar laminectomy with formation of a pseudomeningocele superficial and deep to the lumbodorsal fascia. The fluid collection impinges on the thecal sac from posterior. The paraspinal muscle is edematous at the surgical site. **B,** Contrast-enhanced T1-weighted image shows inflammatory enhancement of the paraspinal muscle, outlining the fluid collections. *(From Naidich TP. Thoracolumbar spine decompression for spinal stenosis and disk disease: Complications of surgery. In Castillo M, Koeller KK, Mukherji SK. Neuroradiology Categorical Course Syllabus, pp 297-305. American Roentgen Ray Society, 107th Annual Meeting, Orlando, FL, 2007.)*

Significant perioperative and delayed infection may require removal of the grafts and hardware, destabilizing the back. Pappou and colleagues analyzed the need to remove hardware in 326 consecutive patients with 13 early infections after anterior and posterior interbody fusions with instrumentation.[94] These physicians were able to salvage 92.3% of the infected grafts during a mean follow-up period of 18 months (range: 12-38 months) without adversely affecting patient outcome.[94]

Pathophysiology

In acute postoperative infections, the organism is most often *Staphylococcus*, followed by "gram-negative organisms" and *Enterococcus*.[87,93] In delayed spinal infections, the organisms are predominantly low-virulence skin organisms, most commonly *Staphylococcus epidermidis* and *Propionibacterium acnes*, then *Micrococcus varians*, coagulase-negative *Staphylococcus* species, and "negative culture."[86,89,93] *Peptococcus, Enterobacter cloacae*, and *Bacteroides* are also common. Successful culture and identification of these low-virulence organisms may require prolonged incubation of the culture plates (7-10 days).[86] Delayed infection is thought to result from true *intraoperative* seeding followed by a long quiescent period and then growth. Delayed infection may also result from seeding of the operative site by later, unrelated infections acquired at remote sites.[86] Histopathologic analysis of the soft tissue and hardware recovered at revision surgery for infection shows local fibrinoid necrosis and nonspecific inflammatory granulation tissue with epithelial-like "membrane" surfaces.[95] Late inflammatory reaction is thought to result from micro-motion between the metal implant and the bone, causing metal debris, foreign-body reaction, formation of the pseudomembrane, implant loosening, and creation of a draining sinus.[95]

Imaging

Contrast-enhanced CT or MRI can depict soft tissue edema and enhancing collections (a hallmark for most infections)

(Figs. 25-22 and 25-23). The imaging provides key data on the deep extent of the infection, any extension to paraspinal soft tissue, and the relation to the instrumentation and the dural sac.

Iliac Crest Donor Site Pain and Infection

The iliac crest is a site from which bone is frequently harvested to perform autologous bone grafting during spinal procedures.

Epidemiology

In Sasso and colleagues' study of 208 patients undergoing anterior lumbar discectomy with autologous iliac bone fusion, only 67% of patients were free of iliac pain at 1 year.[96]

Clinical Presentation

The donor site is subject to hematoma. Harvest of bone at the iliac donor site has led to postoperative hemorrhage that required return to surgery in 7.7% of patients.[21] Persistent postoperative pain (30% or more) is a major limitation of using autologous grafts. In Sasso and colleagues' series, significant pain was present at the harvest site in 33% of all patients at 1 year and persisted through the second year in 31%.[96] Postoperative infection is uncommon (0.9%). Such infection may be separate from the spinal wound or may be confluent with it when both sites are exposed through the same skin incision.[97] These infections may require long-term intravenous antibiotics and re-exploration for débridement.[97]

Pathophysiology

Donor site iliac pain occurred equally often whether the bone harvested was unicortical or bicortical bone, whether it was from the left or right iliac crest, and whether it was from the anterior or posterior iliac crest.[52] With time, the donor cavity gradually fills in with new bone. Recent dem-

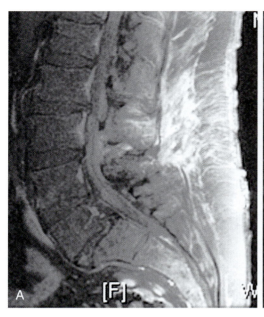

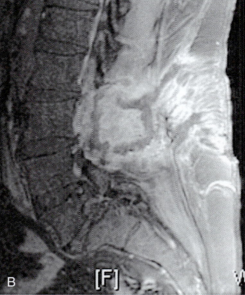

■ **FIGURE 25-23** Sagittal contrast-enhanced fat-suppressed T1-weighted MR images through the spinal canal (**A**) and lateral to it (**B**) show abnormal contrast enhancement, representing inflammation within the spinal canal, the surgical incision, and the paraspinal soft tissue. There is exaggerated lumbar lordosis with anterior listhesis of L5 forward on S1. *(From Naidich TP. Thoracolumbar spine decompression for spinal stenosis and disk disease: Complications of surgery. In Castillo M, Koeller KK, Mukherji SK. Neuroradiology Categorical Course Syllabus, pp 297-305. American Roentgen Ray Society, 107th Annual Meeting, Orlando, FL, 2007.)*

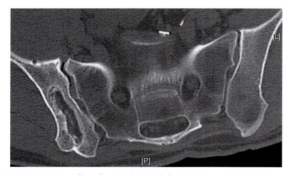

■ **FIGURE 25-24** Iliac donor site. Axial noncontrast CT section. Years after harvest of iliac bone for lumbar fusion, the right ilium shows beginning of filling in of bone within a well-corticated cavity with no evidence of soft tissue edema or inflammation.

onstration that autogenous bone grafts harvested from the local surgical site (e.g., spinous processes and laminae) fuse as well as autogenous bone harvested from the iliac crest may eliminate these complications in the future.[98]

Imaging

The iliac crest shows defects in the cortical and medullary bone, typically extending to the superior surface of the iliac crest (Fig. 25-24). The surrounding soft tissue shows edema (acutely) or scar (chronic). Additional full-thickness breaks suggest inadvertent iliac fracture. Defined soft tissue "masses" adjacent to the donor site suggest seroma, hematoma, or abscess. Ring enhancement of the mass and/or of a linear sinus tract may be found with both sterile inflammation and frank infection.

Specific Complications of Anterior Thoracolumbar Surgery

Anterior exposure for thoracic and lumbar spine surgery carries a total mortality of 0.7% (30 of 4,074 patients).[99]

Complications occur in 11.5% of all anterior thoracic and lumbar surgeries and include aortic laceration (0.08%), superficial wound infection (0.98%), deep wound infection (0.57%), and nerve root injury (0.54%).[78] At lumbar levels, the overall complication rate is 30% to 40%, including arterial thrombosis (<1% of cases), venous hemorrhage (2%-15%), ureteral injury (0.3%-8%), neurogenic deficits (e.g., retrograde ejaculation, groin nerve injury, and warm leg), and local wound problems (e.g., infection, disruption, herniation, and denervation).[99]

Nonfusion (pseudarthrosis) of the spine is often associated with persistent pain and lingering disability. Thin-section CT shows the fusion rate for stand-alone ALIFs is 51%; for ALIF stabilized by translaminar screws, 58%; for ALIF stabilized by unilateral pedicle screws, 89%; and for ALIF stabilized by bilateral pedicle screws, 88%.[100] Use of recombinant human bone morphogenic protein (rhBMP-2) is reported to promote fusion in patients undergoing ALIF with cages and threaded allograft.[101] However, prospective evaluation of rhBMP-2 for ALIFs with femoral ring allografts demonstrated a very low fusion rate (44%) compared with the same procedure not using rhBMP-2 (64%).[101]

Major Vascular Injury

A major vascular injury is an intraoperative injury to the aorta, vena cava, or iliac arteries and veins.[102]

Epidemiology

Major vascular complications occur in approximately 2.9% of *anterior* lumbar surgeries.[102] The mean number of levels exposed, patient gender, and patient age did not correlate with risk of vascular injury.[102] Most frequently, the injury affects the veins (2.6%), primarily the left common iliac vein, then the inferior vena cava and the iliolumbar vein.[52] Most venous injuries occur at L4-L5.[52] Risk factors include current or prior osteomyelitis/disc

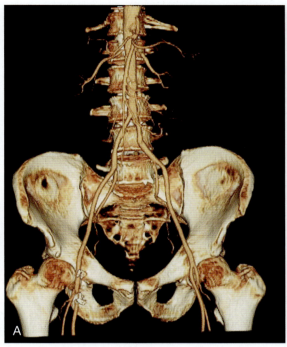

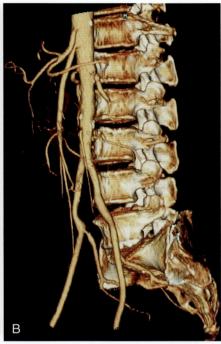

■ FIGURE 25-25 Aortic bifurcation. 3D-color reformatted CT angiograms of the distal aorta and iliac arteries in frontal (**A**) and lateral (**B**) projections show the relationships of the aortic bifurcation and iliac arteries to the intervertebral disc spaces L4-L5 and L5-S1. The left iliac artery is especially vulnerable to injury by surgery at the L4-L5 level. *(From Naidich TP. Thoracolumbar spine decompression for spinal stenosis and disk disease: Complications of surgery. In Castillo M, Koeller KK, Mukherji SK. Neuroradiology Categorical Course Syllabus, pp 297-305. American Roentgen Ray Society, 107th Annual Meeting, Orlando, FL, 2007.)*

infection, prior anterior spinal surgery, spondylolisthesis, large anterior osteophyte, transitional lumbosacral vertebra, and anterior migration of an interbody device.[102] Arterial injuries are less common (0.3%), probably because the aorta and iliac vessels are more elastic and better able to tolerate the stretching and displacement caused by mobilization and retraction.[52,102] The left iliac artery is injured most frequently (0%-0.9%).[52] Injury to the thoracic aorta is rare, but delayed rupture of a calcified descending thoracic aorta at the site of retraction with consequent patient death has been reported.[102] Thrombosis of the left common iliac artery may result from prolonged retraction of the common iliac arteries to the right side with consequent stagnation of arterial flow on the left.[52] Of 16 cases of postoperative common iliac artery thrombosis reported in the literature, 15 (94%) were on the left side.[52]

Clinical Presentation

Vascular injuries typically cause immediate hemorrhage when the injury occurs in the surgical field. Smaller injuries or those not in the field commonly present as hypotension and tachycardia. Venous injuries are associated with substantial blood loss (average: 1500 ± 850 mL, up to massive hemorrhage of 5 L).[52] The injuries are treated by compression proximal and distal to the defect and application of topical agents.[102] Arterial injuries can cause massive life-threatening hemorrhage and are typically managed with arterial repair, usually by a vascular surgeon.

Pathophysiology

ALIF requires the surgeon to approach the intervertebral disc level through the prevertebral tissue, mobilize the prevertebral vessels, resect tissue and bone, and then distract the adjacent vertebrae to place the graft. Anterior surgery at L4-L5 and L5-S1 requires mobilization of the left common iliac vessels.[102] Because the left common iliac vein is situated most dorsally, it is injured most frequently.[102] Because the vessels are tethered to the vertebrae by segmental branches, they also may be injured secondarily during distraction of the vertebrae. In Fantini and associates' series,[102] all vascular injuries occurred during attempts to mobilize or maintain mobilization of major vessels entrapped within dense inflammatory reaction caused by the risk factors just mentioned.

Venous injuries most commonly occur during retraction of the great vessels with tear of the main vein or avulsion of a branch. Less commonly, the veins are injured during the discectomy, placement of the interbody graft, and removal of the Steinmann pin (used to secure venous retraction). Threaded fusion devices cause venous injury more commonly than do unthreaded devices (11.5% vs. 3.2%), probably because the tools needed to introduce them into the interspace are larger and require greater retraction.[52]

Inamasu and coworkers documented the relationships of the great abdominal vessels to the intervertebral disc levels using 3D CT.[103] In 100 studies, the bifurcation of the aorta lay above L4 in 4%, at L4 in 55%, at L4-L5 in 23%, and at L5 in 18% (Figs. 25-25 and 25-26).[103] The iliac veins joined to form the inferior vena cava at L4 in 17%, at L4-L5 in 14%, at L5 in 68%, and below L5 in 1%.[103] In most patients, the aortic bifurcation lay one to two segments superior to the origin of the inferior vena cava.[103] 3D CT also successfully displayed the positions of the middle sacral artery (79%) and the L4 radicular artery (83%) in most patients.[103] Brau and colleagues[104] have reported six cases (0.45%) of iliac artery thrombosis. Kulkarni and associates[105] reported 8 cases (2.4%) of arterial injury, including thromboembolism, intimal tear, and vasospasm of the iliac artery, with one fatality secondary to rhabdomyolysis.

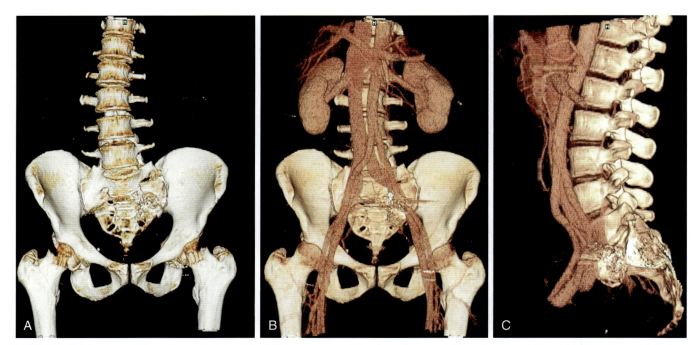

■ **FIGURE 25-26**   Aortic bifurcation and origin of the inferior vena cava. 3D-color reformatted CT angiograms in frontal (**A-B**) and lateral (**C**) views. Comparing the frontal "bare bone" view of the lumbosacral spine (**A**) with the vascular images (**B** and **C**) shows the relationships of the vertebrae and discs to the distal aorta, iliac arteries, common iliac veins, and origin of the inferior vena cava. *(From Naidich TP. Thoracolumbar spine decompression for spinal stenosis and disk disease: Complications of surgery. In Castillo M, Koeller KK, Mukherji SK. Neuroradiology Categorical Course Syllabus pp 297-305. American Roentgen Ray Society, 107th Annual Meeting, Orlando, FL, 2007.)*

Imaging

Duplex ultrasonography should be used to assess the lower extremities for venous thromboses. MR venography or CT venography should be used to assess patency of the pelvic veins after repair of venous injury.[102]

Specific Complications of Posterior Thoracolumbar Surgery

The rate of pseudarthrosis varies widely from about 5% up to 94% for one- and two-level posterior surgical procedures.[97,106] Autografts are incorporated more rapidly and completely than allografts.[106] Fresh-frozen grafts are stronger, more immunogenic, and more completely incorporated in the fusion than freeze-dried grafts.[106] Combining allografts with autografts decreases the fusion rate versus autografts alone.[106] Use of recombinant human bone morphogenic protein (rhBMP-2) has been reported to increase the rate and robustness of lumbar spinal fusions with instrumentation (97%) versus the same procedure without rhBMP-2 (77%).[107] However, experience with rhBMP-2 has not been uniformly good.[101]

Pseudarthroses are often related to spinal infection. In the series of Abbey and associates of 34 spinal infections after posterior fusion with instrumentation, 12 patients (35.3%) had to have their instrumentation removed to treat the infection.[87] Of these 12, 5 had solid fusions but 2 had solid fusion at one level with limited motion at another level, 3 did not have solid fusion, 1 had nonfusion, and in 1 the fusion status was not determined.[87] In Viola and coworkers' series of eight delayed infections, 5 patients (63%) had pseudarthrosis at one or more levels.[89]

Incidental Durotomy and Pseudomeningocele

Incidental durotomy is an unintended tear or injury to the dura during surgery or other invasive procedure such as epidural injection.[108] The underlying arachnoid may or may not be injured.

Epidemiology

Incidental durotomy occurs in 1% to 14% of spinal surgeries (9.9% in a meta-analysis of 1,091 lumbar decompressions).[108] Durotomy occurred in 7.6% of 2,024 primary surgical procedures for lumbar degenerative disease and 15.9% of 1,159 revision surgeries for lumbar degenerative disease, average 10.6%.[109] In 2,144 surgeries at all levels, incidental durotomy occurred in 3.1% after simple decompression, 1.0% after decompression and fusion without instrumentation, and 2.0% after decompression and fusion with instrumentation.[108] Six of 3,183 lumbar decompression surgeries (0.2%), that is, 6 of 383 durotomies (1.8%), led to reoperation for repair of the leak despite initial conservative management.[109]

Clinical Presentation

Most durotomies are recognized and repaired during surgery. Approximately 0.3% of incidental durotomies are not recognized at surgery and lead to significant complications.[108] In Camissa and coworkers' series, six durotomies that were not recognized and treated during surgery led to persistent headache (2 patients), persistent postural headache with meningeal irritation and fluctuance at the operative site (1 patient), neurologic deficit (2 patients), and

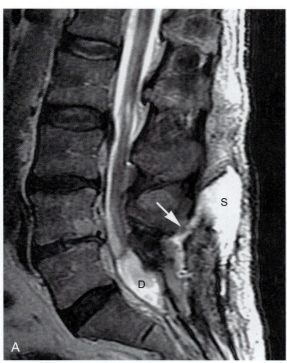

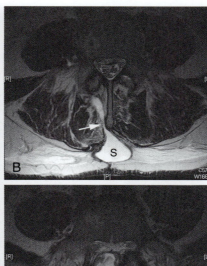

■ **FIGURE 25-27** Pseudomeningocele after posterior lumbar surgery. T2-weighted images in the sagittal (**A**) and axial (**B-C**) planes show loss of disc height at L4-L5, surgical approach to the L5-S1 level, and a large well-defined pseudomeningocele with superficial (S) and deep (D) compartments connected through a narrow isthmus (*arrow*) along the right side of the residual L5 spinous process.

visible CSF leak (1 patient).[108] Five of these six patients developed pseudomeningoceles, while the sixth showed CSF leak alone. Clinically, one can readily test for even a few drops of CSF on gauze by immunofixation electrophoresis for β_2-transferrin. This protein is produced by cerebral neuraminidase and is found only in the CSF and perilymph.[110] The incidence of deep wound infection may be higher in patients with durotomies.[108] Repair of the durotomies may be achieved by primary surgical closure, application of tissue sealants, blood patches, and tissue grafting.[109]

Pathophysiology

Inadvertent durotomy may result from direct full-thickness incision of the dura or from nicking or attenuation of the dura leading to later dehiscence. Pulsations of the arachnoid may then lead to bulging and puncture of the protruding arachnoid with CSF leak. Factors predisposing to durotomy include epidural adhesions to the dura, dural scarring and fibrosis, redundant dura in patients with severe spinal stenosis, large disc herniations causing difficult dissections, occult spina bifida, excessive nerve root traction, implantation of instruments, and the use of transpedicle screws, plates, and/or cross-links between vertical members of the constructs.[110] Dural breakdown due to infection, severe coughing, violent awakening from anesthesia, and postoperative seizures may also contribute.

In dogs, experimental durotomies begin to repair spontaneously by fibroblastic bridging on day 6 and are complete by approximately day 10.[110] In humans, any defects found are repaired directly, often with 4-0 nylon sutures. Unrepaired durotomies may lead to dural-cutaneous fistulas, meningitis, arachnoiditis, and epidural/paraspinal abscesses.[110] The subcutaneous fluid collection may prevent proper wound healing, leading to incisional infection, wound breakdown, or pseudomeningocele. Pseudomeningoceles may trap nerve roots to cause sciatica and may form a pool of CSF that leads to postural shifts of CSF and headaches.[110]

Imaging

Both CT and MRI successfully detect focal collections of fluid and demonstrate the superficial and deep extents of the collections (Fig. 25-27).[111] Imaging typically displays the sometimes narrow connection between the two compartments but may fail when the connection is very narrow. Both CT and MRI have difficulty in distinguishing simple seroma from CSF-filled pseudomeningocele and sterile collections from infected cavities. When there is suspicion of occult leak, nuclear scintigraphy or myelographic CT may prove helpful.

Misplacement of Pedicle Screws and Nerve Root Irritation

Misplacement occurs when the screw is positioned at an unwanted site or in a manner that causes secondary complications.

Epidemiology

Lonstein and associates analyzed 4,790 pedicle screws inserted in 875 patients during 915 spinal procedures of all types (76.3% lumbosacral arthrodesis) and followed the patients for a mean of 3 years[112]: 94.9% of screws were placed correctly. Screws penetrated the anterior cortex of the vertebrae in 2.8%, mostly in the sacral region, where anterior penetration was intentional to enhance screw fixation. Screws penetrated the pedicular cortex in 108 of 4,790 screw placements (2.3%) (see Fig. 25-20).[112] Screw breakage was found in 25 screws (2.2%), all of an early design. Six screws (0.1%) bent on insertion, reducing their structural integrity. Three screws (0.1%) were associated with pedicular fracture, and 4 screws (0.1%) were associated with dural tear.[112] Pseudarthrosis occurred in 65% of patients with broken screws. Overall, approximately 25% of the screws used in this study were later removed for diverse causes.[112] Later removal of interbody fusions and fixation hardware via anterior exposure carries significant risks. Nguyen and colleagues reported complications in 71% of patients undergoing anterior revision lumbar surgery to remove interbody devices.[113] Vascular complications occurred in 57% of the cases, including 100% of prior posterior lumbar interbody fusions and 80% of prior anterior lumbar interbody fusions.[113] The complication rate varied with the level operated and was twice as high at L4-L5 (89%) as at L5-S1 (40%). One patient died.[113]

Pedicle screws may also be misplaced into the facet joints, especially at the uppermost pair of pedicle screws.[114] Shah and associates reported pedicle screw violations of the facets at the uppermost instrumented level in 32% to 35% of patients (20%-23% of the uppermost pedicle screws).[115] Moshirfar and coworkers analyzed 204 patients with posterior lumbar interbody fusions performed via a midline incision and found that pedicle screws violated the most superior instrumented level in 24% of patients. The violations were bilateral in 7%, unilateral in 17%, twice as common on the left side when unilateral, and more common with single-level fusions (38%) than multilevel interbody fusions (14%).[114] Overall, the L5-S1 facet joint was affected most often (48% of single level L5-S1 fusions).[114]

Clinical Presentation

In Lonstein and colleagues' series of 915 spinal procedures with pedicle screw insertion, the most common postoperative problem (23% of screws, 24.3% of procedures) was late-onset discomfort or pain due to pseudarthrosis or perhaps to the instrumentation, necessitating removal of the hardware (with or without repair of the pseudarthrosis).[112] Specific nerve root irritation with pain or weakness occurred with 11 screws (0.2%) used in nine procedures (1%). In seven patients with 9 misplaced screws, surgical exploration of the level showed that the nerve was displaced but not transfixed nor lacerated by the screw. Eight of the 9 symptomatic screws were removed, with relief of deficit after removal of 7 of the 8. Even though the eighth (inferiorly misplaced) screw was removed on the day of surgery, the patient still had marked residual weakness. One additional screw, placed too far anteriorly in a sixth lumbar vertebra, caused definite weakness. This screw was withdrawn and replaced with a shorter screw, but the weakness persisted.[112]

Pathophysiology

Because thoracic and lumbar roots hug the medial and inferior surfaces of the pedicles as they exit the neural foramina, nerve root irritation occurs more commonly with screws that are misplaced medially (36.8%) and infe-

riorly (10%) than with those that are misplaced anteriorly (1%).[112]

Imaging

Direct axial and reconstructed coronal and sagittal CT images are most helpful for evaluating placement of the instrumentation. However, the artifact from the instrumentation can sometimes obscure the anatomy.

Vascular Injury

Vascular injury is any alteration in the lumen or wall of a blood vessel leading to narrowing, occlusion, intravascular clot with progressive thrombosis or embolization, dissection, pseudoaneurysm, and/or rupture.

Epidemiology

The incidence and nature of vascular injury from the posterior lumbar approach differ from those seen with anterior lumbar surgery.[52] No major vessel injuries have been reported to occur during the instrumentation phase itself, including pedicle screw placement.[52] From the posterior approach, "ventral perforation" causes prevertebral vascular injuries in only 0.01% to 0.05% of cases and, when it does, carries an overall mortality of 15% to 65%.[116,117]

Clinical Presentation

The most frequent injury is laceration of the left common iliac artery, because that vessel lies immediately anterior to the L4-L5 interspace.[116] Such arterial lacerations are detected rapidly. The next most frequent injury is arteriovenous fistula, which carries a mortality rate of approximately 10%.[117] Arteriovenous fistulas usually develop between the left common iliac artery and the left common iliac vein and are rare at L3-L4 or L5-S1.[117,113] They are usually detected late: 10% within 24 hours after surgery, 20% during the first year after disc removal, and some after very long delay (e.g., 8 years).[117] Pseudoaneurysms may also go undetected for long periods. Both arteriovenous fistulas and pseudoaneurysms may cause regional venous hypertension with swelling and pain in the abdomen and leg.[116]

Pathophysiology

With the posterior lumbar approach, vascular injuries usually result from situations that provide unexpected access to the prevertebral space or that cause adhesions between the spinal column and the vascular tree. These include degeneration/defect in the annulus fibrosus or anterior longitudinal ligament, prior adhesion of prevertebral structures to the anterior longitudinal ligament, difficult operative conditions such as revision surgery, aggressive exploration, and complex patient position such as knee-elbow position.[117]

Imaging

For acute injury with clinical decline, there may be no time for diagnostic imaging. Emergent surgical exploration may be warranted. Time permitting, CT can assess the presence and size of any hematoma. Catheter angiography typically provides the best assessment for vascular anatomy and may provide access for potential intravascular repair in select cases.

Delayed Epidural Hematoma

Delayed epidural hematoma is a collection of blood in the epidural space intraoperatively and postoperatively.

Epidemiology

Symptomatic postoperative epidural hemorrhages are found in 0.1% to 0.22% of patients.[119,120] Delayed symptomatic postoperative epidural hemorrhages are found in 0.17% of patients.[120] Asymptomatic postoperative epidural hemorrhages that compress the thecal sac are found in 58% of patients, commonly extend cephalic and/or caudal to the operative defect, and reduce the cross-sectional area of the canal by an average of 32% (range, 12%-56%).[119] The site of maximal compression lies deep to an adjacent unoperated level in 28% of patients with asymptomatic compressive hematomas. Risk factors for spinal epidural hemorrhage include use of nonsteroidal anti-inflammatory medications, preoperative coagulopathy, international normalized ratio (INR) greater than 2.0 within the first 48 hours after surgery, multilevel spinal procedures, posterior approach with laminectomy/laminoplasty versus anterior surgical approach, prior surgery at the same site, and large intraoperative blood loss.[119]

Pathophysiology

Spinal epidural hemorrhages are believed to originate from the rich venous plexus of the epidural space and are most frequent in the thoracic spine, where the epidural space is most prominent.[120] Disruption of the epidural vasculature and decreased coagulation ability lead to enlarging hemorrhage in this space.

Clinical Presentation

Patients with symptomatic epidural hemorrhages usually present within 24 hours after surgery but may present first after a multi-day symptom-free postoperative period (average, 3.8 days).[120] Patients commonly complain of intense sharp pain at the surgical site, followed by dysesthesias, radicular symptoms, and, finally, motor weakness. Seventy-one percent of patients improve after surgical evacuation of the hematoma.[120]

Imaging

Early on, the epidural hemorrhages appear as well-defined dorsally situated lentiform masses with heterogeneously variable signal intensity (acutely) and increased signal intensity on both T1- and T2-weighted images (subacutely).[119] The lesions may extend to each side. In sagittal view, they often show variable thickness with an undulant anterior border. Seromas, especially partially hemorrhagic seromas may have similar appearance but often have lower, more homogeneous signal intensity.[119]

Gelfoamoma

Gelfoamoma is a "mass" created by expansion of a Gelfoam pledget placed in situ before preliminary soaking in solution has allowed it to expand to its full "wet" size.

Epidemiology

The reported incidence is rare and anecdotal, but the actual incidence may be higher.

Clinical Presentation

Friedman and Whitecloud reported one patient who underwent decompressive laminectomies and posterior instrumentation/fusion using pedicle screws from L2 to L5.[121] At closing, a Gelfoam pad approximately the size of the laminectomy defect was placed over the exposed dura to provide hemostasis and protect the dura during irrigation. Immediately after surgery the patient reported right L5 radiculopathy. By postoperative day 13, symptoms progressed to bilateral cauda equina syndrome. Re-exploration revealed hard epidural fibrosis at L2-L5 with acute and chronic inflammation, granulation tissue, and reactive-degenerative change admixed with Gelfoam. After removal of this material, the patient quickly regained normal motor strength and sensation in the lower extremities and full bowel and bladder control.[121]

Pathophysiology

Dry Gelfoam imbibes fluid and swells as it becomes wet. Soaking in a solution of hemostatic agent typically brings the Gelfoam pad to full volume before placement into the wound. Gelfoam pads that are incompletely soaked may swell within the closed spinal canal after surgery, leading to compression of the thecal sac and nerve roots.

Imaging

Both CT and MRI may prove helpful to delineate the lesion and assess the degree of mass effect and potential associated hematoma.

Transforaminal Lumbar Interbody Fusion

Unilateral TLIF is an increasingly popular alternative to standard anterior and posterior approaches.[122] Study of 52 consecutive patients who were operated at one level (39 patients), two levels (11 patients), or three levels (2 patients) and observed for at least 3 years postoperatively disclosed relief of pain and disability equal to standard approaches and a fusion rate of 89%. There were four serious complications (7.7%): deep infection, persistent radiculopathy, symptomatic contralateral disc herniation, and pseudarthrosis with loosening of the implants.[122] Houten and coworkers studied 33 consecutive TLIFs in patients observed for a mean of 37 months after surgery.[123] Postoperatively, back pain was improved in 67%, unchanged in 27%, and worsened in 7%.[123] Leg pain was improved in 80%, unchanged in 10%, and worsened in 10%.[123] Fusion was successful in all cases.

Combined Anteroposterior "Circumferential" Cervical Spinal Decompression and Fusion

For selected complex lumbar problems, especially those with instability, surgeons may undertake combined anterior and posterior spinal decompression and fusion at the same session. Snell and colleagues reported single-stage, four- to eight-level, circumferential thoracolumbar vertebrectomy with circumferential reconstruction and arthrodesis via a midline posterior approach.[124] Four of 15 patients had complications: delayed transient neurologic deficit, infection, postoperative myocardial infarction, and hardware failure.[124]

ANALYSIS

For most purposes, CT is the preferred method for assessing the vertebral column for the extent of spondylosis/disc disease and for detecting anatomic variations that could increase the risk of surgical complications. MRI is the preferred method for assessing the spinal cord.

In the preoperative assessment, beyond the typical description of specific level and pathology, the imager should assess and report any conditions that might increase the risk of perioperative complications. Thus, the presence of right aortic arch or aberrant origin of the subclavian artery should be indicated, because they increase the likelihood of direct-origin laryngeal nerves and the risk of causing laryngeal dysfunction. In selected circumstances, it may be wise to assess the vocal apparatus before surgery to ensure that no unilateral vocal cord dysfunction already exists and predisposes the patient to the risk of bilateral vocal cord paralysis and permanent tracheostomy. The foramina transversaria should be assessed to predict the entry point of the vertebral arteries, because high entry of the vertebral artery into the foramina increases the risk of arterial damage during low cervical surgery. Any medially directed loops of the vertebral artery and any unusually narrow uncinate processes should also be reported as further protection against potential vertebral artery injury during resection of osteophytic spurs. In the lumbar region, the positions of the aortic bifurcation and the union of the iliac veins to form the inferior vena cava should be noted as a guide to the risk of vascular injury for anterior lumbar discectomy and fusion.

In the immediate postoperative period, the images should be assessed for correct level of surgery, proper alignment of the vertebral elements, safe positioning of the hardware and bony plugs (struts, cages), and successful decompression of the portions of the spinal canal or neural foramina addressed. Specific analysis should be made of potential complications of the surgery such as fractured bony elements, vascular injury, spinal cord or nerve root injury, and increased compression of the spinal canal and neural elements by hemorrhage, Gelfoam, or the instrumentation itself. The prevertebral soft tissue including the upper airway and larynx should be assessed and described to help detect esophageal perforation, laryngeal dysfunction, and hematoma.

Follow-up studies reassess these features and then analyze the images for evidence of spinal stability, (un)successful fusion, interval development of kyphosis, breakdown or migration of instrumentation and bone grafts, interval development of infection, and successful wound healing versus development of seroma or pseudomeningocele. Specific attention is directed to whether the surgical decompression remains adequate and whether the adjacent levels now show increased disease. Direct comparison with preoperative and with immediate postoperative studies helps to determine the stability of the surgical construct and to detect new problems. CT angiography or direct catheter angiography is most useful for defining any vascular injury or complication.

For specific question of spinal cord injury and detailed analysis of nerve roots, MRI is preferred. Although MR images are degraded by artifacts arising from the hardware utilized for fixation, new pulse sequences now coming into practice help to reduce the severity of these artifacts. MRI can also be used to study the relative positions of the spinal cord and roots within the canal and neural foramina at each level in flexion, neutral, and extension. These "motion" studies help to determine the stability of the fusion and any recurrent or new impingements on the neural tissue by bony, discal, or ligamentous pathology.

Sample reports are presented in Boxes 25-1 and 25-2.

BOX 25-1   Complications after C3-C4 Discectomy

PATIENT HISTORY

A 62-year-old man underwent single-level anterior C3-C4 discectomy with interbody fusion and anterior cervical fixation for cervical spondylosis.

TECHNIQUE

The cervical spine was studied by serial axial CT scans obtained from the skull base through T1 and processed with separate bone and soft tissue algorithms. The serial axial bone algorithm images were then reformatted into stacks of sagittal and coronal plane images. No contrast agent was administrated. No other study was available for comparison.

FINDINGS

There is an anterior cervical discectomy at C3-C4 with decortication of the apposing end plates, placement of an interbody bone plug, and screw fixation of an anterior cervical plate (Fig. 25-28A, B). The C3 vertebra lies slightly anterior to C4. The fixation plate stands away from the anterior surface of the C3 vertebra owing to the prominent residual anterior osteophytes (see Fig. 25-28B-D). The bone plug lies partially anterior to C4 and angles caudad at the anterior margin of C4. The upper screw traverses the C3 vertebra close to the inferior margin of the residual bone. The lower screws are placed within the center of the C4 vertebra and cinch together posteriorly (see Fig. 25-28D). There are residual osteophytes at C5-C6. The remainder of the study is unremarkable.

IMPRESSION

There is an anterior position of C3 forward on C4 with offset of the anterior cervical plate at C3 and anterior position of the C3-C4 interbody plug.

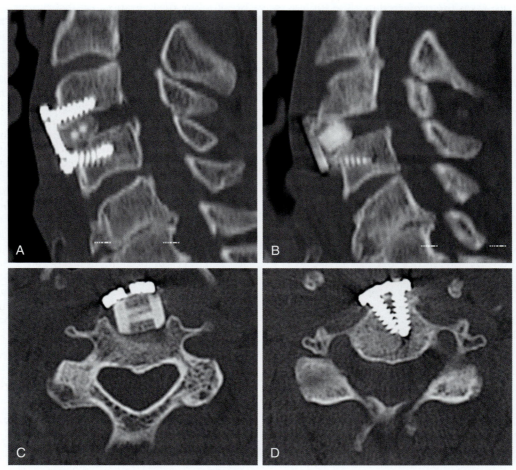

■ **FIGURE 25-28**   Complications after C3-C4 discectomy. See Box 25-1.

BOX 25-2 Complications after Two-Level Anterior Cervical Discectomy

PATIENT HISTORY

A 36-year-old man underwent two-level anterior cervical discectomy with interbody fusion and anterior cervical fixation 1 year ago. He complains of hoarseness that has persisted since the immediate postoperative period.

TECHNIQUE

The cervical spine was studied by serial axial CT sections obtained from the skull base through T1 and processed with separate bone and soft tissue algorithms. The serial axial bone algorithm images were then reformatted into stacks of sagittal and coronal plane images. No contrast agent was administrated. The present study was compared with the 3-month follow-up study.

FINDINGS

The serial axial and sagittal reformatted images show anterior cervical discectomy and fusion at C5-C6-C7, with placement of interbody bone plugs at C5-C6 and C6-C7 and internal fixation by anterior cervical plate and screws (Fig. 25-29). There is main-tenance of normal cervical lordosis. The alignment of the verte-brae is unchanged from the 3-month control study. The anterior cervical plate sits flush with the anterior surfaces of the vertebral bodies. The fixation screws are well positioned in the centers of the vertebral bodies with good bony purchase. There is now direct continuity of bony trabeculae through the fusion plugs across the C5-C6 and C6-C7 interspaces, indicating complete bony fusion. Small posterior osteophytes remain at C5-C6.

The prevertebral soft tissue shows thickening and medializa-tion of the right aryepiglottic fold, asymmetric widening of the ipsilateral pyriform sinus, and distorsion/medialization of the right vocal cord (see Fig. 25-29B). These imaging features are found with laryngeal dysfunction.

The remainder of the study is unremarkable.

IMPRESSION

There is complete bony fusion at C5-C7 with maintenance of normal cervical lordosis. Imaging features are consistent with laryngeal dysfunction on the right.

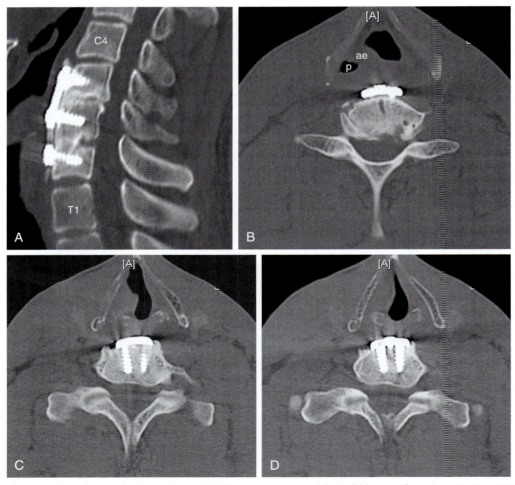

■ **FIGURE 25-29** Complications after two-level anterior cervical discectomy. ae, aryepiglottic fold; p, pyriform sinu . See Box 25-2.

KEY POINTS

- *Fusion:* Successful fusion may be inferred when the images show continuous bony trabeculae across the interspace or facet joint, motion of less than 3 degrees between flexion and extension images, and resorption of previously existing osteophytes.
- *Adjacent level disease:* Postoperatively, imaging signs of increasing "adjacent level" disease include progressive loss of disc height cephalad and caudad to the fusion zone, increasing luxation of adjacent interspaces on flexion-extension views, increasing size of osteophytes at the adjacent levels, and greater impingement of the bony and ligamentous elements of the spine upon adjacent neural structures.
- *Hardware failure:* Imaging signs of hardware failure include angulation and fracture of the screws, hooks, and rods; separation of the screws, rods, and fixation plate from the vertebrae; and progressive loss of height and angulation of bony elements and cages at the site of the construct.
- *Spinal cord injury:* Imaging signs of acute and subacute spinal cord injury include detection of hemorrhage or infarction within the cord, new or increasing T2 signal intensity within the cord, and increased compression of the spinal cord by external elements. Signs of prior, now-chronic spinal cord injury include loss of cord contour and volume, hemosiderin staining within the cord, and increased T2 signal in ascending tracts cephalad to the surgical level and descending tracts and caudad to the surgical level (i.e., a pattern of wallerian degeneration).
- *Esophageal perforation:* Imaging signs of esophageal perforation include advancing mediastinitis with acute edema and inflammation in the prevertebral soft tissue, air bubbles within this soft tissue, infection extending from the prevertebral soft tissue around the surgical hardware into the spinal column and spinal epidural space, and progressive deterioration of the construct with kyphosis.
- *Laryngeal dysfunction:* Imaging signs of laryngeal dysfunction include asymmetries of the pharynx and larynx, especially thickening and medialization of the aryepiglottic folds, widening of the ipsilateral pyriform sinus, medialization of the vocal cord, and dilatation of the ipsilateral laryngeal ventricle.
- *Vascular injury:* Imaging signs of vascular injury include narrowing of the affected vessel, thrombosis of the vessel, formation of pseudoaneurysm(s), operative site hematoma, and infarction or hemorrhage within the territory downstream of the vessel, including the spinal cord and brain.
- *Infection:* Infection may be simple superficial wound infection not extending down to the dura or it may be deeply seated infection involving the paraspinal musculature, spinal column, epidural space, and/or spinal cord. Spinal infection typically results from implantation of low-virulence organisms at the operative site *at the time of surgery* and smoldering growth over a long period, perhaps years, until the original infection becomes manifest. Imaging signs of infection include formation of local fluid collections in the wound or adjacent soft tissue, permeation of the bone, formation of intracanalicular or paraspinal masses, collapse of the surgical constructs, and draining fistulas. Fat-suppressed contrast-enhanced MR images typically display these signs of infection best.
- *Hematoma:* Imaging signs of hematoma include early formation of an unexpected mass in or near the surgical bed and compression and displacement of the esophagus, airway, and/or spinal cord by a mass. The hemorrhage may have lower density or different signal than expected due to admixed elements.
- *Pseudomeningocele:* Imaging signs of inadvertent durotomy with formation of pseudomeningocele include formation of a (usually) large fluid collection within the operative defect extending cephalad and caudad along the midline, laterally along the superficial fascia, and deeply toward the dura at the operative level.

SUGGESTED READINGS

Barker FG. Efficacy of prophylactic antibiotic therapy in spinal surgery: a meta-analysis. Neurosurgery 2002; 51:391-401.

Fountas KS, Kapsalaki EZ, Nikolakakos LG, et al. Anterior cervical discectomy and fusion associated complications. Spine 2007; 32:2310-2317.

Fraser JF, Härtl R. Anterior approaches to fusion of the cervical spine: a meta-analysis of fusion rates. J Neurosurg Spine 2007; 6:298-303.

Hannallah D, Lee J, Khan M, et al. Cerebrospinal fluid leaks following cervical spine surgery. J Bone Joint Surg Am 2008; 90:1101-1105.

Lee MJ, Bazaz R, Furey CG, Yoo J. Clinical studies: risk factors for dysphagia after anterior cervical spine surgery: a two-year prospective cohort study. Spine J 2007; 7:141-147.

Naidich TP. Cervical spine decompression for spinal stenosis and disk disease: Complications of surgery. In Castillo M, Koeller KK, Mukherji SK. Neuroradiology Categorical Course Syllabus, pp 289-296. American Roentgen Ray Society, 107th Annual Meeting, Orlando, FL, 2007.

Naidich TP. Thoracolumbar spine decompression for spinal stenosis and disk disease: Complications of surgery. In Castillo M, Koeller KK, Mukherji SK. Neuroradiology Categorical Course Syllabus, pp 297-305. American Roentgen Ray Society, 107th Annual Meeting, Orlando, FL, 2007.

Peng CW, Chou BT, Bendo JA, Spivak JM. Vertebral artery injury in cervical spine surgery—anatomical considerations, management and preventive measures. Spine J 2009;9:70-76.

Sagi HC, Beutler W, Carroll E, Connolly PJ. Airway complications associated with surgery on the anterior cervical spine. Spine 2002; 27:949-953.

Samartzis D, Shen FH, Matthews DK, et al. Comparison of allograft to autograft in multilevel anterior cervical discectomy and fusion with rigid plate fixation. Spine J 2003; 3:451-459.

Sasso RC, Garrido BJ. Postoperative spinal wound infections. J Am Acad Orthop Surg 2008; 16:330-337.

Suk KS, Kim KT, Lee SH, Park SW. Prevertebral soft tissue swelling after anterior cervical discectomy and fusion with plate fixation. Int Orthop 2006; 30:290-294.

Terao Y, Masumoto S, Yamashita K, et al. Increased Incidence of emergency airway management after combined anterior-posterior cervical spine surgery. J Neurosurg Anesthesiol 2004; 16:282-286.

Wang JC, Hart RA, Emery SE, Bohlman HH. Graft migration or displacement after multilevel cervical corpectomy and strut grafting. Spine 2003; 10:1016-1022.

Xie, J-C, Hurlbert RJ. Discectomy versus discectomy with fusion versus discectomy with fusion and instrumentation: a prospective randomized study. Neurosurgery 2007; 61:107-117.

Young PM, Berquist TH, Bancroft LW, Peterson JJ. Complications of spinal instrumentation. RadioGraphics 2007; 27:775-789.

REFERENCES

1. Baig MN, et al. Vision loss after spine surgery: review of the literature and recommendations. Neurosurg Focus 2007; 23:E15.
2. Cowan JA Jr, et al. Changes in the utilization of spinal fusion in the United States. Neurosurgery 2006; 59:15-20; discussion 15-20.
3. Zeidman SM, Ducker TB, Raycroft J. Trends and complications in cervical spine surgery: 1989-1993. J Spinal Disord 1997; 10:523-526.
4. Fountas KN, et al. Anterior cervical discectomy and fusion associated complications. Spine 2007; 32:2310-2317.
5. Edwards CC 2nd, et al. Accurate identification of adverse outcomes after cervical spine surgery. J Bone Joint Surg Am 2004; 86:251-256.
6. Abumi K, et al. Complications of pedicle screw fixation in reconstructive surgery of the cervical spine. Spine 2000; 25:962-969.
7. Salcman M. Complications of cervical spine surgery. Crit Care Med 2001; 29:2027-2028.
8. Sakaura H, et al. Long-term outcome of laminoplasty for cervical myelopathy due to disc herniation: a comparative study of laminoplasty and anterior spinal fusion. Spine 2005; 30:756-759.
9. Peolsson A, Peolsson M. Predictive factors for long-term outcome of anterior cervical decompression and fusion: a multivariate data analysis. Eur Spine J 2008; 17:406-414.
10. Wang JC, et al. Graft migration or displacement after multilevel cervical corpectomy and strut grafting. Spine 2003; 28:1016-1021; discussion 1021-1022.
11. Bose B. Anterior cervical instrumentation enhances fusion rates in multilevel reconstruction in smokers. J Spinal Disord 2001; 14:3-9.
12. Samartzis D, et al. Is autograft the gold standard in achieving radiographic fusion in one-level anterior cervical discectomy and fusion with rigid anterior plate fixation? Spine 2005; 30:1756-1761.
13. Jacobs WC, et al. Single or double-level anterior interbody fusion techniques for cervical degenerative disc disease. Cochrane Database Syst Rev 2004; (4):CD004958.
14. Hilibrand AS, et al. Increased rate of arthrodesis with strut grafting after multilevel anterior cervical decompression. Spine 2002; 27:146-151.
15. Samartzis D, et al. Does rigid instrumentation increase the fusion rate in one-level anterior cervical discectomy and fusion? Spine J 2004; 4:636-643.
16. Hughes SS, et al. Settling of fibula strut grafts following multilevel anterior cervical corpectomy: a radiographic evaluation. Spine 2006; 31:1911-1915.
17. Fraser JF, Härtl R. Anterior approaches to fusion of the cervical spine: a meta-analysis of fusion rates. J Neurosurg Spine 2007; 6:298-303.
18. Bolesta MJ, Rechtine GR 2nd, Chrin AM. Three- and four-level anterior cervical discectomy and fusion with plate fixation: a prospective study. Spine 2000; 25:2040-2044; discussion 2045-2046.
19. Ray CD. Threaded titanium cages for lumbar interbody fusions. Spine 1997; 22:667-679; discussion 679-680.
20. Uchida K, et al. Multivariate analysis of the neurological outcome of surgery for cervical compressive myelopathy. J Orthop Sci 2005; 10:564-573.
21. Koller H, et al. 4- and 5-level anterior fusions of the cervical spine: review of literature and clinical results. Eur Spine J 2007; 16:2055-2071.
22. Xie JC, Hurlbert RJ. Discectomy versus discectomy with fusion versus discectomy with fusion and instrumentation: a prospective randomized study. Neurosurgery 2007; 61:107-116; discussion 116-117.
23. Ashkenazi E, et al. Anterior decompression combined with corpectomies and discectomies in the management of multilevel cervical myelopathy: a hybrid decompression and fixation technique. J Neurosurg Spine 2005; 3:205-209.
24. Ikenaga M, Shikata J, Tanaka C. Anterior corpectomy and fusion with fibular strut grafts for multilevel cervical myelopathy. J Neurosurg Spine 2005; 3:79-85.
25. Lowery GL, McDonough RF. The significance of hardware failure in anterior cervical plate fixation: patients with 2- to 7-year follow-up. Spine 1998; 23:181-186; discussion 186-187.
26. Seichi A, et al. Postoperative expansion of intramedullary high-intensity areas on T2-weighted magnetic resonance imaging after cervical laminoplasty. Spine 2004; 29 1478-1482; discussion 1482.
27. Kraus DR, Stauffer ES. Spinal cord injury as a complication of elective anterior cervical fusion. Clin Orthop Relat Res 1975; (112):130-141.
28. Sagi HC, et al. Airway complications associated with surgery on the anterior cervical spine. Spine 2002; 27:949-953.
29. Lee MJ, et al. Risk factors for dysphagia after anterior cervical spine surgery: a two-year prospective cohort study. Spine J 2007; 7:141-147.
30. Heese O, et al. Intraoperative measurement of pharynx/esophagus retraction during anterior cervical surgery: II. Perfusion. Eur Spine J 2006; 15:1839-1843.
31. Heese O, et al. Intraoperative measurement of pharynx/esophagus retraction during anterior cervical surgery: I. Pressure. Eur Spine J 2006; 15:1833-1837.
32. Cloward RB. Complications of anterior cervical disc operation and their treatment. Surgery 1971; 69:175-182.
33. Eleraky MA, Llanos C, Sonntag VK. Cervical corpectomy: report of 185 cases and review of the literature J Neurosurg 1999; 90(1 Suppl):35-41.
34. Orlando ER, Caroli E, Ferrante L. Management of the cervical esophagus and hypopharynx perforations complicating anterior cervical spine surgery. Spine 2003; 28:E290-E295.
35. Patel NP, et al. Esophageal injury associated with anterior cervical spine surgery. Surg Neurol 2008; 69:20-24; discission 24.
36. Newhouse KE, et al. Esophageal perforation following anterior cervical spine surgery. Spine 1989; 14:1051-1053.
37. Jones WG 2nd, Ginsberg RJ. Esophageal perforation: a continuing challenge. Ann Thorac Surg 1992; 53:534-543.
38. Shenoy SN, Raja A. Delayed pharyngo-esophageal perforation: rare complication of anterior cervical spine surgery. Neurol India 2003; 51:534-536.
39. Fountas KN, et al. Extrusion of a screw into the gastrointestinal tract after anterior cervical spine plating. J Spinal Disord Tech 2006; 19:199-203.
40. Fujibayashi S, et al. Missing anterior cervical plate and screws: a case report. Spine 2000; 25:2258-2261.
41. Terao Y, et al. Increased incidence of emergency airway management after combined anterior-posterior cervical spine surgery. J Neurosurg Anesthesiol 2004; 16:282-286.
42. Epstein NE, et al. Can airway complications following multilevel anterior cervical surgery be avoided? J Neurosurg 2001; 94(2 Suppl):185-188.
43. Suk KS, et al. Prevertebral soft tissue swelling after anterior cervical discectomy and fusion with plate fixation. Int Orthop 2006; 30:290-294.
44. Sanfilippo JA Jr, et al. "Normal" prevertebral soft tissue swelling following elective anterior cervical decompression and fusion. J Spinal Disord Tech 2006; 19:399-401.
45. Beutler WJ, Sweeney CA, Connolly PJ. Recurrent laryngeal nerve injury with anterior cervical spine surgery risk with laterality of surgical approach. Spine 2001; 26:1337-1342.
46. Apfelbaum RI, Kriskovich MD Haller JR. On the incidence, cause, and prevention of recurrent laryngeal nerve palsies during anterior cervical spine surgery. Spine 2000; 25:2906-2912.
47. Morpeth JF, Williams MF. Vocal fold paralysis after anterior cervical diskectomy and fusion. Laryngoscope 2000; 110:43-46.
48. Audu P, et al. Recurrent laryngeal nerve palsy after anterior cervical spine surgery: the impact of endotracheal tube cuff deflation, reinflation, and pressure adjustment. Anesthesiology 2006; 105:898-901.
49. Chin SC, et al. Using CT to localize side and level of vocal cord paralysis. AJR Am J Roentgenol 2003; 180:1165-1170.
50. Manski TJ, Wood MD, Dunsker SB. Bilateral vocal cord paralysis following anterior cervical discectomy and fusion: case report. J Neurosurg 1998; 89:839-843.
51. Daentzer D, Deinsberger W, Boker DK. Vertebral artery complications in anterior approaches to the cervical spine: report of two cases and review of literature. Surg Neurol 2003; 59:300-309; discussion 309.

52. Inamasu J, Guiot BH. Vascular injury and complication in neurosurgical spine surgery. Acta Neurochir (Wien) 2006; 148:375-387.

53. Neo M, et al. The clinical risk of vertebral artery injury from cervical pedicle screws inserted in degenerative vertebrae. Spine 2005; 30:2800-2805.

54. Peng CW, et al. Vertebral artery injury in cervical spine surgery—anatomical considerations, management, and preventive measures. Spine J 2009; 9:70-76.

55. Pait TG, Killefer JA, Arnautovic KI. Surgical anatomy of the anterior cervical spine: the disc space, vertebral artery, and associated bony structures. Neurosurgery 1996; 39:769-776.

56. Bruneau M, et al. Anatomical variations of the V2 segment of the vertebral artery. Neurosurgery 2006; 59(Suppl 1):ONS20-S24; discussion ONS20-S24.

57. Adachi B. Das arterien System der Japaner. Kyoto, Verlagr der Kaiserlich Japanischen Universitat, col 1, 1928.

58. Newton T, Mani RL. The vertebral artery in radiology of the skull and brain. In: Newton T, Potts DG (eds). Angiography. St. Louis, CV Mosby, 1974, pp 1659-1709.

59. Daseler EH, Anson BJ. Surgical anatomy of the subclavian artery and its branches. Surg Gynecol Obstet 1959; 108:149-174.

60. Curylo LJ, et al. Tortuous course of the vertebral artery and anterior cervical decompression: a cadaveric and clinical case study. Spine 2000; 25:2860-2864.

61. Ebraheim NA, et al. Vulnerability of the sympathetic trunk during the anterior approach to the lower cervical spine. Spine 2000; 25:1603-1606.

62. Barker FG 2nd. Efficacy of prophylactic antibiotic therapy in spinal surgery: a meta-analysis. Neurosurgery 2002; 51:391-400; discussion 400-401.

63. Sasso RC, Garrido BJ. Postoperative spinal wound infections. J Am Acad Orthop Surg 2008; 16:330-337.

64. Hannallah D, et al. Cerebrospinal fluid leaks following cervical spine surgery. J Bone Joint Surg Am 2008; 90:1101-1105.

65. Sciubba DM, et al. Factors associated with cervical instability requiring fusion after cervical laminectomy for intradural tumor resection. J Neurosurg Spine 2008; 8:413-419.

66. Dai L, et al. Radiculopathy after laminectomy for cervical compression myelopathy. J Bone Joint Surg Br 1998; 80:846-549.

67. Heller JG, Silcox DH 3rd, Sutterlin CE 3rd. Complications of posterior cervical plating. Spine 1995; 20:2442-2448.

68. Sekhon LH. Posterior cervical decompression and fusion for circumferential spondylotic stenosis: review of 50 consecutive cases. J Clin Neurosci 2006; 13:23-30.

69. Hale JJ, Gruson KI, Spivak JM. Laminoplasty: a review of its role in compressive cervical myelopathy. Spine J 2006; 6(Suppl):289S-298S.

70. Kast E, et al. Complications of transpedicular screw fixation in the cervical spine. Eur Spine J 2006; 15:327-334.

71. Kim PK, Alexander JT. Indications for circumferential surgery for cervical spondylotic myelopathy. Spine J 2006; 6(Suppl):299S-307S.

72. Yoshimoto H, et al. Spinal reconstruction using a cervical pedicle screw system. Clin Orthop Relat Res 2005; (431):111-119.

73. Kwon B, et al. Risk factors for delayed extubation after single-stage, multi-level anterior cervical decompression and posterior fusion. J Spinal Disord Tech 2006; 19:389-393.

74. Postacchini F. Surgical management of lumbar spinal stenosis. Spine 1999; 24:1043-1047.

75. Jansson KA, et al. Health-related quality of life in patients before and after surgery for a herniated lumbar disc. J Bone Joint Surg Br 2005; 87:959-964.

76. McAfee PC, et al. Symposium: a critical discrepancy—a criteria of successful arthrodesis following interbody spinal fusions. Spine 2001; 26(3):320-334.

77. Kroner AH, et al. Magnetic resonance imaging evaluation of posterior lumbar interbody fusion. Spine 2006; 31:1365-1371.

78. Faciszewski T, et al. The surgical and medical perioperative complications of anterior spinal fusion surgery in the thoracic and lumbar spine in adults: a review of 1223 procedures. Spine 1995; 20:1592-1599.

79. Mummaneni PV, Haid RW, Rodts GE. Lumbar interbody fusion: state-of-the-art technical advances. Invited submission from the Joint Section Meeting on Disorders of the Spine and Peripheral Nerves, March 2004. J Neurosurg Spine 2004; 1:24-30.

80. Jansson KA, et al. Surgery for herniation of a lumbar disc in Sweden between 1987 and 1999: an analysis of 27,576 operations. J Bone Joint Surg Br 2004; 86:841-847.

81. Fritzell P, Hagg O, Nordwall A. Complications in lumbar fusion surgery for chronic low back pain: comparison of three surgical techniques used in a prospective randomized study. A report from the Swedish Lumbar Spine Study Group. Eur Spine J 2003; 12:178-189.

82. Bernsmann K, et al. Lumbar micro disc surgery with and without autologous fat graft: a prospective randomized trial evaluated with reference to clinical and social factors. Arch Orthop Trauma Surg 2001; 121:476-480.

83. Gejo R, et al. Serial changes in trunk muscle performance after posterior lumbar surgery. Spine 1999; 24:1023-1028.

84. Gambardella G, et al. Prevention of recurrent radicular pain after lumbar disc surgery: a prospective study. Acta Neurochir Suppl 2005; 92:151-154.

85. Valentini LG, et al. Surgical site infections after elective neurosurgery: a survey of 1747 patients. Neurosurgery 2008; 62:88-95; discussion 95-96.

86. Richards BR, Emara KM. Delayed infections after posterior TSRH spinal instrumentation for idiopathic scoliosis: revisited. Spine 2001; 26:1990-1996.

87. Abbey DM, et al. Treatment of postoperative wound infections following spinal fusion with instrumentation. J Spinal Disord 1995; 8:278-283.

88. Perry JW, et al. Wound infections following spinal fusion with posterior segmental spinal instrumentation. Clin Infect Dis 1997; 24:558-561.

89. Viola RW, et al. Delayed infection after elective spinal instrumentation and fusion: a retrospective analysis of eight cases. Spine 1997; 22:2444-2450; discussion 2450-2451.

90. Clark CE, Shufflebarger HL: Late-developing infection in instrumented idiopathic scoliosis. Spine 1999; 24:1909-1912.

91. Heggeness MH, et al. Late infection of spinal instrumentation by hematogenous seeding. Spine 1993; 18:492-496.

92. Richards BS. Delayed infections following posterior spinal instrumentation for the treatment of idiopathic scoliosis. J Bone Joint Surg Am 1995; 77:524-529.

93. Beiner JM, et al. Postoperative wound infections of the spine. Neurosurg Focus 2003; 15:E14.

94. Pappou IP, et al. Postoperative infections in interbody fusion for degenerative spinal disease. Clin Orthop Relat Res 2006; 444:120-128.

95. Wimmer C, Gluch H. Management of postoperative wound infection in posterior spinal fusion with instrumentation. J Spinal Disord 1996; 9:505-508.

96. Sasso RC, LeHuec JC, Shaffrey C. Iliac crest bone graft donor site pain after anterior lumbar interbody fusion: a prospective patient satisfaction outcome assessment. J Spinal Disord Tech 2005; 18(Suppl):S77-S81.

97. Davne SH, Myers DL. Complications of lumbar spinal fusion with transpedicular instrumentation. Spine 1992; 17(Suppl):S184-S189.

98. Sengupta DK, et al. Outcome of local bone versus autogenous iliac crest bone graft in the instrumented posterolateral fusion of the lumbar spine. Spine 2006; 31:985-991.

99. Ikard RW. Methods and complications of anterior exposure of the thoracic and lumbar spine. Arch Surg 2006; 141:1025-1034.

100. Anjarwalla NK, Morcom RK, Fraser RD. Supplementary stabilization with anterior lumbar intervertebral fusion—a radiologic review. Spine 2006; 31:1281-1287.

101. Pradhan BB, et al. Graft resorption with the use of bone morphogenetic protein: lessons from anterior lumbar interbody fusion using femoral ring allografts and recombinant human bone morphogenetic protein-2. Spine 2006; 31:E277-E284.

102. Fantini GA, et al. Major vascular injury during anterior lumbar spinal surgery: incidence, risk factors, and management. Spine 2007; 32:2751-2758.

103. Inamasu J, Kim DH, Logan L. Three-dimensional computed tomographic anatomy of the abdominal great vessels pertinent to L4-L5 anterior lumbar interbody fusion. Minim Invasive Neurosurg 2005; 48:127-131.

104. Brau SA, et al. Vascular injury during anterior lumbar surgery. Spine J 2004; 4:409-412.

105. Kulkarni SS, et al. Arterial complications following anterior lumbar interbody fusion: report of eight cases. Eur Spine J 2003; 12: 48-54.
106. Ehrler DM, Vaccaro AR. The use of allograft bone in lumbar spine surgery. Clin Orthop Relat Res 2000; (371):38-45.
107. Singh K, et al. Use of recombinant human bone morphogenetic protein-2 as an adjunct in posterolateral lumbar spine fusion: a prospective CT-scan analysis at one and two years. J Spinal Disord Tech 2006; 19:416-423.
108. Cammisa FP Jr, et al. Incidental durotomy in spine surgery. Spine 2000; 25:2663-2667.
109. Khan MH, et al. Postoperative management protocol for incidental dural tears during degenerative lumbar spine surgery: a review of 3,183 consecutive degenerative lumbar cases. Spine 2006; 31:2609-2613.
110. Bosacco SJ, Gardner MJ, Guille JT. Evaluation and treatment of dural tears in lumbar spine surgery: a review. Clin Orthop Relat Res 2001; (389):238-247.
111. Vakharia SB, et al. Magnetic resonance imaging of cerebrospinal fluid leak and tamponade effect of blood patch in postdural puncture headache. Anesth Analg 1997; 84:585-590.
112. Lonstein JE, et al. Complications associated with pedicle screws. J Bone Joint Surg Am 1999; 81(11):1519-1528.
113. Nguyen HV, et al. Anterior exposure of the spine for removal of lumbar interbody devices and implants. Spine 2006; 31:2449-2453.
114. Moshirfar A, et al. Computed tomography evaluation of superior-segment facet-joint violation after pedicle instrumentation of the lumbar spine with a midline surgical approach. Spine 2006; 31:2624-2629.
115. Shah RR, et al. Radiologic evaluation of adjacent superior segment facet joint violation following transpedicular instrumentation of the lumbar spine. Spine 2003; 28:272-275.
116. Dosoglu M, et al. Nightmare of lumbar disc surgery: iliac artery injury. Clin Neurol Neurosurg 2006; 108:174-177.
117. Szolar DH, et al. Vascular complications in lumbar disk surgery: report of four cases. Neuroradiology 1996; 38:521-525.
118. Prabhakar H, et al. Rupture of aorta and inferior vena cava during lumbar disc surgery. Acta Neurochir (Wien) 2005; 147:327-329; discussion 329.
119. Sokolowski MJ, et al. Postoperative lumbar epidural hematoma: does size really matter? Spine 2008; 33:114-119.
120. Uribe J, et al. Delayed postoperative spinal epidural hematomas. Spine J 2003; 3:125-129.
121. Friedman J, Whitecloud TS 3rd. Lumbar cauda equina syndrome associated with the use of gelfoam: case report. Spine 2001; 26: E485-E487.
122. Hackenberg L, et al. Transforaminal lumbar interbody fusion: a safe technique with satisfactory three to five year results. Eur Spine J 2005; 14:551-558.
123. Houten JK, et al. Clinical and radiographically/neuroimaging documented outcome in transforaminal lumbar interbody fusion. Neurosurg Focus 2006; 20:E8.
124. Snell BE, Nasr FF, Wolfla CE. Single-stage thoracolumbar vertebrectomy with circumferential reconstruction and arthrodesis: surgical technique and results in 15 patients. Neurosurgery 2006; 58(4 Suppl 2):ONS-263-268; discussion ONS-269.

PART THIRTEEN

The Brachial and Sacral Plexuses

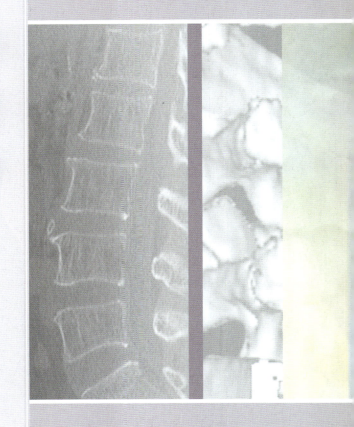

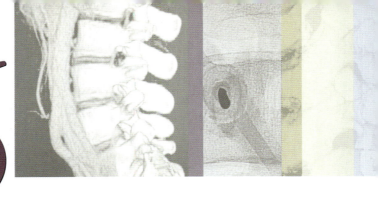

26

Imaging of the Brachial Plexus

Marta Martínez Schmickrath and Mauricio Castillo

The brachial plexus is the name given to the plexus of nerves formed by the lower four ventral cervical roots (C5-C8) and the first thoracic ventral root (T1) as they emerge from the spinal cord, intermingle, realign, and emerge from the plexus as defined distal nerves. C4 and T2 may contribute axons to the plexus with little effect on the clinical location of the lesion.[1] The brachial plexus is responsible for the motility and sensitivity in the upper extremities.

At each spinal level, the ventral and dorsal rootlets emerge from the spinal cord and unite distal to the dorsal ganglia to form the root proper. This root then divides into dorsal and ventral portions designated the dorsal and ventral roots of each level. The dorsal portions of the lower cervical roots do not contribute to the brachial plexus; they pass dorsally to innervate the skin and muscles of the neck and upper back.[2] The ventral roots form the brachial plexus. First, the ventral roots realign into three trunks. The ventral root of C5 joins the ventral root of C6 to form the upper trunk. The ventral root of C7 remains alone and forms the middle trunk. The ventral root of C8 joins the ventral root of T1 to form the lower trunk. Each trunk then splits into an anterior and a posterior division, which reunite to form three cords (posterior, lateral, and medial) that finally end as the branches (peripheral nerves) (Fig. 26-1).

The ventral cervical roots descend toward the first rib, whereas the ventral T1 root ascends over the first rib to form the brachial plexus. The brachial plexus emerges between the anterior and middle scalene muscles (the interscalenic triangle), where sympathetic fibers controlling vasoconstriction and sweat gland activity join the nerve roots. The sympathetic contributions to C5 and C6 arise from the inferior cervical ganglion. The sympathetic contributions to C7, C8, and T1 arise from the stellate

ganglion.[2] T1 nerve roots also contribute parasympathetic fibers to the ganglion, which, when injured, cause Horner syndrome (Fig. 26-2).[2,3]

TECHNIQUE

MRI is the most widely accepted imaging modality used to evaluate the brachial plexus. Sequences that are usually employed include the following:

- T1-weighted (T1W) imaging is used to evaluate the regional anatomy and fatty post-traumatic denervation changes of the muscle.[4]
- T2-weighted (T2W) imaging with fat suppression can highlight the pathologic signal changes within the nerves. Fat suppression sequences such as short tau inversion recovery (STIR) or frequency-selective fat saturation are necessary so that abnormal signal is not obscured by adjacent fat.[4] STIR offers a consistent and uniform suppression of fat signal with excellent T2 contrast but has a low signal-to-noise ratio (SNR), greater sensitivity to blood flow artifacts, and no T1 tissue contrast images. Frequency-selective fat saturation methods have a higher SNR (resulting in better image quality), have fewer blood-flow–related artifacts, and can generate T1W images. The greatest disadvantage of frequency-selective fat saturation is the variable completeness of fat suppression across the field of view and consequent signal inhomogeneity.[4]
- Constructive interference in steady-state (CISS)/fast imaging employing steady-state acquisition (FIESTA) show pools of cerebrospinal fluid (CSF) associated with nerve root avulsions and small schwannomas.[5,6]
- Contrast-enhanced T1W imaging is done with a standard dose of 0.1 mmol/kg of gadolinium-based contrast

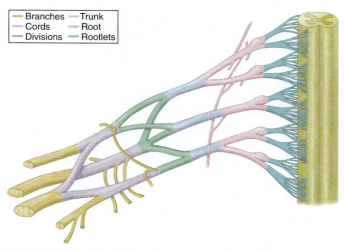

■ FIGURE 26-1 The different elements of the brachial plexus and their relationships to highlighted anatomic landmarks. The roots are within the neural foramina and medial to the scalene muscles. The trunks are located between the anterior and middle scalene muscles. The cords are below the clavicle. Thus, the divisions are slightly superior and posterior to the clavicle. The branches or nerves are in the axilla.

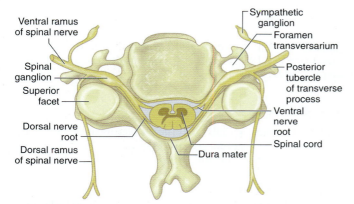

■ FIGURE 26-2 Formation of spinal nerves in the cervical region. As they exit the spinal cord, the ventral and dorsal rootlets join to form the spinal or dorsal root ganglion. These ganglia then split into ventral and dorsal rami. Sympathetic fibers originate from the ventral rami. *(Redrawn from Middleditch A, Oliver J. Functional Anatomy of the Spine, 2nd ed. Edinburgh, Butterworth-Heinemann, 2006, p 234.)*

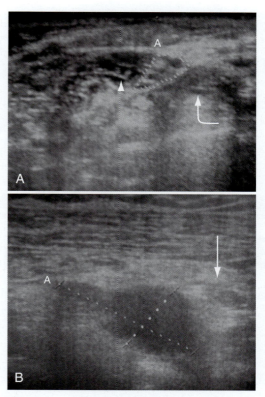

■ FIGURE 26-3 A, Normal ultrasonographic appearance of the trunks (*dotted lines*) of a brachial plexus, localized under the sternocleidomastoid muscle and between the anterior scalene (*arrowhead*) and middle scalene (*curved arrow*) muscles. B, Ultrasonographic study for a supraclavicular "lump" felt by the patient. The mass (*dotted lines*) does not have the typical hyperechoic hilum of a lymph node and demonstrated no flow with Doppler technique (not shown). The mass has a solid appearance suggesting a neural sheath tumor arising from the posterior cord. *Arrow* indicates a normal medial cord.

material to display neoplasms, radiation injury, inflammation/abscess, or other enhancing disease processes. Contrast enhancement is not indicated in trauma,[6] although acute denervated muscles enhance.[6] Contrast-enhanced studies must be performed with frequency-selective fat saturation to better visualize enhancing structures.

The study is performed to maximize information from the symptomatic side and obtain basic information from the normal side for comparison.

Imaging planes and methods include the following:

- Symptomatic side
  - T1, T2, CISS/FIESTA true or oblique coronal
  - T1 true or oblique sagittal
  - T1 and T2 axial
  - T1 images repeated after gadolinium administration with fat suppression
- Asymptomatic side (to enable comparison with normal structures)
  - T1 and T2 true or oblique coronal
- CT cannot visualize the brachial plexus directly, but it is helpful for evaluating neighboring structures to detect post-traumatic clavicle fractures, cervical ribs, lung masses, and so on.
- CT myelography may be helpful when nerve root avulsion is suspected. It has greater sensitivity and specificity than a simple myelogram but is less sensitive than MRI for identification of pseudomeningoceles.
- Ultrasonography is highly useful for guiding placement of local anesthesia and evaluating the echo texture of a mass before biopsy (e.g., subclavian aneurysm vs. nerve sheath tumor vs. adenopathy) (Fig. 26-3).

Indications for the different techniques are as follows:

- *Trauma:* radiography, MRI, and CT myelography
- *Tumor:* MRI and CT

● *Thoracic outlet syndrome:* radiography, MRI, CT, and angiography
● *Plexitis and suspected inflammatory processes:* MRI

NORMAL APPEARANCE

The components of the brachial plexus normally have intermediate signal intensity, similar to muscle in both T1W and T2W images. Distal to the dorsal root ganglia there is no normal enhancement. All of the portions of the brachial plexus (roots, trunks, divisions, cord, and branches) are uniform in size (within groups) and are separated by fat. The roots are located in the neural foramina, the trunks within the fat of the interscalene triangle (between the anterior and middle scalene muscles), and the divisions behind (posterior to) the clavicle. The lateral and medial cords lie anterior to the subclavian artery, whereas the posterior cord lies dorsal to the artery. Their branches wrap around the axillary artery.

Artifacts may be associated with this technique:

● Inhomogeneity of fat saturation in frequency-selective fat saturation images may lead to varying signal intensities in the brachial plexus, simulating edema.[4]
● The "magic angle" effect in STIR images results in an isolated hyperintensity of portions of the plexus. It results from T2 anisotropy attributed to densely packed and hydrated collagen and from the fact that the brachial plexus is oriented at 55 degrees to the main B° magnetic field (the magic angle).[4]
● Flow artifacts arise from the artery or aneurysms.

SPECIFIC USES

Trauma

Obstetric trauma to the brachial plexus occurs in 0.4 to 2.5 per 1000 live births. Plexus injuries are mainly associated with shoulder dystocias, which are the most frequent cause of obstetric brachial plexus palsies. There are two major presentations of obstetric trauma to the brachial plexus: an upper root injury at C5-C6 (Erb's palsy), which is more frequent, and an isolated lower root injury at C8-T1 (Dejerine-Klumpke palsy). The typical posture of Erb's palsy consists of shoulder adduction and internal rotation, elbow extension, forearm pronation, wrist flexion, and finger flexion (Fig. 26-4). Extended Erb's palsy includes C7, leading to additional paralysis of elbow and finger extension. Klumpke's palsy should be suspected if Horner syndrome is present.[1] Because limited external rotation may also be due to a concomitant shoulder dislocation and the humeral head of a newborn is neither ossified nor visible on radiographs, ultrasonography or MRI may be required to rule out this differential possibility.[1]

Stab wounds or gunshot wounds can transect portions of the brachial plexus directly or produce vascular injuries with expanding hematomas or pseudoaneurysms that compress the nerves secondarily (Fig. 26-5).[1] In these conditions, brachial plexus imaging is necessary to sort out which lesions are present, which specific therapies they require, and their prognoses.

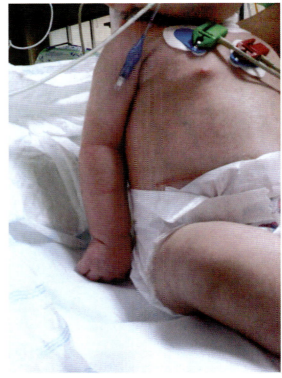

■ **FIGURE 26-4** A 3-month-old presented with the typical clinical finding of Erb's brachial plexus obstetric palsy. The right upper extremity is held in a "waiter's tip" position (shoulder adduction with internal rotation, elbow extension, forearm pronation, wrist flexion and finger flexion). Most of these palsies resolve spontaneously without any surgical procedures. *(Courtesy of Drs. Alfredo García-Alix and Marta Benito, Hospital La Paz, Madrid.)*

Traction injuries are the most common cause of brachial plexus injury in young adults, with most of them resulting from motorcycle accidents in males. Some call these injuries "burners or stingers" when they are due to minor stretch traumas common in contact sports such as football. Clinically, they cause a burning pain and paresthesias that radiate from the supraclavicular area into the arm with transient weakness and sensory abnormalities. They usually resolve spontaneously over a few minutes and do not require imaging. If there is incomplete recovery or restricted neck motion, diagnostic imaging is required to rule out a cervical spine injury or other important pathology.[1]

All traumatic lesions of the brachial plexus may be classified as postganglionic or preganglionic. The prognosis and treatment planning are different for the two types, so it is essential to differentiate between them.

Postganglionic injuries are treated surgically to reestablish local nerve continuity and afford a better prognosis. Preganglionic avulsions are usually irreparable and require alternative techniques to restore function or to at least decrease the patient's pain (nerve transfer and more recent reimplantation or graft insertion).[1]

Preganglionic lesions may be root stretches or partial/complete root avulsions. The most common pattern of injury (69% of partial avulsions) is partial avulsion of a ventral rootlet with an intact dorsal rootlet.[3] If the motor rootlet is avulsed, the motor cell body in the spinal cord

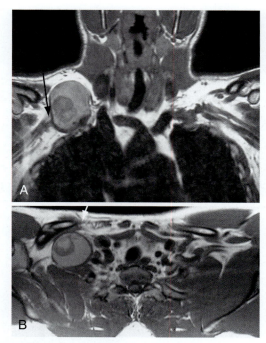

■ FIGURE 26-5 Coronal (**A**) and axial (**B**) T1W contrast-enhanced MR images show the right brachial plexus displaced anteriorly and compressed against the clavicle (*arrows*) by a traumatic subclavian artery pseudoaneurysm. The patient reported symptoms compatible with a compressive plexopathy, and the aneurysm was treated with a subclavian artery stent placed across its neck. With time, the aneurysm became smaller and the symptoms resolved.

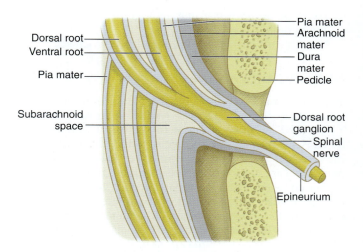

■ FIGURE 26-6 As the ventral and dorsal rootlets leave the spinal cord, they carry with them an extension of the arachnoid and dura that forms the nerve root sleeve. The sleeve attaches to the ventral and dorsal rootlets and spinal ganglion to form the sheath of the spinal nerve. CSF does not usually extend beyond the intervertebral foramen. This explains the close association of preganglionic rootlet avulsion with dural tear and subsequent pseudomeningocele formation, a lesion that does not commonly occur with more distal tears. *(Redrawn from Middleditch A, Oliver J. Functional Anatomy of the Spine, 2nd ed. Edinburgh, Butterworth-Heinemann, 2006, p 277.)*

is separated from its axons. The axons then undergo wallerian degeneration.[1] If the dorsal rootlet is avulsed, the sensory cell bodies in the dorsal root ganglia remain connected to their axons, so sensory fibers are spared from wallerian degeneration. In these cases, therefore, electrodiagnostic studies reveal abnormal motor findings with intact sensory conduction.[1] Avulsion occurs more frequently at the C8-T1 rootlets. These rootlets lack fibrous attachments to the transverse processes, so they are prone to avulsions.[3]

MRI and CT myelography may both help to identify fluid-filled pseudomeningoceles.[3,6,7] Traumatic tears of the meningeal sleeves of brachial plexus rootlets permit CSF to leak into the soft tissue, forming fluid pouches termed *pseudomeningoceles*. Pseudomeningoceles are almost pathognomonic preganglionic rootlet avulsions (Fig. 26-6).[3,5-7] MRI demonstrates pseudomeningoceles better than CT, simple myelography, or even CT-myelography, because swelling and early granulation tissues may block free communication between the intraspinal CSF and the pseudomeningoceles. In this situation, no contrast agent fills the pouch, so the pouch will not be demonstrated. However, MRI demonstrates even noncommunicating fluid collections in the paraspinal soft tissue and often shows an alignment of their long axes that defines the specific rootlets affected.[3] The T2 signal intensity of pseudomeningoceles is characteristically higher than normal CSF, owing to absent CSF pulsations or higher protein/blood content (Fig. 26-7).[8] Complications associated with pseudomeningoceles include spinal cord herniation and displacement (Fig. 26-8), hematoma formation, and even

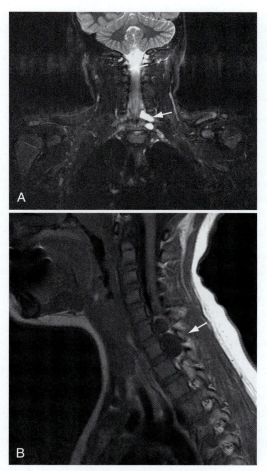

■ FIGURE 26-7 Coronal STIR (**A**) and parasagittal T1 (**B**) images demonstrate left pseudomeningoceles (*arrows*) compatible with nerve root avulsions.

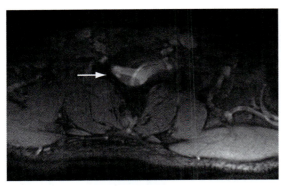

■ **FIGURE 26-8** Axial STIR MR image with the spinal cord (*arrow*) displaced posterolaterally due to compression of a left pseudomeningocele that is mostly located inside the thecal sac. This generally implies avulsion of the roots in their intraspinal course. The compression of the cord may result in a compressive myelopathy.

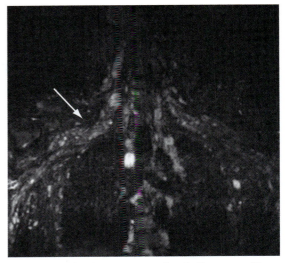

■ **FIGURE 26-9** Classic appearance of a plexiform neurofibroma in a patient with neurofibromatosis type 2. The brachial plexuses are bilaterally irregular, enlarged, and hyperintense in this coronal STIR MR sequence, resembling a "bag of worms" (*arrow*).

superficial siderosis.[9] Twenty percent of patients with root avulsions show abnormal signal intensity within the spinal cord. Areas of T2 hyperintensity suggest edema in the acute phase and myelomalacia in the chronic phase. T2 hypointensity suggests hemorrhage in the acute phase and siderosis from repeated hemorrhages in the chronic phase.[6] Enhancement of intradural nerve rootlets and paraspinal muscles suggests functional impairment.

In postganglionic injuries, the stretching or tearing of the nerves may separate them from the cell bodies of the motor and sensory neurons, leading to wallerian degeneration.

For surgical purposes, postganglionic lesions can be classified by their relationships to the clavicle. Supraclavicular lesions involve the roots and trunks of the brachial plexus. Seventy-five percent of these are Erb-Duchenne (extended upper brachial plexus) palsies, Dejerine-Klumpke (lower brachial plexus) palsies, or complete palsies. Retroclavicular lesions predominantly affect the divisions of the brachial plexus. They are relatively rare and generally result from clavicular fracture (acute period) or prominent callus formation (chronic period). Infraclavicular lesions predominantly affect the cords and branches. The axillary nerve is particularly susceptible to traction injury as it traverses the quadrangular space because this tight space anchors or fixes it in position.[1]

Tumors

Tumors are an important cause of brachial plexopathies, particularly in older individuals.[10] They cause sensory deficits with patchy and incomplete distribution more frequently than motor symptoms (which tend to be related to trauma).[7] Tumors may be primary or secondary (typically metastases). Primary neurogenic tumors are rare but usually treatable. They consist of neurofibromas (most frequent), schwannomas, malignant peripheral nerve sheath tumors, and post-traumatic neuromas.[10]

One third of patients with neurofibromas have localized or plexiform neurofibromas, associated with neurofibromatosis type 1. In these patients the nerves of the brachial plexus show diffuse and gross enlargement resembling a "bag of worms" (Fig. 26-9).[11] Sporadic neurofibromas are typically solitary and more commonly found in the supraclavicular region. They are more often seen in females than males (3:1).[7] Histologically, these lesions are unencapsulated tumors that appear to arise from the nerve fascicles. The tumor cells penetrated into the nerve deeply and diffusely (Fig. 26-10). Complete resection is not possible and results in neurologic deficits.[7]

The second most common neural tumors of the brachial plexus are encapsulated eccentric nerve sheath masses that arise from Schwann cells. Schwannomas are slightly more common in the upper brachial plexus and tend to displace the nerve fascicles instead of invading them. Therefore, surgical excision is often complete and is not associated with a high level of neurologic deficits.[7] Multiple schwannomas suggest the diagnosis of neurofibromatosis type 2. When they are malignant (very rare) they may also be associated with neurofibromatosis type 1.

The imaging features of neurofibromas and schwannomas may be very similar, so they may be very difficult to differentiate successfully. Plain radiographs show foraminal enlargement and well-defined bony remodeling. Ultrasonography demonstrates well-defined oval hypoechoic masses with posterior acoustic enhancement. Absence of a central echogenic hilum differentiates these lesions from cervical lymph nodes (see Fig. 26-3B). On CT, neurofibromas and schwannomas both have attenuations similar to muscle and both enhance variably after administration of a contrast agent. On MRI, both appear isointense to muscle on T1W imaging, have a characteristic high signal on T2W imaging, and enhance intensely after gadolinium is given intravenously.[7] Neurofibromas often show a central area of low signal intensity within the area of high T2 signal, giving the appearance of a "target" sign.[7] On histology, the "target sign" is created by a central core of nonenhancing collagenous and fibrillary tissue and a peripheral, less densely cellular, enhancing myxoid tissue (Fig. 26-11). Cystic and necrotic regions exhibit high T2 signal but do not enhance after contrast agent administration.[11]

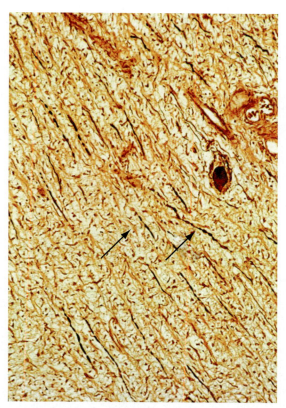

■ **FIGURE 26-10**   Histologic specimen of a neurofibroma, with "Glees technique" (silver impregnation for axons) that highlights a nerve axon's myelin (*darker lines shown by arrows*) embedded in neoplastic cells. (*Courtesy of Dr. Luciano Queiroz, Brazil.*)

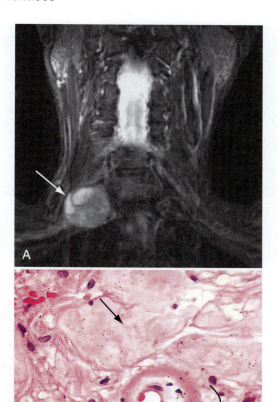

■ **FIGURE 26-11**   **A,** Schwannoma arising from the right brachial plexus shows heterogeneous signal in this coronal STIR image. The hyperintense areas correspond with cystic or necrotic components (*arrow*). This is explained by the tendency of the vessels to hyalinize. This phenomenon does not occur in neurofibromas where the hyperintense sign corresponds to less dense cellular myxoid tissue. **B,** Hematoxylin-eosin histologic preparation. *Straight arrow* shows a cystic area within a schwannoma and a hyalinized vessel (*curved arrow*) in the center of the image. (*Histologic preparation with kind permission of Dr. Luciano Queiroz, Brazil.*)

Malignant nerve tumors are less common than neurofibromas and schwannomas and mostly consist of fibrosarcomas and neurogenic sarcomas. They are more frequent in patients with neurofibromatosis type 1, especially after radiation therapy. Their imaging features are similar to their benign counterparts, which makes it difficult to differentiate between them.[7] The diagnosis of a malignant nerve sheath tumor is suggested by a progressively enlarging mass in a patient with neurofibromatosis, concurrent bone destruction, poorly defined margins with infiltration into neighboring soft tissues, heterogeneous contrast enhancement, and a lack of the "target sign."[7,12] Although diffusion-weighted MRI and fluorodeoxyglucose-labeled positron emission tomography (FDG-PET) have been used with some success for diagnosing malignant change in plexiform neurofibromas, a biopsy should always be performed whenever the question of a malignancy is considered.[7]

The main primary tumors that affect the brachial plexus are lymphoma, lung apex carcinoma, and skeletal soft tissue tumors, especially desmoid tumors and lipomas (Fig. 26-12). Head and neck tumors may also extend to involve the brachial plexus.[10] Primary cancers arising from the apex of the lung may invade into the brachial plexus and other para-apical structures to cause Pancoast syndrome. This syndrome consists of pain around the shoulder and arm (the most common initial symptom) produced by neoplastic involvement of C8 and T1-T2 nerve roots. Horner syndrome is seen in 20% of patients and muscle atrophy of the hand and rib destruction are also common.[7] MRI displays these tumors and their relationship to the brachial plexus well (Fig. 26-13). Tumor invasion of the brachial plexus may preclude surgery.

Secondary tumors involve the brachial plexus more often than primary nerve tumors do. The most common lesions to metastasize to the region of the brachial plexus are breast carcinoma (from axillary drainage of metastases), lung carcinoma, and head and neck tumors. True hematogenous metastases are rare.

MRI evaluation of tumors affecting the brachial plexus must define two important factors: (1) does the tumor lie adjacent to the brachial plexus or actually invade it; and (2) are the findings observed the result of prior therapy, particularly surgery and radiation therapy, or are they due to residual or recurrent tumor?[7,10]

The most reliable signs to differentiate tumor from radiation fibrosis are the presence of a soft tissue mass and clinical and imaging evidence of a progressive abnormality.[10] Clinical features suggestive of radiation-induced brachial plexopathy are little or no pain, lymphedema, cutaneous radiation changes, and known radiation doses

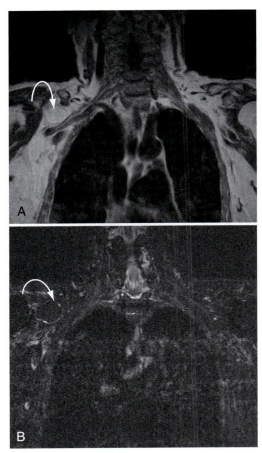

■ FIGURE 26-12 Noncontrast T1W (**A**) and STIR (**B**) coronal MR images show a lipoma compressing the right brachial plexus cords. The mass (*curved arrows*) is hyperintense on **A** similar to the subcutaneous and surrounding fat, and its signal suppresses on **B**. Note the lesion is well encapsulated.

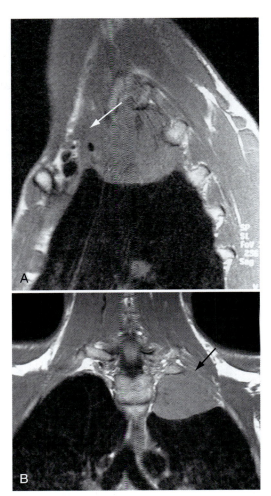

■ FIGURE 26-13 T1W noncontrast parasagittal (**A**) and coronal (**B**) MR images show a lung apical mass invading the adjacent soft tissues and in close proximity to the trunks and divisions of the brachial plexus. The lack of fat planes between them (*arrows*) suggests tumor invasion.

of more than 60 Gy.[13] Imaging features suggestive of radiation-induced brachial plexopathy include upper trunk involvement (from its longer course through the radiation field and lesser protection by thinner layers of soft tissue within the occipital triangle), thickening of the brachial plexus and stranding of the neighboring fat within the irradiated field, and low signal intensity on both T1W and T2W images. However, radiation therapy can also cause high T2 signal intensity (edema) in the brachial plexus and enhancement after gadolinium administration.

Thoracic Outlet Syndrome

Thoracic outlet syndrome refers to clinical manifestations attributable to impingement on the brachial plexus and the subclavian vessels as they pass from the thoracic cavity to the axilla. Congenital bony or fibromuscular anomalies, trauma, and posture may contribute to the compression or elongation of the neurovascular bundle. Movements such as raising the arms above the head may further compromise the thoracic outlet. Symptoms are variable and nonspecific. Whereas nearly all patients with thoracic outlet syndrome have compression of the brachial plexus, only a minority have symptoms or sequelae due to arterial or venous impingement.[14]

One frequent cause of brachial plexus compression in thoracic outlet syndrome is a cervical rib (or hypertrophied C7 transverse process), sometimes with an associated fibrous band. Cervical ribs are present in 6% of the normal population and in 13% of patients with thoracic outlet syndrome (Fig. 26-14).[14] The rib or transverse process can be diagnosed with plain radiographs. MRI better displays the fibrous bands that attach to the first rib and narrow the thoracic outlet. MRI also helps to display hypertrophied musculature, such as the scalene muscles, which may also cause thoracic outlet syndrome.[14] Hyperabduction of the ipsilateral upper extremity accentuates the degree of compression on the neurovascular structures. Therefore, it can be important to image the thoracic outlet during hyperabduction of the ipsilateral extremity to detect subtle cases and define the severity of the rest.[14] The hyperabduction maneuver can by employed during conventional angiography, CT, CT angiography, MRI, and MR angiography. Ultrasonography and Doppler sonography may also be helpful, particularly when venous obstruction is suspected.[14] Positive electrophysiologic nerve conduction studies are useful in selecting patients for surgical decompression of neurogenic thoracic outlet syn-

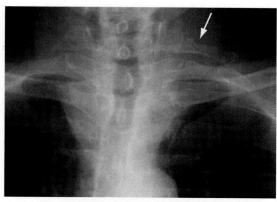

■ **FIGURE 26-14** Close-up of a frontal chest radiograph showing the presence of a left cervical rib (*arrow*) in a patient with ipsilateral thoracic outlet syndrome.

drome. Resection of the first rib—the standard surgical treatment for thoracic outlet syndrome—usually fails to improve long-term function in neurogenic thoracic outlet syndrome but helps patients with vascular thoracic outlet syndrome.[14]

Miscellaneous Conditions

Hypertrophic polyneuropathies may result in a grossly enlarged brachial plexus with expansion of the intervertebral foramina and scalloping of the vertebral bodies. The hypertrophic polyneuropathies are a heterogeneous group of diseases that include the hereditary motor-sensory neuropathies (HMSN type I or Charcot-Marie-Tooth, HMSN II, and HMSN III or Dejerine-Sotas), amyloidosis, leprosy, sarcoidosis, chronic inflammatory demyelinating polyradiculoneuropathy, and acromegaly.[15] The clinical presentation, CSF analysis, nerve conduction studies, sural nerve biopsies, and genetic studies are needed to make an exact diagnosis because the imaging features of these disorders overlap and may even be confused with neurofibromatosis.[16] MRI reveals abnormal thickening and enhancement of all components of the brachial plexus. Their signal intensity may remain normal on T1W imaging (Fig. 26-15A) but slightly hyperintense on T2W imaging (see Fig. 26-15B).

Sudden, unexplained brachial plexus plexopathy may be called neuralgic amyotrophy, Parsonage-Turner syndrome, brachial neuritis, or brachial plexitis. Patients usually experience sudden onset of severe, constant pain in the lateral neck, shoulder, and upper arm, followed by a profound weakness and atrophy of the painful muscles. The serratus anterior is most frequently affected.[4] The condition may (1) be idiopathic, (2) be the result of a primary viral infection, especially in older individuals, (3) be a complication of prior infection (herpes) or serum vaccine, antibiotic, or other drug administration, or (4) have a heredofamilial prevalence.[7] Symptoms usually resolve, partially or completely, but recovery may not begin until 6 months after the onset of symptoms and may require up to 3 years.[4] The MRI findings are frequently normal, but MRI may also show diffusely enlarged brachial plexus nerves with increased T2 signal (Fig. 26-16).[4] Newer MRI techniques such as MR neurography are particularly useful for confirming the diagnosis of this entity, which has previously been a diagnosis of exclusion.[17]

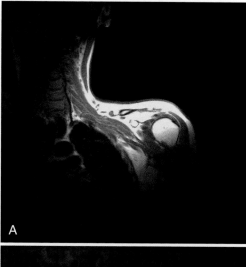

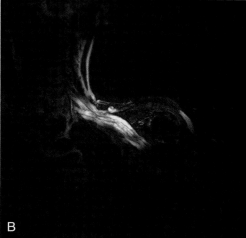

■ **FIGURE 26-15** **A,** Coronal T1W MR image showing normal signal intensity in an abnormally thickened left brachial plexus in a patient with Charcot-Marie-Tooth disease. **B,** Corresponding STIR image. The enlarged brachial plexus is hyperintense.

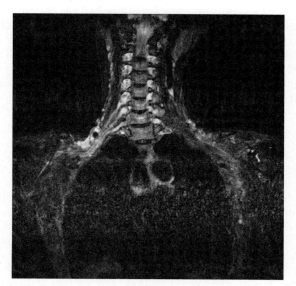

■ **FIGURE 26-16** Coronal STIR image shows a diffusely enlarged and hyperintense right brachial plexus in a patient with a sudden onset of weakness in ipsilateral upper extremity. Symptoms resolved spontaneously 12 weeks later and thus were thought to be viral.

ANALYSIS

Sample reports are presented in Boxes 26-1 to 26-3. See also Box 26-4 for pitfalls and limitations of the brachial plexus imaging and Figures 26-17 to 26-19 for examples.

MR neurography is a technique that offers higher-resolution imaging of the brachial plexus and a guide to selection of surgical entry sites (Fig. 26-20).[17] It requires specifically designed surface coils and sequences that may not be immediately available from all of the manufactur-ers. Diffusion-weighted imaging of the brachial plexus is hampered by lower resolution and by artifacts inherent to the magnetic susceptibility of the sequence but may be helpful in assessing a variety of injuries whose end result is ischemia.[6] Diffusion-tensor imaging may permit MR display of the continuity of the brachial plexus and depict any injury to it.[18] Figure 26-21 shows an anatomic dissection of the right brachial plexus. Part A shows the dissection without labels. Part B shows the dissection with anatomic structures labeled.

BOX 26-1   MRI for Traumatic Avulsion of the Brachial Plexus

PATIENT HISTORY

A young male adult involved in a motorcycle accident presented with upper arm and shoulder palsy and pain.

TECHNIQUE

Bilateral noncontrast T1W spin-echo axial MR study (Fig. 26-17A) was done with a large field of view. Axial (see Fig. 26-17B) and left parasagittal (see Fig. 26-17C) T2W spin-echo MR studies were also obtained.

FINDINGS

At the level of the C7 and T1 vertebral bodies on the right (see Fig. 26-17C) there are two well-defined T1-hypointense and T2-hyperintense lesions (see Fig. 26-17A and B). These have higher signal intensity than the CSF in the neighboring spinal canal and show a low signal rim cue to flow voids. No nerve root is visualized within these lesions, although nerve roots are well defined in the contralateral neural foramen.

IMPRESSION

Traumatic nerve root avulsion with pseudomeningocele is suggested.

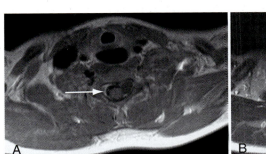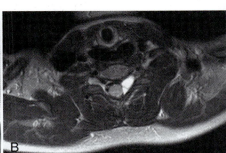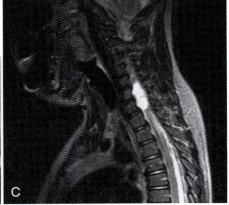

■ FIGURE 26-17   Left nerve root avulsion with pseudomeningocele formation. **A,** Axial T1W study at the level of C7-T1 shows a hypointense well-defined lesion left of the medullary canal that corresponds to a post-traumatic pseudomeningocele. Notice on the right (*arrow*) a linear structure that exits the neuroforamina that is well visible by the contrast agent with its neighboring fat, consisting of a normal right nerve root. **B,** Axial T2W spin-echo MR study at the level of C7-T1. The well-defined ovoid structure left of the medullary canal has an hyperintense signal that shows a fluid-filled collection corresponding to a pseudomeningocele; no root can be seen at this side. On the right, however, a nonavulsed right root can be identified against the dark sign of the CSF (which is dark in this case because of flow voids; be aware that CSF in T2W imaging has a hyperintense sign). **C,** Right parasagittal T2W study of the same patient shows at the level of C7-T1 two ovoid and well-defined fluid-filled collections that are more hyperintense than the neighboring CSF; they correspond to pseudomeningoceles.

BOX 26-2   MRI for Suggested Neurofibromas

PATIENT HISTORY

A patient with a known history of phakomatosis presented for routine follow-up.

TECHNIQUE

Parasagittal with a large field of view and axial STIR MRI studies were done. A contrast-enhanced T1W axial MRI study was obtained through the same level as the axial STIR image.

FINDINGS

Multiple fusiform and well-delineated masses enlarge the neural foramina bilaterally and surround the nerve roots at nearly all spinal levels. The masses appear heterogeneously hyperintense on STIR MR images (Fig. 26-18A, B) and enhance avidly on the T1W contrast-enhanced axial study (see Fig. 26-18C). These imaging features are consistent with nerve sheath tumors. Numerous hyperintense nodules are seen in the subcutaneous fat on STIR images, likely corresponding to subcutaneous neurofibromas.

IMPRESSION

Of the nerve sheath tumors, therefore, the most likely diagnosis is neurofibromas in the context of neurofibromatosis type 1.

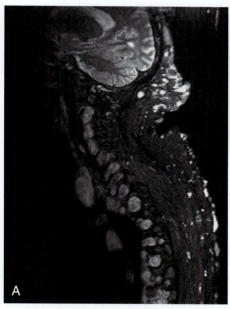
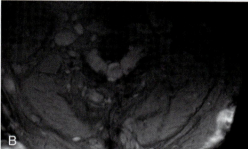
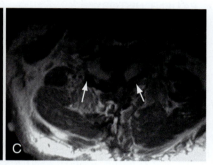

■ **FIGURE 26-18**   **A,** Right parasagittal STIR MR study of a patient with neurofibromatosis type 1. At multiple neuroforaminal levels there are ovoid and well-defined masses with a heterogeneous, but mostly hyperintense signal. They correspond to nerve sheath tumors, most likely neurofibromas. Also, there are numerous small and hyperintense lesions in the subcutaneous tissue, representing cutaneous fibromas typical of this disease. **B,** Axial STIR MR study at the C7 level of the same patient. Bilateral, well-defined, ovoid masses follow the cervical roots as they exit the medullary canal throughout bilaterally enlarged neuroforamina. Taking into account the clinical history of the patient, and the heterogeneous but mostly hyperintense signal of these lesions in STIR, they are highly suggestive of nerve sheath tumors, most likely neurofibromas. **C,** Axial T1W postcontrast image at the C7 level. The previously described bilateral neuroforaminal lesions enhance avidly after intravenous gadolinium administration (*arrows*), a typical characteristic of neural sheath tumors.

BOX 26-3   MRI for Radiation-Induced Inflammation

PATIENT HISTORY

A 45-year-old woman with breast cancer treated with local radiation therapy 8 months previously presented with slight pain and reduced mobility of her left upper arm.

TECHNIQUE

Coronal STIR and contrast-enhanced T1W MR images were obtained.

FINDINGS

Compared with the contralateral right brachial plexus, there is a diffuse and homogeneous enlargement of the whole left brachial plexus. The left cords appear discretely hyperintense against the fat-suppressed neighboring tissues on STIR MRI (Fig. 26-19A). This portion of the brachial plexus also enhances homogenously on coronal T1W post-contrast study (see Fig. 26-19B). No focal mass or stranding is identified.

IMPRESSION

The findings were consistent with radiation-induced plexopathy.

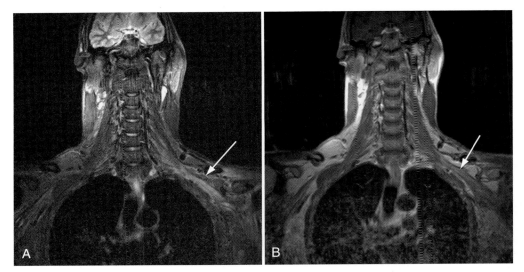

■ **FIGURE 26-19** **A,** Coronal, large field of view STIR MR study at the level of the interscalenic triangle of a patient who presented with pain in the upper arm and a past history of breast cancer. The left brachial plexus is diffusely and homogeneously enlarged compared with the contralateral one. Note the hyperintensity (*arrow*) of the cords against the darker signal of the fat-suppressed neighboring tissues. Taking into account that the patient received radiation therapy 8 months previously, these findings are compatible with brachial plexitis secondary to radiation therapy and not with tumor recurrence. **B,** Coronal, large field of view T1W MR study after contrast agent administration. At the level of the signal hyperintensity in the STIR study there is a moderate homogeneous enhancement of the cords of the left brachial plexus (*arrow*). No focal mass is identified. This imaging finding strongly suggests that the patient´s pain is produced by radiation-induced plexopathy due to her local radiation therapy.

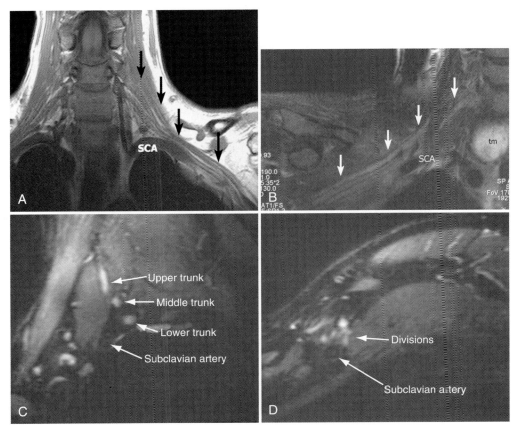

■ **FIGURE 26-20** Normal brachial plexus. **A,** Coronal T1W MR image of a normal brachial plexus obtained using dedicated phased array of radiofrequency receiver coils. The *arrows* indicate the approximate sagittal locations for the roots, trunks, divisions, and cords. SCA, subclavian artery. **B,** Coronal fat-saturated T2-weighted image obtained using an integrated array of coils. The *arrows* indicate the approximate sagittal locations for the roots, trunks, divisions, and cords. Note the hyperintensity of the intermuscular fat in the lower neck on the right. This results from incomplete fat saturation due to magnetic susceptibility variation in the region being imaged. SCA, subclavian artery; tm, thyroid mass. **C,** Sagittal STIR image of the trunks. The trunks are located superior to the subclavian artery. With fat suppression, the trunks are distinguished by their mild hyperintensity relative to muscle and fat. **D,** Sagittal STIR image of the divisions. The divisions are located primarily superior to the subclavian artery in the retroclavicular region. The plane of the image is near the lateral border of the first rib. (*A, C,* and *D* reprinted from Maravilla KR, Bowen BC. Imaging of the peripheral nervous system: evaluation of peripheral neuropathy and plexopathy. AJNR Am J Neuroradiol 1998; 19:1011-1023; and *B* reprinted from Bowen BC, Pattany PM, Saraf-Lavi E, Maravilla KR. The brachial plexus: normal anatomy, pathology, and MR imaging. Neuroimag Clin North Am 2004; 14:59-85.)

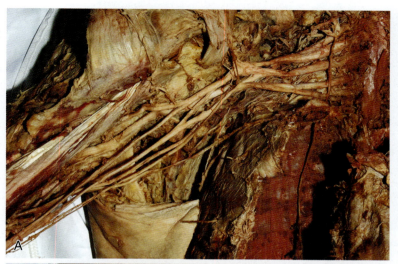

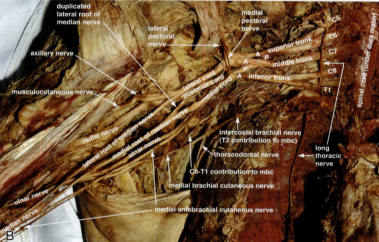

duplicated lateral root of median nerve

lateral pectoral nerve

medial pectoral nerve

axillary nerve

C5

C6

superior trunk

C7

middle trunk

A P

A P

C8

inferior trunk

A

T1

musculocutaneous nerve

lateral cord
posterior cord
medial cord

spinal cord (under dura mater)

radial nerve

intercostal brachial nerve
(T2 contribution to mbc)

lateral root of median nerve
medial root of median nerve
ulnar nerve

thoracodorsal nerve

long thoracic nerve

C8-T1 contribution to mbc

medial brachial cutaneous nerve

ulnar nerve

medial antebrachial cutaneous nerve

median nerve

B

■ **FIGURE 26-21** Anatomic dissection of the right brachial plexus. **A,** Dissection. **B,** Dissection with structures labeled. In **B,** C5-T1 indicate the ventral rami of the spinal nerves that form the brachial plexus. A and P indicate the anterior and posterior divisions of the three trunks, except that the posterior division of the inferior trunk is not visible. There is duplication of the lateral root of the median nerve (a common variation). Two contributions to the medial brachial cutaneous (mbc) nerve are shown: C8-T1 and T2. The dorsal scapular and suprascapular branches of C5 and the superior trunk are not clearly visible. The upper and lower subscapular branches of the posterior cord are not clearly visible. The ventral ramus of spinal nerve C4 and its contribution to the cervical plexus is visible above the C5 ventral ramus. *(Dissection courtesy of Professor Joy S. Reidenberg, PhD, Ms. Nancy Hoo, and Mr. Jeremy Tietjens, Center for Anatomy and Functional Morphology, Mount Sinai School of Medicine, New York, NY.)*

BOX 26-4   Pitfalls and Limitations of Brachial Plexus Imaging

NONINVASIVE TECHNIQUES

MRI

Limitations of MRI include difficulty in obtaining studies from claustrophobic patients, from patients with metallic devices such as pacemakers, and, if contrast is to be used, from patients with severe renal failure. Protocols tend to be long (about 60 minutes) and lead to patient intolerance and motion. Multiple planes are needed to display the downward oblique course of the brachial plexus. Pulsation artifacts from arteries may result in artifacts. Fat suppression is indispensable in the postcontrast studies but may lead to artifacts when it is inhomogeneous throughout the field of view. Metal and blood products may cause blooming artifacts in gradient-echo images. Specifically designed surface coils may be needed. Use of the standard body coil make images of lower quality.

Ultrasonography

This technique offers very low specificity and a limited window of exploration. The study results depend on the patient's body habitus and the ability of the operator. Nonetheless, ultrasonog-raphy does visualize superficial structures, generally limited to the cords of the brachial plexus.

CT

Simple CT has poor soft tissue contrast and limited utility for evaluating the brachial plexus. CT is useful for displaying the neighboring bone structures.

CT Angiography

CT angiography is useful for patients with possible vascular abnormalities and thoracic outlet syndrome. Large-bore venous access and a fast rate of contrast agent delivery are imperative for good quality studies. In large patients, visualization of the shoulder structures may be limited. CT angiography may not be used in patients with renal failure.

CT Myelography

This technique requires a spinal tap and myelogram, with the usual complications associated with both. CT myelography visu-alizes the spinal canal and its contents but fills only those pseu-

BOX 26-4 Pitfalls and Limitations of Brachial Plexus Imaging—cont'd

domeningoceles that communicate with the subarachnoid space. Noncommunicating pseudomeningoceles may easily be overlooked. As with simple CT, the visualization of the remainder of the brachial plexus is limited.

INVASIVE TECHNIQUES

Catheter Angiography

Catheter studies may be used to document vascular compression in patients with thoracic outlet syndrome. They may also be used to study patients with suspected subclavian and axillary artery injuries. Demonstration of vascular compression increases the likelihood of neural compression but does not document its presence or location(s). Catheter angiography carries all the risks traditionally associated with any angiographic procedure.

Myelography

Traditional myelography provides a limited evaluation of the spinal cord and intraspinal nerve roots. It may display features consistent with traumatic avulsion of nerve roots, neuritis, and tumor. It can only display those post-traumatic pseudomeningoceles that communicate with the rest of the subarachnoid space and fill with contrast agent. Severe allergies to iodinated contrast agent and coagulopathies that increase the risk of performing a spinal tap limit the utility of this technique. In addition, there are all of the risks traditionally associated with this technique.

SUGGESTED READINGS

Anatomical Pathology/Neuroimaging website of the Department of Pathology and Radiology at Sate University of Campinas, School of Medicine (FCM-UNICAMP), Campinas, Brazil. Available in English at http://www.fcm.unicamp.br/deptos/anatomia/epathenglish.html.

Demondion X, Herbinet P, Van Sint JS, et al. Imaging assessment of thoracic outlet syndrome. RadioGraphics 2006; 26:1735-1750.

Kaplan PA, Helms CA, Dussault R, et al. Musculoskeletal MRI. Philadelphia, WB Saunders, 2001, p 95.

Maravilla KR, Bowen BC. Imaging of the peripheral nervous system: evaluation of peripheral neuropathy and plexopathy. AJNR Am J Neuroradiol 1998; 19:1011-1023.

Mukherji SK, Castillo M, Wagle AG. The brachial plexus. Semin Ultrasound CT MR 1996; 17:519-538.

Spinner RJ, Shin AY, Bishop AT. Update on brachial plexus surgery in adults. Curr Opin Orthop 2004; 15:203-214.

REFERENCES

1. Kozin SH. Injuries of the brachial plexus. In Ianotti JP, Williams GR (eds). Disorders of the Shoulder. Diagnosis and Management. Philadelphia, Lippincott Williams & Wilkins, 2006, pp 1111-1113.

2. Van Es HW. Anatomy and imaging techniques. In: MR Imaging of the Brachial Plexus, thesis. Sate University, Utrecht, The Netherlands, 1997. Available at www.library.uu.nl/proefsch/01825445/inhoud.htm.

3. Rankine RR. Adult traumatic brachial plexus injury. Clin Radiol 2004; 59:767-774.

4. Bowen BC, Pattany P, Saraf-Lavi E, Maravilla KR. The brachial plexus: normal anatomy, pathology and MR imaging. Neuroimag Clin North Am 2004; 14:59-85.

5. Petit Lacour MC, Ducreux D, Adams D. IRM du plexus brachial. J Neuroradiol 2004; 31:198-206.

6. Yoshikawa T, Hayashi N, Yamamoto S, et al. Brachial plexus injury: clinical manifestations, conventional imaging findings, and the latest imaging techniques. RadioGraphics 2006; 26:S133-S143.

7. Todd M, Shah GS, Mukherji SK. MR imaging of brachial plexus. Top Magn Reson Imaging 2004; 15:113-125.

8. Gasparotti R, Ferraresi S, Pinelli L, et al. Three-dimensional MR myelography of traumatic injuries of the brachial plexus. AJNR Am J Neuroradiol 1997; 18:1733-1742.

9. Cohen-Gadol AA, Krauss WE, Spinner RJ. Delayed central nervous system superficial siderosis following brachial plexus avulsion injury. Neurosurg Focus 2004; 16:1-8.

10. Van Es HW. Tumours. In: MR Imaging of the Brachial Plexus, thesis. Sate University, Utrecht, The Netherlands, 1997. Available at www.library.uu.nl/proefsch/01825445/inhoud.htm.

11. Wilkinson LM, Manson D, Smith R. Plexiform neurofibroma of the bladder. RadioGraphics 2004; 21:S237-S242.

12. Bhargava R, Parham DM, Lasater OE, et al. MR imaging differentiation of benign and malignant peripheral nerve sheath tumors: use of the target sign. Pediatr Radiol 1997; 27:124-129.

13. Gosk J, Rutowski R, Reichert P, Rabczynski J. Radiation-induced brachial plexus neuropathy: aetiopathogenesis, risk factors, differential diagnostics, symptoms and treatment. Folia Neuropathol 2007; 45:26-30.

14. Charon J-P, Milne W, Sheppard DC, Houston JG. Evaluation of MR angiographic technique in the assessment of thoracic outlet syndrome. Clin Radiol 2004; 59:588-595.

15. Maki DD, Yousem DM, Corcoran C, Galetta SL. MR imaging of Dejerine-Sottas disease. Am J Neuroradiol 1999; 20:378-380.

16. Fletcher GP, Roberts CC. AJR teaching file: progressive polyradiculopathy. AJR Am J Roentgenol 2006 186:S230-S232.

17. Zhou L, Yousem DM, Chaudhry V. Role of magnetic resonance neurography in brachial plexus lesions. Muscle Nerve 2004; 30:305-309.

18. Dicreux D, Fillard P, Facon D, et al. Diffusion tensor magnetic resonance imaging and fiber tracking in spinal cord lesions: current and future indications. Neuroimag Clin North Am 2007; 17:137-147.

27

Imaging of the Sacral Plexus

Sumit Pruthi and Kenneth R. Maravilla

The sacral plexus and sciatic nerve are formed within the pelvis from contributions of the ventral nerve roots of L4 through S4. The sciatic nerve originates from the sacral plexus within the pelvis and then exits the pelvis through the greater sciatic foramen. Technical advances in the surface coils and pulse sequences used for MRI now make it possible to display the normal anatomy and pathology of the sacral plexus and sciatic nerve in great detail. Introduction of the surgical operating microscope and improved surgical technique have opened the possibility of surgical, medical, or combined therapy for pathologic processes involving this plexus. Successful therapy will then depend on accurate display of the anatomy and pathology of this region.

ANATOMY

The sacral plexus is formed by the ventral rami of nerve roots L4 to S4. A variable portion of the L4 ramus joins with L5 to form the lumbosacral trunk. The lumbosacral trunk consistently courses medial to the psoas muscle and enters the pelvis just anterior to the sacral ala and medial to the sacroiliac joint. The ventral rami of S1 to S4 enter the pelvis through the anterior sacral foramina S1 to S4. As the lumbosacral trunk enters the pelvis, it joins the ventral ramus of S1 to form a large upper band. The rami of S2, S3, and S4 join together to form a small inferior band. These bands pursue an inferior, posterior, and lateral course within the pelvis, pass between the internal iliac vessels anteriorly and the piriformis muscle posteriorly, and converge at the greater sciatic foramen to form the sciatic nerve (Fig. 27-1).

The piriformis muscle is the key landmark for identifying the anatomy of the sacral plexus and sciatic nerve. The piriformis originates from the anterolateral aspect of the sacrum at S3 to S5 and passes through the greater sciatic foramen to insert on the greater trochanter of the femur. The nerve roots that comprise the sacral plexus come together on the ventral surface of the piriformis. The piriformis muscle divides the sacral plexus into three anatomic sections. The preplexal portion of the sacral plexus includes the lumbosacral trunk and the portion of S1 situated cranial to the superior border of the piriformis muscle. The plexal segment of the sacral plexus is the portion that lies anterior to the piriformis muscle. The sciatic nerve originates at the inferior margin of the pyriformis. The postplexal segment of the sacral plexus includes the proximal sciatic nerve caudal to the inferior margin of the piriformis muscle in the greater sciatic foramen.

The sciatic nerve is the largest nerve in the body and measures 10 to 20 mm in its largest cross-sectional dimension. It contains contributions from the L4 through S3 nerve roots. The sciatic nerve arises at the anteroinferior surface of the piriformis muscle and exits the pelvis through the anterior third of the greater sciatic foramen, posterior to the ischial spine.

Other important branches of the sacral plexus include the superior gluteal nerve (L4-S1), the inferior gluteal nerve (L5-S2), the pudendal nerve (S2-S4), the nerve to the quadratus femoris and inferior gemellus muscles (L4-S1), the nerve to the internal obturator and superior gemellus muscles (L5-S2), the posterior femoral cutaneous nerve (S1-S3), and the parasympathetic splanchnic nerves of the pelvis (S2-S4). Many important vascular landmarks are present in this region. The common iliac vessels and bifurcations are situated anteromedial to the lumbosacral trunk at the level of the sacral promontory. The superior gluteal vessels pass between the lumbosacral trunk and the S1 (or S1 and S2) nerve(s), exiting the pelvis by turning laterally just inferior to the sacroiliac joint. The inferior gluteal vessels pass between S1 and S2 (or S2 and S3) to lie adjacent to the medial aspect of the sciatic nerve and accompany the sciatic nerve through the greater sciatic foramen. The internal pudendal vessels are located between the pudendal nerve and ischial spine. After coursing through the greater sciatic foramen, the nerve and vessels turn

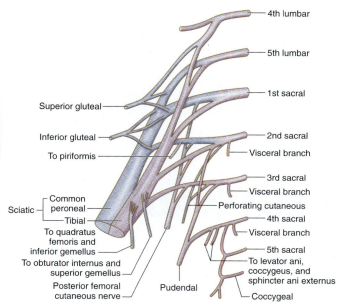

■ FIGURE 27-1 Anatomy of the sacral plexus.

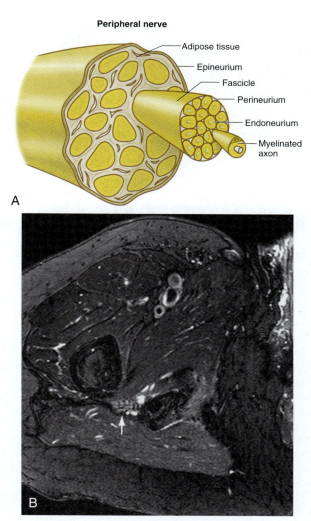

■ FIGURE 27-2 **A,** Schematic diagram of a peripheral nerve showing the various compartments bounded by three connective tissue sheaths that support and protect the complex. Multiple fascicles are seen interspersed with variable amount of adipose tissue bounded by epineurium. The fascicles are in turn encompassed by a dense perineurial sheath. The inner endoneurial sheath invests the Schwann cell/axon complex. **B,** Axial STIR image of the sciatic nerve shows the same fascicular pattern (*arrow*) easily depicted on this high-resolution MR neurogram.

through the lesser sciatic foramen to enter the pudendal canal.

MICROSCOPY

The basic unit of the peripheral nerve is the axon. This axon may be myelinated or unmyelinated and may carry efferent (motor) or afferent (sensory) electrical impulses. Bundles of axons form the individual peripheral nerves in the extremities, as well as the nerves composing the sacral plexus. Large peripheral nerves like the sciatic nerve consist of compartments bounded by three connective tissue sheaths, which support and protect the complex (Fig. 27-2). The innermost compartment is the endoneurium. It consists of loose vascular connective tissue and extracellular fluid. The endoneurial sheath invests the Schwann cell/axon complex. Its inner border is the basement membrane of the Schwann cell. Its outer border is the second connective tissue sheath, the perineurium. The axons, Schwann cells, and endoneurium are bundled together into fascicles, each of which is encompassed by a dense perineurial sheath. The endoneurial fluid within each fascicle is isolated from the general extracellular space by tightly adherent epithelial-like cells, which form the perineurium. The endoneurial space within each fascicle is isolated from the circulating blood by the tight junctions between endothelial cells of the endoneurial capillaries. The perineurium normally acts as a protective barrier against infectious or toxic agents. However, once this barrier is penetrated, there is the potential for spread of disease along the fascicle. The epineurium is the outermost connective tissue sheath. It envelops the nerve and has extensions that encompass each of the perineurial-lined fascicles. This arrangement provides mechanical support for the axons when they are subjected to stretching forces. The epineurium consists of dense, irregular connective tissue, with thick collagen and elastin fibers.

Variable amounts of interfascicular adipose tissue are present within the larger nerves. At the central or proximal end of the spinal nerves, the epineurium is continuous with the dura mater. At the distal or peripheral end of the peripheral nerves, the epineurium is progressively reduced in thickness, eventually becoming incorporated into the perineurium.

INDICATIONS

The diagnosis of plexal involvement has traditionally relied on information obtained from the clinical history, physical and neurologic examinations, and electrophysiologic studies. Clinical evidence of nerve involvement is generally based on dermatomal assessment (areas of anesthesia or hyperesthesia), changes in reflexes, patterns of muscle weakness, and points of tenderness.

Electrophysiologic and nerve conduction studies are widely used and have high sensitivity for detecting a conduction abnormality and hence are an important part of assessing nerve abnormality. These studies aid in confirming the presence of disease and may also help to localize it. However, these studies have significant shortcomings. Nerve conduction measurements reflect the status of the best surviving nerve fibers, so test results may be normal even if a few fibers remain unaffected by the disease process. Focal compression of the nerve may produce localized slowing of conduction; however, presence of normal conduction time does not exclude the compression. Conditions that affect extended portions of the nerve such as segmental demyelination may also cause slowed velocities and are poorly evaluated.[1] Lastly, conduction studies lack specificity and cannot display the anatomic detail needed for precise localization and treatment planning.

Before the advent of ultrasonography, CT, and MRI, radiologic examination of sacral plexus lesions was largely limited to demonstration of the secondary skeletal changes caused by a plexal lesion. Expansion of neural foramina, periosteal reaction, and scoliosis of the lower spine were a few of the indirect signs of plexal involvement.

IMAGING

Ultrasonography

Ultrasonography has been applied to visualize and evaluate the sacral plexuses and the sciatic nerve. On ultrasonography, the normal nerve appears as a tubular echogenic structure with parallel linear internal echoes on longitudinal sonograms and as a round echogenic structure with punctate echoes on transverse scans (Fig. 27-3).[1] The internal echogenic structure presumably represents fascicles within the nerve. Ultrasonography may demonstrate early changes in neural architecture with peripheral compressive neuropathies similar to those seen with compression of the median nerve in the carpal tunnel.[2] However, the major limitation to using ultrasound in the evaluation of the sacral plexus is its inability to demonstrate the intrapelvic segment of the sacral plexus and the sciatic nerve.[1] Ultrasonography also has inherent limitations with operator dependency, lack of the multiplanar capability, and inferior contrast resolution.

CT

CT has had limited success in demonstrating the detailed anatomy of the sacral plexus. The sciatic nerve itself can readily be identified on axial CT images of the lower pelvis, but the individual extradural peripheral nerves (L4 to S4) that form the sacral plexus and the sciatic nerve cannot be distinguished reliably from adjacent normal intrapelvic soft tissues such as the piriformis muscle, blood vessels, and lymph nodes (Fig. 27-4).[3] In the future, multidetector CT scanners that can image large areas rapidly and that achieve isotropic voxels suitable for multiplanar display may permit the use of CT for imaging the sacral plexus.

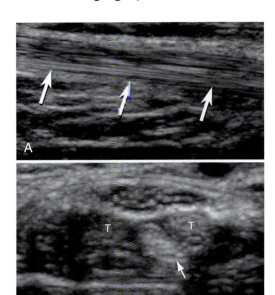

■ **FIGURE 27-3** Ultrasound images of the normal median nerve (*arrows*) obtained at the wrist. Note the parallel linear internal echoes on the longitudinal scans (**A**) and the punctate echoes on the transverse scans (**B**) of the nerve surrounded by the tendons (**T**). It is easier to image superficial nerves such as the median nerve on ultrasonography but very difficult to image the intrapelvic segment of the sciatic nerve and the sacral plexus.

MRI

MRI of the peripheral nerves (MR neurography) is now the modality of choice for evaluating peripheral nerves and the sacral plexus.[4] MR neurography enables the physician to examine major peripheral nerves for the presence, extent, and localization of structural abnormalities.[5] The ultimate goal of MR neurography is to generate tissue-specific images of nerves analogous to angiograms. To date, this is still a work in progress.[6]

T2-based MR neurography can be applied reliably using existing top-of-the-line clinical MR scanners of 1.5 to 3.0 T with only minor modifications to technique and to radio-frequency coils used for these studies. The predominant technique for MR neurography uses T2-weighted (T2W) techniques. Nerves contain multiple different "types" of tissue water. Evidence suggests that the low-protein endoneurial fluid is what is seen most prominently on T2W MR neurograms.[5] Although endoneurial fluid is responsible for only a fraction of the protons in a nerve that can be imaged, it has distinct properties that increase its detectability and display by T2W MRI. The low protein endoneurial fluid lies within the privileged space of the endoneurium. It is confined by the perineurial blood/nerve barrier and bathes the axons. It exhibits bulk flow directed from proximal to distal along the nerve, and that bulk flow can be disrupted by nerve compression and edema. Technically, by applying a chemical shift-selective pulse, it is possible to suppress the signal from the fat around the nerve and from much of the fat from within the nerve. By selecting an echo time longer than 90 ms,

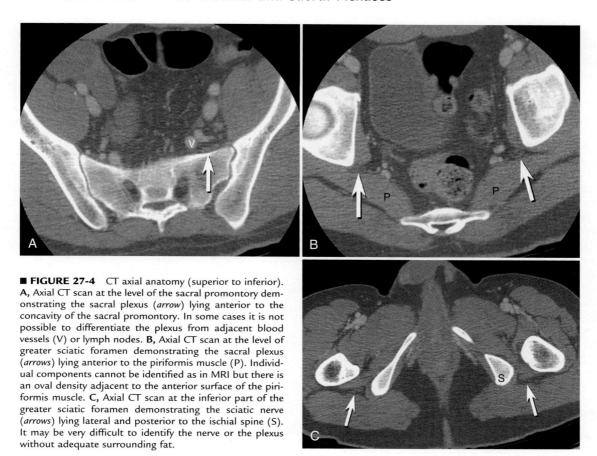

■ FIGURE 27-4 CT axial anatomy (superior to inferior). **A,** Axial CT scan at the level of the sacral promontory demonstrating the sacral plexus (*arrow*) lying anterior to the concavity of the sacral promontory. In some cases it is not possible to differentiate the plexus from adjacent blood vessels (V) or lymph nodes. **B,** Axial CT scan at the level of greater sciatic foramen demonstrating the sacral plexus (*arrows*) lying anterior to the piriformis muscle (P). Individual components cannot be identified as in MRI but there is an oval density adjacent to the anterior surface of the piriformis muscle. **C,** Axial CT scan at the inferior part of the greater sciatic foramen demonstrating the sciatic nerve (*arrows*) lying lateral and posterior to the ischial spine (S). It may be very difficult to identify the nerve or the plexus without adequate surrounding fat.

it is possible to achieve a T2 weighting that results in relative suppression of muscle signal. By employing flow suppression techniques, it is possible to eliminate the high signal of flowing blood. Use of all three measures—fat suppression, T2W, and flow suppression—together creates the conditions that allow the generation of peripheral nerve images.[5]

A newer technique, described by Filler and colleagues, utilizes diffusion-weighted imaging to visualize the nerves.[4] To date, diffusion-weighted neurography has shown limited resolution and no clear advantage over T2W neurography.[7]

Muscle Imaging

Imaging of the regional musculature innervated by the sacral plexus contributes little to the diagnosis of sacral plexus neuropathy because most of the muscles innervated by the plexus lie in the lower extremity outside the imaging field of view (FOV). Within the pelvic FOV the gluteal muscles and the piriformis are the most important muscles innervated by the sacral plexus. When detected, increased T2 signal intensity within denervated muscle can help to confirm the presence of, and to localize the specific segments of, nerve injury or disease (Fig. 27-5).

The major change seen with acute or subacute denervation is increased T2 signal in the affected muscle(s) on either T2W or short tau inversion recovery (STIR) images. These changes begin between 4 and 14 days after onset

of nerve abnormality or after nerve injury. They may persist for weeks or months if the nerve does not recover. T1W images can also be helpful for diagnosis, by identifying atrophy and fatty infiltration of the musculature, which occur in later stages of denervation (Fig. 27-6). The specific imaging features of denervation atrophy evolve with time, so the pattern of change observed may also help to identify the chronicity of the lesion.

Improvement or normalization of signal intensity within a denervated muscle correlates with re-innervation of the musculature. In our experience, improvement of muscle signal toward normal in the absence of fatty infiltration correlates with recovery of nerve function.

Optimal Imaging Planes and Technique

Good visualization of small nerve structures within the sacral plexus requires very highly detailed images. The combination of thin slices, the smallest imaging FOV required, and a matrix size adequate to yield small, submillimeter pixel sizes are all necessary to obtain good images of the nerves. Clinically, diagnostic nerve imaging, therefore, requires an MR scanner of 1.5 T or higher, good magnetic field homogeneity over a relatively large volume, steep gradients to provide high-resolution imaging, and multi-element phased-array surface coils. Sacral plexus imaging typically requires an FOV in the range of 20 to 25 cm and a matrix of 512 × 512.

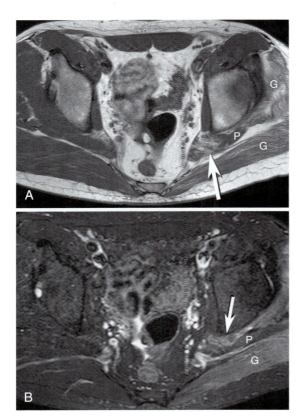

■ **FIGURE 27-5** Muscle denervation. Axial T1W (**A**) and STIR (**B**) MR images in a patient with lung carcinoma showing focal soft tissue mass surrounding and infiltrating the left sacral plexus (*arrows*). The nerve is hyperintense with loss of normal fascicular architecture. Note adjacent muscle changes suggestive of muscle denervation. The left gluteal (G) and piriformis muscles (P) appear hyperintense and show atrophy with fatty infiltration compared with the normal contralateral right side.

Pulse Sequences

The imaging protocol for sacral plexus evaluation should include a set of T1-weighted (T1W) images to provide good anatomic definition of (1) nerves outlined by perineural fat, (2) regional muscles, (3) bony landmarks, and (4) regional blood vessels. A fat-saturated T2W imaging sequence is also obtained as a conventional T2W turbo spin-echo image with selective fat saturation, a STIR series, or both. T2W images with fat saturation have the advantage of providing higher signal-to-noise ratio (SNR) compared with STIR images. However, T2W spin-echo imaging sometimes shows a lower sensitivity for detection of abnormal signal change within the nerve and the T2W images can also demonstrate inhomogeneous and inadequate fat saturation due to magnetic susceptibility changes. In such situations STIR imaging is preferred.

In cases in which contrast enhancement is utilized, additional postcontrast fat-saturated T1W series are also obtained to detect subtle enhancement within and around the nerves. In difficult cases a set of precontrast, fat-saturated T1W images may be obtained just before contrast injection to enable direct comparison with the postcontrast images. Having both sets of images improves the sensitivity for detection for contrast enhancement and permits an increased level of confidence for the interpreting physician.

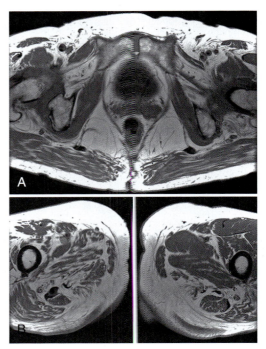

■ **FIGURE 27-6** Chronic denervation. **A,** Axial T1W MR image at the level inferior to the greater sciatic foramen shows fatty replacement of the gluteal muscles bilaterally. **B,** Axial T1W MR images at the mid-thigh level show extensive fatty replacement and atrophy of the muscles in the distribution of the sciatic nerve bilaterally consistent with chronic denervation. Note the right side is affected more than the left. These changes indicate long-standing nerve involvement.

The most reliable imaging plane for assessing nerve pathology is the plane that is orthogonal to the longitudinal axis of the nerve under study. Orthogonal images provide cross-sectional full-thickness images of the nerve, which are free of partial volume artifacts. In-plane imaging oriented parallel or nearly parallel to the long axis of the nerve can help to display the course of the nerve and possible changes in nerve caliber. Because it courses obliquely, the sacral plexus is best imaged with a combination of true coronal and axial plane images through the pelvis. In suspected cases of piriformis syndrome, additional oblique coronal plane images oriented perpendicular to the long axis of the piriformis muscle can be used to accurately assess the sciatic nerve and its relation to the piriformis (Fig. 27-7).

Image Interpretation

Interpretation of the sacral plexus requires direct comparison of the T1W and fat-saturated T2W or STIR images. The T1W images are needed to see the anatomic detail of the regional nerves, muscles, and bones, because fat-saturated T2W images tend to obscure anatomic landmarks and render all structures a relatively uniform intensity of gray. By comparing T1W and fat-saturated T2W images obtained in the same plane with the same centering and the same FOV, one can visually co-register any two images to identify the nerves and other key structures on the fat-saturated T2W images. In sequential images obtained perpendicular to the long axis of the nerve the course and continuity of the nerve can be readily

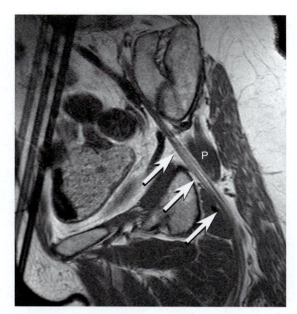

■ **FIGURE 27-7** T1W oblique coronal MR image obtained perpendicular to the piriformis muscle (P) demonstrating the sciatic nerve (*arrows*) exiting the greater sciatic foramen anterior to the piriformis muscle. This plane is essential for assessment of patients with suspected piriformis syndrome.

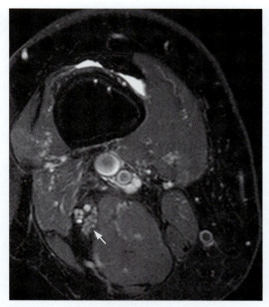

■ **FIGURE 27-8** Axial STIR MR image of a sciatic nerve showing the characteristic dot-like or honeycomb pattern, which represents rod-like collections of fascicles within the nerve that are easily seen end-on (*arrow*). Note that the adjacent vessels appear more hyperintense than the normal, minimally hyperintense nerve.

followed. In some cases multiplanar reformatting is done in oblique planes to obtain an image that provides better visualization of nerve continuity.

Maximum intensity projection (MIP) algorithms have been advocated to provide an image of the nerve distinct from adjacent structures.[6] This is analogous to blood vessel visualization with MR angiography. In our experience, however, this technique works well in only a limited number of cases, when the nerve has abnormally high signal intensity due to intrinsic signal abnormality of the nerve. Use of this technique typically also requires editing of the source images to eliminate high signal from blood vessels and other high signal structures before obtaining the MIP, so this methodology is not often used.

Gadolinium-enhanced imaging is used selectively in sacral plexus imaging based on clinical indications. For most cases, including traumatic nerve injury or compressive neuropathy, a noncontrast examination is sufficient. Nevertheless, contrast material has proved useful—assessment of unexplained nerve enlargement, mass lesions, presence of signs or symptoms suggestive of inflammation or abscess formation, and postoperative evaluations. A standard dose of 0.1 mmol/kg of a gadolinium contrast agent is used and is administered as an intravenous bolus. T1W spin-echo images, with frequency-selective fat saturation, are acquired within 3 to 5 minutes after injection.

Imaging Appearance

Normal Findings

Understanding the normal appearance of nerves on MR neurography is the key for accurate and correct interpretation of these studies. In most cases, the only finding on MR neurography is hyperintensity of the nerve or the plexus, which can be subjective. There are no objective criteria to assess the degree or amount of hyperintensity. In interpretation, one first assesses the size, shape, and location of the nerve on T1W images. In some cases, all or part of the course of the nerve may be obscured by surrounding muscle tissue, because of a lack of intervening fat. In these cases, correlative assessment of T1W and T2W images is done to trace the course of the nerve and to monitor its appearance. The normal nerve is oval or round. The size of a sacral plexus and sciatic nerve can vary along the length of the nerve and from person to person, but they tend to be symmetric from side to side. On MR neurograms, the nerve displays a characteristic "dot-like" or honeycomb pattern, which represents the cut cross-section of rod-like collections of fascicles within the nerve (Fig. 27-8). In cross section, the fascicular pattern is more easily discernible on T2W images than on corresponding T1W images. The fascicles are uniform in size and generally mildly hyperintense relative to adjacent muscle on T2W images. The signal intensity seems to vary slightly among nerves, with larger, centrally located nerves having a higher nerve/muscle signal intensity ratio than do smaller, more peripheral nerves. In-plane sections along the length of a nerve typically show uniform appearance and signal intensity within the nerve over the full extent of the FOV.

The anatomy of the sacral plexus and sciatic nerve can be effectively demonstrated with high resolution MRI in the axial and coronal planes (Figs. 27-9 and 27-10). The normal lumbosacral trunk and the sacral plexus have signal intensity similar to that of muscle on T1W sequences and slightly increased signal on T2W sequences. Within

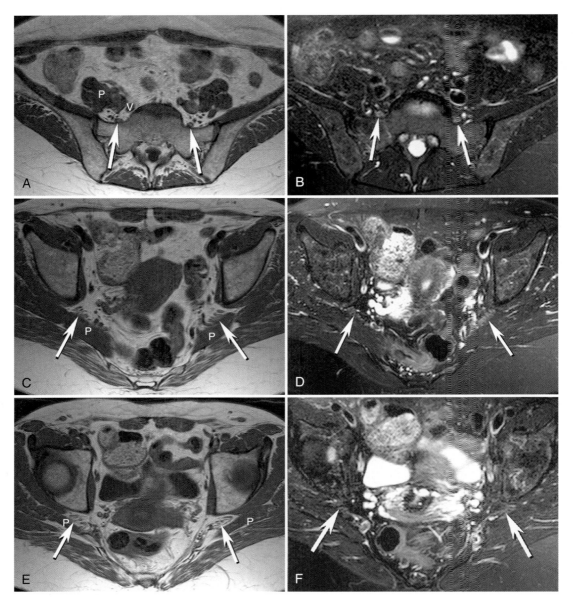

■ **FIGURE 27-9** MRI axial anatomy (superior to inferior). T1W (**A**) and T2W fat-suppressed (**B**) MR images at the level of the sacrum demonstrating the normal lumbosacral trunk (*arrows*) lying medial and posterior to the psoas muscle (P) and iliac vessels (V). The normal lumbosacral trunk and the sacral plexus have signal intensity similar to that of muscle on T1W sequences and are slightly hyperintense on T2W sequences. T1W (**C**) and T2W (**D**) fat-suppressed MR images at the level of the greater sciatic foramen demonstrating the sacral plexus (*arrows*) lying anteromedial and in close relation to the piriformis muscle (P) at the greater sciatic foramen. Note the elongated, dot-dash configuration of the sacral plexus on T1W images within the fat anterior to the piriformis muscle. T1W (**E**) and T2W (**F**) fat-suppressed MR images clearly demonstrating the normal size and fascicular morphology of the sciatic nerve (*arrows*) outlined by the surrounding fat. Note that the normal nerve is less hyperintense than the adjacent pelvic vessels and minimally hyperintense relative to the muscle.

the pelvis the sacral plexus and sciatic nerve are surrounded by fat, improving visualization, particularly on T1W sequences. At the level of the greater sciatic foramen, the sacral plexus is identified by its elongated, dot-dash configuration within the fat anterior to the piriformis muscle. If the S2 and S3 nerves are situated on, or interdigitate with, serrations in the piriformis muscle and are not surrounded by fat, these nerves can be difficult to

distinguish from the muscle on T1W images. From its position at the apex of the plexus, the sciatic nerve courses laterally and inferiorly through the greater sciatic foramen into the gluteal region. The medially located inferior gluteal vessels can usually be identified by their brighter T2W signal intensity and contour as compared with the sacral plexus and sciatic nerve.

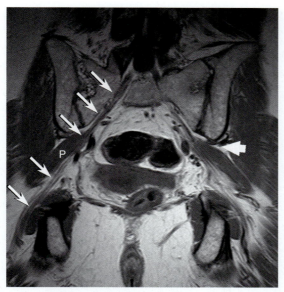

■ **FIGURE 27-10** MR coronal anatomy. T1W MR image obtained roughly parallel to the sacral plexus (*arrows*) as it courses obliquely and inferiorly, exiting the pelvis through the greater sciatic foramen (*arrowhead*) as the sciatic nerve. The nerve/plexus lies anterior/medial to the piriformis (P) muscle. Note the normal longitudinal fascicular appearance of the pelvic sciatic nerve. It is very easy to trace the entire nerve and compare it with the opposite side for changes in size, morphology and signal intensity.

Abnormal Findings

Loss of fat planes on T1W images is one of the abnormal findings associated with infiltrating or compressive lesions, but this appearance may be normal in younger, thinner patients, who have a low percentage of body fat.

Diffuse or focal enlargement of a nerve is definitely an abnormal finding. However, it is difficult to assess mild enlargement of the nerve, especially bilateral enlargement, without substantial clinical expertise. Marked diffuse or focal T2 hyperintensity of the nerve is also an abnormal finding, but assessment of lesser degrees of signal intensity is clearly subjective (Fig. 27-11). At present, there are no reliable quantitative parameters for evaluating the signal intensity of normal versus abnormal nerves. In some compressive neuropathies, focal hyperintense areas are observed in the affected nerve at the site of compression, while normal or nearly normal T2 signal intensity is present both proximal and distal to that region. The exact pathogenesis of this focal change in signal intensity is not known, but it may represent localized edema or increased fluid accumulation within the endoneurial spaces at the site of compression. An altered fascicular pattern is another finding indicative of an abnormal nerve. In some cases, individual fascicles are not resolved even though the MR images are of sufficient quality to do so. In other cases, some fascicles are markedly enlarged and/or hyperintense relative to adjacent fascicles, resulting in a decidedly nonuniform pattern. Changes in the fascicular pattern are almost always accompanied by a marked increase in signal intensity within the abnormal nerve on T2W images.

Limitations of MR Neurography

MR neurography has definite limitations. It cannot distinguish reversible from irreversible nerve injuries in the acute or early subacute stages when surgical treatment of reversible injuries would be most useful. In cases of diffuse peripheral neuropathies, MR neurography often does not achieve a specific diagnosis when the clinical features are not specific.

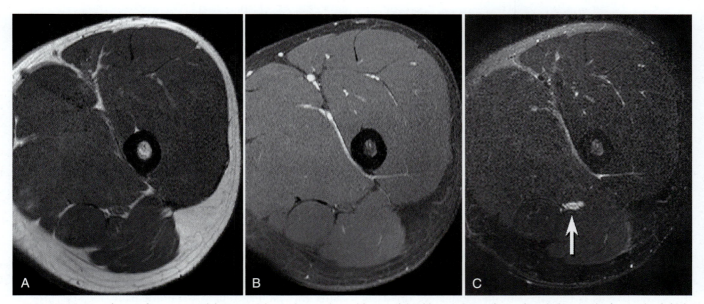

■ **FIGURE 27-11** Abnormal nerve. **A,** Axial T1W MR image in a patient with unexplained leg weakness shows the sciatic nerve in the proximal thigh. The nerve is of normal size and fascicular morphology. **B,** Axial contrast-enhanced T1W MR image at the same level. There is no abnormal enhancement of the nerve or of the adjacent tissues. **C,** Axial T2W fat-suppressed MR image at the same level shows abnormally increased nerve hyperintensity (*arrow*) that is very bright compared with the surrounding muscle and approaches that of the regional vessel signal intensity. Hyperintensity without nerve enlargement, enhancement, or associated mass can be easily overlooked without adequate experience.

Neurography involves high-resolution imaging; the individual views are relatively time consuming (several minutes per sequence) and subject to degradation by patient motion. Despite the use of saturation pulses to suppress flow, artifacts from blood flow in regional vessels can propagate as phase-shift artifacts across an image and interfere with nerve identification and evaluation. This is most often encountered with slowly flowing blood in regional veins on STIR imaging. Inhomogeneous fat suppression due to magnetic susceptibility effects may obscure fine detail and T2 signal changes in portions of a nerve. Although the use of STIR imaging results in more homogeneous and reproducible fat suppression, its lower SNR and higher propensity for flow artifacts may limit the utility of this sequence. Finally, there is an inverse relationship between the imaging FOV and the image resolution obtainable. Because high detail is needed, a targeted FOV that encompasses only a localized portion of a nerve must be utilized. This means that the most likely segment of abnormal nerve must be identified clinically before the MR neurographic examination and this information provided to the MR physician. Long segments of nerve cannot be imaged in sufficient detail to provide an adequate MR neurography examination.

The "magic angle" effect previously described in imaging of tendons can also be seen in peripheral nerve imaging. In peripheral nerves, these effects typically occur with STIR or heavily T2W fast spin-echo (long echo time) sequences and are seen against a background of detectable signal intensity. They may appear as a more gradual transition over a wider range of angles rather than just those closely related to an angle of 55 degrees in relation to the long axis of the magnet bore as seen in tendon imaging. However, abrupt changes in signal intensity may be seen where a nerve is sharply angulated. The increase in signal intensity in nerves (relative to muscle) produced by "magic angle" effects may simulate disease. Although it is less likely to be seen with sacral plexus imaging versus brachial plexus, median nerve, or ulnar nerve imaging, this phenomenon must be recognized and differentiated from pathologic changes to improve the diagnostic accuracy of MR neurography.[8]

Future Directions

Introduction of higher field magnets (3 T) and parallel imaging techniques have improved SNR and reduced imaging time, resulting in improved image quality. Continued improvements in this area may lead to better application of MR neurography in the future.

Improvements in the number and bandwidth of radiofrequency channels available in newer MR scanners will allow for further improvements in radiofrequency imaging coil design. The increased number of channels will provide increased flexibility in the area of coverage and in fitting coils to the different anatomic contours of the body without sacrificing SNR.

Advanced MRI techniques can potentially apply physiologic imaging sequences to peripheral nerve studies. Injury to white matter tracts results in loss of the anisotropy of diffusion through the damaged tissue. Application of diffusion techniques to peripheral nerve imaging could improve the sensitivity and specificity of MR neurographic diagnosis. If so, one may in the future expect clinical indications for peripheral nerve diffusion tensor imaging with fiber tracking.[7]

An additional approach under active development is the use of black blood contrast agents. These are typically iron oxide–based contrast agents that are designed to remain within the circulating bloodstream during the image session and to obliterate the signal from intravascular blood by virtue of their high susceptibility effects. These agents are also taken up by the bone marrow and therefore suppress bone marrow signal as well. This further improves the conspicuity of nerves.[5] As MR technology evolves we will see further advances in sacral plexus imaging.

NEOPLASM/MALIGNANT INFILTRATION

Masses involving the sacral plexuses can be broadly divided into intrinsic and extrinsic tumors and subdivided into benign and malignant categories. Benign nerve sheath tumors include neurofibromas, schwannomas, and ganglion cysts. Malignant nerve sheath tumors (malignant peripheral nerve sheath tumors [MPNST]) include malignant schwannoma, malignant neurilemoma, nerve sheath fibrosarcoma, and neurinosarcoma.

Extrinsic masses that affect the sacral plexus generally originate from or secondarily involve the pelvis and the sacrum. Tumor involvement of the piriformis muscle can cause sacral plexopathy, because the muscle is intimately related to the sacral nerves and plexus. Ischial masses can also affect the plexus because they have a close relationship to the inferior plexus and proximal sciatic nerve.

Precise assessment of tumor extension and involvement is essential for surgical planning to facilitate resection. Early excision of a benign tumor may lead to permanent nerve damage. Late excision may be incomplete owing to larger tumor size and prevent cure of a coexistent malignant tumor.

Intrinsic Lesions

All neurogenic tumors exhibit a similar morphology. They typically show a fusiform shape oriented longitudinally along the length of the nerve and tapered ends that are contiguous with the parent nerve. This relationship is usually easy to detect on MRI owing to its large FOV and multiplanar capability.

Benign Lesions

Neurofibromas

Neurofibromas are common tumors of the peripheral nerves. They typically occur in patients who are 20 to 30 years old, and there is no sex predilection. They may present as either a solitary localized lesion or as multiple lesions in association with neurofibromatosis. Neurofibromas are unencapsulated tumors that tend to infiltrate along the nerve, become inseparable from the fascicles of the nerve, and therefore become unresectable without sacrifice of the entire nerve.

On noncontrast CT, a neurofibroma appears as a well-defined mass that is hypodense relative to muscle due to the presence of Schwann cells, neural elements, and adipocytes.[9] On contrast-enhanced CT scans, neurofibromas usually show mild or no contrast enhancement. More than half of neurofibromas remain hypodense after injection of a contrast agent.[10]

On MRI neurofibromas show low to intermediate signal intensity on T1W images and moderately high signal intensity on T2W images. Inhomogeneous contrast enhancement is seen in two third of cases, although uniform enhancement may be noticed. Signal on T2W images can be homogeneously hyperintense or show a characteristic target sign, consisting of a central hypointense region with surrounding hyperintensity. This pattern corresponds to a distinctive zonal histologic appearance that is only found in neurofibromas. The central area of low signal intensity probably reflects the concentration of dense collagen and fibrillary tissue, which causes T2 shortening. The high signal intensity in the peripheral zone may reflect more myxoid tissue with higher water content.

Although the target sign has been described as being nearly pathognomonic for neurofibroma, it can still be seen in schwannoma and MPNST. The split-fat sign represents a rim of fat surrounding the tumor, which originates from the nerve in an intramuscular location and is much easier to appreciate on T1W images. The split fat sign is more common in benign PNSTs and lesions of large nerves.[11]

Schwannoma

Schwannoma (also designated neurilemoma or neurinoma) is an encapsulated nerve sheath tumor seen at all ages but most common in persons between the ages of 20 and 50 years. Men and women are equally affected. Most lesions are solitary and present as a slowly growing soft-tissue mass.[9] Pain and neurologic symptoms are uncommon unless the tumor becomes large. Deep schwannomas become symptomatic by virtue of their large size and impingement on neighboring structures

Because schwannomas arise within the nerve sheath, they are surrounded by a true capsule consisting of epineurium. Smaller tumors are generally fusiform and relatively homogeneous in texture and histology. Larger tumors typically present as eccentric masses over which the nerve fibers are splayed and manifest secondary degenerative changes, such as cysts, hemorrhage, and calcification. Most schwannomas are unilobular masses surrounded by fibrous capsules consisting of epineurium and residual nerve fibers.[11]

Histologically, schwannomas are characterized by a pattern of alternating areas of Antoni A and B pathology. Antoni A areas are composed of compact spindle cells. Antoni B areas are far less orderly and less cellular and exhibit signs of secondary degeneration.

CT shows a well-defined mass that is isodense to hypodense relative to muscle and that enhances uniformly after contrast agent administration. Nonenhancing cystic or necrotic areas are often found in schwannomas and help to differentiate schwannomas from neurofibromas.

On T1W images schwannomas have intermediate signal intensity similar to that of muscles. Sometimes they are barely visible. On T2W images schwannomas show markedly increased signal intensity. Cystic areas within them show low signal intensity on T1W images and high signal intensity on T2W images. Small schwannomas tend to enhance uniformly after gadolinium administration, whereas larger lesions show a far more heterogeneous enhancement. A low-intensity rim-like capsule is detectable in 70% of schwannomas but only 30% of neurofibromas.[11]

Neurofibromas and schwannomas may be indistinguishable by MRI criteria alone. The fusiform shape, split-fat sign, and target sign can be seen in either of the lesions.[12] However, some features do help to differentiate these two entities. Schwannomas are generally eccentrically positioned in relation to the parent nerve, whereas neurofibromas tend to be centrally located within the nerve. Schwannomas tend to be small or moderate in size, sharply demarcated from adjacent tissues, and localized to a single nerve. Schwannomas also generally show a very marked increase in T2 signal and intense homogeneous contrast enhancement (but may show areas of heterogeneity reflecting necrosis and cyst formation within the schwannoma).

Neurofibromas are generally larger and demonstrate moderate or patchy contrast enhancement. In the presence of known neurofibromatosis the probability that the lesion represents a neurofibroma is greatly increased, especially if the lesion has a plexiform appearance. The plexiform neurofibromas that involve the sacral plexus generally appear as large lobular masses that encompass multiple nerves of the plexus in continuity (Fig. 27-12). The presence of necrosis within a neurofibroma raises the question of malignant degeneration of the tumor, especially when the lesion is large, is poorly demarcated from surrounding structures, and shows an inhomogeneous pattern of increased T2 signal.[11,12]

Ganglion Cyst

Ganglion cysts appear as low-intensity lesions with well-defined margins on the T1W images and show marked hyperintensity on the T2W images. There is no contrast enhancement within the cystic portion of the mass, but there may be mild enhancement along the thin wall of the cyst capsule.[13]

Extrinsic Tumors Causing Plexopathy

Neoplastic lumbosacral plexopathy is an infrequent complication associated with advanced systemic cancer and local or regional progression of the primary tumor. Lumbosacral plexus involvement occurs most commonly with intra-abdominal tumor extension (73% of cases) and less commonly with growth from metastases, lymph nodes, or bone structures. A tumor may invade the plexus directly or track along the connective tissue or epineurium of nerve trunks.[14]

The lower sacral plexus is involved most frequently (50%), followed by the upper plexus (33%) and panplexopathy (18%). Bilateral plexopathy occurs in 25% of cases and is usually caused by metastases from breast cancer. Involvement of the lower (sacral) plexus generally

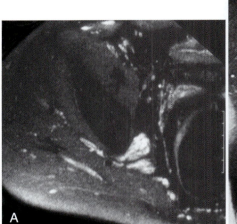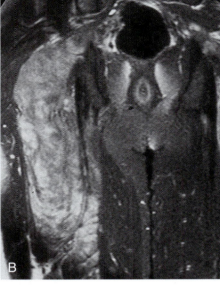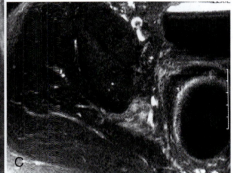

■ **FIGURE 27-12** Neurofibroma. Axial (**A**) and coronal (**B**) STIR MR images with postcontrast T1W fat-saturated (**C**) image show a large hyperintense plexiform neurofibroma originating from the right sacral plexus and extending along the course of the sciatic nerve that enhances inhomogenously with administration of a contrast agent.

occurs with colorectal and cervical neoplasms. Involvement of the sacral sympathetic nerves is less common (10%).[14]

The most prevalent types of tumors are colorectal tumors (20%), sarcomas (16%), breast tumors (11%), lymphoma (9%), and cervical tumors (9%). Other tumors, including multiple myeloma, account for another 37% of cases. The most common distant metastatic lesions are caused by breast cancer.[14]

Pain is the most prominent symptom. It usually occurs early in the course of the disease and is the initial symptom in most patients. Pain is often located over the costovertebral angle when the lumbar plexus in involved and in the hip or buttock, radiating down to the toes of the affected leg when the lower sacral plexus is involved. The pain may worsen after a bowel movement and is usually worse when the patient is supine. Pain that worsens with movement suggests underlying involvement of bone.[15]

Areflexia, weakness, and sensory loss are other common manifestations. Involvement of the sacral sympathetic nerves is less common, being reported in about only 10% of patients. Vegetative sympathetic symptoms, particularly hot and dry feet, have been suggested as indicators of neoplastic involvement of the lumbosacral plexus. Patients with metastatic lumbosacral plexopathy have a poor prognosis.[15,16]

CT is useful for imaging patients with suspected lumbosacral plexopathy and easily characterizes the mass, delineates its extent, and documents any involvement of the plexus. The correlation between clinical and radiologic findings on CT is good; however, clinical findings and CT scan levels do not always demonstrate positive correlation. MRI may offer better anatomic resolution and better tissue discrimination and is superior to CT for imaging lumbosacral plexopathy.

Both MRI and CT demonstrate thickening or enlargement of the plexus itself and/or show a mass that directly involves the plexus (Fig. 27-13). Some data suggest that MRI may be more sensitive than CT in detecting tumor and distinguishing it from radiation-induced plexopathy. CT scan of the abdomen and pelvis is probably more valuable in the diagnosis of the primary tumor and gives more information on tumor and bony erosion and can help guide in biopsy.[16]

Radiation-Induced Plexopathy

Radiation-induced sacral plexopathy can result from radiation therapy or radiation exposure. The symptoms include loss of function, strength, and balance and possible incontinence. The onset of the symptoms is generally insidious and progresses gradually with variable rapidity.

The time range of symptoms varies widely from 3 months to 22 years after the completion of radiation therapy. Jaeckle and coworkers[15] found that 20% of patients developed moderate or severe weakness over 6 months. Others were found to have mild weakness at 4 to 5 years after the onset of neurologic symptoms. Electromyographic findings of decreased conduction also have variable onset, ranging from 4 months to 5 years after irradiation.

Radiation plexopathy is most commonly noted with uterine, cervical, ovarian, and testicular cancers, as well as lymphomas.

The pathophysiology of radiation injury to peripheral nerves or the sacral plexus is still debatable. Radiation fibrosis is believed to be the most likely initial inciting event, eventually causing entrapment of the nerves with secondary demyelination.[17] Experimental studies in rats suggest that the target cell may be the Schwann cell,

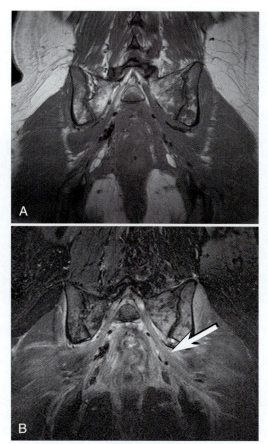

■ **FIGURE 27-13**   Extrinsic tumor. Coronal T1W (**A**) and STIR (**B**) MR images in a patient with carcinoma of the cervix showing an extensive soft tissue mass surrounding and infiltrating the entire pelvis and the sacral plexus bilaterally (*arrow,* **B**) that is enlarged with loss of fat planes and normal fascicular architecture. Note the hyperintense signal consistent with extensive marrow infiltration by the mass lesion.

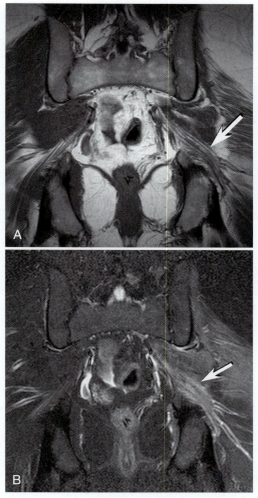

■ **FIGURE 27-14**   Neoplastic plexopathy. **A,** Coronal T1W MR image showing focal unilateral enlargement of the left sacral plexus (*arrow*) at the greater sciatic foramen. **B,** Coronal T1W fat-suppressed postcontrast MR image demonstrates a focal enhancing mass (*arrow*) representing metastasis from lung carcinoma encasing the sacral plexus with associated nerve enhancement. Note adjacent muscle changes suggestive of muscle denervation.

which produces myelin in the spinal roots and nerves of the peripheral nervous system.

Postirradiation plexopathy is relatively uncommon but must be differentiated from recurrent malignancy, because recurrent malignancy is much more common. Both entities may present as similar clinical pictures but require very different treatment regimens. Nerve imaging often helps to differentiate between these two.

Clinically, the pain associated with malignancy is more severe and more difficult to treat than the pain associated with radiation plexopathy. Bilateral involvement is more common with radiation-induced plexopathy than metastatic plexopathy. Bilateral involvement of metastatic plexopathy can occur in 25% of patients (frequently caused by metastasis of breast cancer), but bilateral involvement is more common with radiation-induced plexopathy that presents in the form of bilateral muscle weakness as opposed to unilateral weakness.[18]

Lymphedema is more common with metastatic sacral plexopathy than with radiation-induced sacral plexopathy, even though the reverse is true for brachial plexopathy. About 40% of patients with metastatic plexopathy show hydronephrosis or hydroureter.[15] Myokymia is often found in radiation-induced plexopathy but is usually absent in metastatic plexopathy. Nerve conduction studies cannot distinguish between metastatic and radiation-induced plexopathy. The electromyogram is more useful, because myokymia is a common finding of radiation change.[18]

MRI can be a very useful tool in differentiating postirradiation plexopathy from recurrent tumor. Detection of a discrete mass in relation to the plexus is the most common finding in patients with metastatic plexopathy, although similar findings have been occasionally reported in radiation plexopathy.

Focal and irregular enlargement of the nerve with increased signal on T2W and STIR images and contrast enhancement is generally seen with tumor (Fig. 27-14). Radiation-induced plexitis on the other hand results in more uniform enlargement and diffuse abnormal signal of the nerve without contrast enhancement (Fig. 27-15).

Fluorodeoxyglucose (FDG)-labeled positron emission tomographic (PET) studies may show increased uptake in

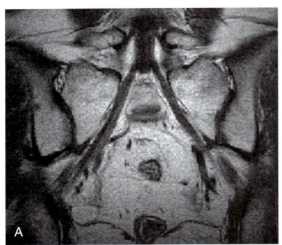

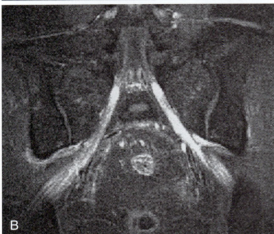

■ **FIGURE 27-15** Radiation injury. Coronal T1W (**A**) and STIR (**B**) MR images showing uniform mild diffuse enlargement and abnormal signal of the entire sacral plexus. The presence of bilateral symmetry with lack of focal enlargement, focal abnormal signal, and/or an associated mass lesion helps differentiate it from tumor-related plexopathy.

the involved region of metastatic plexopathy but are usually negative in radiation-induced plexopathy. Therefore, FDG-PET may help to differentiate between tumor and radiation-induced plexopathy, although the normal excretion of radioisotope by the kidney and bladder may limit the interpretation of the findings in sacral plexopathy.[19]

Miscellaneous Causes

Retroperitoneal Hemorrhage

Retroperitoneal hemorrhage can compress the lumbar plexus, the entire lumbosacral plexus, or the femoral nerve. It usually results from supertherapeutic anticoagulation and less commonly from hemophilia, disseminated intravascular coagulopathy, thrombocytopenia, or, rarely, rupture of an abdominal aortic aneurysm. In cancer patients with thrombocytopenia, retroperitoneal bleeding can cause plexopathy with rapid onset of pain and neurologic signs within 24 hours.

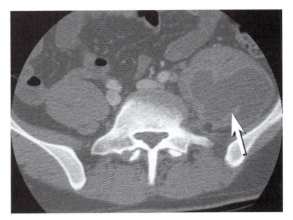

■ **FIGURE 27-16** Infection. CT scan of the pelvis showing a left iliopsoas abscess (*arrow*) that originated from tuberculous osteomyelitis. CT is very useful in assessing the extent of the abscess, associated bone involvement, destruction and in guiding drainage.

Infection and Inflammation

Soft tissue abscesses can spread along the psoas muscle, iliacus muscle, and iliac vessels to affect the sacral plexus. Gluteal abscesses can affect the proximal sciatic nerve directly and can reach the sacral plexus secondarily via the greater sciatic foramen. Retroperitoneal abscess may arise from infection in the vertebral bodies, perinephric tissues, or gastrointestinal tract. Human immunodeficiency virus immunosuppression with rectal abscess and pelvic cellulitis can also affect the plexus. Tuberculosis (Fig. 27-16), syphilis, and schistosomiasis (a recurring syndrome) are recognized causes of sacral plexitis.[20] Noninfectious inflammations such as sarcoid can also cause painful lumbosacral plexopathy.

Pregnancy and Complications of Delivery

Lumbosacral plexopathy can also result from prolonged labor and cephalopelvic disproportion when pressure from the fetal head and forceps injure the nerves. Damage to the lumbar nerve roots by epidural analgesia can also lead to plexopathy.

Diabetic Radiculoplexopathy

Diabetic radiculoplexopathy, also erroneously termed *diabetic femoral neuropathy*, is a syndrome of pain and weakness due to diffuse involvement of the lumbosacral plexus. The pathophysiology of this disorder is not clear. Multiple infarcts in the lumbosacral plexus and proximal obturator and femoral nerves have been implicated in its pathogenesis. Potential toxic effects of metabolites peculiar to diabetics have been postulated. Electromyographic evidence implicates the spinal nerves, hence the designation radiculoplexopathy. Clinically, there may be sudden or gradual onset with severe pain in the back, hips, and thighs and weakness. Commonly, the pain is relentless, worse at night and worse at rest (distinguishing it from mechanical low back pain). The pain and weakness are usually asymmetric.[20] Rarely, there is little or no pain. The weakness is generally progressive and often continues or even worsens after the pain subsides. Partial recovery of at least a mild degree is seen in 60% of patients and this may take from 3 to 18 months.

Idiopathic Lumbosacral Plexopathies

Rarely, a syndrome resembling diabetic plexopathy with acute or insidious onset of severe pain and subsequent weakness is seen in patients with no diabetes mellitus. There is no age predilection. Children have been reported with this syndrome. Electromyography shows widespread involvement of the plexus but sparing of the paraspinal muscles (unlike diabetic plexopathy). Painful lumbosacral plexopathy may be seen with an elevated erythrocyte sedimentation rate responsive to immunosuppressive therapy. This condition can be classified with the idiopathic group as well as the inflammatory group. Heroin addicts have also been reported to have intense pain and relatively mild weakness, usually with good resolution. Rhabdomyolysis with a compartment-elevated pressure is usually imputed as the likely pathophysiology. Injections, intravenous administration of a chemotherapeutic agent, and viral infections have all been implicated in the production of lumbosacral plexitis. The viral infections are usually herpes zoster, although genital herpes may produce a syndrome of urinary retention, constipation, and sacral pain.[20]

ENTRAPMENTS AND COMPRESSIONS

Compressive neuropathies and plexopathies are among the most common indications for performing peripheral nerve imaging. Compression may be acute or chronic and may result from nerve entrapment or repetitive stress injury. In the sciatic plexus the most commonly searched for site of entrapment is at the level of the piriformis muscle where the distal sacral plexus and the proximal sciatic nerve come together and normally pass anterior and inferior to the belly of the piriformis.

A patient with compressive neuropathy affecting the sacral plexus generally presents with low back or extremity pain, weakness, sensory loss or paresthesias, and abnormal reflexes. Less common symptoms include incontinence and impotence. These symptoms are not specific for sacral plexopathy, so cauda equina or cord compression should be ruled out with lumbar spine MRI.

MR neurography may also be useful in sciatica of nondisc origin when the cause of compression is other than disc or piriformis muscle. MR neurography may identify a causative lesion in some patients in whom routine diagnostic modalities have failed to establish a structural etiology for their back or radicular pain. These include a variety of pathologic processes that may result in compression or irritation of adjacent nerve plexus structures, such as enlarged lymph nodes, pelvic masses, seeding from a primary carcinoma located elsewhere, or a localized abscess or myositis. This can help resolve the diagnosis in many of these patients and can help differentiate among the cases that should be directed toward reoperation, radiofrequency neurolysis, or medical treatments directed at inflammation.

On imaging, acute and chronic compressive neuropathies demonstrate increased T2 signal intensity within the nerve. Increased T2 signal is seen focally at the site of nerve compression but, with severe or long-standing compression, may extend distally to involve a variable length of the nerve. Detection of short segment involvement, as short as 1 or 2 cm, helps to implicate entrapment as the most likely etiology for the nerve dysfunction. In some cases the abnormal nerve segment may be elongated over a few centimeters. It has been shown by Jarvik and colleagues[2] that the length of abnormal nerve signal roughly correlates with the severity and duration of the entrapment symptoms, as well as the degree of nerve conduction slowing seen on electrodiagnostic testing. There may also be nerve enlargement with accompanying change of the normal fascicular pattern. This swelling may occur both proximal and distal to the site of maximal compression. The fascicular swelling is often heterogeneous, with some fascicles being quite swollen while others remain relatively normal. The MR appearance of hyperintensity within nerves in acute or chronic compressive processes reflects an alteration in the endoneurial free water. The hypothesis, extrapolated from work done in nerve injury models, is that an increase in permeability of endothelial tight junctions within the endoneurium allows increased transmission of water into the endoneurial space. The subsequent edema raises pressure within the nerve, eventually leading to axonal loss from ischemia. Changes are first apparent at the site of known compression and may subsequently extend to the distal axons as wallerian degeneration occurs. MR neurography can also be a valuable tool in assessing recovery because it also shows restoration of normal signal with nerve regeneration.

Piriformis Muscle Syndrome

Piriformis syndrome is a rare cause of myofascial pain syndrome characterized by low back pain and sciatica secondary to sciatic nerve entrapment at the greater sciatic notch.

Piriformis muscle syndrome is still a controversial and debatable entity. Since its first description in 1928 by Yeoman as periarthritis of the anterior sacroiliac joint, there is still no general consensus about the etiology and pathophysiology of this entity.[21] The end point is neuritis of the proximal sciatic nerve resulting from either irritation or compression by the piriformis muscle.

Given the lack of general consensus, the exact frequency of this clinical entity is still debatable and ranges from rare to approximately 6% in different studies, with female preponderance.[22]

Understanding the basic functional anatomy is very important for better understanding of the entity. The piriformis muscle originates from the anterior surface of the S2-S4 vertebrae, the sacrotuberous ligament, and the upper margin of the greater sciatic foramen. This muscle passes through the greater sciatic notch and inserts onto the superior surface of the greater trochanter of the femur. The function of the piriformis muscle is to externally rotate the hip in extension and to abduct the thigh in flexion. The sacral plexus is closely associated with the anterior surface of the piriformis muscle. The sciatic nerve passes inferior to the piriformis muscle.

The sciatic nerve may exit the pelvis via four different routes:

1. The nerve passes anterior to the piriformis between the rims of the greater sciatic foramen.
2. The peroneal portion of the sciatic nerve passes through the piriformis muscle while the tibial portion passes anterior to the piriformis muscle.
3. The peroneal branch of the sciatic nerve loops above and posterior to the piriformis muscle, whereas the tibial branch passes anterior to the piriformis muscle.
4. The undivided sciatic nerve penetrates the piriformis muscle.

Involvement of the superior gluteal nerve usually is not seen in cases of piriformis syndrome. This nerve leaves the sciatic nerve trunk and passes through the sciatic foramen above the piriformis muscle.

The etiology of piriformis syndrome can be subdivided as follows[22]:

- Hyperlordosis
- Muscle anomalies with hypertrophy
- Fibrosis (due to trauma)
- Partial or total nerve anatomic abnormalities
- Muscle hematoma (due to trauma)

Other causes of piriformis syndrome include:

- Pseudoaneurysms of the inferior gluteal artery adjacent to the piriformis syndrome
- Bilateral piriformis syndrome due to prolonged sitting during an extended neurosurgical procedure
- Cerebral palsy
- Total hip arthroplasty
- Myositis ossificans
- Vigorous physical activity
- Altered biomechanics resulting from leg-length discrepancy

Papadopoulos and associates[23] proposed a new classification of piriformis syndrome. Primary piriformis syndrome includes cases caused by all intrinsic pathology of the piriformis muscle itself, such as myofascial pain, anatomic variations, and myositis ossificans. Secondary piriformis syndrome (pelvic outlet syndrome) includes all other causes of piriformis syndrome, with the exclusion of lumbar spinal pathology.

Clinically, piriformis syndrome is characterized by pain and paresthesias in the unilateral gluteal region radiating to the hip and posterior thigh in a sciatic radicular distribution. Pain increases on prolonged sitting. At physical examination, the patient's symptoms can be reproduced by digital pressure over the belly of the piriformis muscle in the gluteal region and by digital pressure on the lateral pelvic wall of the affected side during rectal or pelvic examination.

The diagnosis of piriformis syndrome was previously thought to be purely clinical and the role of imaging techniques largely ignored. In most of the centers the diagnosis is made by clinical examination and electromyography after ruling out other causes of pain. However, MR neurography can be a valuable noninvasive diagnostic method that provides a reliable diagnosis of piriformis syndrome. In some patients with severe symptoms, hyperintensity, shape changes, and asymmetric enlargement of the piriformis muscle are seen. The asymmetry may reflect either hypertrophy on one side or atrophy and spasm on the other. Muscle spasm may change the shape and hardness of a muscle without altering its total volume. Altered fascicular pattern within the nerve may be seen along with signal intensity changes. MRI can also help to differentiate piriformis syndrome from other possible causes of lower lumbar pain and sciatica, such as lumbar disc herniation, lumbar stenosis, and mass lesions in the region of the piriformis muscle.

Imaging can easily depict the abnormal course of the sciatic nerve through the muscle (when the nerve passes through the substance of the muscle) or through the split (bifid) piriformis tendon (Fig. 27-17). Familiarity with the appearance of piriformis syndrome on MRI is important to facilitate appropriate diagnosis and treatment.

Botulinum Toxin Injection for Piriformis Syndrome

Traditional methods for relief of piriformis muscle syndrome include slow stretch exercise, massage, heat, ultrasound, surgical division of the muscle, and injection of the muscular trigger point with local anesthetic and corticosteroids.[24] There has been increasing use of image-guided botulinum toxin injection into the piriformis muscle.

The introduction of botulinum toxin type A has allowed a new therapeutic approach. The degree of symptom improvement correlates with weakness in the offending muscle secondary to blockade of neuromuscular transmission. The role of highly accurate imaging-guided injection in the pelvis is critical. Both electromyographic and fluoroscopic guidance can help to localize the injection to the target muscle, but they do little to mitigate the risk of nerve or bowel injury and do not provide the direct vision and precise localization CT and MRI guidance do. Ultrasonography provides a very low level of target reliability and few means of confirming the ultimate distribution of the injectate. Open MRI or CT guidance nearly eliminates the risk of penetrating the nerve or bowel with the needle and allows for documentation of the selective presence of the injectate within the piriformis muscle. Hence CT-guided or open MRI-guided botulinum toxin injection is an emerging and feasible technique. Radiographic exposure to the unshielded pelvis during a procedure involving CT guidance could be a significant concern, but the accuracy of CT has been documented more than MRI because blind transvaginal piriformis injection technique conducted in the design phase of this study revealed that these injections do not reliably reach the piriformis muscle. Moreover, the presence of implanted metallic device and less availability can prompt for more CT-guided procedures.[25]

POSTSURGICAL RADICULOPATHY

MR neurography is very useful for evaluating persistent, exacerbated, or altered radiculopathy after lumbar spinal surgery.[5] It allows clear differentiation among

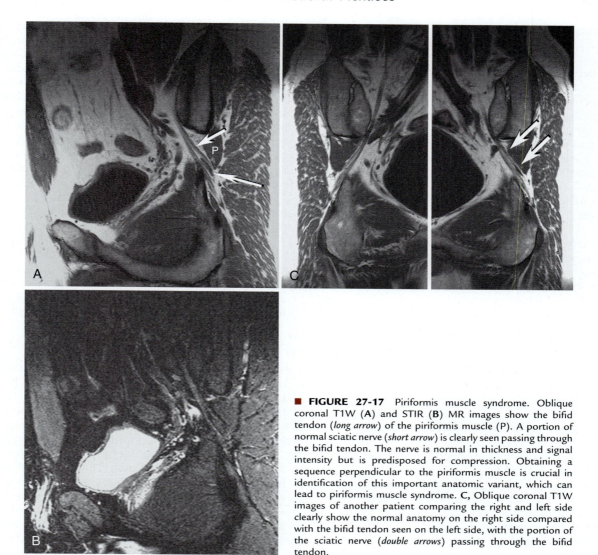

■ **FIGURE 27-17** Piriformis muscle syndrome. Oblique coronal T1W (**A**) and STIR (**B**) MR images show the bifid tendon (*long arrow*) of the piriformis muscle (P). A portion of normal sciatic nerve (*short arrow*) is clearly seen passing through the bifid tendon. The nerve is normal in thickness and signal intensity but is predisposed for compression. Obtaining a sequence perpendicular to the piriformis muscle is crucial in identification of this important anatomic variant, which can lead to piriformis muscle syndrome. **C,** Oblique coronal T1W images of another patient comparing the right and left side clearly show the normal anatomy on the right side compared with the bifid tendon seen on the left side, with the portion of the sciatic nerve (*double arrows*) passing through the bifid tendon.

several different causes of this problem and identifies cases that are best treated by reoperation, by allowing additional time to elapse, or by referral for electronic stimulators or other treatments for chronic, irremediable pain. In a number of common situations, MR neurography can provide a specific diagnosis and determine treatment by revealing pathology that cannot be detected by any other methodology. Postoperative hyperintensity in the ganglion can be connected with a specific anatomic feature not adequately treated by the surgery, such as a persistent bone spur.

Another diagnosis made possible by neurography is lumbar monoradiculitis, a condition that is easily mistaken for a herniated disc syndrome if any disc abnormality happens to be seen in the patient's MR image.[5]

TRAUMA

Injury to the sacral plexus can result from blunt or penetrating trauma. Because of the stability of the pelvic girdle and lumbar spine, blunt traumatic injury to the sacral plexus is relatively uncommon.

Lumbosacral plexopathy due to blunt trauma usually results in severe neurologic deficit. Many post-traumatic cases remain undiagnosed owing to the high mortality in this patient population and because survivors of multiple trauma, including pelvic fractures, frequently have incomplete work-up because no significant intervention can be offered. In several series of trauma patients, a correlation was seen between occurrence of lumbosacral plexopathy and type of pelvic fracture. The proximity of the lumbosacral plexus to the sacral bone and the sacroiliac joint suggests a higher incidence of lumbosacral plexopathy with injury to these structures. Patients with unstable pelvic fractures completely disrupting the sacroiliac complex are more susceptible to sacral plexus injury. Therefore, it is not surprising that the highest incidence of lumbosacral plexopathy is found among patients with sacral fractures. The occurrence of lumbosacral plexopathy in patients with acetabular fractures is also common, but its association is more difficult to understand.[26]

Hemorrhage and edema immediately after an acute trauma may obscure details of the nerve image. In many

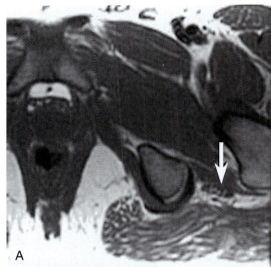

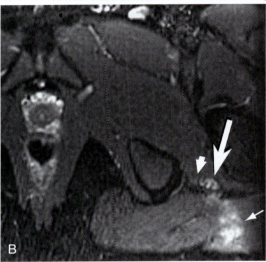

■ **FIGURE 27-18** Trauma. Axial T1W (**A**) and STIR (**B**) MR images in a patient with a stab wound to the gluteal region show marked hyperintense T2 signal with mild enlargement (*large arrow,* **A**) of the left sciatic nerve indicating associated sciatic nerve injury. There is associated soft tissue hyperintensity (*small arrow,* **B**), indicating the tract of the stab wound. Note only the lateral portion of the nerve is bright (*large arrow,* **B**) as opposed to the normal medial portion (*arrowhead*), indicating injury only to the peroneal component of the sciatic nerve. Clinically, the patient only had peroneal signs. This clearly depicts how MR neurography can easily identify the presence of partial nerve injury in such cases.

cases, the nerve structures are completely indistinguishable from surrounding edematous tissues and the MR neurography study is of no diagnostic help. This highly limits the utility of MR neurography in the acute post-traumatic period. Delayed imaging after 3 to 4 weeks is recommended for traumatic nerve evaluation in these cases. This coincides with delays in surgical treatment for most traumatic nerve injuries other than complete disruption by laceration of a nerve, in which case the mechanism of trauma is usually sufficient to indicate the diagnosis and surgical exploration is undertaken without imaging. It is possible that improvement in MR technology in the future may enable diagnostically useful diffusion-weighted

nerve imaging and that this may be applicable in acute traumatic nerve injury in the future. The proximal sciatic nerve in the buttocks beginning with the point where it emerges from the greater sciatic foramen is well visualized and easily evaluated with sacral plexus imaging.

Following acute trauma and severe nerve injury, MRN may help define disruption and discontinuity of the nerve. Disruption of nerve continuity is generally associated with extensive swelling and increased T2 signal (Fig. 27-18) within the disrupted nerve and the surrounding soft tissue structures. At times, pseudomeningeal formation may occur. There is still no completely reliable means of confirming a true nerve root avulsion by imaging.

On the other hand, severe nerve injuries more often occur without complete loss of anatomic continuity of the nerve. In such cases, severe stretch injuries to the nerve can still result in axonal disruption and complete loss of distal function. The MR neurographic study shows continuity of the nerve, although there is usually swelling and markedly increased T2 signal at the site of injury that may propagate distally. At present it is difficult on imaging and electrophysiologic studies to assess reversible versus nonreversible change after injury. Serial MRI may help in this differential diagnosis (Fig. 27-19). We have observed normalization of abnormal signal intensity within injured nerves of the brachial plexus and within denervated muscles as nerve function recovers. In some cases, these imaging improvements have preceded changes demonstrated by electrical studies or clinical examination. At the same time, we have seen persistence of abnormal signal intensity in irreversibly injured nerves well beyond 1 year after injury. Whereas our series is small and relates mainly to the brachial plexus and is anecdotal rather than based on rigorous scientific analysis, it does provide encouraging evidence for improved earlier assessment of severely injured nerves. With future advances in physiologic MRI techniques, such as diffusion-weighted imaging, further improvements may be made in earlier diagnosis of reversible versus irreversible nerve injury affecting the peripheral nerves.

In addition to defining nerve injuries in the acute and subacute stages, late complications of nerve injury can also be seen. Diagnosis of post-traumatic neuromas, which represent disordered attempts at regrowth of axons that are misdirected into a tangled mass of disorganized tissue, can be made on MR neurography. The exact location, size, and extent of the lesion can be seen. In addition to their mass-like appearance, these masses usually show mild to moderate contrast enhancement, which further helps to establish the correct diagnosis.[5]

PERIPHERAL NEUROPATHIES

In patients with peripheral neuropathies, MR neurography can confirm the presence, extent, and morphologic appearance of an abnormal nerve by demonstrating nerve swelling and hyperintense T2 signal within the nerve. MRN can readily define the hyperintense swollen fascicles of a nerve and therefore identify an unknown "mass" as a swollen nerve. The abnormal signal usually extends over

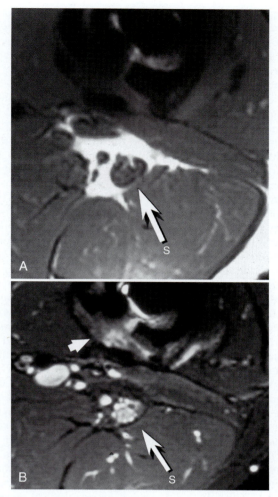

■ FIGURE 27-19 Trauma. Axial T1W (**A**) and STIR (**B**) MR images at mid-thigh level in a patient with a gunshot wound. The images were obtained 3 weeks after the incident. The study shows continuity of the sciatic nerve (S), although there is still swelling and markedly increased T2 signal at the site of injury. These findings indicate either nonreversible injury or inadequate recovery. Note residual associated soft tissue edema and injury (*arrowhead*). Serial MR neurography is very useful for follow-up of nerve trauma and in assessing recovery.

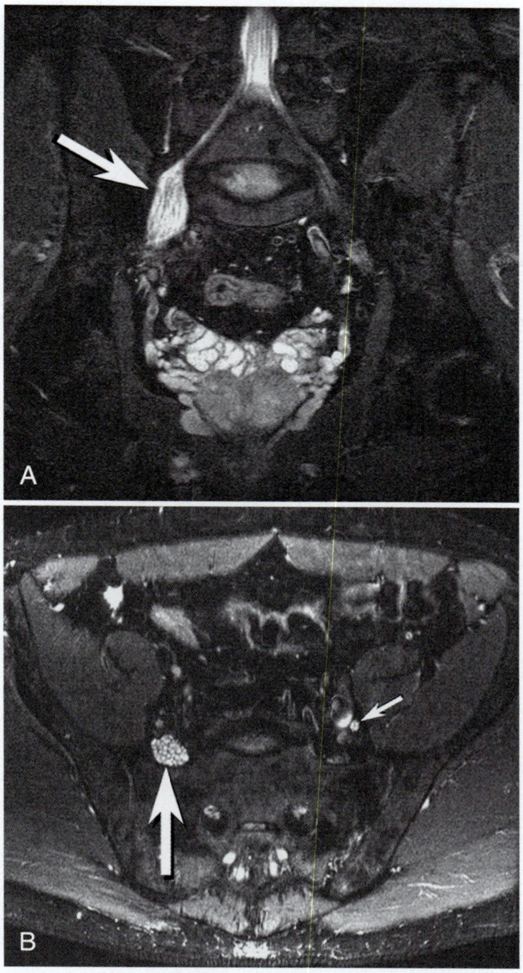

■ FIGURE 27-20 Neuropathy. Coronal (**A**) and axial (**B**) STIR MR images show the abnormal lumbosacral trunk. The nerve is markedly enlarged with swollen fascicles (*large arrow*) showing heterogeneity in the size of the fascicles. There is marked hyperintense signal within the nerve relative to surrounding structures. These findings are highly suggestive of a hypertrophic neuropathy. The contralateral sacral plexus is normal for comparison. Note the contralateral abnormal obturator nerve (*small arrow*, **B**) in this patient with polyneuropathy.

a long segment of nerve, generally the entire length of a peripheral nerve. The lesions are remarkable for the absence of a focal mass and (usual) preservation of the fascicular pattern (Fig. 27-20). The pathologic appearance may involve a single nerve (mononeuropathy) or multiple nerves throughout the body (polyneuropathy). The determination of single or multiple nerve involvement is usually made by clinical examination, although the presence of multiple abnormal nerves within a single MR neurographic study may make a diagnosis of previously unsuspected polyneuropathy.

These neuropathies can be hereditary, owing to demyelinating, inflammatory, or infectious cause, or idiopathic. MR neurography can help to guide a nerve biopsy when the nerve selected is not just the sural nerve. Finally, the absence of any abnormal findings in an area thought to have nerve involvement may indicate that the lesion is not

peripheral nerve in origin and obviate the need for biopsy.

Hereditary Motor and Sensory Neuropathies

At present, diagnosis of HMSN is based on information derived from its mode of inheritance, clinical course, neuropathologic, neurophysiologic, and molecular genetic findings. Because MRI can provide insight into CNS pathology in a noninvasive manner, its inclusion in the assessment of HMSN is being contemplated. Preliminary case reports have shown that MRI has the potential to detect enlarged nerve roots in those types of HMSN that are known to cause nerve hypertrophy.[27] Nerve root enlargement on MR images is, however, a disease-nonspecific sign, and, as a consequence, the detection of nerve root enlargement on MR images does not modify the "classic"

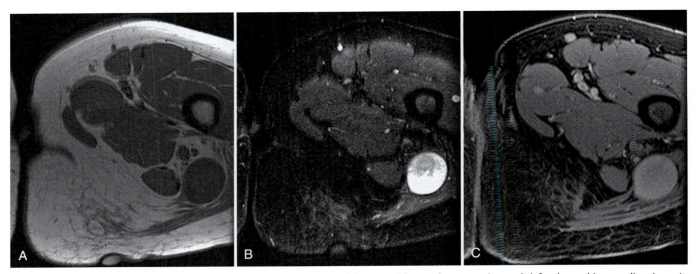

■ **FIGURE 27-21** Neoplasm. Schwannoma of the left sacral nerve. **A,** Axial T1W MR image shows a typical well-defined round intermediate-intensity mass, delineated by signal from fat, in the gluteal region. **B,** Axial T2W fat-suppressed image shows the lesion has homogeneous high signal intensity. **C,** Axial postcontrast T1W image shows intense inhomogeneous enhancement of the lesion.

approach to diagnosis and classification of HMSN. Thus, the role of MRI in the assessment of patients with HMSN is likely to remain modest.[28]

ANALYSIS

The sacral plexus can be involved by diverse pathologic processes, including primary involvement of the nerve plexus and secondary involvement by pathologic processes originating from adjacent structures. Although clinical history, physical examination, and electrodiagnostic studies play a crucial role, the complex anatomy in this region makes it difficult to precisely locate the level of pathologic involvement by these means alone.

MR neurography is the only imaging technique capable of providing high-quality information about nerve compression, nerve inflammation, nerve trauma, systemic neuropathies, nerve tumors, and recovery of nerve from prior pathologic states. MR neurography not only increases the conspicuity of peripheral nerve lesions but also allows differentiation of the nerves of the sacral plexus from adjacent pelvic viscera, adipose tissue, muscle, and vascular structures.

Thorough understanding of the anatomy and imaging appearance of the normal sacral plexus is an absolute prerequisite for properly performing and interpreting studies of the sacral plexus. Technically, excellent imaging of the sacral plexus and sciatic nerve requires a high-field MR scanner (1.5 T or 3 T) with good magnetic-field homogeneity; performance of both large area survey imaging and high-resolution, small FOV studies; correct choice of image plane; and postprocessing of data into multiplanar images. Taken in isolation, the MRI findings may be nonspecific and redundant, so careful clinical correlation plays an important role in interpreting radiologic studies.

Imaging features that are helpful in narrowing the differential diagnosis of sacral plexus pathologic processes are listed below:

1. Neoplasm (Fig. 27-21)
   - Mass in or along the nerve
   - Generally round or fusiform
   - No diffuse nerve enlargement
   - Contrast enhancement often present within the mass
2. Entrapment or compressive neuropathies (Fig. 27-22)
   - Mild to moderate localized nerve swelling/enlargement
   - T2 hyperintensity over short segment, in the area of entrapment
   - No contrast enhancement
   - Follow-up nerve imaging helpful in assessing recovery after treatment
3. Trauma (Fig. 27-23)
   - Usually diagnosed by clinical history
   - Variable nerve swelling and T2 hyperintensity
   - Often associated with extensive surrounding tissue signal changes
   - Variable contrast enhancement
   - Possible discontinuity of the nerve
   - Follow-up nerve and muscle denervation imaging helpful in assessing recovery
4. Infection/inflammation (Fig. 27-24)
   - Reactive changes involving the adjacent soft tissues, vessels, musculature, and bones
   - Diffuse moderate swelling of the nerve
   - Diffuse or long segment hyperintensity
   - Contrast enhancement of both nerves and adjacent tissues
5. Neuropathies (Fig. 27-25)
   - Classified as mononeuropathy versus polyneuropathy
   - Long segment enlarged nerves with swollen fascicles
   - Long segment T2 hyperintensity
   - Usually no contrast enhancement

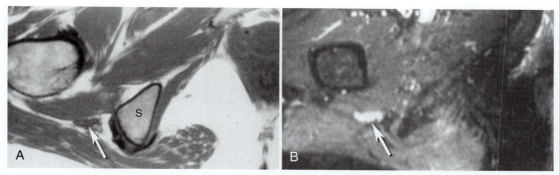

■ **FIGURE 27-22** Entrapment. Axial T1W (**A**) and STIR (**B**) MR images in a patient with clinical suspicion of piriformis syndrome reveal focal enlargement and hyperintensity of the right sciatic nerve (*arrows*) lying lateral and posterior to the ischial spine (S). A short segment of nerve involvement, like in this case, likely suggests compressive neuropathy.

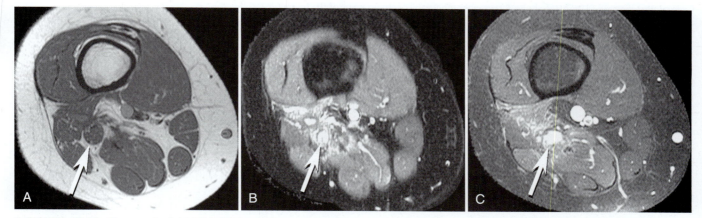

■ **FIGURE 27-23** Trauma. **A**, Axial T1W MR image in a patient with a gunshot wound shows an enlarged sciatic nerve in the proximal thigh. **B**, Axial STIR image at the same level shows abnormally increased nerve hyperintensity (*arrow*) with surrounding adjacent soft tissue signal changes consistent with tissue edema and nerve injury. **C**, Axial contrast-enhanced T1W image at the same level. There is abnormal enhancement (*arrow*) of the nerve and of the adjacent tissues. There is no obvious nerve disruption.

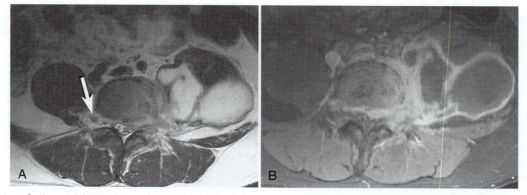

■ **FIGURE 27-24** Infection. Axial T2W (**A**) and T1W fat-suppressed postcontrast (**B**) MR images demonstrate a large left psoas abscess extending into the paraspinous region with foraminal and epidural extension. The peripheral enhancing abscess completely encases and effaces the left L5 nerve root. Note the normal exiting right L5 nerve root (*arrow*, **A**). MRI is very good in assessing intraspinal extension and nerve compression.

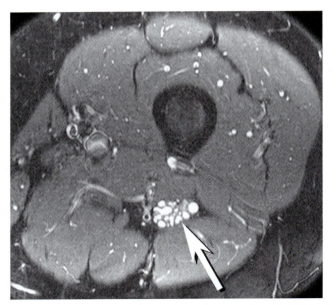

■ **FIGURE 27-25** Neuropathy. Axial STIR image at the mid-thigh level reveals an abnormal hyperintense sciatic nerve, which is enlarged with swollen fascicles of different sizes (*arrow*) with preserved fascicular architecture. These findings are generally characteristics of neuropathy in the appropriate clinical setting.

BOX 27-1 MRI Evaluation of Sacral Plexus

PATIENT HISTORY

A patient presented with buttock pain that was worse on the left than on the right.

TECHNIQUE

MR neurography of the sacral plexus and the proximal sciatic nerves was done without intravenous administration of a contrast agent. Coronal STIR, coronal T1W, axial T1W, axial STIR, axial T2W fat-saturated, and coronal T1W oblique images were obtained.

FINDINGS

The sacral plexus and the proximal third of the sciatic nerves bilaterally are visualized through the pelvis and deep to the gluteal muscles. There is no evidence of enlargement, altered fascicular pattern, abnormal signal, or entrapment bilaterally. No evidence for any mass lesion is seen along the course of the nerve, and no muscle denervation is noted.

IMPRESSION

This is a normal study of the sacral plexus and proximal sciatic nerves.

KEY POINTS

- MR neurography is the modality of choice in the imaging of sacral plexopathy.
- MRI shows that the abnormal nerve responds in one or more of four ways: nerve enlargement, altered fascicular pattern, T2 hyperintensity, and/or abnormal contrast enhancement.
- MRI is valuable for defining the presence of nerve pathology and for assessing the extent and severity of involvement, even guiding nerve biopsy in some cases.

- MRI can be very helpful in planning treatment and assessing its response.
- MRI may not be conclusive and should always be used in conjunction with detailed clinical history and physical examination.
- Adequate knowledge of anatomy, normal and abnormal MRI appearance, and optimal technique for MR neurography is crucial for achieving good diagnostic accuracy.

SUGGESTED READINGS

Blake LC, Robertson WD, Hayes CE. Sacral plexus: optimal imaging planes for MR assessment. Radiology 1996; 199:767-772.

Filler AG, Hayes CE, Howe FA, et al. MR neurography for improved characterization of peripheral nerve pathology [Abstract]. Proc Soc Magn Reson Med 1993; 1:101.

Filler AG, Kliot M, Howe FA, et al: Application of magnetic resonance neurography in the evaluation of patients with peripheral nerve pathology. J Neurosurg 1996; 85:299-309.

Gierada DS, Erickson SJ, Haughton VM, et al. MR imaging of sacral plexus: Normal findings. AJR Am J Roentgenol 1993; 60:1059-1065.

Gierada DS, Erickson SJ. MR imaging of sacral plexus: Abnormal findings. AJR Am J Roentgenol 1993; 60:1067-1071.

Howe FA, Filler AG, Bell BA, et al: Magnetic resonance neurography: optimizing imaging techniques for peripheral nerve identification [Abstract]. Proc Soc Magn Reson Med 1992; 1:1701.

Moore KR, Tsuruda JS, Dailey AD. The value of MR neurography for evaluating extraspinal neuropathic leg pain: a pictorial essay. AJNR Am J Neuroradiol 2001; 22:786-794.

REFERENCES

1. Graif M, Seton A, Nerubai J, et al. Sciatic nerve: sonographic evaluation and anatomic-pathologic considerations. Radiology 1991; 181:405-408.

2. Scroop R, Maravilla KR, Jarvik J, Kliot M. Magnetic Resonance Neurography. Spinal Imaging: State of the Art. Philadelphia, Hanley & Belfus, 2001, pp 65-79.

3. Lanzieri CF, Hilal SK. Computed tomography of the sacral plexus and sciatic nerve in the greater sciatic foramen. AJR Am J Roentgenol 1984; 143:165-168.
4. Howe FA, Filler AG, Bell BA, et al. Magnetic resonance neurography. Magn Reson Med 1992; 28:328-38.
5. Filler AG, Maravilla KR, Tsuruda JS. MR neurography and muscle MR imaging for image diagnosis of disorders affecting the peripheral nerves and musculature. Neurol Clin 2004; 22:643-682.
6. Filler AG, Howe FA, Hayes CE, et al. Magnetic resonance neurography. Lancet 1993; 341:659-661.
7. Skorpil M, Karlsson M, Nordell A. Peripheral nerve diffusion tensor imaging. Magn Reson Imaging 2004; 22:743-745.
8. Chappell KE, Robson MD, Stonebridge-Foster A, et al. Magic angle effects in MR neurography. Am J Neuroradiol 2004; 25:431-440.
9. Resnick D, Niwayama G. Soft tissues. In Resnick D (ed). Diagnosis of Bone and Joint Disorders, 3rd ed. Philadelphia, WB Saunders, 1995, pp 4552-4554.
10. Chui MC, Bird BL, Rogers J. Extracranial and extraspinal nerve sheath tumors: computed tomographic evaluation. Neuroradiology 1988; 30:47-53.
11. Pilavaki M, Chourmouzi D, Kiziridou A, et al. Imaging of peripheral nerve sheath tumors with pathologic correlation: pictorial review. Eur J Radiol 2004; 52:229-239.
12. Murphey MD, Smith WS, Smith SE, et al. From the archives of the AFIP. Imaging of musculoskeletal neurogenic tumors: radiologic-pathologic correlation. RadioGraphics 1999; 19:1253-1280.
13. Maravilla KR, Bowen BC. Imaging of the peripheral nervous system: evaluation of peripheral neuropathy and plexopathy. AJNR Am J Neuroradiol 1998; 19:1011-1023.
14. Yadav RR. Neoplastic lumbosacral plexopathy. eMedicine Specialities. Available at www.eMedicine.com. Last updated Feb. 7, 2007.
15. Jaeckle KA, Young DF, Foley KM. The natural history of lumbosacral plexopathy in cancer. Neurology 1985; 35:8-15.
16. Taylor BV, Kimmel DW, Krecke KN, Cascino TL. Magnetic reso- nance imaging in cancer-related lumbosacral plexopathy. Mayo Clin Proc 1997; 72: 823-829.
17. Stryker JA, Sommerville K, Perez R, Velkley DE. Sacral plexus injury after radiotherapy for carcinoma of cervix. Cancer 1990; 66:1488-1492.
18. Thomas JE, Cascino TL, Earle JD. Differential diagnosis between radiation and tumor plexopathy of the pelvis. Neurology 1985; 35:1-7.
19. Ramchandren S, Dalmau J. Metastases to the peripheral nervous system. J Neurooncol 2005; 75:101-110.
20. Bernard A. Lumbosacral plexopathy and femoral neuropathy. CME/CE article. Available at http://www.pain.com/sections/professional/cme_article/article.cfm?id=256
21. Yeoman W. The relation of arthritis of the sacroiliac joint to sciatica. Lancet 1928; 2:1119-1122.
22. Klien JM. Piriformis syndrome. Emedicine specialities. Available at www.emedicine.com/pmr/topic106.htm.
23. Papadopoulos EC, Khan SN. Piriformis syndrome and low back pain: a new classification and review of the literature. Orthop Clin North Am 2004; 35:65-71.
24. Hanania M, Kitain E. Peri-sciatic injection of steroid for the treatment of sciatica due to piriformis syndrome. Reg Anesth Pain Med 1998; 23:223-228.
25. Filler AG, Haynes J, Jordan SE, et al. Sciatica of nondisc origin and piriformis syndrome: diagnosis by magnetic resonance neurography and interventional magnetic resonance imaging with outcome study of resulting treatment. J Neurosurg Spine 2005; 2:99-115.
26. Stoehr M. Traumatic and postoperative lesions of the lumbosacral plexus. Arch Neurol 1978; 35:757-760.
27. Cellerini M, Salti S, Desideri M, Marconi G. MR imaging of the cauda equina in hereditary motor sensory neuropathies: correlations with sural nerve biopsy. Am J Neuroradiol 2000; 21:1793-1798.
28. Fillipi M. Is there room for MR imaging in the assessment of hereditary motor and sensory neuropathies? Am J Neuroradiol 2000; 21:1779-1780.

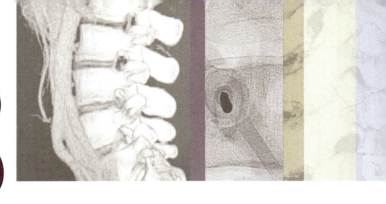

28

Peripheral Nerve Imaging: The Carpal Tunnel

Sundar Jayaraman

The most common peripheral nerve compression syndrome is compression neuropathy of the median nerve at the carpal tunnel. The median nerve innervates the wrist and sends cutaneous sensory branches to innervate the palm, the palmar aspect of the first three digits, and the radial half of the fourth digit. The median nerve also innervates the superficial flexors of the first three rays, as well as the pronator teres, the flexor pollicis longus and brevis, the abductor pollicis, the lateral aspect of the flexor digitorum profundus, the pronator quadratus, the first and second lumbricals, and the interossei of the hand. Compression of the median nerve within the carpal tunnel causes median nerve dysfunction, including numbness and paresthesias of the tips of the thumb, index, and middle finger. The condition is frequently bilateral.[1] Women are affected more often than men.[2]

The diagnosis of carpal tunnel syndrome is typically made using the history and physical examination along with electrophysiologic testing. Imaging techniques, specifically ultrasonography and MRI, are used in equivocal cases to provide anatomic information not achievable by electrophysiologic testing alone. Current ultrasound techniques using high-frequency linear-array transducers of 7 to 15 MHz provide exquisite display of the carpal tunnel, the contained tendons and vessels, and the superficially situated median nerve.

ANATOMY

The carpal tunnel is a fibro-osseous tunnel on the volar aspect of the wrist. The volar border of the carpal tunnel is formed by the flexor retinaculum. The flexor retinaculum extends from the scaphoid and the tubercle of the trapezium on the radial aspect of the wrist to the pisiform and the hook of the hamate on the ulnar aspect. Normally, the flexor retinaculum is nearly straight or slightly convex ventrally.[1] The floor of the carpal tunnel is formed by the carpal bones, predominantly the capitate, trapezoid, and part of the hamate (Fig. 28-1).

The 10 structures that traverse the carpal tunnel include the four tendons of the flexor digitorum superficialis, the four tendons of the flexor digitorum profundus, the tendon for the flexor pollicis longus, and the median nerve. The eight digital flexor tendons are enclosed within a common synovial sheath. The single tendon for the flexor pollicis longus is contained within its own synovial sheath along the radial aspect of the other flexor tendons within the carpal tunnel. The median nerve resides just deep to the flexor retinaculum and abuts upon its inner surface. It is usually located on the radial side of the flexor digitorum superficialis.

Guyon's canal is a separate fibro-osseous canal formed by the transverse and palmar carpal ligaments at the ulnar aspect of the wrist. It lies adjacent to, but separate from, the carpal tunnel and contains the ulnar artery, ulnar vein, and ulnar nerve.

IMAGING

Ultrasonography

Ultrasound exquisitely displays the median nerve at the wrist and distinguishes it from the adjacent tendons on the basis of four features: (1) the nerve's intrinsic echotexture, (2) persistence of that texture in all planes (isotropy), (3) superficial position of the median nerve within the carpal tunnel, and (4) ready differentiation between the moving tendons and the relatively nonmoving median nerve during finger flexion.

Intrinsic Echotexture

In-vitro studies at 15 MHz document that peripheral nerves display a distinct "speckled" fascicular pattern that derives from their internal structure.[3] Each nerve fiber is invested by the endoneurium. These fibers group into fascicles that are invested by perineurium. The fascicles then group into nerve trunks that are invested by epineurium. The

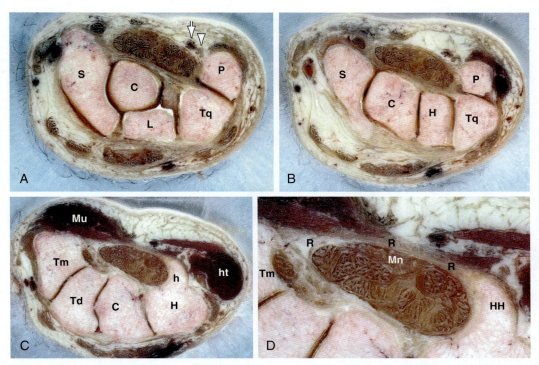

■ **FIGURE 28-1** Transverse cryomicrotome sections of a formalin-fixed adult human cadaver wrist. **A,** Proximal carpal tunnel: the scaphoid (S) forms the proximal radial border of the carpal tunnel. The pisiform (P) forms the proximal ulnar border. The capitate (C), lunate (L), and triquetrum (Tq) form the floor. Guyon's canal, containing the ulnar artery (*arrow*), ulnar vein, and ulnar nerve (*arrowhead*), lies just radial to the pisiform. **B,** Carpal tunnel, just distal to section in A: In this plane, the scaphoid and the pisiform still form the side walls of the carpal tunnel but the capitate and the hamate (H) now form the floor. **C,** Distal carpal tunnel: the tuberosity of the trapezium (Tm) forms the distal radial border of the carpal tunnel, whereas the hook of the hamate (h) forms the distal ulnar border. The trapezoid (Td), capitate (C), and body of the hamate (H) comprise the floor of the carpal tunnel. The thenar muscles (Mu) form the radial aspect of the palm ventral to the trapezium, whereas the hypothenar muscles (ht) form the ulnar aspect of the palm, ventral to the hamate. **D,** Magnified view of the distal carpal tunnel. The elliptic median nerve (MN) lies just deep to the flexor retinaculum (R) at the most superficial aspect of the carpal tunnel. HH, hook of the hamate.

epineurium surrounds the entire nerve and extends inward, around the fascicles, as the interfascicular epineurium, binding the nerve together. The endoneurium and perineurium are too thin for ultrasound to resolve as separate structures. The epineurium, however, is a thick sheath containing loose connective tissue, elastic fibers, and vessels.[4] Ultrasound resolves the epineurium well and thereby delineates the size, position, and configuration of the median nerve within the carpal tunnel.

In longitudinal sonographic sections the median nerve shows multiple hypoechoic, parallel-but-discontinuous lines separated by echogenic bands. In transverse sections, the nerve shows a round to elliptical contour and exhibits round hypoechoic spaces within an echogenic background.[4] Correlation of ultrasound images with histologic sections demonstrates that the hypoechoic spaces correspond to the nerve fascicles whereas the echogenic background corresponds to the interfascicular epineurium.[3] This ultrasound appearance is reproduced in clinical studies[1] using high-frequency linear-array transducers of 10 to 15 MHz (Fig. 28-2).

In ultrasound studies performed with lower-frequency transducers, the hypoechoic spaces within the nerves appear less defined and less numerous (i.e., blurred). This blurring may be due to poor lateral resolution with "coalescence" of adjacent structures of similar echogenicity, to reverberation artifact from hyperechoic stroma, and/or to

inability to depict the nerve fascicles unless they are oriented perpendicular to the direction of the ultrasound beam.[3]

Normal tendons display a fibrillar echotexture. When the tendon is insonated at right angles to its fibers, it shows strong, bright, highly ordered echoes reflecting from its fibers. In longitudinal section, these fibers form thick bands of tightly packed, parallel, linear echos.[3] In transverse section, the fibers form round arrays of closely grouped, dot-like echoes (see Fig. 28-2). The differing echotextures of nerve and tendon enable the sonographer to distinguish the speckled fascicular median nerve from the hyperechoic fibrillar tendon in both transverse and longitudinal ultrasound sections.

Isotropy

In this context, isotropy signifies the unchanging appearance of a structure when the structure is examined from different directions. Anisotropy signifies that the appearance of the structure changes significantly with changing direction of examination. The median nerve is isotropic. Longitudinal and transverse sections through the median nerve display the same fascicular sonographic pattern. Naturally, that pattern appears "speckled" in transverse section and more linear in longitudinal section, but both planes of study show the fascicular pattern. Tendons are

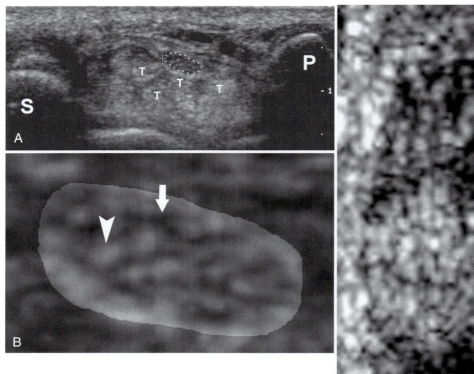

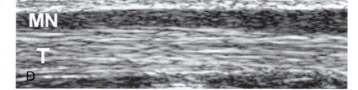

■ **FIGURE 28-2** Ultrasonography of the tendons and nerves: echotexture. **A,** High-frequency transverse ultrasound image of the proximal carpal tunnel in a healthy 30-year-old man demonstrates the normal median nerve (*trace marks*), the flexor tendons (T), the scaphoid (S), and the pisiform (P). **B,** Ultrasound image of the median nerve, magnified from image **A,** demonstrates hypoechoic foci corresponding to the nerve fascicles (*arrow*) and echogenic foci corresponding to the interfascicular epineurium (*arrowhead*). Magnified ultrasound images display the superficially situated median nerve (MN) and one deep flexor tendon (T) in transverse (**C**) and longitudinal (**D**) planes.

strongly anisotropic. Their echotexture changes markedly with changing sonographic sections. Because the tendon has a highly ordered structure with superimposed planes of collagen and septa, the characteristic fibrillar pattern is demonstrated only when the ultrasound beam is oriented perpendicular to the structural planes.[4] Changing the angle of insonation by angling ("rocking") the transducer to and fro causes great variability in the intensity and the sonographic pattern of the fibrillar echoes. As the angle of insonation deviates from perpendicular, the fibrillar structure becomes less intense and less distinct. At too great an angle of insonation, the sonostructure almost disappears, leaving "hollow cylinders" designated tendon ghosts (Fig. 28-3). These differences in (an)isotropy enable the sonographer to distinguish the isotropic median nerve from the strongly anisotropic tendon.

Superficial Position of the Median Nerve

Within the carpal tunnel, the flexor tendons for the fingers and thumb are situated dorsally, close to the radius, ulna, and carpal bones. The median nerve is situated ventrally, just deep to the flexor retinaculum, toward the radial aspect of the tunnel. In the supinated, volar position used for ultrasonographic examination of the carpal tunnel, the median nerve characteristically lies "superficial" to the tendons, immediately deep to the flexor retinaculum (Fig. 28-4).

Motion with Finger Flexion

Finger flexion is achieved by muscle contractions that pull on the tendons within the carpal tunnel. During finger flexion, the tendons move within their sheaths and tend to shift ventrally, then dorsally, as the tension pulls them more or less tightly against the flexor retinaculum. Tendon motion is readily apparent. The median nerve remains relatively motionless and exhibits only a slight "rocking" caused by the shifting positions of the subjacent tendons. This difference enables the sonographer to distinguish the moving tendons from the relatively static median nerve during finger flexion.

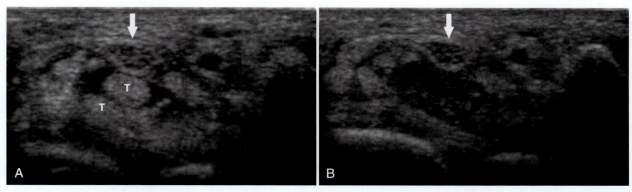

■ FIGURE 28-3 Ultrasonography of the tendons and nerves: anisotropy. **A,** With the transducer oriented perpendicular to the carpal tunnel, the ultrasound image demonstrates the normal median nerve (*arrow*) and echogenic flexor tendons (T). **B,** When the angle of insonation is shifted slightly away from perpendicular, the tendon's fibrillar structure appears less intense and less distinct whereas the echotexture of the median nerve (*arrow*) remains relatively stable. The change in echotexture with changing angle of insonation (anisotropy) is characteristic of tendons and serves to distinguish them from the median nerve.

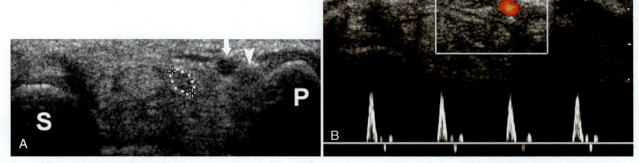

■ FIGURE 28-4 Ultrasonography of the proximal carpal tunnel. **A,** Ultrasound image of the proximal carpal tunnel demonstrates the pisiform bone (P) forming the ulnar aspect of the wrist, the ulnar artery (*arrow*), and the ulnar nerve (*arrowhead*) within Guyon's canal just radial to the pisiform and the median nerve (*trace marks*) at the superficial aspect of the carpal tunnel. Osseous structures, such as the scaphoid (S) and pisiform, are identified on ultrasound by their strong surface echoes and posterior acoustic shadowing (see also Fig. 28-1A). **B,** With Doppler ultrasound, the anechoic ulnar artery seen in **A** (*arrow*) now demonstrates bright coloration and a characteristic arterial waveform, confirming the identification of the ulnar artery.

The ulnar artery shows an anechoic lumen with arterial waveform in response to color Doppler interrogation (see Fig. 28-4). When irritated due to compression in the carpal tunnel, the median nerve may show peripheral coloration due to surface hyperemia, but this appearance is distinct from that of the artery.[4] Veins are recognized by their course adjacent to the artery and are easily compressed with light ultrasound pressure, owing to their compliant walls.

Ultrasound demonstrates the thenar and hypothenar muscles (Fig. 28-5). In transverse sections, the muscles show large hypoechoic spaces surrounding echogenic foci. This pattern is designated "starry night" for its resemblance to Van Gogh's painting.[5] In longitudinal sections, muscles exhibit a number of angled echogenic lines, which converge toward a central or peripheral aponeurosis that ends in a tendon.[5] This appearance resembles a "blade of grass." The muscles lie external to the carpal tunnel itself, external to the flexor retinaculum.

Bones are easily identified on sonography by their strong surface echoes, their posterior acoustic shadowing, and their position at the periphery of the carpal tunnel (see Fig. 28-4).

Identification of the Structures within Guyon's Canal

The ulnar nerve enters the wrist through Guyon's canal, accompanied by the ulnar artery and vein (see Figs. 28-1 and 28-4). The contents of Guyon's canal are bordered on the ulnar aspect by the pisiform. The dorsal surface (floor) of the canal is formed by the flexor retinaculum. The ventral surface (roof) is formed by the palmar carpal ligament.[6] The ulnar artery lies anterolateral to the nerve. In the distal canal, the ulnar nerve bifurcates into a superficial sensory branch and a deep motor branch. The sensory branch supplies the hypothenar eminence, the fifth digit, and the medial half of the fourth digit. The deep motor branch supplies the hypothenar muscles and then passes across the palm to other intrinsic hand muscles. At the level of the pisiform, high-resolution ultrasonography demonstrates the ulnar nerve as a thin, rounded structure situated medial to the ulnar artery. Distally, at the level of the hook of the hamate, ultrasonography displays the two terminal divisions of the nerve. The sensory branch continues to run in proximity to the ulnar artery. The motor branch courses

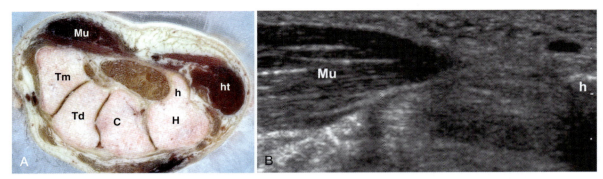

■ FIGURE 28-5 Ultrasonography of the distal carpal tunnel. **A,** Transverse cryomicrotome section of the distal carpal tunnel shows the thenar muscles (Mu), hypothenar muscles (ht), trapezium (Tm), trapezoid (Td), capitate (C), and hook of the hamate (h). **B,** Magnified ultrasound image through the distal carpal tunnel displays the thenar muscles as a "blade of grass" formed by angled echogenic lines converging to a central point.

more deeply, adjacent to the medial surface of the hamate hook.

Ulnar neuropathies in Guyon's canal are rare. Ultrasound can accurately detect extrinsic causes of ulnar nerve compression within Guyon's canal, including ganglion cysts related to the pisotriquetral joint space, anomalous muscles (accessory abductor digiti minimi, anomalous hypothenar adductor), pseudoaneurysms of the ulnar artery, and fracture fragments, all of which can compress the nerve.[5,6]

CT

CT is not routinely used in the diagnosis of carpal tunnel syndrome. CT can be performed for specific indications such as evaluation for osseous spurring, tophaceous gout,[7] or fracture fragment.[8]

MRI

On high-resolution axial T1-weighted (T1W) spin-echo images, the normal peripheral nerve is isointense to normal muscle. On axial T2-weighted (T2W) short tau inversion recovery (STIR) images, the normal nerve is isointense to slightly hyperintense to normal muscle. Typical abnormalities in patients with carpal tunnel syndrome include high signal of the median nerve on T2W images, flattening of the nerve within the tunnel, swelling of the nerve proximal to the tunnel, and bowing of the flexor retinaclum.[9]

How Pathology Alters Normal Appearance

The classic triad of median nerve compression comprises (1) nerve flattening in the distal carpal tunnel, (2) nerve swelling within the proximal tunnel itself, and (3) palmar bowing of the flexor retinaculum.[1,6] Because the shape of the median nerve varies as it passes through the tunnel, indexes have been introduced to quantify abnormality. The cross-sectional area of the median nerve can be measured directly by tracing its boundary with electronic calipers at the time of ultrasonography. Eight separate ultrasonographic measurements have been analyzed in patients with carpal tunnel syndrome and in asymptomatic controls.[10] These eight criteria are four measures of the cross-sectional area of the median nerve: (1) at the distal forearm, (2) immediately proximal to the tunnel, (3) at the tunnel inlet, and (4) at the tunnel outlet; two determinations of a "flattening ratio" for the median nerve (defined as the ratio of the transverse axis of the nerve to the anteroposterior axis of the nerve) (5) at the tunnel inlet and (6) at the tunnel outlet; and two measurements of the flexor retinaculum: (7) the degree of ventral retinacular bowing and (8) the thickness of the retinaculum itself.[10]

Three of these eight measurements prove to be the most predictive of carpal tunnel syndrome and the most accurate for distinguishing symptomatic patients from normal control subjects.[10] These three were the cross-sectional areas of the median nerve (1) proximal to the tunnel inlet, (2) at the tunnel inlet, and (3) at the tunnel outlet. One study established that a cutoff value of more than $0.098 \ cm^2$ for the cross-sectional area of the median nerve at the tunnel inlet provided a diagnostic sensitivity of 89% and a specificity of 83%. Another study obtained similar results, showing that a cross-sectional area of the median nerve greater than $0.09 \ cm^2$ at the level of the proximal tunnel was the best criterion for diagnosing carpal tunnel syndrome.[8] This criterion provided a sensitivity of 82%, specificity of 97%, and accuracy of 88%.[11]

Comparative studies have shown good correlation between the measurements of the cross-sectional area of the median nerve obtained by ultrasonography and those obtained by MRI in vivo and good correlation between ultrasonographic measurements and anatomic measurements made in unfixed human cadavers at postmortem study.[12,13]

In routine practice, transverse sections of the median nerve are obtained at four sequential levels: (1) in the distal forearm at the level of the distal radioulnar joint, (2) in the proximal carpal tunnel at the level of the pisiform bone, (3) in the midcarpal tunnel, and (4) in the distal carpal tunnel at the level of the hook of the hamate. At each level, the cross-sectional area of the median nerve is measured by tracing around the margin of the nerve with electronic calipers (Figs. 28-6 and 28-7). For standardization, the "margin of the nerve" is defined as the margin outside the hypoechoic nerve fascicles and inside the hyperechoic nerve sheath.[10]

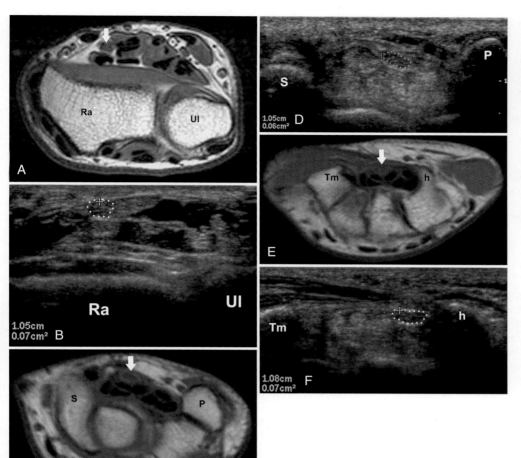

■ **FIGURE 28-6** Paired T1W MR and ultrasound images of the carpal tunnel in a healthy 28-year-old man. Cross-sectional areas of the median nerve at three levels. **A** and **B,** Distal radioulnar joint. The cross-sectional area of the median nerve (*arrow* in **A,** *trace marks* in **B**) measures 0.07 cm². **C** and **D,** Proximal carpal tunnel. The cross-sectional area of the median nerve (*arrow* in **C,** *trace marks* in **D**) measures 0.06 cm². **E** and **F,** Distal carpal tunnel. The cross-sectional area of the median nerve (*arrow* in **E,** *trace marks* in **F**) measures 0.07 cm². h, hook of hamate; P, pisiform; Ra, radius; S, scaphoid, Tm, trapezium; Ul, ulna.

The swelling ratio is determined by dividing the cross-sectional area of the median nerve at the proximal carpal tunnel by the cross-sectional area of the median nerve at the distal forearm. This ratio provides an internal control for assessing swelling of the median nerve, because it compares the affected median nerve inside the carpal tunnel against its own unaffected proximal portion (see Fig. 28-7). The normal swelling ratio is less than 1.3.[14]

Palmar bowing is determined by drawing a straight line from the tubercle of the trapezium to the hook of the hamate (T-H line) and measuring the anteroposterior displacement of the posterior border of the flexor retinaculum from this line (Fig. 28-8). In normal patients the retinaculum is relatively flat to minimally convex and lies within 2.5 mm anterior to the T-H line.[10] In patients with carpal tunnel syndrome, the retinaculum often appears bowed and displaced more than 2.5 mm anterior to the T-H line.

Anatomic Variations

The carpal tunnel exhibits anatomic variations that may influence diagnosis or surgery. The median nerve may display accessory branches or show premature proximal bifurcation.[4,15] Approximately 10% of patients have vascular anomalies such as a persistent median artery of the forearm.[16] The persistent median artery appears as a small anechoic structure running parallel to the median nerve and is readily identified by its bright coloration and arterial waveform on color Doppler evaluation (Fig. 28-9). Another variation of the median nerve is the bifid median nerve, defined as a high division of the median nerve proximal to the carpal tunnel.[17,18] In a dissection study of 246 hands, the incidence of bifid median nerve was 2.8%.[19] On ultrasound, the bifid median nerve appears as two small nerve trunks with an interposed persistent median artery (Fig. 28-10). These variations are important to recognize, especially in the preoperative setting, because they may influence decisions whether to inject anti-inflammatory medication percutaneously and decisions whether to perform open or endoscopic release of the median nerve.[19,20]

Other Causes of Carpal Tunnel Pathology

The imaging study must also evaluate, and exclude, other causes of nerve compression. Extrinsic causes for nerve entrapment include tenosynovitis of the flexor tendons, traumatic neuromas, neurogenic tumors such as schwannoma and neurofibroma, ganglia, soft tissue masses, deposits of amyloid, and accessory muscles.[6]

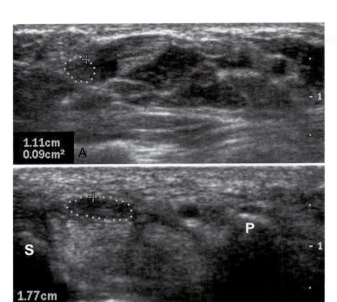

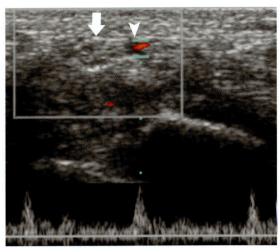

■ FIGURE 28-9 Normal anatomic variation: persistent median artery in a healthy 29-year-old man. The persistent median artery (*arrowhead*) appears as a pulsatile vessel coursing with the median nerve (*arrow*).

■ FIGURE 28-7 Ultrasonographic diagnosis of carpal tunnel syndrome in a 58-year-old woman. **A,** Distal radioulnar joint. The cross-sectional area of the median nerve (*trace marks*) measures 0.09 cm². **B,** Proximal carpal tunnel. The cross-sectional area of the median nerve (*trace marks*) measures 0.16 cm². This finding is abnormal. The swelling ratio is 1.8 (normal, <1.3). These findings are sufficient to confirm the diagnosis of median nerve compression within the carpal tunnel. P, pisiform; S, scaphoid.

displays the surgical incision as a cleft in the flexor retinaculum and demonstrates improvement in the appearance and the mobility of the nerve.[22] After surgical reconstruction of the nerve, ultrasonography provides reliable postoperative evaluation of the continuity of the nerve at the anastomosis and can rule out any perineural collections.[4]

ANALYSIS

A sample report for ultrasound evaluation of median nerve compression is presented in Box 28-1.

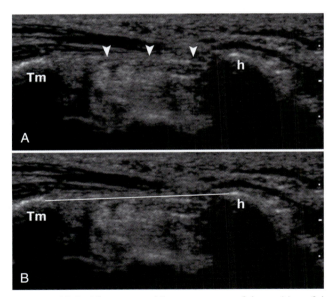

■ FIGURE 28-8 Ultrasonographic measurement of the position of the flexor retinaculum. **A,** The flexor retinaculum (*arrowheads*) normally lies no more than 2.5 mm anterior to the T-H line drawn between the tuberosity of the trapezium (Tm) and the hook of the hamate (h). **B,** In this healthy volunteer, the flexor retinaculum shows no significant bowing or displacement relative to the T-H line.

Follow-up Studies

Ultrasonographic examination of the wrist may also be performed after carpal tunnel release to ensure complete decompression of the nerve and to evaluate any other causes of clinical concern.[21] Typically, ultrasonography

---

BOX 28-1 Ultrasound Evaluation for Median Nerve Compression

PATIENT HISTORY

A 46-year-old typist presented with numbness of the first two digits of the right hand.

TECHNIQUE

Focused high-frequency ultrasonography of the right carpal tunnel was performed.

FINDINGS

The cross-sectional area of median nerve at the distal radioulnar joint is 0.09 cm². The cross-sectional area of the median nerve at the proximal carpal tunnel is 0.16 cm². The swelling ratio is 1.8 (normal <1.3). No mass or abnormal fluid collection is seen.

IMPRESSION

The findings confirm the diagnosis of median nerve compression within the carpal tunnel.

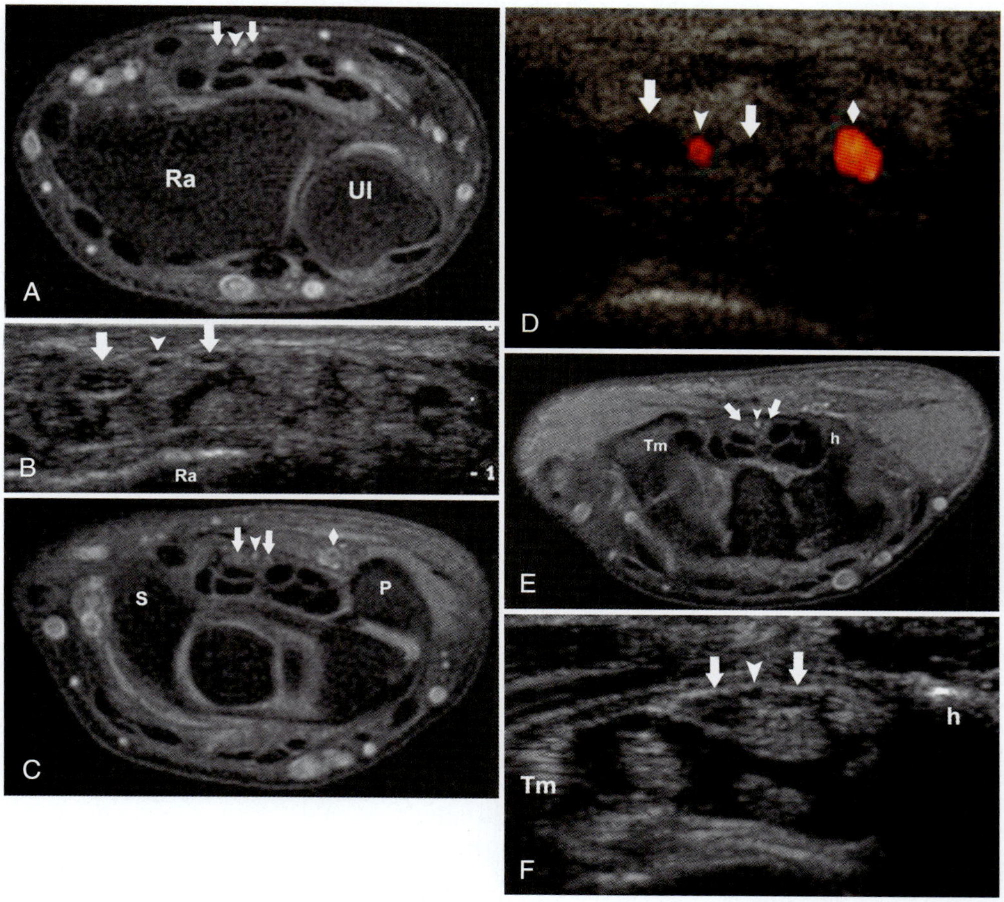

FIGURE 28-10 Normal anatomic variation: bifid median nerve in a healthy 28-year-old man. Paired proton density MR and ultrasound images. The two nerve trunks of the bifid median nerve (*arrows*) flank the intervening persistent median artery (*arrowhead*) at all levels of the wrist and carpal tunnel. **A** and **B**, Distal forearm at the distal radioulnar joint. **C** and **D**, Proximal carpal tunnel at the pisiform bone (the ulnar artery is represented by a *diamond*). **E** and **F**, Distal carpal tunnel at the hook of the hamate. Ra, radius; Ul, ulna; S, scaphoid; P, pisiform; Tm, tuberosity of the trapezium; h, hook of the hamate.

KEY POINTS

- The most common peripheral nerve compression syndrome is compression neuropathy of the median nerve at the carpal tunnel. The diagnosis of carpal tunnel syndrome is typically made using history and physical examination along with electrophysiologic testing. However, ultrasonography has advantages over nerve conduction studies and MRI and promises to be the most comfortable, inexpensive, and precise test for the diagnosis of carpal tunnel syndrome.
- Ultrasonography successfully distinguishes the median nerve from the adjacent tendons in the carpal tunnel on the basis of (1) the nerve's intrinsic echotexture, (2) persistence of that texture in all planes (isotropy), (3) superficial position of the median nerve within the carpal tunnel, and (4) ready differentiation between the moving tendons and the relatively nonmoving median nerve during finger flexion.
- The classic triad of median nerve compression comprises (1) nerve flattening within the distal carpal tunnel, (2) nerve swelling at the proximal tunnel, and (3) palmar bowing of the flexor retinaculum. A cutoff value of 0.10 cm^2 for the cross-sectional area of the swollen median nerve at the proximal tunnel inlet is a sensitive and specific criterion for the diagnosis of carpal tunnel syndrome.

SUGGESTED READINGS

Andreisek G, Crook DW, Burg D, et al. Peripheral neuropathies of the median, radial, and ulnar nerves: MR imaging features. RadioGraphics 2006; 26:1267-1287.

Beekman R, Visser LH. Sonography in the diagnosis of carpal tunnel syndrome: a critical review of the literature. Muscle Nerve 2003; 27:26-33.

Bland JD. Carpal tunnel syndrome. Curr Opin Neurol 2005; 18:581-585.

Hochman MG, Zilberfarb JL. Nerves in a pinch: imaging of nerve compression syndromes. Radiol Clin North Am 2004; 42:221-245.

Jarvik JG, Yuen E, Kliot M. Diagnosis of carpal tunnel syndrome: electrodiagnostic and MR imaging evaluation. Neuroimaging Clin North Am 2004; 14:93-102, viii.

REFERENCES

1. Buchberger W. Radiologic imaging of the carpal tunnel. Eur J Radiol 1997; 25:112-117.
2. Chen P, Maklad N, Redwine M, Zelitt D. Dynamic high-resolution sonography of the carpal tunnel. AJR Am J Roentgenol 1997; 168:533-537.
3. Silvestri E, Martinoli C, Derchi LE, et al. Echotexture of peripheral nerves: correlation between US and histologic findings and criteria to differentiate tendons. Radiology 1995; 197:291-296.
4. Martinoli C, Bianchi S, Derchi LE. Tendon and nerve sonography. Radiol Clin North Am 1999; 37:691-711.
5. Loewy J. Sonoanatomy of the median, ulnar and radial nerves. Can Assoc Radiol J 2002; 53:33-38.
6. Martinoli C, Bianchi S, Gandolfo N, et al. US of nerve entrapments in osteofibrous tunnels of the upper and lower limbs. RadioGraphics 2000; 20:S199-S213.
7. Andresen R, Radmer S, Sparmann M, et al. Imaging of hamate bone fractures in conventional X-rays and high-resolution computed tomography: an in vitro study. Invest Radiol 1999; 34:46-50.
8. Chen CK, Chung CB, Yeh L, et al. Carpal tunnel syndrome caused by tophaceous gout: CT and MR imaging features in 20 patients. AJR Am J Roentgenol 2000; 175:655-659.
9. Jarvik JG, Yuen E, Kliot M. Diagnosis of carpal tunnel syndrome: electrodiagnostic and MR imaging evaluation. Neuroimaging Clin North Am 2004; 14:93-102.
10. Wong SM, Griffith JF, Hui AC, et al. Discriminatory sonographic criteria for the diagnosis of carpal tunnel syndrome. Arthritis Rheum 2002; 46:1914-1921.
11. Duncan I, Sullivan P, Lomas F. Sonography in the diagnosis of carpal tunnel syndrome. AJR Am J Roentgenol 1999; 173:681-684.
12. Buchberger W, Judmaier W, Birbamer G, et al. Carpal tunnel syndrome: diagnosis with high-resolution sonography. AJR Am J Roentgenol 1992; 159:793-798.
13. Kamolz LP, Schrogendorfer KF, Rab M, et al. The precision of ultrasound imaging and its relevance for carpal tunnel syndrome. Surg Radiol Anat 2001; 23:117-121.
14. Keberle M, Jenett M, Kenn W, et al. Technical advances in ultrasound and MR imaging of carpal tunnel syndrome. Eur Radiol 2000; 10:1043-1050.
15. Lanz U. Anatomical variations of the median nerve in the carpal tunnel. J Hand Surg [Am] 1977; 2A:44-53.
16. Coleman SS, Anson BJ. Arterial patterns in the hand based upon a study of 650 specimens. Surg Gynecol Obstet 1961; 113:409-424.
17. Propeck T, Quinn TJ, Jacobson JA, et al. Sonography and MR imaging of bifid median nerve with anatomic and histologic correlation. AJR Am J Roentgenol 2000; 175:1721-1725.
18. Iannicelli E, Chianta GA, Salvini V, et al. Evaluation of bifid median nerve with sonography and MR imaging. J Ultrasound Med 2000; 19:481-485.
19. Lindley SG, Kleinert JM. Prevalence of anatomic variations encountered in elective carpal tunnel release. J Hand Surg [Am] 2003; 28:849-855.
20. Russell SM, Kline DG. Complication avoidance in peripheral nerve surgery: injuries, entrapments, and tumors of the extremities—part 2. Neurosurgery 2006; 59(4 Suppl 2):ONS449-57.
21. Lee CH, Kim TK, Yoon ES, Dhong ES. Postoperative morphologic analysis of carpal tunnel syndrome using high-resolution ultrasonography. Ann Plast Surg 2005; 54:143-146.
22. El-Karabaty H, Hetzel A, Galla TJ, et al. The effect of carpal tunnel release on median nerve flattening and nerve conduction. Electromyogr Clin Neurophysiol 2005; 45:223-227.

Index